MANUAL OF
EQUINE
REPRODUCTION

MANUAL OF
EQUINE
REPRODUCTION

THIRD EDITION

Steven P. Brinsko, DVM, MS, PhD, Dipl ACT
Associate Professor and Chief of Theriogenology
Department of Large Animal Clinical Sciences
College of Veterinary Medicine and Biomedical Sciences
Texas A&M University, College Station, Texas

Terry L. Blanchard, DVM, MS, Dipl ACT
Professor
Department of Large Animal Clinical Sciences
College of Veterinary Medicine and Biomedical Sciences
Texas A&M University, College Station, Texas

Dickson D. Varner, DVM, MS, Dipl ACT
Professor
Department of Large Animal Clinical Sciences
College of Veterinary Medicine and Biomedical Sciences
Texas A&M University, College Station, Texas

James Schumacher, DVM, MS, Dipl ACVS, MRCVS
Professor
Department of Large Animal Clinical Sciences
College of Veterinary Medicine
University of Tennessee, Knoxville, Tennessee

Charles C. Love, DVM, PhD, Dipl ACT
Associate Professor
Department of Large Animal Clinical Sciences
College of Veterinary Medicine and Biomedical Sciences
Texas A&M University, College Station, Texas

Katrin Hinrichs, DVM, PhD, Dipl ACT
Professor
Department of Physiology & Pharmacology
College of Veterinary Medicine and Biomedical Sciences
Texas A&M University, College Station, Texas

David L. Hartman, DVM
Hartman Equine Reproduction Center
Whitesboro, Texas

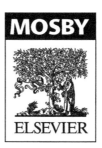

MOSBY

ELSEVIER

3251 Riverport Lane
Maryland Heights, Missouri 63043

MANUAL OF EQUINE REPRODUCTION   ISBN: 978-0-323-06482-8

Notice

Knowledge and best practice in this field are constantly changing. As new research and experience broaden our knowledge, changes in practice, treatment and drug therapy may become necessary or appropriate. Readers are advised to check the most current information provided (i) on procedures featured or (ii) by the manufacturer of each product to be administered, to verify the recommended dose or formula, the method and duration of administration, and contraindications. It is the responsibility of the practitioner, relying on their own experience and knowledge of the patient, to make diagnoses, to determine dosages and the best treatment for each individual patient, and to take all appropriate safety precautions. To the fullest extent of the law, neither the Publisher nor the Authors assumes any liability for any injury and/or damage to persons or property arising out of or related to any use of the material contained in this book.

The Publisher

Library of Congress Cataloging-in-Publication Data

Manual of equine reproduction / Steven P. Brinsko . . . [et al.]. – 3rd ed.
        p. ; cm.
    Includes bibliographical references and index.
    ISBN-13: 978-0-323-06482-8 (pbk. : alk. paper)
    ISBN-10: 0-323-06482-5 (pbk. : alk. paper) 1. Horses–Reproduction.
2. Horses–Breeding. I. Brinsko, Steven P. II. Blanchard, Terry L. III. Title: Equine reproduction.
    [DNLM: 1. Horses–physiology. 2. Reproduction–physiology. 3. Genital Diseases,
Female–veterinary. 4. Genital Diseases, Male–veterinary. 5. Horse Diseases–therapy. 6. Reproductive
Techniques, Assisted–veterinary. SF 768.2.H67 M294 2011]
    SF768.2.H67M36 2011
    636.1'08982–dc22

                                                                                          2009044342

Vice President and Publisher: Linda Duncan
Acquisitions Editor: Penny Rudolph
Associate Developmental Editor: Lauren Harms
Publishing Services Manager: Catherine Jackson
Project Manager: Jennifer Boudreau
Design Direction: Paula Catalano

Printed in the United States of America
Last digit is the print number: 12 11 10

Dedication

This textbook is dedicated to Dr. Robert M. Kenney, Professor Emeritus of Reproduction in the Section of Reproductive Studies, New Bolton Center, University of Pennsylvania School of Veterinary Medicine, and Dr. O.J. Ginther, Professor of Veterinary Science in the Department of Veterinary Science, University of Wisconsin-Madison. These two individuals have devoted their entire professional lives to advancements in equine reproduction and have served as invaluable resources and mentors for countless veterinary students, graduate students, clinical residents, university faculty, and practicing veterinarians. They can be considered true fathers of the modern-day discipline of equine reproduction.

We also wish to dedicate this third edition to the late Drs. John P. Hurtgen and John Steiner, Diplomates of the American College of Theriogenologists. These two individuals were lost tragically to our profession, but were devoted colleagues, valued mentors, and friends of many who practice the discipline.

Preface

We originally wrote this manual to serve as a textbook for veterinary students studying clinical reproduction in horses. We quickly found that the manual became a popular resource for veterinarians practicing equine reproduction.

In the third edition, we have updated and expanded many of the chapters while maintaining the manual's readability and clinical emphasis. The figures have been colorized and many new figures have been added to the expanded chapters. We have also added a new chapter that focuses on the use of assisted reproductive technologies.

Each chapter begins with a listing of important learning objectives, along with questions to guide self-study. Numerous figures are included in each chapter to enhance the reader's ability to grasp the material discussed.

The manual was written with the target audience of veterinary students, practicing veterinarians, and animal scientists teaching equine reproductive physiology and artificial insemination in mind. As such, a background in reproductive physiology would be helpful to fully comprehend the text in its entirety. However, horse owners and breeders will also find useful information regarding reproductive management, breeding with transported cooled or frozen semen, and management of the pregnant/foaling mare and newborn foal.

Steven P. Brinsko, DVM, MS, PhD, Dipl ACT
Terry L. Blanchard, DVM, MS, Dipl ACT
Dickson D. Varner, DVM, MS, Dipl ACT
James Schumacher, DVM, MS, Dipl ACVS, MRCVS
Charles C. Love, DVM, PhD, Dipl ACT
Katrin Hinrichs, DVM, PhD, Dipl ACT
David L. Hartman, DVM

About the Covers:

FRONT COVER

Photograph of American Quarter Horse champion race mare, *Your First Moon*, owned by Frank "Scoop" Vessels III, Vessels Stallion Farm, Bonsall, CA, with foal. The foal, *Stray Cat*, owned by Lyle Lovett and Scoop Vessels, was sired by the great Thoroughbred stallion, *Storm Cat*, Overbrook Farm, Lexington, KY, after the stallion's retirement from Thoroughbred breeding. The successful breeding was achieved by transrectally-guided low-dose insemination of semen that was first centrifuged though a silica-particle solution, EquiPure (Nidacon International AB, Mölndal, Sweden) to enhance semen quality in the inseminate.

BACK COVER

Photograph of American Quarter Horse performance champion and elite sire, *Shining Spark*, owned by Carol Rose, Carol Rose Quarter Horses, Gainesville, TX. *Shining Spark's* foals have earned more than $7.3 million, and over 32,881 AQHA points. He is a $3 million dollar NRHA sire, and the only $3 million dollar NRCHA sire. He is also the sire of 20 AQHA World or Reserve World champions, numerous NRCHA world champions, NRCHA Snaffle Bit Futurity champions, an AQHA World Show Super Horse, and a NRHA Open Futurity champion. In the past 10 years, the stallion has sired foals through transrectally-guided low-dose insemination, and in recent years, with EquiPure-processed semen.

Table of Contents

Reproductive Anatomy of the Mare

CHAPTER 1

OBJECTIVES

While studying the information covered in this chapter, the reader should attempt to:
- Acquire a working understanding of the anatomy of the reproductive organs of the mare.
- Acquire a working understanding of how defects in anatomic development of the reproductive tract of the mare, or changes in anatomy that occur with injury or age, may adversely affect fertility.
- Acquire a working understanding of procedures to be used for safe examination of the reproductive tract of the mare per rectum.

STUDY QUESTIONS

1. Describe the normal nonpregnant equine reproductive tract, including location and shape of the ovaries, ovulation fossa, oviducts, uterus, cervix, vagina, vestibule, and vulva.
2. Describe normal equine ovarian structures, the process of ovulation and oocyte entry into the oviduct, the process of sperm entry into the oviduct, and the site of fertilization.
3. List structures that are physically isolated from the reproductive tract but play a central role in regulation of reproductive events in the mare.
4. List three major physical barriers to contamination of the mare's uterus.
5. Describe important guidelines for examination of the mare reproductive tract per rectum, including restraint, protective wear, lubrication, manure removal, guards against rectal perforation, and anatomic orientation.
6. Discuss congenital and acquired defects of the mare reproductive tract that may affect reproductive performance.

The reproductive system is made up of two groups of organs: (1) those structures that are intrinsic to the reproductive tract (ovaries and tubular genitalia) and (2) those structures that are physically isolated from the reproductive tract but play a role in the regulation of reproductive events (e.g., pineal gland, retina, hypothalamus, pituitary gland).

The reproductive tract (Figures 1-1 through 1-7) consists of two ovaries and a tubular tract, including the paired oviducts and uterine horns, and a single uterine body, cervix, vagina, vestibule, and vulva. The lumen of the female reproductive tract is the only channel in the body that communicates between the abdominal cavity and the external environment. More than half of the reproductive tract lies within the abdominal cavity, with the remainder confined to the pelvic cavity. When the **ovum** is discharged from the follicle at ovulation, it is received at the level of the **ovarian bursa,** which is thought to assist the passage of the ovum into the **oviduct.** The oviduct is responsible for movement of sperm and ova to a common site (the **ampullary-isthmic junction**) for fertilization. After fertilization, the developing equine embryo travels down the oviduct; and after 4.5 to 5 days, it secretes increasing amounts of

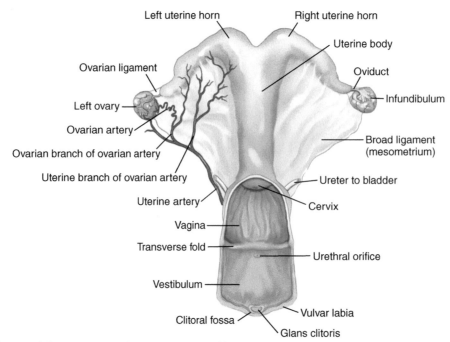

Figure 1-1   Dorsal view of the mare reproductive tract. Broad ligament attachments to the abdominal and pelvic walls are not depicted, and the dorsal vaginal wall has been omitted to reveal the mucosal surface of the external cervical os, vagina, and vestibule.

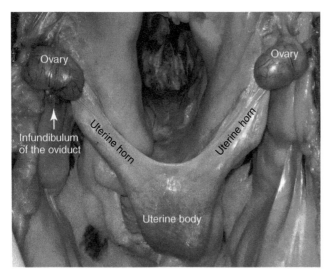
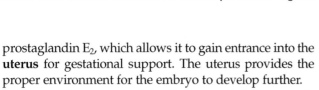

Figure 1-2   Frontal aspect of the suspended ovaries and uterus in situ. The rectum and abdominal viscera have been removed to facilitate visualization of the reproductive organs.

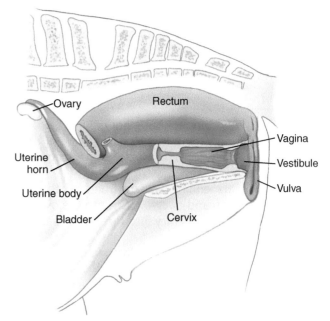

Figure 1-3   Lateral view of the reproductive organs and adjacent structures of the mare. Abdominal viscera are not depicted to facilitate visualization of the reproductive organs.

prostaglandin E_2, which allows it to gain entrance into the **uterus** for gestational support. The uterus provides the proper environment for the embryo to develop further.

The **cervix** accommodates the expanded glans penis of the stallion at estrus to allow intrauterine deposition of sperm and closes tightly during pregnancy to prevent ascending bacterial or fungal infection from the posterior tract. The cervix also expands considerably at the time of parturition to accommodate passage of the foal. The caudal portion of the cervix projects into the lumen of the vagina (Figure 1-8). Longitudinal folds comprise the lining of the cervix and are continuous with the

endometrial folds that line the uterine body. The cervix secretes two types of mucus: a thin mucus to lubricate the posterior genital tract in preparation for coitus and a more viscid mucus to help seal the cervical lumen during pregnancy.

The vagina is a potential space that expands to permit penile and foal passage. A transverse fold (remnant of the hymen) overlies the external urethral orifice and is the anatomic division between the **vagina,** which is

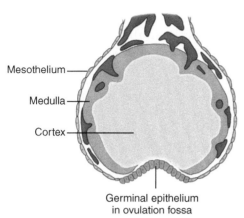

Figure 1-4 Schematic drawing of cortical and medullary areas of equine ovary. Germinal epithelium lines the surface of the ovulation fossa, where all ovulations take place. The oviductal fimbriae (not pictured) pick up the ovulated oocyte and move it to the site where fertilization takes place.

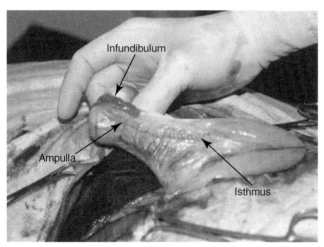

Figure 1-5 Lateral surface of ovary, oviduct, and end of uterine horn exposed through laparotomy site. The portions of the oviduct (infundibulum, ampulla, and isthmus) are identified.

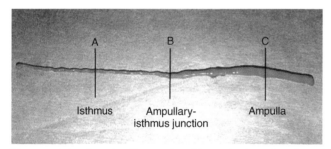

Figures 1-6 Grossly dissected oviduct depicts the site of fertilization near the end of the ampulla (ampullary-isthmic junction). *A* to *C* correspond with photomicrographs *A* to *C* in Figure 1-7.

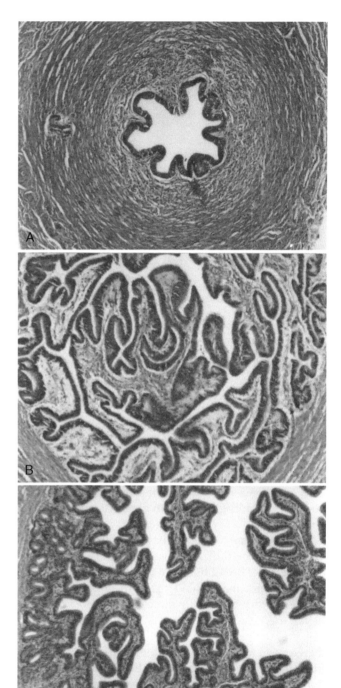

Figure 1-7 Corresponding histologic cross sections of the dissected oviduct in Figure 1-6. Note the smaller lumen and highly muscular component of the isthmus and the larger stellate lumen/diameter of the ampulla.

OVARIES

anterior, and the **vestibule,** which is posterior. The juncture between the vestibule and vagina is referred to as the **vestibulovaginal ring.** When closed, this ring restricts entry of air and debris into the upper tubular tract. The **vulva** is limited to the external opening of the tubular tract.

The ovaries of the mare are usually the most anterior part of the reproductive tract in the nonpregnant mare (see Figure 1-3). The noncoiled and dorsally suspended uterus of the mare (as compared with the coiled tract and more posterior [flank] broad ligament attachment in other farm animal species) accounts for the more cranial location of the ovaries. So, in the mare, the ovaries are in the

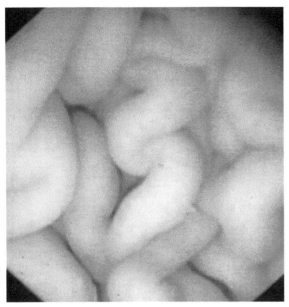

Figure 1-8 Endoscopic view of endometrial folds within collapsed uterine horn.

cranial-most transverse plane, whereas in other farm animal species, a portion of the uterus is cranial to the ovaries. The ovaries and the follicles are larger in the mare than in other farm animal species (see Figure 2-5). Equine ovaries are bean-shaped and vary in size according to ovarian activity; they are largest during the breeding season (spring and summer) and smallest during the nonbreeding season (winter anestrus). Average ovaries are 6 to 8 cm in length, 3 to 4 cm in height, and 70 to 80 g in weight.

The ovaries are located in the sublumbar area (ventral to the fourth or fifth lumbar vertebra), suspended by long sheet-like **broad ligaments,** and are usually located several centimeters behind the corresponding kidney. The right ovary is typically more cranial (2 to 3 cm) than the left. Because the ovaries may be lifted by the intestines, their actual location in the body is quite variable. Therefore, to facilitate locating the ovaries during palpation per rectum, we recommend tracing the tip of each uterine horn to the associated ovary (as the ovary may be in contact with, to within 5 cm of, the tip of the ipsilateral uterine horn). Each ovary consists of two surfaces (medial and lateral), two borders (attached [dorsal] and free [ventral]), and two poles (cranial [tubal] and caudal [uterine]). The caudal border is connected to the uterine horn by the ovarian ligament. Each ovary is kidney-bean shaped, with a prominent depression on the free or ventral border. The convex dorsal border is sometimes called the greater curvature.

The ovarian surface is largely covered by peritoneum except at the attached border where nerves and vessels enter. The relationship between ovarian cortical and medullary areas is unusual in the mare (see Figure 1-4). The ovary of the mare is "inside-out" compared with those of other farm animal species. In other words, the medullary or vascular zone is superficial and the

cortical zone (which contains the follicles) is in the interior of the gland. The cortical tissue reaches the surface only at the depression of the ventral or free border. This, therefore, is the only area from which normal ovulation occurs and is appropriately termed the **ovulation fossa.** The ovulation fossa is covered by a layer of short polygonal cells, which are a remnant of the primitive germinal epithelium. The ovulation papilla of the corpus luteum does not project from the convex surface of the ovary as it does in other species but rather protrudes into the ovulation fossa.

The ovary has both exocrine and endocrine functions. The **exocrine function** is development of gametes, and the **endocrine function** is production of hormones.

OVIDUCTS

The oviducts (Fallopian tubes, uterine tubes) are long tortuous ducts that measure 20 to 30 cm in length when fully extended in horse mares. Cilia are present on the epithelium of the oviduct and produce a current directed toward the uterus. The oviduct is divided into three parts: the **infundibulum** (funnel-shaped portion nearest the ovary), the **ampulla** (expanded middle portion), and the **isthmus** (narrowed portion that connects the ampulla to the uterine horn). The cranial edge of the infundibulum attaches to the lateral surface of the mare's ovary (see Figures 1-5 and 4-7). At ovulation, this fan-shaped structure envelopes the ovulation fossa to facilitate ovum entry into the oviduct. Cannulation of the infundibulum is possible through a flank approach, which has been used for such clinical and research procedures as **oocyte transfer** to a recipient mare, gamete intrafallopian transfer (GIFT) (instillation of both sperm and oocyte into a recipient mare), and flushing to determine oviductal patency. The ampulla is the middle part of the oviduct (see Figure 1-6) where fertilization and early cleavage of fertilized ovum occur. The highly muscular isthmus (see Figure 1-7) serves both as sperm reservoir and as a conduit to transport sperm from the uterus to the ampulla and fertilized ova (embryos) from the site of fertilization into the uterine lumen (see Figure 1-6). The oviduct enters the uterus just caudal to the blunt end of the uterine horn through a distinct papilla **(oviductal papilla)** that is easily visualized from the uterine lumen (see Figure 4-35). Normal oviducts are not usually palpable per rectum.

Sperm gain access to the oviduct through the **uterotubal junction (UTJ),** which is located in the center of the oviductal papilla that projects into the uterine lumen near the blunt end of the uterine horn. Deep edematous longitudinal folds are present in the UTJ during estrus, and numerous sperm can be found "bound" to epithelial cells or "trapped" in these folds within 4 hours of breeding. The UTJ may play a role in the selection of morphologically normal sperm (i.e., allowing only normal sperm to access the oviduct) and may also act as a storage site for sperm awaiting transport into the oviduct. The muscular isthmus is believed to contract rhythmically after breeding in a fashion that propels sperm to the fertilization site in the ampulla (near its end at the ampullary-isthmic junction). Adhesion of sperm to epithelial cells in this area is thought to prevent premature capacitation and increase the lifespan of the sperm, resulting in a sperm reservoir awaiting the opportunity for release to fertilize the ovum. Because mares may become pregnant (albeit at a lower rate) when ovulation occurs as late as 6 to 7 days after breeding, the sperm attached to the oviductal epithelium are thought to be gradually released in waves so as to continuously supply capacitated sperm that can fertilize the ovum.

UTERUS

The uterus consists of two horns and a singular body. The uterus has been described as T-shaped in the mare, but Y-shaped (see Figures 1-1 and 1-2) is probably a more accurate description of the organ when viewed dorsally in its natural position in the mare. The uterus is suspended within the pelvic cavity and abdomen by the broad ligament. These suspensory attachments also serve as sheaths that contain blood vessels, lymphatics, and nerves; the serous layer is continuous with the serous lining of the abdominal cavity. The portion of the broad ligament that attaches to the uterus is called the **mesometrium**. In the mare, the mesometrium attaches to the dorsal surface of the uterine horns, whereas in the cow, the attachment is on the ventrolateral surface. Therefore, in mares, the free (unattached) surface of the uterus is ventral to the broad ligament, whereas in cattle, the free surface is dorsal to the broad ligament. This arrangement hinders digital evaluation of the uterine body and likewise prevents retraction of the uterus into the pelvic cavity during palpation of the mare per rectum, in contrast with the cow, in which these procedures are easily accomplished. The uterine horns of the mare are entirely in the abdominal cavity and "float" on, or are intermingled with, intestinal viscera.

The serosal layer of the uterus and the vascular layer plus longitudinal muscular layer are continuous with that of the broad ligament. The **myometrium** is composed of an inner circular layer and an outer longitudinal layer, with the outer longitudinal layer continuous with that in the oviducts. Finally, the innermost layer of the uterus consists of the **endometrium**, which is glandular and secretory (see Figure 4-26).

The uterine lumen in the normal nonpregnant state is nearly obliterated by the collapsed wall and prominent **endometrial folds** (see Figure 1-8). The endometrial folds are arranged longitudinally in the uterus and are usually palpable per rectum when the uterus is "strummed" between the thumb and forefingers. The myometrium is quite thick and is responsible for variation in uterine tone of the mare during estrus versus diestrus or early pregnancy. In contrast with the cow, the uterus of the mare is not coiled, the intercornual ligament is not prominent, the internal bifurcation is marked by a short uterine septum (see Figure 4-33), and the body of the uterus is longer.

The vasculature of the uterus is supplied on each side by three arteries and veins (see Figure 1-1) that weave their way through the broad ligament: the uterine branch of the **vaginal artery** and corresponding vein, the **uterine artery** (sometimes called **middle uterine artery**) and corresponding vein, and the uterine branch of the ovarian artery and corresponding vein. Rupture of these arteries or veins sometimes occurs during parturition in aged mares, leading either to hematoma formation within the broad ligament or fatal hemorrhage into the abdomen (see Chapter 10). The **ovarian artery** is located in the cranial portion of the broad ligament and follows the course of the ovarian vein and the uterine branch of the ovarian vein; in contrast to ruminant species, the ovarian artery is not as closely attached or applied to the ovarian vein. This has important functional considerations, namely for countercurrent transport of prostaglandin-$F_2\alpha$ ($PGF_2\alpha$) from the veins draining the uterus into the ovarian artery. Because this countercurrent exchange is not efficient in the mare, regression of the corpus luteum is induced by $PGF_2\alpha$ that reaches the ovary via the systemic circulation, as opposed to ruminants, in which $PGF_2\alpha$ reaches the ovary in higher concentrations via the ovarian artery because of countercurrent exchange from the closely entwined uterine venous drainage.

CERVIX

The cervix is a dynamic organ in the mare. It is lined internally by epithelium-containing secretory cells that produce a thin mucus to serve as a lubricant during estrus and a thick mucus to occlude the cervical lumen during diestrus and pregnancy so that it is less permeable to bacteria and foreign material. The longitudinal folds of the cervix are continuous with the endometrial folds present in the body of the uterus. The cervix expands to accommodate the stallion's penis during estrus and the foal during parturition, and it closes tightly during diestrus and even more so during pregnancy.

The thick-walled cervix is usually identifiable via palpation per rectum, particularly during diestrus or pregnancy, and is typically 5 to 7.5 cm in length and 2 to 4 cm in diameter. During estrus, the cervix is quite flaccid and thus more difficult to feel via palpation per rectum.

The cervix of the mare has two features that differ from the cow: (1) the cervical lumen greatly expands and contracts during the estrous cycle as a result of a thick layer of circular muscle rich in elastic fibers; and (2) the cervix has only longitudinal folds with no obstructing transverse cervical rings. Therefore, the cervical changes are readily palpable throughout the estrous cycle in the mare, and the uterus is more easily accessed through the cervix than in the cow. The **external os of the cervix** protrudes into the vaginal lumen (Figure 1-9) and is surrounded by the **vaginal fornix**

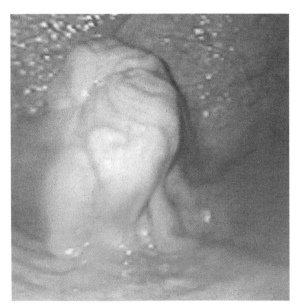

Figure 1-9   Per vagina view of external cervical os protruding into vaginal lumen.

(i.e., the area of reflection of vaginal mucous membrane onto the cervix).

VAGINA

The vagina is a tubular organ that extends horizontally for 15 to 20 cm through the pelvic cavity from the external os of the cervix to the **transverse fold** overlying the **external urethral orifice** (see Figure 1-1). In maiden mares, this transverse fold is often continued on either side of the vagina and forms the hymen. Occasionally, the hymen completely encircles the vestibulovaginal junction and is imperforate (**persistent hymen**) (Figure 1-10), precluding breeding until it is removed. The vagina continues caudally as the vestibule.

The lumen of the vagina is normally collapsed except during breeding and passage of the foal at parturition. The vagina, including its mucosa, is highly elastic and expands considerably to accommodate the passage of the foal. It becomes distended with air when the abnormal condition of **pneumovagina** exists. The lumen of the vagina is covered with stratified squamous epithelium. The cranial vagina is covered with serosa and lies within the peritoneal cavity. The posterior vagina is in a retroperitoneal position and is therefore not covered with serosa. Because **most of the vagina is retroperitoneal**, vaginal injuries (such as tearing during breeding) usually do not perforate into the peritoneal space, although this sometimes occurs. Puncturing the vaginal wall near the cervix does provide a surgical approach into the abdomen (**colpotomy**) for procedures such as ovariectomy. Unlike the uterus, cervix, and vestibule, the vagina contains no glandular structures.

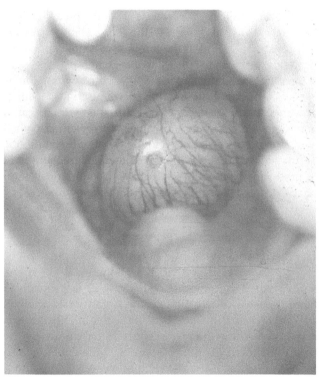

Figure 1-10   Persistent hymen in a maiden mare.

VESTIBULE

The vestibule extends 10 to 12 cm from the transverse fold overlying the external urethral orifice to the vulva. A vestibulovaginal ring exists at the junction of the vestibule and vagina and, because of vulvar and vaginal constrictor muscles that encircle this area, forms a seal, thereby minimizing entry of foreign material into the upper tubular tract. This ring oftentimes is incompetent (weak or incapable of closing) when pneumovagina exists, allowing entry of air into the vaginal space. The vestibule contains vestibular glands ventrally that secrete mucus to provide lubrication of the posterior tubular tract.

VULVA

The vulva (Figure 1-11) refers to the external opening of the female reproductive tract and the structures that surround it. The vertical vulvar opening normally begins 5 to 7 cm directly under the anus and is 12 to 15 cm in length. The dorsal commissure of the vulva normally is less than 5 cm above the ischium (floor of the pelvis). The mare is prone to aspiration of air into the vagina (**pneumovagina**) if the dorsal commissure is greater than 5 cm above the ischium, particularly if the anus is recessed (sunken) and the vulvar lips are tipped horizontally so the vulva is no longer vertical (Figure 1-12). The labia of the vulva contain underlying musculature that functions to close the vulvar opening, providing a further barrier to the entrance of foreign material into the tubular tract. The vulva contains much elastic tissue and expands

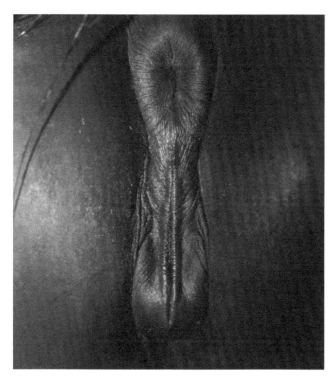

Figure 1-11 Normal vulva and anus of a mare.

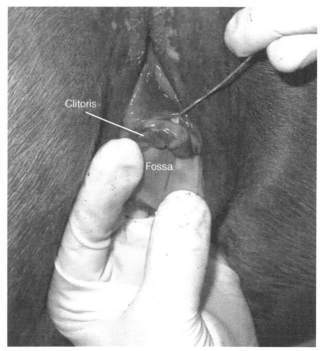

Figure 1-13 The clitoris is located in a cavity just cranial to the ventral commissure of the vulva. A wire is placed within one of the clitoral sinuses, and the edges of the clitoral fossa are retracted to expose the glans clitoris.

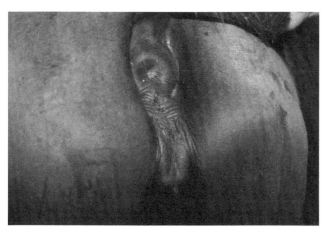

Figure 1-12 Sunken anus and tipped vulva in an aged mare.

EXAMINATION OF THE REPRODUCTIVE TRACT OF THE MARE PER RECTUM

Mare Restraint

The mare must be adequately restrained before examination of the reproductive tract. Such precautions protect both the mare and the examiner from severe injury. Minimal but effective restraint is the key to a safe examination and varies from mare to mare. The disposition of the mare should be determined before the examination begins. Mares accustomed to frequent examinations per rectum tend to need little restraint, whereas mares not accustomed to such practices often become anxious and sometimes explosive during the examination. In any case, one should never be careless and should always use caution. A strategically placed kick can quickly terminate a career! If available, all mares should be placed in stocks (Figure 1-14) before the examination. Ideally, the stocks should be equipped with a solid padded rear door to help prevent leg extension if the mare does decide to kick and to afford some protection against injury to the lower legs of the mare. The height of the door should not be higher than the mid-upper gaskin region of the mare's hindquarters. Higher doors could damage the examiner's arm if the mare abruptly squats while the arm is in the rectum. If stocks are not available, the mare should be examined in a doorway with the hindquarters remaining 2 feet beyond the doorway. The examiner, when

greatly during passage of the fetus at parturition. The **clitoris**, a homologue of the penis, is located in a cavity just cranial to the ventral commissure of the vulvar opening (Figure 1-13). The **glans clitoris** is more prominent in the mare than in other farm animal species. Three **clitoral sinuses** are located on the dorsal aspect of the clitoris, and a large singular **clitoral fossa** is located ventral to the glans clitoris. The clitoral sinuses and fossa must be swabbed for bacteriologic culture to document freedom from infection with *Taylorella equigenitalis* (formerly *Haemophilus equigenitalum)*, the causative organism of contagious equine metritis.

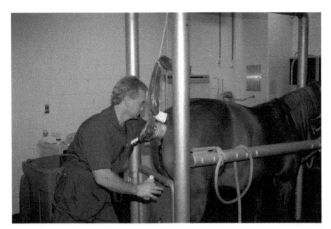

Figure 1-14 Mare being palpated in a stock with padded kickboard.

standing to the side, is thus protected by the door frame. If a mare must be examined in an open area, breeding hobbles can be properly secured to the mare's hind legs to reduce the range of limb motion, should she decide to kick. A leg strap can also be applied to a flexed front leg. Lifting the tail directly over the back of the mare also helps distract her from the examiner's activities. If necessary a twitch can also be placed on the mare's muzzle as an additional means of physical restraint. Tranquilization or sedation may be necessary to adequately restrain an anxious mare. Remember, overrestraint can be as dangerous to the mare and the examiner as underrestraint.

Never develop a false sense of security through the use of protective devices. Always take special precautions when walking around the hindquarters of a mare. Approach the mare from the front and work your way back to the hindquarters while quietly talking to her so she is aware of your location. Never surprise her. Minimize time spent directly behind the mare. Rather, stand to one side when possible. Stand close to the mare to reduce concussion, should you be in the line of fire if she decides to kick.

Technique

The first question that comes to mind is which arm to use to perform the examination. Ambidexterity may provide some advantage, but both hands are probably equally clumsy at the onset. Therefore, a general recommendation is to teach the off hand to palpate per rectum. The more frequently used hand can then be used to perform other duties (i.e., operating an ultrasound machine) during the examination.

Shoulder-length rubber obstetric sleeves or disposable plastic sleeves can be used to protect the arm during the examination. Soft pliable sleeves increase sensitivity. Alternatively, the fingers can be removed from the plastic sleeve and replaced with a latex surgical glove. To minimize horizontal disease transmission, sleeves should be changed between mares.

The protected hand should be well lubricated before use. A water-based lubricant such as methylcellulose can be used. The lubricated hand should then be shaped into a cone and gently inserted into the rectum through the tight anal sphincter. Slow rotation of the arm in conjunction with gentle forward pressure enhances advancement into the rectum. *Do not rush.* Rectal perforation is a common cause of malpractice claims against equine practitioners. Use extreme caution, and never perform forceful manipulations in the rectum against peristaltic waves or a tense rectal wall. If necessary, products such as propantheline bromide (Pro-Banthine, Schiapparelli Searle, Chicago, Ill.) or N-butylscopolammonium bromide (Buscopan, Boehringer Ingelheim Pharmaceuticals, Ridgefield, Conn.) can be administered to the mare to relax the rectum and reduce straining.

As much fecal material as possible should be removed from the rectum and distal colon before evaluation of abdominal and pelvic structures. This task is accomplished by passing the coned hand past a small amount of feces and then cupping the hand to facilitate removal when the arm is withdrawn.

Two established principles for examination of the female reproductive tract per rectum are (1) establish normal anatomic orientation and (2) follow a thorough methodical approach. Adherence to these principles reduces the chance of error.

Before emphasis is placed on detection of the reproductive tract, the examiner should first become properly oriented by identifying topographic landmarks that are in a constant position, such as the outlines of the pelvic cavity (the pelvic floor, sacrum, wings of the ilia, and pelvic brim). Once the examiner is confident of the location in the pelvic and abdominal cavities, specific examination of reproductive structures may begin.

Three initial landmarks for locating the reproductive tract in the mare have been described by various authorities on the subject: the cervix, the leading edge of the uterus, and the ovary. All of the structures have a relatively inconstant position. The cervix of the nonpregnant mare is located in the pelvic cavity, whereas the leading edge of the uterus and the ovaries are always in the abdominal cavity. To locate the cervix of a nonpregnant mare, one should produce a side-to-side motion with the extended hand in the pelvic cavity, with downward pressure with the fingers held together and the palm facing downward (Figure 1-15). The cervix can be palpated in almost all instances but may relax during estrus to the point of becoming barely perceptible. However, even in this relaxed state, it can be identified when the fingers slip caudally off the shelf formed by the external os. Uterine contents (e.g., fetus or pyometra) may pull the cervix into an abdominal position, making palpation more difficult. Palpation of the dilated cervix per rectum is also difficult in the early postpartum period.

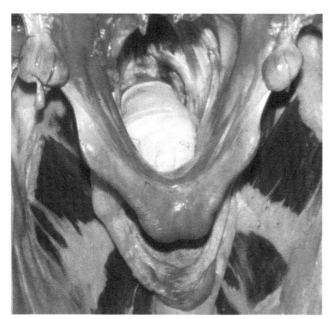

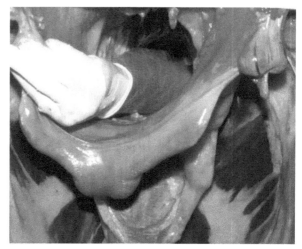

Figure 1-17 Palpation of an ovary per rectum. The ovary is gently grasped with the finger tips, to enable the examiner to identify raised or softened follicles. The rectum and abdominal viscera have been removed to facilitate visualization.

Figure 1-15 Procedure used to locate cervix during palpation per rectum. A side-to-side motion is made with the extended hand in the pelvic cavity, with downward pressure with the fingers held together and the palm facing downward. The rectum and abdominal viscera have been removed to facilitate visualization.

The leading edge of the uterus can be detected by first inserting the arm deeply into the rectum, cupping the hand downward, then slowly retracting the arm (Figure 1-16). Alternatively, the hand can be gently pressed downward as the arm is advanced into the rectum until a potential space is felt beyond the brim of the pelvis, whereupon the hand is cupped and retracted. The cupped hand "hooks" the uterus if the technique is properly applied and if the uterus is of a normal nonpregnant size and in the usual location. Enlarged uteri that have begun descent into the lower abdomen are difficult to identify with this method.

The ovaries are located in the sublumbar area, caudoventral to the corresponding kidney. By following the leading edge of the uterus laterally and slightly cranially, the ovary can usually be located with the fingertips. Gently retracting the ipsilateral uterine horn or broad ligament often helps bring the ovary to a more readily palpable location. If the rectal wall is relaxed, gentle grasping motions can be used to pick up the ovary (Figure 1-17). The ovaries are pulled downward and toward the midline when the uterus becomes greatly enlarged (i.e., in the early postpartum period, in advanced pregnancy [see Figure 7-11], or in some cases of pyometra).

Once any of these landmarks is located, the practitioner should proceed with a methodical examination of the accessible reproductive tract. The examination should include both ovaries, the uterus, and the cervix. Structures caudal to the cervix do not lend themselves to palpation per rectum but rather are evaluated via the vulvar opening.

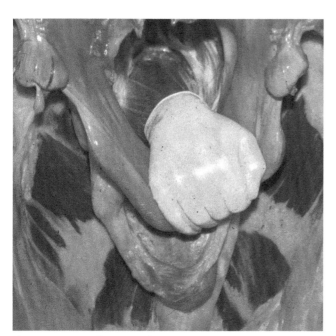

Figure 1-16 Palpation of uterine horns per rectum. The cupped hand is used to grasp the leading edge of the uterine horn. The rectum and abdominal viscera have been removed to facilitate visualization.

BIBLIOGRAPHY

Ginther OJ: *Reproductive biology of the mare: basic and applied aspects,* ed 2, Cross Plains, WI, 1992, Equiservices, 1-40.

Greenhoff GR, Kenney RM: Evaluation of reproductive status of non-pregnant mares, *JAVMA* 167:449-458, 1975.

Sisson S, Grossman JD: *The anatomy of domestic animals,* ed 4, Philadelphia, 1953, Saunders, 606-614.

Reproductive Physiology of the Nonpregnant Mare

2

CHAPTER

OBJECTIVES

While studying the information covered in this chapter, the reader should attempt to:
- Acquire a working understanding of the physiology of the estrous cycle of the mare.
- Acquire a working knowledge of the criteria used for staging the estrous cycle of the mare.
- Acquire a working understanding of seasonal control of reproductive function of the mare.

STUDY QUESTIONS

1. List the length of the estrous cycle, estrus, and diestrus in the mare.
2. Explain the endocrine events that occur during estrus, ovulation, formation of the corpus luteum, and luteolysis in the mare.
3. Explain why determination of the presence of a large follicle on an ovary is a poor predictor of estrus in the mare.
4. List the criteria that are useful in staging the estrous cycle via palpation per rectum in the mare.
5. Describe the ultrasonographic changes that occur in the dominant follicles as ovulation approaches.
6. Describe the effects of long and short photoperiods on control of reproductive function of the mare.
7. Describe the seasonal effects on incidence of ovulation in mare populations in the Northern Hemisphere.
8. Discuss effects of season on duration of estrus in the mare, including the first postpartum estrus (foal heat).

THE ESTROUS CYCLE

The mare is a **seasonal polyestrous** animal. During the breeding season (spring and summer), the nonpregnant mare has recurring estrous cycles. The length of the estrous cycle can be defined as the period from one ovulation to a subsequent ovulation (interovulatory interval). Each ovulation is accompanied by a period of behavioral signs of estrus while plasma progesterone concentrations remain low (<1 ng/mL). The estrous cycle is divided into the ovulation process and an interovulatory period. The estrous cycle may also be considered to consist of a **follicular phase** (**estrus**) (in which

the mare is sexually receptive to the stallion, and the genital tract is prepared to accept and transport sperm to the oviducts for fertilization) that involves the ovulation process and a **luteal phase** (**diestrus**) (in which the mare is not receptive to the stallion, and the genital tract is prepared to accept and nurture the conceptus). The diestrous period ends with regression of the corpus luteum, initiation of the next follicular phase, and onset of estrous behavior. The average length of the estrous cycle in mares during the physiologic breeding season is 21 to 22 days (range, approximately 18 to 24 days), with estrus comprising 4 to 7 of these days (Figure 2-1). The length of diestrus remains relatively

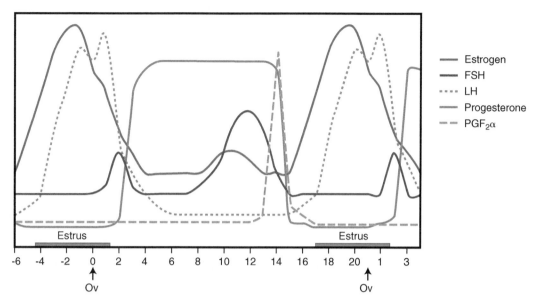

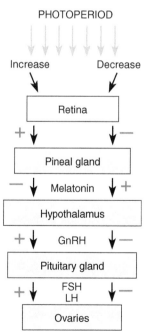

Figure 2-1 The estrous cycle of the mare averages 21 to 22 days, with 4 to 7 days of estrus (sexual receptivity) and 14 to 15 days of diestrus (during which the mare is not sexually receptive to the stallion). Ovulation generally occurs 1 to 2 days before the end of estrus. (Modified from Irvine CHG: Endocrinology of the estrous cycle of the mare: applications to embryo transfer, *Theriogenology* 15:85, 1981; and Neely DP, et al: *Equine reproduction*, Princeton, NJ, 1983, Veterinary Learning Systems Co)

constant at 14 to 15 days and is less affected by season than is the length of estrus. The length of estrus is more variable (range, 2 to 12 days, or more), typically with a longer duration early in the breeding season, perhaps as the result of a less prominent **luteinizing hormone (LH)** surge during this time period. The diameter of the largest follicle at the time of luteolysis affects the interval from onset of estrus to ovulation; larger follicles present at **corpus luteum (CL)** regression typically ovulate sooner, thus shortening the associated estrous period.

The regular pattern of the estrous cycle relies on the delicate balance among hormones produced by the pineal gland, hypothalamus, pituitary gland, ovaries, and endometrium (Figures 2-2 and 2-3). The neurosecretory cells in the hypothalamus produce **gonadotropin-releasing hormone (GnRH).** Axons of these cells project into the perivascular space in the median eminence at the origin of the pituitary stalk and *episodically* release GnRH into the hypothalamic-hypophyseal (hypothalamic-pituitary) portal system, which transports the hormone to the anterior pituitary. GnRH stimulates the synthesis and release of the gonadotropin **follicle-stimulating hormone (FSH)** and LH from the anterior pituitary gland. These hormones enter the systemic circulation, and at the level of the ovaries, FSH is responsible for follicular recruitment whereas LH is responsible for follicular maturation and production of estrogen, ovulation, and luteinization. The estrogen produced by maturing follicles (particularly the dominant follicle) has a positive feedback on LH release (i.e., it promotes further LH release) in the

presence of low circulating progesterone concentration. **Inhibin** and estrogen produced by growing follicles have a negative feedback effect on release of FSH (i.e., they inhibit FSH release). Progesterone produced by the CL has a negative feedback effect on release of LH from the anterior pituitary.

Figure 2-2 A simplified version of hormonal regulation of the estrous cycle of the mare. The regular pattern of the estrous cycle of the mare is controlled by the interplay among the pineal gland, hypothalamus, pituitary, ovaries, and endometrium. The role of the endometrium is depicted in Figure 2-3.

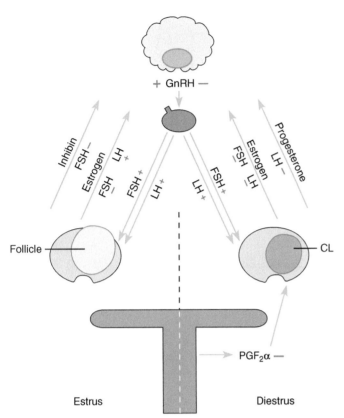

Figure 2-3 Schematic depiction of hormonal control of ovarian activity in the mare.

The follicular phase of the estrous cycle is characterized by follicular growth with **estrogen** production, which results in behavioral estrus (Figure 2-4). Many follicles start the maturation process, but usually only one follicle becomes dominant and ovulates. Follicular development typically occurs in one or two major waves during the estrous cycle. The term **follicular wave** has been used to describe the initially synchronous growth of a group of follicles until one or perhaps two, or rarely more, follicles begin preferential growth (i.e., become dominant) to the remaining follicles. The selected follicle continues to grow (>30 mm diameter) (Figure 2-5) until it either ovulates or regresses. For mares with one follicular wave during the estrous cycle, the wave emerges at midcycle (approximately day 10 after ovulation). This **primary follicular wave** results in an ultrasonographically identifiable dominant follicle approximately 7 days before ovulation. For mares with two follicular waves during the estrous cycle, the dominant follicle selected during the first follicular wave that begins during late estrus or early diestrus sometimes ovulates **(diestrous ovulation)**. The incidence of **secondary follicular waves** and diestrous ovulations is currently thought to be higher in Thoroughbreds than in Quarter Horses and ponies and may contribute (when ovulation occurs) to longer diestrous intervals within a breed when compared with mares of the same breed that do not have diestrous ovulations.

At the onset of luteolysis, the largest follicle is typically the one to enlarge and ovulate. Ovulation is a rapid process, with most of the follicular fluid being released within 2 minutes (50% to 90% evacuation within 60 seconds) and with complete evacuation typically requiring 2 to 7 minutes. The remainder of the follicles that have already become atretic eventually regress. In light breed horse mares, follicular diameter at ovulation normally ranges from 30 to 50 mm (seldom <35 mm) and usually approximates 40 to 45 mm, although smaller or larger follicles sometime ovulate. Smaller breeds (e.g., ponies and miniatures) tend to ovulate smaller (≤30 mm) follicles, and larger breeds such as draft mares, especially Friesians, tend to ovulate larger (>45-mm follicles). Ovulatory follicles are often larger early in the breeding season (March to May) compared with those that ovulate in the peak of

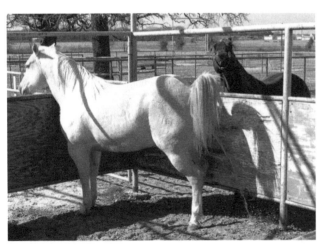

Figure 2-4 Mare shows typical signs of estrus: squatting with tail raised, urinating, and everting clitoris.

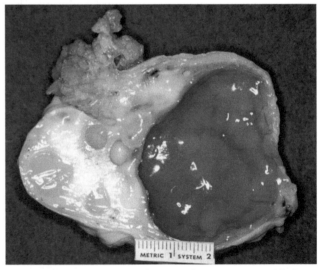

Figure 2-5 Cross-sectional view of mare ovary with large preovulatory follicle.

the season (June and July). Most mares ovulate within 48 hours before the end of estrus; occasionally mares ovulate after the end of estrus (usually on the day when intensity of estrous signs is decreasing). The incidence of double (multiple) ovulations averages 16%, with Thoroughbred, Warmblood, and draft mares having the highest incidence of multiple ovulations and Quarter Horse, Appaloosa, and pony mares having the lowest incidence.

The luteal phase is initiated at ovulation by the formation of a progesterone-secreting CL (Figure 2-6), which causes the mare to cease showing signs of behavioral estrus (Figure 2-8). Maximum circulating progesterone concentrations are reached by 6 days after ovulation. A mare rarely shows behavioral signs of estrus when plasma progesterone concentrations exceed 1 to 2 ng/mL, even when large follicles are present on the ovaries. The life span of the corpus luteum is dependent on the endogenous release of **prostaglandin-$F_2\alpha$ ($PGF_2\alpha$)** from the endometrium, which occurs in bursts between days 13 and 16 after ovulation. The $PGF_2\alpha$ is absorbed into the uterine venous drainage and, unlike in the cow, enters the circulation and

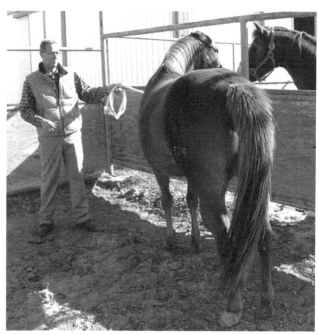

Figure 2-8 Mare shows typical signs of nonestrus: laid-back ears, switching tail, and kicking.

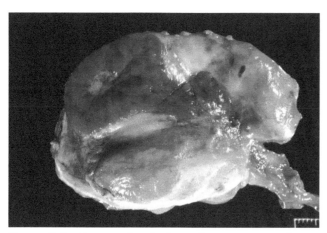

Figure 2-6 Cross-sectional view of mare ovary. Corpus luteum protrudes into ovulation fossa. (Photo courtesy of Dr. John Edwards.)

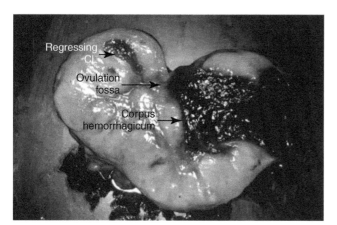

Regressing CL
Ovulation fossa
Corpus hemorrhagicum

Figure 2-7 Cross section of mare ovary depicting recent ovulation (corpus hemorrhagicum).

reaches the ovaries primarily via systemic circulation. Rapid luteolysis is caused by the $PGF_2\alpha$, resulting in a decline in circulating progesterone concentration (a detectable decline occurs within 4 hours, with concentrations less than 1 ng/mL occurring within 40 hours of the initial $PGF_2\alpha$ release), which, in turn, removes the block to LH secretion. Follicular maturation and behavioral signs characteristic of the follicular phase of the estrous cycle then ensue. Deviations (of several days) in the length of the luteal phase are usually the result of uterine disorders that lead to spurious secretion of $PGF_2\alpha$, such as acute endometritis (which shortens diestrus) or persistent luteal function (which prolongs diestrus) from failure of the luteolytic mechanism (perhaps from failure of the endometrium to release sufficient amounts of $PGF_2\alpha$ in late diestrus).

STAGING THE ESTROUS CYCLE VIA EXAMINATION

Determination of the stage of the estrous cycle can be made via examination of the reproductive tract. Criteria that are used for determining the stage of the cycle include the size and softness of ovarian follicles and relaxation of the uterus and cervix, via palpation per rectum. With the exception of determination of a recent ovulation (i.e., typically within 0 to 3 days) (see Figure 2-7), palpation for presence of a CL is not possible in the mare (e.g., the follicle ovulates into the ovulation fossa and the CL does not protrude from the surface of the ovary). Use of transrectal ultrasonography is also helpful for staging the estrous cycle because the size and character of the follicles can be determined, corpora lutea can be visualized, and the degree of endometrial edema can be determined. Determination of whether the cervix is tight and closed or relaxed and open is typically made via palpation per rectum. Determination of whether the cervix is closed and dry or relaxed, edematous, and moist with cervical mucus can also be made via palpation per vagina or via visualization per vagina with a speculum. Finally, accurate teasing information, including the dates on which signs of estrus or nonestrus were determined when the mare was presented to the stallion, is helpful in staging the cycle (see Figures 2-4 and 2-8 to 2-11).

Large follicles can be present during any stage of the estrous cycle, so *follicular size alone is not a reliable indicator of estrus or diestrus*. When a mare shows signs of estrus during teasing with a stallion, one or more large follicles are present on an ovary, and the uterus and cervix are soft and relaxed (edematous endometrial folds may also be seen on ultrasound examination), a determination of estrus can be made. The same criteria are used to predict time of ovulation for breeding of a mare in estrus. If the mare does not exhibit positive behavioral signs of estrus when teased by a stallion, the uterus is firm ("toned up"), and the cervix is narrow and tightly closed on palpation, a determination of diestrus can be made. In the diestrous mare, a corpus luteum can be visualized on an ovary with ultrasound examination, and the endometrium exhibits uniform echodensity without visualization of edema. A summary of criteria used to stage the estrous cycle in the mare is presented in Table 2-1. Note that in some maiden mares, the cervix may not completely relax and

the mares may not be receptive to the stallion when in estrus despite the presence of a large preovulatory follicle.

Prediction of Time of Ovulation

Although not foolproof, a number of criteria can be used to predict the expected time of ovulation occurrence in mares that are in estrus. Criteria typically used by veterinary practitioners include day of estrus, intensity of signs of estrus, degree of uterine edema and cervical relaxation, size of dominant follicles, softness of dominant follicles, size and shape of dominant follicles on ultrasound examination, and ultrasonographic characteristics of the dominant follicular wall and fluid. If good teasing procedures are practiced, and if regular estrous cycles are occurring, the length of estrus tends to be somewhat repeatable within a mare. For example, if a mare ovulated on day 4 of estrus during the last estrous cycle, she is likely to ovulate near this time during her next estrous cycle. Likewise, maximum intensity of estrous behavior tends to occur near the end of estrus as a mare approaches ovulation. Relaxation of the cervix and uterus, along with intensity of edema noted within endometrial folds on ultrasound examination, progressively increases throughout estrus until 1 to 2 days before ovulation, when endometrial edema begins to decline.

Wisconsin workers recently performed frequent ultrasonographic assessments of the dominant follicle of mares until ovulation occurred. When follicles reached 35 mm in diameter and prominent uterine edema was present, examinations at 12-hour intervals for 36 hours were instituted. After this 36-hour observation period, examinations were continued once

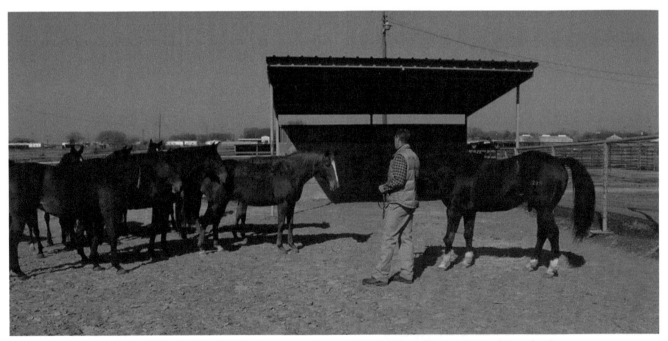

Figure 2-9 Method for teasing mares in a paddock with stallion restrained on a lead.

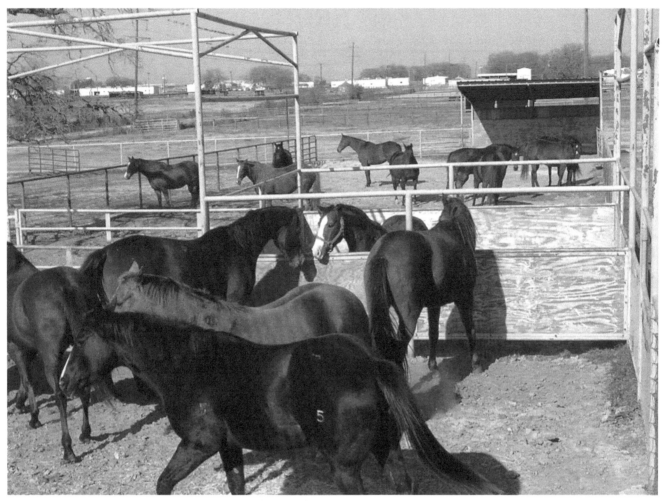

Figure 2-10 Method for teasing mares with stallion in a box, allowing unrestrained mares in adjoining paddocks to approach the stallion at will.

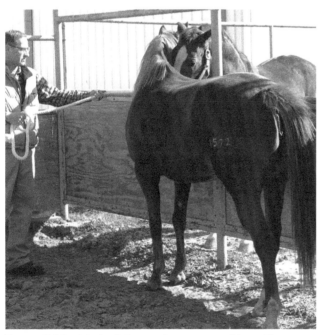

Figure 2-11 Method for teasing mares with stallion unrestrained in a box and mare on a lead taken to stallion.

hourly for 12 hours or until ovulation occurred. The investigators specifically noted degree of serration of the granulosa layer (i.e., irregular or notched appearance of inner follicular wall); assessment of the turgidity of the follicular wall (via palpation per rectum); loss of spherical shape; development of an apex, sometimes with a nipple area representing the stigma; and presence of echoic spots within the follicular antrum. They found that no single criterion approached 100% as a predictor of impending ovulation when mares were examined at 12- to 24-hour intervals. However, with once- or twice-daily examination frequencies, the best predictor of ovulation occurring within the next 12-hour period was development of serration of the granulosa (i.e., 59% ovulated within 12 hours). When they aligned hourly examinations to the time of ovulation, they found that serration, decreased turgidity, loss of spherical shape, and development of an apex reached 100% within 1 hour before ovulation. Echoic spots appeared in only 50% of follicles within the 1 to 2 hours before ovulation. The investigators concluded that when examinations are performed only

TABLE 2-1

Criteria Used to Stage the Estrous Cycle of the Mare

Criteria	Estrus	Diestrus
Teasing with stallion	1. Tail raise	1. Switch tail
	2. Squat, tip pelvis	2. Kick, squeal
	3. Urinate	3. Attempt to bite stallion
	4. Evert clitoris	4. Move away from stallion
Examination of ovaries	1. Large follicle(s) that may be soft	1. Presence of corpus luteum on ultrasound examination
	2. Follicle may be triangular with scalloped edges on ultrasound examination if mare is nearing ovulation	2. Follicles of varying sizes, may be large
	3. No corpus luteum on ultrasound examination	
Examination of uterus	1. Relaxed with soft texture	1. Firm texture (good tone)
	2. Edematous endometrial folds visible on ultrasound examination	2. Uniform echogenicity on ultrasound examination
Examination of cervix	1. Shortening, widening	1. Long and narrow with firm texture
	2. Relaxed with soft texture	2. Pale, dry, and centrally located in cranial vagina when visualized through speculum
	3. Pink and drooping on vaginal floor when visualized through speculum	3. Closed lumen on digital examination per vagina
	4. Lumen open 1 to 3+ fingers on digital examination per vagina	

daily, serration of the granulosa is detected in only 30% of mares before ovulation. If examinations are performed twice daily, serration of the granulosa is detected in 60% of mares, of which two thirds ovulate within 12 hours and one third ovulate within 24 hours. However, if echoic spots are detected within the follicular antrum, ovulation usually occurs within 1 to 2 hours.

SEASONALITY

Seasonal variation in the duration of daylight has a profound influence on mare reproductive performance. The horse is a seasonal breeder, and this pattern is regulated by day length or **photoperiod.** The horse responds positively (with improved reproductive efficiency) to increasing amounts of daylight and negatively (with reduced reproductive efficiency) to decreasing amounts of daylight. Length of photoperiod modulates reproductive activity through regulation of GnRH secretion. Although modulation of pineal activity in the mare remains speculative, the **pineal gland** is thought to signal the hypothalamus through secretion of **melatonin.** Kentucky workers have shown that in most but not all mares,

melatonin secretion is increased during nighttime hours. When day length is short, melatonin released by the pineal is thought to suppress GnRH synthesis and release. When day length is long, melatonin secretion is reduced and the inhibitory influence on GnRH synthesis and secretion is removed (see Figure 2-2). These concepts are supported by Florida pinealectomy studies in equids. In addition, French workers have shown that melatonin administration during winter months can block the stimulatory effect of artificially increased photoperiod and thus delay the onset of the breeding season. However, Kentucky workers found the presence or absence of nighttime rises in melatonin concentrations was not predictive of whether mares would continue to have regular estrous cycles in winter and suggested melatonin secretion during this time plays a limited role in controlling the onset of winter anestrus.

Opioids may participate in regulation of seasonal reproduction by modulating LH secretion during winter anestrus. Endogenous opioids are known to suppress gonadotropin secretion in farm animals, presumably by dampening the **GnRH pulse generator** (synchronous activation of GnRH neurons). New Zealand workers showed that "opioid tone" was higher in mares during deep winter anestrus than during the breeding season, but the use of opioid antagonists in mares has failed to alter seasonality. Research on the role of endogenous opioids in reproductive seasonality in mares is continuing.

Although transition between seasons is a gradual progressive process, the reproductive year for the mare population can be divided for descriptive purposes into four seasons that correspond with changes in day length. Pennsylvania workers have summarized these seasons as follows: The period of peak fertility (i.e., the physiologic breeding season or period of **ovulatory receptivity**) surrounds the longest day of the year, or summer solstice (June 21 to 22), The mare then moves into a transitional period of **anovulatory receptivity** that coincides with the autumnal equinox (September 21 to 22), when day and night are of equal length. During this period, the mare exhibits erratic estrous behavior often without corresponding ovulation. If ovulation does occur, CL function is not maintained. Mares then enter a state of **anestrus,** or sexual quiescence, that centers on and after the shortest day of the year, or winter solstice (December 21 to 22). After this period, the mare enters another transitional period of **anovulatory receptivity** that corresponds with the vernal equinox (March 21 to 22). This period is characterized by a long and erratic heat period that finally culminates in an ovulation, thus initiating the period of ovulatory receptivity. This cyclic pattern is a trend and does not include all mares because a small percentage (approximately 15% to 20%) cycle regularly throughout the year. Even mare populations near the equator tend to show a seasonal pattern of reproductive cyclicity. Interestingly, Kentucky workers have recently shown that, within a mare, the seasonal pattern of reproductive activity can vary considerably from year to year.

Reproductive seasonality effectively results in foals being delivered in the spring, when environmental conditions are favorable for foal survival. The role of seasonality on several aspects of reproductive performance helps exemplify this point. For instance, the initiation of estrus is under the direct influence of day length. As day length increases, the length of estrus decreases and the incidence of ovulation increases, both of which result in more conceptions for less work. The shortest heat periods and highest ovulation rates occur in June, thereby producing May foals. Furthermore, some poorly understood factors encourage a pregnant mare to foal during the physiologic breeding season. Mares with foals born near the first of the year tend to have a longer gestation length than mares with foals born late in the season. Another factor that favors May and June breeding occurs in mares that undergo **foal heat** (first postpartum estrus) near the first of the year; they tend to ovulate at a longer interval from parturition than those mares that enter foal heat later in the year. In addition, Texas workers recently showed that the incidence rate of postpartum anestrus (i.e., first

postpartum estrus delayed to more than 30 days after foaling) was higher in early than in late-foaling mares (28% in January-foaling mares to less than 3% in April-foaling mares). All these phenomena suggest that an inherent mechanism is present that pushes breeding and foaling toward the physiologic breeding season (May through July).

Physiologic Changes That Occur During Transition from Seasonal Anestrus Through the Onset of the Breeding Season

Most mares in the Northern Hemisphere (approximately 85%) enter a period of reproductive quiescence (winter or seasonal anestrus) during the late fall or winter (period of shortened day length). During the period of seasonal anestrus, the hypothalamic-pituitary-ovarian axis is relatively inactive, with GnRH content of the hypothalamus, LH content of the pituitary, and circulating concentrations of gonadotropin (LH and FSH) and ovarian steroids (progesterone and estrogen) being decreased. In response to the cue of increasing day length, this axis becomes progressively more active, and pituitary stores of gonadotropin gradually increase. GnRH is released more frequently from the hypothalamus, resulting in concurrent episodes of gonadotropin secretion. In mid to late transition, FSH concentrations are elevated, and LH concentrations remain comparatively low. Follicular growth occurs, resulting in development of several follicles 20 to 35 mm in diameter that do not ovulate. Evidence shows that the increased follicular activity may not be attributable to changes in circulating concentrations of FSH and LH, but perhaps a change in the responsiveness of the growing follicles to gonadotropin occurs instead. Nevertheless, as ovulation approaches, a reciprocal relationship between the gonadotropins develops, with mean concentrations of LH increasing and mean concentrations of FSH decreasing. Apparently, once a dominant follicle develops (35 mm in diameter and capable of producing significant amounts of estrogen) in concert with an increased pituitary store of LH, LH release is enhanced, causing ovulation to occur. In general, once a mare ovulates and forms a corpus luteum, regular estrous cycles ensue (e.g., 14- to 16-day periods of diestrus; followed by a variable period of estrus, which may exceed 10 days early in the spring but eventually averages 4 to 7 days in late spring or summer). The physiologic breeding season, when the preponderance of mares is ovulating in concurrence with regular estrous cycles **(ovulatory estrus),** typically is achieved during the late spring and summer months in the northern hemisphere (reviewed in Ginther 1992).

As follicular growth and regression begins during the spring transitional period (last 1 to 2 months of the anovulatory period), mares typically show erratic signs of estrous behavior toward the stallion. This **transitional estrus** is variable in length and intensity but frequently is of prolonged duration (i.e., sometimes a month or more in length). Because estrogen production by large follicles is an indication of competence, some workers have proposed that the concurrent development of prominent endometrial edema might indicate follicular maturation with impending ovulation. However, English workers recently showed that several such follicular waves occur (on average, 3 to 5) during the late transition period (each with development of large follicles exceeding 30 mm in diameter and significant estradiol production, with the appearance of marked endometrial edema) before culmination in the first ovulation of the year. Therefore, prediction that a mare will ovulate during this late transition period remains fraught with difficulty, as does determining the precise time the mare should be bred to maximize the opportunity to establish pregnancy.

Interestingly, although this first ovulation is unpredictable, it is fertile. Colorado workers achieved normal pregnancy rates by breeding mares in transitional estrus every other day until the first ovulation of the year, even though some mares were bred more than 10 times during this estrus. Because it is not efficient stallion usage to breed mares during this long transitional estrus, efforts can be directed at (1) hastening the onset of regular estrous cycles by providing an **artificial photoperiod;** (2) shortening the duration of the late transition period by administering hormones; (3) hastening, or ensuring, ovulation of a dominant follicle within 48 hours after breeding by the stallion; or (4) waiting to breed the mare until regular estrous cycles occur naturally.

OPERATIONAL BREEDING SEASON

Horses have been described as inefficient breeders in comparison with other domestic species. This description, however, is a fallacy and stems from man's attempt to redesign the breeding season of the horse to meet his own needs. The operational breeding season for horses with a universal birthday of January 1 is often precariously assigned as the period from February 15 to the first week of July. This modified breeding season overlaps into the period of anovulatory receptivity that is characterized by prolonged heats and delayed ovulation, thus indicating that the mares have not yet obtained their optimum reproductive potential. Breeding inefficiency in horses evolves when they are bred out of the physiologic breeding season. Otherwise, intrinsic fertility is quite acceptable in the horse.

BIBLIOGRAPHY

Blanchard TL, Thompson JA, Brinsko SP, et al: Mating mares on foal heat: a five-year retrospective study, *Proc 50th Ann Mtg Am Assoc Equine Pract* 525-530, 2004.

Daels PF, Hughes JP: The normal estrous cycle. In McKinnon AO, Voss JL, editors: *Equine reproduction,* Philadelphia, 1993, Lea & Febiger, 121-132.

Daels PF, Fatone S, Hansen BS, et al: Dopamine antagonist-induced reproductive function in anoestrous mares: gonadotropin secretion and effect of environmental cues, University of Pretoria, South Africa, 1998, *Proc 7th Int Symp Equine Reprod*, 45-46.

Fitzgerald BP, Schmidt MJ: Absence of an association between melatonin and reproductive activity in mares during the nonbreeding season, *Biol Reprod* (Mono 1):425-434, 1995.

Gastal EL, Gastal MO, Ginther OJ: Serrated gransulosa and other discrete ultrasound indicators of impending ovulation in mares, *J Equine Vet Sci* 26:67-73, 2006.

Ginther OJ: *Reproductive biology of the mare: basic and applied aspects,* ed 2, Cross Plains, WI, 1992, Equiservices, 41-74, 105-290, 158-161.

Greenhoff GR, Kenney RM: Evaluation of reproductive status of nonpregnant mares, *JAVMA* 167:449-458, 1975.

Grubaugh W, Sharp DC, Berglund LA, et al: Effects of pinealectomy in pony mares, *J Reprod Fertil* 32(Suppl):293-295, 1982.

Guillaume D, Arnaud G, Camillo F, et al: Effect of melatonin implants on reproductive status of mares, *Biol Reprod Mono* 1:435-442, 1995.

Nagy P, Guillame D, Daels PF: Seasonality in mares, *Anim Reprod Sci* 60/61:245-262, 2000.

Nishikawa Y, Hafez ESE: Horses. In Hafez ESE, editor: *Reproduction in farm animals,* Philadelphia, 1975, Lea & Febiger, 288-300.

Sharp DL, et al: Photoperiod. In McKinnon AO, Voss JL, editors: *Equine reproduction,* Philadelphia, 1993, Lea & Febiger, 179-185.

Squires EL, et al: Relationship of altrenogest to ovarian activity, hormone concentrations and fertility of mares, *J Anim Sci* 56:901-910, 1983.

Turner JE, Irvine CHG, Alexander S: Regulation of seasonal breeding by endogenous opioids in mares, *Biol Reprod Mono* 1:443-448, 1995.

Watson ED, Thomassen R, Nikolakopoulos E: Association of uterine edema with follicle waves around the onset of the breeding season in pony mares, *Theriogenology* 59:1181-1187, 2003.

Manipulation of Estrus in the Mare

3

OBJECTIVES

While studying the information covered in this chapter, the reader should attempt to:
- Understand potential advantages for manipulating estrus in broodmares.
- Acquire a working understanding of the principles by which manipulation of the photoperiod advances the onset of the breeding season in mares.
- Acquire a working knowledge of the rationale for, and efficacy of, hormone administration for hastening the onset of the breeding season in mares.
- Acquire a working knowledge of the use of various hormones for manipulating estrus in the cyclic mare, including the first postpartum estrus.

STUDY QUESTIONS

1. Describe the physiologic changes that occur during transition from seasonal anestrus through onset of the breeding season in mares in the northern hemisphere.
2. Define the following terms:
   a. Seasonal (winter) anestrus
   b. Transitional estrus
   c. Ovulatory estrus
   d. Artificial photoperiod
3. List guidelines to be followed when designing an artificial lighting program for broodmares in the Northern Hemisphere.
4. Discuss the rationale for use of progestogen/progesterone to hasten (synchronize) the onset of ovulatory estrus in mares.
5. Outline a program (and include expected responses) for treating mares with altrenogest to:
   a. Hasten (synchronize) the onset of ovulatory estrus early in the breeding season.
   b. Synchronize estrus in cyclic mares.

6. Outline a program (and include expected responses) for treating mares with progesterone and estradiol-17β plus prostaglandin-F$_2\alpha$ (PGF$_2\alpha$) to synchronize estrus and ovulation in cyclic mares.
7. Outline a program (and include expected responses) for use of human chorionic gonadotropin (hCG) (Chorulon, Intervet/Shering-Plough Animal Health, Whitehouse Station, N.J.) or deslorelin (Ovuplant, Fort Dodge Laboratories, Kalamazoo, MI) to induce ovulation in mares:
   a. In late transitional estrus.
   b. That have regular estrous cycles but are to be bred at a precise time.
8. Outline a program (and include expected responses) for use of PGF$_2\alpha$ to:
   a. Induce estrus in a mare with a functional corpus luteum.
   b. Synchronize estrus in a group of cyclic mares.
   c. Induce earlier estrus in mares after foal-heat ovulation.
9. Explain the rationale for the use of hormones to improve fertility in the early postpartum period.

Registry-derived time constraints, in conjunction with a seasonal breeding pattern, result in use of a narrowly confined breeding season to produce most equine offspring. In the operational breeding season (mid February through the first week in July), the veterinarian is often called on to assist in breeding mares early in this time period to facilitate birth of foals as soon after January 1 as possible. In addition, to maximally utilize genetically superior, popular stallions, veterinary management schemes have been developed to limit the number of services per estrus to the minimum necessary to establish pregnancy. The ascribed goal is one pregnancy per service per mare. To these ends, artificial lighting programs and hormone administration are used to (1) hasten the onset of the breeding season; (2) induce ovulation in cyclic mares being bred; (3) synchronize estrus and ovulation in individual mares or groups of mares; and (4) increase the opportunity for establishment of pregnancy in foaling mares bred early in the postpartum period. Table 3-1 presents a summary of hormones commonly used in broodmare practice. This table also lists hormones used for purposes other than manipulation of estrus (e.g., induced abortion, induced parturition), which are discussed in later chapters.

ARTIFICIAL LIGHTING

The physiologic breeding season can be successfully manipulated to fit into the operational breeding season by *artificially increasing the photoperiod*. The minimal length of light exposure necessary has not been critically established, but field experience indicates that 14 to 16 hours of light stimulus (artificial plus natural) per day is adequate. A recent French study provided evidence that high light intensities may not require as many days of lighting to induce cyclicity in anestrous mares and that low light intensities may not be as efficacious in stimulating desired responses. Nevertheless, because lighting programs have traditionally been thought to require a minimum of 8 to 10 weeks for response, mares in the northern hemisphere are exposed to the lighting system by December 1 to establish normal cyclic activity by mid-February. Various methods of light administration have been used successfully, the most common of which are (1) use of a light source that is held steady at 14 to 16 hours/day throughout the entire stimulation period; or alternatively, (2) increasing light by small increments (similar to that which occurs naturally), usually by adding 30 minutes of daily light stimulation at weekly intervals until 14 to 16 hours of light exposure is achieved (e.g., 10 hours December 1, 10.5 hours December 8, and so on). After summarizing results of various lighting programs, Sharp et al. (1993) suggested best results are obtained when the supplemental light is either added to the end of the day or split and added to both the beginning and

the end of the day, instead of adding the supplemental light only at the beginning of the day. Palmer and coworkers (1982) have described a technique for providing a 1-hour pulse of light 18.5 hours after the onset of daylight. This dark-phase light pulse has reportedly resulted in resumption of reproductive cyclicity similar to that observed with the more traditional lighting techniques. The efficacy of this lighting technique should probably be studied further before being applied to commercial operations.

For individual stall-lighting systems, Kenney et al. (1975) recommended the mare should be within 7 to 8 feet of a 200-watt incandescent light bulb to provide adequate light exposure and the stall should have sufficient window space to permit the same exposure during daylight. Minimal light intensities have not been adequately determined. Sharp et al. (1993) recommend a minimum intensity of 10 foot-candles at mare eye level. The presence of shadows can prevent achievement of desired results, so care should be taken to eliminate them. Paddock lighting systems are also successful if light exposure is sufficient in all areas of the paddock. Guidelines for ensuring adequate light exposure in paddock lighting programs have been reviewed by Ginther (1992). A practical method for measuring light intensity has been described by Sharp et al. (1993) wherein the American Standards Association (ASA) reading of a 35-mm single-lens reflex camera is set to 400 and the shutter speed to 1/4 second. The bottom of a Styrofoam cup is cut off, and the cup is fitted over the lens to gather diffused light. If the aperture reading is f4, light intensity is 10 foot-candles.

With artificial lighting systems, a widely held belief is that pregnant mares should also be exposed to lights because early-foaling mares that are not exposed to lights are thought to be at risk for entering seasonal anestrus. Kentucky workers recently showed that no consistency exists regarding when mares enter anestrus (e.g., an individual mare may enter seasonal anestrus in November of one year and in December or January of the next year; and an individual mare that cycled throughout one year may enter seasonal anestrus the next year), so provision of artificial lighting to all mares to be bred on the farm may be critical if consistent responses to lighting are to be expected.

DOPAMINE D2 ANTAGONISTS

Although the mechanism of ovarian stimulation remains unclear, evidence shows that inhibition of dopamine activity in mares in late anestrus can shorten the interval to first ovulation of the year. Cornell workers have postulated that dopamine exerts a tonic inhibition of reproductive activity during the anovulatory season of the mare. Dopamine may mediate its effects through prolactin (PRL) secretion (PRL increases during the ovulatory season in relation to increasing day length),

TABLE 3-1

Hormones Commonly Used in Broodmare Practice in the United States

Compound	Actions	Indications	Product	Source	Dosage	Comments
GnRH (gonadotropin-releasing hormone)	Release of FSH and LH from anterior pituitary gland	Stimulation of follicular growth Ovulation induction (?)	Cystorelin (synthesized native GnRH) Fertagyl (Gonadorelin)	Ceva Intervet/Schering-Plough	Suggested dosages of 500 μg twice daily or 250 μg 4 times daily; IM or SQ	Not licensed for use in horses. Long/term exogenous GnRH stimulates follicular growth in seasonally anestrous mares but may not be cost effective. Mares treated late in the transition period (larger follicles) are more likely to respond with follicular growth, ovulation and formation of a normal CL, and in less time, than mares with static ovaries (winter anestrus) or in early transition (smaller follicles).
Deslorelin (GnRH analog)	Same, longer action, more potent	Ovulation induction	Ovuplant (deslorelin implant)	Fort Dodge	Sustained release SQ implant containing 2.1 mg deslorelin acetate	Administer 1 implant once estral mare has a follicle ≥30 mm (35 mm may be better) in diameter; more than 80% of mares ovulate within 48 hours. Extended interovulatory intervals occur in some mares that fail to become pregnant due to gonadotroph downregulation. Placing in vulvar mucosa allows easy removal after ovulation, and will avoid subsequent follicular suppression.
			Bio Release Deslorelin Injectable	BET Pharm	Sustained release IM injection containing 1.5 mg deslorelin	Use as above; no evidence of follicular suppression following its use, so may not result in downregulation of pituitary gonadotrophs.
			Deselorelin injection	Compounding pharmacies	Use as above.	Use as above. Dosages of 63 μg twice daily can hasten onset of first ovulation of year according to Canadian workers.
Oxytocin	Myometrial contractions	Parturition induction	Oxytocin	Several sources	40-100 IU IM (bolus injection or slow IV drip) or 5-15 IU IV or IM q 15 min until 2nd stage of parturition	Can cause premature placental separation. Do not use in dystocia until fetal position/posture is corrected.

TABLE **3-1**

Hormones Commonly Used in Broodmare Practice in the United States—cont'd

Compound	Actions	Indications	Product	Source	Dosage	Comments
Oxytocin (continued)	See previous page	Uterine evacuation (can be done in conjunction with uterine lavage)			20-40 IU IV	Ensure that cervix is patent before use.
		Expulsion of retained placenta			10-20 IU IV or IM, can repeat at 2-4 hr intervals as needed	May cause abdominal cramps or, rarely, uterine prolapse.
		Acceleration of uterine involution after dystocia			10-20 IU IM q 8-24 hr	May cause abdominal cramps or, rarely, uterine prolapse. Will not accelerate uterine involution in normal foaling mares.
	Contraction of myoepithelial cells in mammary gland	Milk letdown			20 IU IV or IM	Generally unsuccessful in mares that are extremely nervous or suffer from agalactia.
Estrogens	Expression of estrus Maturation of reproductive tract and mammary glands Increased uterine circulation Uterine contraction	Expression of estrus in "jump" mare (for semen collection)	Estradiol cypionate (ECP)	Upjohn	1-2 mg IM	Only effective in the absence of progesterone. Do not use in mares to be bred. Not approved for use in the horse.
	Cervical relaxation Resistance to uterine infection	Treatment of infectious endometritis	Estradiol-17β	Compounding pharmacy	10 mg/day IM for 1-3 days	Usefulness questionable.
	Suppression of follicular growth to improve synchrony of ovarian response	Synchronization of ovulation	Estradiol-17β		10 mg/day IM for 10 days	Used in conjunction with progesterone in oil (150 mg/day for 10 days) and prostaglandin (on day 10 only).
		Postponement of "foal heat"	Estradiol-17β		10 mg/day IM for 1-10 days	Use in conjunction with progesterone in oil (150 mg/day).

TABLE 3-1

Hormones Commonly Used in Broodmare Practice in the United States—cont'd

Compound	Actions	Indications	Product	Source	Dosage	Comments
Progestogens	Inhibition of LH release Suppression of estrus Reduce myometrial excitability Increase uterine tone Endometrial gland growth	Shorten duration of transitional season	Progesterone in oil	Compounding pharmacy	150 mg/day IM for 10-15 days	Can use in conjunction with estradiol-17β (10 mg/day IM) for 10-15 days and prostaglandin (on last day of treatment). Effective only in mares during late transitional phase
			Altrenogest (Regu-Mate)	Intervet/Shering-Plough	0.044 mg/kg/day orally for 10-15 days	Effective only in mares during late transitional phase. Administering prostaglandin on the last day of treatment may improve results if the mare(s) ovulated during treatment.
	Cervical closure Mammary gland development	Suppression of estrus	Progesterone in oil		150 mg/day IM	May take 2-3 days for mare to go out of behavioral estrus.
			Altrenogest (Regu-Mate)		0.044 mg/kg/day orally	Does not appear to affect subsequent fertility when given for 30-60 consecutive days.
		Synchronization of ovulation	Progesterone in oil		150 mg/day IM for 10 days	Use in comjunction with estradiol-17β (10 mg/day) and prostaglandins (on day 10 only) for best results.
			Altrenogest (Regu-Mate)		0.044 mg/kg/day orally for 10-15 days	Administer prostaglandin on last day of treatment for best results.
		Maintenance of pregnancy in ovariectomized recipient mares for embryo transfer	Progesterone in oil		300 mg/day IM	Begin injections 5 days before embryo transfer and continue for first 100-120 days of pregnancy.
		Pregnancy maintenance in habitually aborting intact mares.	Progesterone in oil Altrenogest (Regu-Mate)		150-300 mg/day IM 0.044 mg/kg/day orally	Efficacy is controversial. Should be given until at least day 100-120 of pregnancy, regardless of whether giving altrenogest or progesterone in oil; may be some risk of fetal mummification if fetus dies and is not expelled. For late-aborting mares, should be given until just before expected parturition.

Continued

TABLE 3-1						
Hormones Commonly Used in Broodmare Practice in the United States—cont'd						
Compound	**Actions**	**Indications**	**Product**	**Source**	**Dosage**	**Comments**
Progestogens *(continued)*	See previous page	Synchronize estrus	CIDR (controlled intravaginal drug release device)	Contains 1.9 g progesterone; release profile 14 days	Place in vagina for 12-14 days; alternatively, administer 8 days and give $PGF_2\alpha$ on day 8 at removal.	Available in North America for use in cattle; not approved for use in horses. Usually results in mild vaginal discharge that does not affect fertility; use aseptic technique at insertion and at removal to minimize chances of ascending infection. Expect efficacy similar to that of other progesterone/progestogen compounds.
hCG (human chorionic gonadotropin)	Support of the CL of pregnancy in women. Has LH activity in the horse.	Ovulation induction	hCG (Chorulon)	Intervet/Shering-Plough, other sources	1500-3500 IU given IM or IV	Administer hCG once a ≥35-mm follicle is detected on the ovary during estrus. Ovulation usually occurs within 36-48 hr after hCG injection.
		Hasten ovulation in transitional mares	hCG	Same as above	1500-3500 IU given IM or IV	Administer hCG once a 40-mm follicle is detected. Not approved for IV use in the horse, but is most commonly given IV.
Prostaglandins ($PGF_2\alpha$)	Regression of CL — Myometrial contractility — Influence on numerous body functions	Shorten interovulatory period ("short-cycle" or induce estrus in cycling mares)	Dinoprost trometha-mine (Lutalyse)	Upjohn	10 mg/1000 lb IM	Give at least 5-6 days after ovulation is detected. Microdose is 0.5 mg once or twice at 24-hour interval; decline in progesterone is slower, but side-effects are reduced (may not be as effective as microdose of cloprostenol).
			Cloprostenol (Estrumate)	Miles	250 μg/1000 IM	Not approved for use in horses in the U.S., but is commonly used. Microdose is 0.25 μg once or twice at 24-hour interval; decline in progesterone is slower, but side effects are reduced.
		Synchronization of estrus	Same as above	Same as above	Same as above	Give two injections, 14 days apart. Effective only in mares with normal estrous cycles.
		Treatment of persistent luteal function	Same as above	Same as above	Same as above	Synthetics and "natural" prostaglandin (dinoprost) are equally effective in causing CL regression, but synthetics have advantage of fewer side effects, such as sweating and abnormal cramping.

TABLE 3-1

Hormones Commonly Used in Broodmare Practice in the United States—cont'd

Compound	Actions	Indications	Product	Source	Dosage	Comments
Prostaglandins (PGF$_{2\alpha}$) *(continued)*	See previous page	Shorten interval to 2nd postpartum estrus	Same as above	Same as above	Same as above	Give prostaglandin 5-6 days after "foal heat" ovulation.
		Induction of abortion	Same as above	Same as above	Same as above	*Single injection* of prostaglandin is sufficient if given *by 35 days of pregnancy. Multiple injections* of prostaglandin are required once supplementary corpora lutea are formed *(beyond 36-40 days of pregnancy).* Prostaglandins may be ineffective beyond 4 months of gestation.
		Acceleration of uterine involution	Same as above	Miles	1 dose twice daily for first 5-10 days after foaling	Of questionable value in normal foaling mares.
		Uterine clearance of fluid	Cloprostenal	Miles	250 μg IM	For uterine clearance of retained fluid: cloprostenol maintains uterine contractions for 2-4 hours. Should probably not be given after ovulation, as may adversely affect CL function.
		Induction of parturition	Cloprostenal	Miles	250 μg IM twice at 2 hr intervals	Studies (limited) suggest various prostaglandin analogues (not dinoprost) can be safely used to induce parturition; however, oxytocin remains the drug of choice.
Ergonovine	Smooth muscle contractions; also aids contraction of smooth muscle in vascular walls to control hemorrhage	Control of postpartum hemorrhage	Ergonovine maleate or methylergonovine maleate	Several sources	1-3 mg IM/1000 lb mare	Produces strong uterine contractions within 10-20 min after injection. Contractions may continue for up to 2-4 hr. Contractions are continuous rather than rhythmic, oxytocin-like contractions. Also aids in controlling certain types of uterine hemorrhage (i.e., uterine rupture; endometrial lacerations); ecbolics should not be used if uterine artery rupture is suspected.
		Hasten uterine involution	Same as above	Same as above	Same as above	Unproven.

Continued

TABLE 3-1

Hormones Commonly Used in Broodmare Practice in the United States—cont'd

Compound	Actions	Indications	Product	Source	Dosage	Comments
Bromocriptine	Inhibits prolactin secretion	Spurious lactation in non-gravid mares	Bromocriptine mesylate	Several sources	30-60 mg/1000 lb mare orally once daily for 3-7 days	Human product; not licensed for use in horses.
Domperidone	Dopamine D2 receptor antagonist Increases prolactin secretion	Agalactia	Equidone (domperidone paste)	Equitox, Center for Applied Technology	1.1 mg/kg orally once daily	Maintains elevated prolactin concentration for 7-9 hours. Increases prolactin to supra-physiologic levels within 7 days. Should be given daily to postpartum agalactic/hypogalactic mares until full milk production is achieved. Foal may need additional nutritional supplementation. Can be started 10-15 days prior to expected foaling in mares grazing endophyte-infested fescue pastures in attempt to decrease parturient problems and agalactia.
		Anestrus	Same as above	Same as above	Same as above	Has been proposed as a treatment for anestrus, to stimulate ovarian follicular activity and advance the first ovulation of the year. Dopamine is thought to inhibit gonadotropin production; therefore, dopamine antagonism is the rationale for its use. Alternatively, it may act directly at the ovary. 2-4 weeks may be required to increase LH levels, so begin treatment in late December or early January. Contradictory results obtained in various studies.
Sulpiride	Dopamine D-2 receptor antagonist	Anestrus	No commercial preparation	Compounding pharmacy	100-200 mg/454 kg body wt, once daily	Rationale is as proposed for domperidone. May hasten response to lighting program if give 14-16 hr light for 2 weeks, then begin daily sulpiride injections; if respond (60-80%), usually do so by ovulating within 15 days of 1st sulpiride injection (sometimes by 8-11 days). Whether should induce ovulation with hCG or deslorelin remains unstudied, but an ovulation-inducing drug is usually given. Concurrent estrogen administration may further increase prolactin and thus improve response.

TABLE 3-1						

Hormones Commonly Used in Broodmare Practice in the United States—cont'd

Compound	Actions	Indications	Product	Source	Dosage	Comments
eFSH	Stimulate follicular growth	Induction of multiple ovulations	Purified equine FSH	Bioniche Animal Health	12.5 mg eFSH twice daily for 3-5 days	CSU protocol—begin eFSH 5-7 days after ovulation. Administer PGF$_{2\alpha}$ on 2nd day of eFSH treatment, and continue eFSH until follicles reach 32-35 mm in diameter. Allow 36 h of no treatments, then administer hCG to induce ovulations. Attempt embryo recovery 7-8 days after ovulation(s). May no longer be available.
		Hasten onset of ovulatory estrus in transition period			12.5 mg injected IM twice daily once ≥25-mm follicle(s) are present; stop treatment once follicle reaches 35 mm and administer hCG IV	Most ovulations (in responding mares) occur between 5-10 days after beginning treatment; 20-30% failures reported. Caution—can induce multiple ovulations which may result in multiple pregnancies.
reLH	Stimulate follicular maturation and ovulation	Induce ovulation	Recombinant equine LH	Not yet commercially available	750-1500 µg injected IV	Administration to estrual mares once mature follicle reaches 35 mm in diameter results in ovulation response similar to hCG (80-90% ovulations within 2 days).

which could in turn stimulate expression of ovarian gonadotropin receptors. D2 receptor antagonists (sulpiride, domperidone) have been used to stimulate PRL secretion and are of particular use in the treatment of some forms of agalactia. D2 receptor antagonists have also been investigated for their potential to advance the ovulatory season in mares. Their success when used by themselves has been equivocal except in mares in mid to late transition. For example, Cornell University workers administered 200 mg sulpride once daily to anestrous mares beginning February 5 and were able to advance the time of the first ovulation of the year by more than a month (compared with untreated control mares), but mean treatment length was 41 days. However, recent results from the use of D2 receptor antagonists in combination with a lighting program have been encouraging. Duchamp and Daels (2002) reported that subjecting anestrous mares to

14.5 hours of light on January 10, with administration of sulpiride (1 mg/kg intramuscularly [IM] twice daily) beginning 2 weeks later, resulted in advancement of the first ovulation of the season in 86% of mares (17 days earlier than lighted mares not given sulpiride). One of the authors has used this program for noncyclic race-trained maiden mares arriving at the breeding farm in February or March (Figure 3-1). Mares are immediately placed on an artificial lighting program and are examined for ovarian activity 2 weeks later. If follicles 15 mm in diameter or more are present at this time, twice-daily intramuscular injections of sulpiride (200 mg) are begun. Beginning 5 days later, mares are examined every other day until a follicle achieves 30 mm in diameter. Examinations are daily thereafter, and once the dominant follicle reaches at least 35 mm in diameter and endometrial edema is present, an ovulation-inducing drug (hCG or deslorelin) is given and the mare is bred. For a

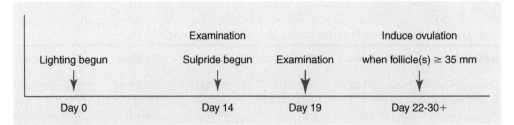

Figure 3-1 Scheme for administration of sulpiride to initiate earlier onset of ovulatory estrus in the mare. Artificial lighting is begun at least 2 weeks before initiation of twice daily intramuscular injections of 200 mg sulpiride. Ovaries should be examined ultrasonographically when starting sulpride injections, and again 5 days later. Once a follicle reaches 30 mm in diameter, examinations should be once daily. An ovulation-inducing drug (e.g., deslorelin or hCG) should be given once the follicle reaches 35 mm in diameter and endometrial edema is present.

group of 16 maiden mares treated in this manner during February and March 2006, 10 responded (64% response rate) to treatment and ovulated 13.4 ± 4.2 days (range, 8 to 22 days) after beginning sulpiride administration (treatment was discontinued in the six mares that showed no significant follicular growth after at least 10 days of treatment). Pregnancy rate was 50% (5 of 10) in the mares that responded to treatment, and all of the mares that did not become pregnant continued to have regular estrous cycles thereafter. Of the six mares that did not respond to sulpiride treatment, ovulation did not occur for 2 to 8 weeks.

SHORTENING THE DURATION OF THE LATE TRANSITION PERIOD WITH ADMINISTRATION OF PROGESTOGENS

Rationale for the use of progestogen/progesterone treatment for hastening the onset of ovulatory estrus is based on insufficient storage or release of luteinizing hormone (LH) from the pituitary in traditional estrus to promote maturation and ovulation of a dominant follicle. **Progestogen** treatment, which generally suppresses LH release during administration, has been postulated to provide for storage and subsequent release of sufficient LH to induce follicular maturation and ovulation once progestogen supplementation ceases. However, Colorado workers have questioned this hypothesis because they recently showed no greater release of LH in response to gonadotropin-releasing hormone (GnRH) (1 mg, pharmacologic dose) administration, and no shortening in mean interval to first ovulation, in six progestogen-treated transitional mares. These workers proposed the main advantage to progestogen treatment of late-transition mares is to synchronize the impending ovulation, thereby facilitating breeding at an opportune and predictable time. Nevertheless, variations of progestogen treatment of mares in transitional estrus remain commonplace in the equine industry.

Progesterone in oil (150 mg each day, IM) or **altrenogest** (0.044 mg/kg each day, orally [PO]) for 10 to 15 days is a common treatment regime for this purpose. Initial experiments with altrenogest, a synthetic progestogen

(Regumate, Intervet/Shering-Plough Animal Health, Whitehouse Station, N.J.) tested efficacy of treatment in mares in early transition (<20-mm diameter follicles) compared with mares treated in late transition (>20-mm diameter follicles) and revealed that mares in early transition did not respond favorably to altrenogest treatment. For best results, current recommendations for the use of progestogen/progesterone are to first examine the mare's ovaries via palpation or ultrasound per rectum to ensure multiple follicles 25 mm or more in diameter are present before instituting therapy. If mares are in early transitional estrus (i.e., only smaller follicles are present), they are unlikely to respond. Although progestogen/progesterone administration is expensive and time-consuming, best results may be achieved by longer (e.g., 2 weeks) durations of treatment, perhaps because of greater storage and subsequent release of LH that occurs as day length increases. Interval to estrus is somewhat variable after cessation of progestogen administration but averages 4 to 7 days, with ovulation usually occurring 7 to 12 days later.

Estradiol, in combination with progesterone, has also been used to shorten (or synchronize) the late transition period. The rationale and guidelines for its use are similar to those stated previously for progestogen/progesterone alone. The addition of estradiol to progesterone results in greater suppression of follicular development than progestogen alone, so follicular size is smaller after cessation of steroid treatment. Therefore, the mean interval to onset of estrus and thus ovulation is typically longer than for progestogen/progesterone treatment alone. Theoretically, the more uniform inhibition of follicular development associated with combined steroid treatment results in less variation in the dynamics of follicular maturation and ovulation after cessation of treatment, thereby providing greater synchrony in mares ovulating on a given day. The dose for estradiol/progesterone is 150 mg progesterone/10 mg estradiol-17β intramuscularly once daily for 10 days. Some practitioners also administer 10 mg PGF$_2$α on the last day of steroid treatment just in case some mares in the group have ovulated and formed a corpus luteum. An ovulation-inducing drug (hCG or deslorelin) is administered to mares once a dominant follicle (≥35 mm in diameter) is achieved, and mares typically ovulate 18 to 23 days after beginning steroid treatment with this regimen. As with altrenogest treatment, mares should be in mid- to late transition for treatment to succeed in initiating regular estrous cycles. To emphasize this point, of 20 2-year-old unlighted anestrous mares in southwest Texas treated as described previously in early February, none responded by initiating regular estrous cycles. None of the mares in that trial had follicles more than 15 mm in diameter at the onset of treatment.

Progestogen/progesterone treatment, with or without estradiol, has also been used at the end of artificial lighting programs (about 60 days after initiation of artificial lighting) and appears to have an additive effect on inducing estrous cycles. A combination of progesterone and estrogen may promote the onset of seasonal cyclicity more efficiently than progestogen/progesterone alone. Practitioners in Thoroughbred broodmare practice commonly use this program to get groups of nonlactating (maiden, barren, not-bred) mares bred during the first week of the season when breeding sheds open. Steroid treatment is generally begun in late January (January 28 to 30), with ovulations expected February 14 to 22 (approximately 3 weeks after starting treatment) (Figure 3-2). Because many of the "programmed" mares become pregnant on this first (synchronized) ovulation in February, this reduces the mating load for Thoroughbred stallions later in the season when most foaling mares are presented for breeding. One precaution for this program in Thoroughbred mares is to ensure that they stand safely for breeding before sending them to the breeding shed to be covered. A number of stallion managers in central Kentucky claim behavioral signs of estrus are less pronounced in those mares treated for 10 days with progesterone/estradiol. Texas workers, using a sustained-release formulation

(steroids released over 12 to 14 days), noted decreased signs of estrus in treated mares just before ovulation. The decreased behavioral signs of estrus were associated with slightly elevated circulating progesterone levels, presumably from the sustained-release formulation used. Whether or not circulating progesterone levels are slightly elevated in mares with progesterone/estradiol treatment at the time of breeding has not been investigated. No commercial preparation containing both progesterone and estradiol is currently licensed and available for use in mares, but practitioners can obtain the formulation from veterinary pharmaceutical compounding companies.

USE OF GnRH TO HASTEN ONSET OF OVULATORY ESTRUS

The integral role of hypothalamic GnRH in controlling recrudescence of ovarian cyclicity in the mare has led to numerous investigations of exogenous administration of native GnRH or its more potent agonists to stimulate follicular development and ovulation. In a review of the use of GnRH regimens used to induce ovulation during the anovulatory season, Ginther (1992) concluded that (1) pulsatile delivery systems may be most effective; (2) the percentage of mares ovulating as a result of treatment increases as day length increases and diameter of the largest follicle increases; (3) not all mares with small follicles respond to treatment; (4) some mares that ovulate as a result of treatment revert to anestrus if they do not become pregnant; and (5) some mares treated when they only have small follicles present may be prone to higher rates of embryonic loss, perhaps because of lower progesterone production from corpora lutea resulting from low LH stimulation. In a recent retrospective study of anestrous and transitional-period mares in central Kentucky, a 79% ovulation rate with a 53% pregnancy

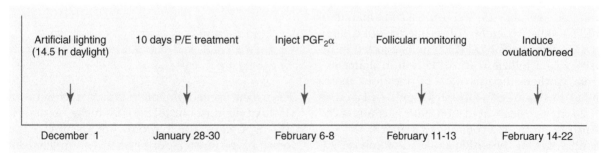

Figure 3-2 Scheme for synchronizing estrus in artificially lighted groups of nonlactating (maiden, barren, not-bred) mares to promote breeding the first week after breeding sheds open and therefore reduce the mating load of stallions later in the year when the preponderance of foaling mares are presented to the stallions. Thoroughbred broodmare practitioners in central Kentucky often refer to this scheme as "programming mares." Artificial lighting is initiated on December 1. Steroid treatment (progesterone and estradiol, P/E) is generally begun in late January (28 to 30); PGF$_2\alpha$ is administered on day 10 of steroid treatment (February 6 to 8); regular examinations via transrectal ultrasound are begun on day 15 (February 11 to 13); and an ovulation-inducing drug (hCG or deslorelin) is given once a 35-mm diameter follicle and endometrial edema are present. Mares should be bred 1 to 2 days before expected ovulation, with ovulations expected during the period of February 14 to 22 (approximately 3 weeks after starting steroid treatment).

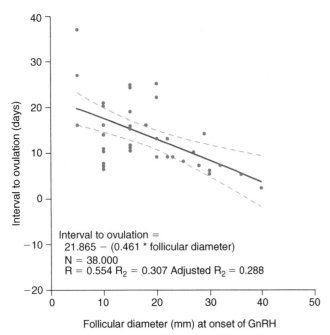

Figure 3-3 Relationship between follicular diameter (in millimeters) at time of onset of native GnRH therapy and interval to ovulation in 38 Thoroughbred or Standardbred mares in central Kentucky. (From Morehead JP, Colon JL, Blanchard TL: Clinical experience with native GnRH therapy to hasten follicular development and first ovulation of the breeding season, *J Eq Vet Sci* 21:54,81-88, 2001.)

rate per cycle was achieved, with ovulation occurring 13.7 ± 7.4 days after beginning twice-daily intramuscular injections of 500 µg native GnRH. Follicular size in that study was an important determinant of interval from onset of native GnRH therapy to ovulation (Figure 3-3), but the use of additional ovulation-inducing drugs (hCG or deslorelin implants) did not improve ovulatory response.

USE OF GnRH ANALOGS FOR ADVANCING ONSET OF OVULATORY ESTRUS

Beginning on February 15, and using a combination of the GnRH agonist buserelin (10 µg injected subcutaneously twice daily) plus hCG (2500 units injected intravenously once a follicle reached 35 mm in diameter), California workers reported 72% of anestrous mares responded to treatment with estrus and ovulation in 10.6 ± 2.2 days. Mean ovulation date was advanced from April 12 (untreated controls) to March 3.

Attempts at using the GnRH-analog deslorelin (Ovuplant) to hasten onset of regular estrous cycles in mares in either deep winter anestrus or early spring transition have mostly been unrewarding. Colorado workers investigated repeated Ovuplant administration (every 3 days for up to 7 treatments) to anestrous mares beginning on February 28 but found only 20% (6 of 30) of mares responded and ovulated. Of the six mares that responded, four were thought to be in transitional

estrus rather than anestrus at the start of the study. Australian researchers showed that once ovarian follicles 35 mm or more in diameter are achieved in mares late in the transition period, treatment with deslorelin implants every other day until ovulation results in approximately 80% of mares ovulating within 3 days of initiating treatment (requiring two implants). Further study of the use of GnRH analogs is warranted to refine methodology of treatment during the transition period.

USE OF hCG IN THE LATE TRANSITION PERIOD

Few studies have been performed on the use of **human chorionic gonadotropin (hCG)** to hasten the first ovulation of the breeding season in mares in the late transition period. Multiple injections of hCG (200 units) given late in the transition period resulted in fertile ovulations unaccompanied by LH surges, but mares tended to relapse into seasonal anestrus after ovulation had been induced. In mares with prolonged estrus early in the breeding season, hCG (1500 to 3500 units, intravenously [IV] or IM) is routinely given when a preovulatory-sized follicle is present to increase the chance that ovulation will occur at a predictable time (approximately 48 hours after injection). Injection of hCG in late-transitional mares can also be done anytime a large preovulatory follicle is thought to be present; however, administration of hCG in this manner does not ensure ovulation will occur at a precise time. California workers found treatment of seasonally anestrous mares with hCG once a dominant follicle developed advanced the mean date for first ovulation by 28 days (March 15 compared with April 12 for untreated control mares). Many practitioners believe prominent edematous endometrial folds must be visible on transrectal ultrasound examination, and for the cervix to be relaxed, for hCG administration to result in ovulation at a predictable time in late transitional estrual mares.

USE OF PURIFIED EQUINE FOLLICLE-STIMULATING HORMONE IN THE LATE TRANSITION PERIOD

The recent development of purified equine follicle-stimulating hormone (eFSH) (Bioniche Animal Health, Athens, Ga.) for use in producing multiple ovulations for embryo transfer purposes has stimulated interest in using the product for stimulating follicular growth in anestrous mares or those in transitional estrus. Colorado workers administered 12.5 mg eFSH (IM) twice daily to anovulatory mares with 25-mm follicles (i.e., late transition) present on their ovaries in February and April. The mares had been under an artificial lighting program since December. When a mare's follicles reached 35 mm in diameter, eFSH treatment was stopped and hCG was administered. Eighty percent of eFSH-treated mares developed large follicles and ovulated in 7.6 ± 2.4 days, which on average was 1 month earlier than in untreated control mares. Similar results were obtained in a Brazilian study with unlighted late-transitional mares. The investigators also noted shortening the interval to first ovulation of the year by almost 2 weeks, but the multiple ovulation rate was higher (average, 5.6 ovulations). Whether this treatment will prove more efficacious or cost effective than other available treatments is currently unknown. Also, because multiple ovulations are induced by eFSH treatment (40% and 86% of transitional mares treated in Colorado and Brazilian studies, respectively), its use in mares intended to carry their own foals may be problematic. As of this writing, eFSH is no longer commercially available.

WAITING TO BREED MARES UNTIL REGULAR ESTROUS CYCLES OCCUR

If teasing practices are good, waiting to breed mares until they have established regular estrous cycles is a viable alternative to using more expensive, labor-intensive practices to induce the onset of ovulatory estrus. This is particularly true with use of hormonal therapy to shorten the late transition period, which sometimes does not result in a significant savings in days to conception. The likelihood of achieving a time savings in this regard must be weighed against the time and expense involved in hormonal treatment and the waiting period after cessation of hormone treatment until ovulation occurs. Another practical approach is to administer **prostaglandin-F₂α (PGF₂α)** 1 week after the mare ceases behavioral estrus, or preferably 1 week after ovulation is confirmed with transrectal palpation and ultrasound examination, when the corpus luteum should be susceptible to the luteolytic effect of prostaglandin. Depending on the size of follicles present at the time of prostaglandin administration, the mare should return to estrus and ovulate within 2 to 10 days.

INDUCTION OF OVULATION IN CYCLIC MARES

To optimize fertility, it is commonly believed that ovulation should occur within 24 to 48 hours after breeding to a fertile stallion. A recent Kentucky study, with records from 902 estrous cycles in 414 Thoroughbred mares mated to 1 of 110 different stallions, showed that mares ovulating more than 2 days after natural cover had significantly reduced pregnancy rates. When cryopreserved semen is used for breeding, or with breeding to certain subfertile stallions, the fertilizable lifespan of sperm may be reduced, thus requiring breeding closer to ovulation to optimize pregnancy rates. At the present time in the United States, administration of either

hCG or deslorelin remains the only reliable practical method for inducing ovulation of a large preovulatory follicle in cyclic mares.

Injection of hCG (1000 to 3500 units, IV or IM) is sufficient to induce ovulation of preovulatory follicles 35 mm or more in diameter in mares having regular estrous cycles. Although we most commonly administer 2500 units, we have achieved similar success rates with intravenous administration of 1000, 1500, and 2500 units of hCG. When hCG is injected on the second or third day of estrus in cyclic mares, most mares so treated ovulate within 48 hours (approximately 65% to 70% ovulation rates between 36 and 48 hours) (Figure 3-4). If the day of estrus is unknown, and the follicle is larger than 35 mm in diameter, the interval to ovulation may be less predictable, sometimes occurring earlier (within 24 hours) after hCG administration. The drug is of most value when used in the early months of the breeding season when criteria used to predict ovulation in cyclic mares (e.g., size and shape of follicle, thickness of follicular wall, softness of follicle, cervical relaxation, day of estrus, and degree of uterine edema) are less reliable indicators of impending ovulation.

Antibodies to hCG are found in serum of mares given repeated injections of the drug. Whether antibodies to hCG interfere with subsequent spontaneous ovulation in treated mares remains controversial. Workers at Ohio State University claim that intravenous injection of hCG is less likely to induce an antibody

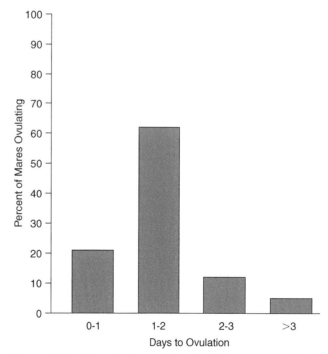

Figure 3-4 Intervals to ovulation in 214 estrous cycles of light breed mares in southwest Texas after intravenous administration of 1000 to 2500 units hCG from March to July 1999. Mares were in estrus with follicles 35-mm or more in diameter present at the time of treatment.

response that delays ovulation than intramuscular injection of the drug. In spite of evidence for antibody formation, we have achieved similar response rates at each injection of hCG in mares treated on up to four different estrous cycles within the same breeding season, or up to seven different estrous cycles in two consecutive breeding seasons (i.e., mares were just as likely to ovulate within 2 days of hCG administration with their third or later injection as they were with their first or second injection). By contrast, Colorado workers have reported less predictable intervals to ovulation after hCG injection in mares that have received the drug in more than two previous estrous periods, particularly late in the season in older mares. Whether the diminished response was truly the result of repeated hCG administration or the result of seasonal effects could not be determined from that study.

Human chorionic gonadotropin can be given in combination with other hormones used to synchronize estrus or shorten the duration of the late transition period. In cyclic mares synchronized with a 10-day regimen of progesterone and estradiol, with $PGF_2\alpha$ given on the 10th day, approximately 80% to 85% of mares ovulate on days 19 to 22 after beginning steroid treatment if hCG is administered on the first day a follicle 35 mm or more in diameter is present (Figure 3-5).

The efficacy of **gonadotropin-releasing hormone (GnRH)** in inducing ovulation in other species, and the ability of GnRH administered in a pulsatile fashion or via constant infusion for prolonged (28-day) periods to stimulate follicular development and ovulation in anestrous

mares (reviewed by Ginther, 1992), stimulated interest in its use to induce ovulation in cyclic mares. Success in inducing ovulation in cyclic mares with administration of single injections of native GnRH has generally been poor. However, more potent GnRH **analogs** with a longer half-life than that of native GnRH have proved to be highly successful for inducing ovulation in cyclic mares. Currently, the only GnRH analog approved for use in horses in the United States is deslorelin. Initially, it was available as a 2.2-mg deslorelin implant (Ovuplant). Subcutaneous administration of implants containing deslorelin on the first day of estrus that a follicle 30 mm or more in diameter is detected results in a shortened time to ovulation and normal pregnancy rates in treated mares (reviewed by Jochle and Trigg, 1994). The implant is not currently available in the United States, although many practitioners import the drug from other countries.

A disadvantage to using Ovuplant has been that of extended interovulatory intervals in mares that fail to become pregnant, thereby delaying rebreeding. Follicular growth is suppressed early in diestrus, resulting in an average delay of 4 to 6 days before the next ovulation. A recent Kentucky study revealed that 10% of interovulatory intervals in deslorelin-treated mares were greater than 30 days, which can be problematic for the practitioner charged with ensuring that mares become pregnant as early as possible in the breeding season. Louisiana researchers recently confirmed this prolonged interovulatory interval was the result of suppressed follicular activity attributable to hyposecretion of gonadotropin from the pituitary,

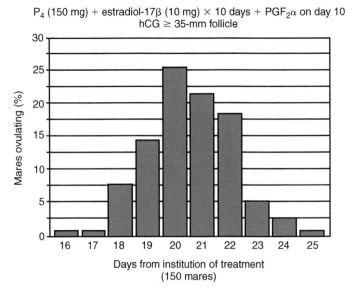

Mare Synchronization

P_4 (150 mg) + estradiol-17β (10 mg) × 10 days + $PGF_2\alpha$ on day 10
hCG ≥ 35-mm follicle

Days from institution of treatment
(150 mares)

Figure 3-5   Intervals to ovulation in 150 estrous cycles of light breed mares in southwest Texas after daily intramuscular injection for 10 days with 150 mg progesterone (P_4)/10 mg estradiol-17β, intramuscular injection of 10 mg $PGF_2\alpha$ on day 10, and intravenous injection of 1500 to 2500 units hCG on the first day a follicle 35 mm or more in diameter was achieved.

presumably from pituitary gonadotroph receptor downregulation. Supporting this concept, Colorado researchers recently showed that gonadotropin response to native GnRH challenge 10 days after ovulation in deslorelin-treated mares is attenuated. Colorado and Texas workers showed that removal of the implant on the day ovulation was confirmed prevents delayed return to estrus. Rather than placing the implant in the neck, many practitioners place it in vulvar mucosa to facilitate its identification and removal (Figures 3-6 and 3-7).

A number of compounding pharmacies in the United States now produce a variety of deslorelin formulations for use in horses. Some preparations, such as Bio-Release Deslorelin Injection (BET Pharm, Lexington, Ky.), have sustained-release characteristics that may improve efficacy. Texas workers reported this drug compared favorably in ovulatory response of foal-heat mares with hCG without any apparent suppression of follicular size 2 weeks after administration. This suggests that delayed return to estrus from follicular suppression that occurs in some mares after Ovuplant administration should not be a problem. Few studies have provided data on direct comparisons between hCG and various deslorelin products, but Texas workers found administration of either Ovuplant or Bio-Release Deslorelin Injection resulted in similar ovulatory responses as did hCG administration (Tables 3-2 to 3-4), and Colorado workers recently found two other compounded deslorelin preparations (compounded by Applied Pharmacy Services, Las Vegas, NV, and Essential Pharmaceuticals, Newtown, Pa.) resulted in similar response rates and intervals to ovulation as did hCG administration. One proposed advantage to using deslorelin is that, unlike with hCG, antibodies that might

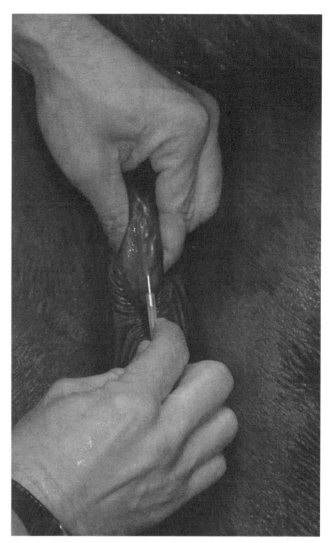

Figure 3-7 Administration of deslorelin (Ovuplant) beneath the mucosa of the dorsal vulvar labium. Before implant insertion, 1 mL of local anesthetic can be injected at the implant site. The needle should be inserted beneath the skin-mucosal junction, the plunger depressed to expel the implant, and the tissue pinched around the needle as the injection device is withdrawn. The implant should be palpable. Removal of the implant on the day of ovulation is recommended.

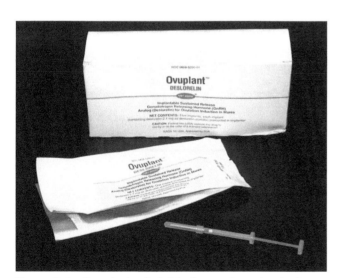

Figure 3-6 Ovuplant administration system. Implant containing deslorelin is contained within the large-bore needle to be inserted subcutaneously.

diminish its effectiveness with repeated use are not formed against the compound. Colorado workers also noted that repeated (up to five times) administration of compounded deslorelin injections did not alter response rates.

Recently, recombinant equine LH (reLH) has become available for research use to induce ovulation in horses. Antibodies directed against the product were not produced after seven injections over a 3-week period. Initial studies suggested the most efficacious dose was 750 μg injected intravenously, and responses have generally been similar to those obtained with hCG administration. Whether this product will prove to be more efficacious or cost-effective requires further study.

TABLE 3-2

Intervals to Ovulation and Interovulatory Intervals in 155 Thoroughbred Mares Receiving Either No Treatment, Deslorelin (Ovuplant) Implants, or Intravenous Injections of 2500 Units hCG During the 1999 Breeding Season in Central Kentucky

	NO TREATMENT		hCG		OVUPLANT	
	n	Mean ± SD	n	Mean ± SD	n	Mean ± SD
Follicular size at treatment	–	–	30	41.0 ± 5.2 mm	204	42.0 ± 5.5 mm
Interval to ovulation	–	–	30	2.4 ± 1.0 days	204	2.1 ± 1.0 days
Interovulatory interval	21	20.8 ± 1.7 days*	13	20.7 ± 2.0 days*	70	24.3±6.2 days†

SD, Standard deviation.
*†Within row, mean values with different superscripts are significantly different (*P* < .01).
Modified from Morehead JP, Blanchard TL: Clinical experience with deslorelin (Ovuplant) in a Kentucky Thoroughbred broodmare practice, *J Eq Vet Sci* 20:358, 2000.

TABLE 3-3

Mean Values (± SD) for Foaling Date, Date of Treatment, Day Post Partum at Treatment and Ovulation, Diameter of Largest Follicle at Time of Treatment, and Outcome in 30 Mares Treated on the First Postpartum Estrus With Either Injection of 1.5 mg Short-Release Deslorelin (Bio-Release Deslorelin Injection) or No Treatment (Control)

Variable	Deslorelin-Treated Mares (n = 16)	Nontreated Control Mares (n = 14)
Foaling date	Feb 6 ± 15 days	Feb 11 ± 14 days
Date of treatment	Feb 16 ±14 days	Feb 22 ± 15 days
Day post partum treated	9.8 ± 2.6 days	9.9 ± 3.7 days
Follicle size at treatment	40 ± 4 mm	39 ± 3 mm
Ovulations within 2 days	75% (12/16)*	7% (1/14)†
Day of postpartum ovulation	12.8 ± 3.3 days‡	15.4 ± 3.2 days§
Date of ovulation	Feb 19 ± 15 days	Feb 27 ± 14 days
Pregnancy rate	69% (11/16)	43% (6/14)
No. of covers after treatment	1.6 ± 1.0*	2.9 ± 0.8†
No. of 20-mm to 29-mm follicles days 14 to 15 after ovulation	2.1 ± 1.7	1.4 ± 1.5
No. of ≥30-mm follicles days 14 to 15 after ovulation	0.4 ± 0.5	0.3 ± 0.5
Interestrous interval in mares not pregnant¶	19.7 ± 4.2 days (n = 3)	23.4 ± 2.4 days (n = 7)

*†Mean values are significantly different (*P* < 0.01).
‡§Mean values are significantly different (*P* < 0.05).
¶Statistical comparisons not made because of low number of mares in each group.

INDUCTION OF MULTIPLE OVULATIONS FOR EMBRYO TRANSFER

A purified eFSH (Bioniche Animal Health) has recently been developed to produce multiple ovulations in mares for embryo transfer purposes. The product is purported to contain 10 times as much FSH as LH. A number of trials have been performed to determine an optimal regimen of treatment to produce not only multiple ovulations but also to result in the production of multiple embryos after breeding eFSH-treated mares. The drug is administered via intramuscular injection, with 12.5 mg twice daily appearing to be an optimal dosage regimen. An ovulation-inducing drug is given once large dominant follicles are present on the ovaries of the mare in estrus. Initial studies suggested more embryos could be obtained if hCG was

TABLE 3-4

Mean Values (± SD) for Interval from Treatment to Ovulation and Percentage of Mares Ovulating Within 2 Days in 112 Estrous Periods of 39 Quarter Horse or Thoroughbred Mares Treated on the First Day a ≥34-mm Diameter Follicle Was Detected With Either Injection of 2500 Units hCG (Group hCG), 1.5 mg Bio-Release Deslorelin Injection (Group DES), or 2.1 mg Deslorelin Implant (Ovuplant; Group OVU)

Variable	hCG (n = 29)	DES (n = 17)	OVU (n = 66)
Interval to ovulation	2.2 ± 0.9 days[*]	2.0 ± 0.4 days[*†]	1.9 ± 0.5 days[†]
Median	2.0 days	2.0 days	2.0 days
Ovulations within 2 days	83%	94%	92%

[*†]Mean values with different superscripts tended to differ ($P = .06$).

used as the ovulation-inducing agent, but recently reLH was found to be at least as, if not more effective in inducing multiple ovulations with maximal embryo production. However, some studies have showed that continuing to administer eFSH until most of the growing follicle cohort reaches 35 mm in diameter may result in suboptimal results. So, at present, Colorado workers recommend administering 12.5 mg of eFSH twice daily beginning 5 to 7 days after ovulation when the diameter of the largest follicle is 22 to 25 mm. Prostaglandin is then administered on the second day of eFSH treatment, and eFSH treatment is continued for 3 to 5 days until follicles reach 32 to 35 mm in diameter, at which time eFSH treatment is stopped. A "coasting period" of 36 hours is then allowed, during which time no drugs are given. Then, hCG is given to induce ovulation and the mare is bred before ovulation at a time conducive to establishing pregnancy based on the type of semen being used (fresh, cooled, frozen). The uterus is then flushed for embryo recovery 7 to 8 days after ovulation is confirmed. At the time of this writing, eFSH is not commercially available.

A recombinant equine FSH (reFSH) has also been produced, but further investigations need to be done before recommendations for its use can be made.

SYNCHRONIZATION OF ESTRUS IN THE CYCLIC MARE

The extended estrus period of the mare, with ovulation occurring variably from 1 to 10 days after the beginning of estrus, necessitates time-consuming, expensive reproductive management of mares. Reproductive management of horses would greatly benefit from development of an accurate, economic method for the precise control of estrus and ovulation in the mare.

Most synchronization methods used to control ovulation in domestic animals modify the **luteal phase** of the estrous cycle. Prostaglandin-$F_2\alpha$ ($PGF_2\alpha$) has been administered to broodmares to shorten the lifespan of the corpus luteum and thus induce estrus. Treatment with $PGF_2\alpha$ is most often used for individual mares when the presence of a mature corpus luteum is suspected or known (e.g., when a breeding was missed or did not result in pregnancy, or mismating has occurred). On average, $PGF_2\alpha$ treatment of mares with a mature corpus luteum results in estrus in 2 to 4 days and ovulation in 7 to 12 days (Table 3-5). The onset of estrus is more synchronized than the day of ovulation. Because of the greater role of the follicular phase in controlling total

TABLE 3-5

Efficacy of Two Intramuscular Injections of 10 mg $PGF_2\alpha$ Given 14 Days Apart to Synchronize Estrus in 33 Nonlactating Quarter Horse Mares; Ovulation Was Induced With 1500 Units hCG Injected Intravenously Once a 35-mm Diameter Follicle Was Detected

Estrus after 1st $PGF_2\alpha$	17/33 (52%)
Estrus after 2nd $PGF_2\alpha$	26/33 (79%)
Mean (± SD) interval to estrus after 2nd $PGF_2\alpha$	4.4 ± 1.7 d
Mean (± SD) duration of estrus after 2nd $PGF_2\alpha$	3.6 ± 1.8 d
Ovulations after 2nd $PGF_2\alpha$	31/33 (94%)
Mean (± SD) interval to ovulation after 2nd $PGF_2\alpha$	7.2 ± 2.6 d (range, 2 to 10 d)
Incidence of silent ovulations	5/31 (16%)
Incidence of treatment failures	2/33 (6%)

length of the estrous cycle in mares, the time of ovulation after PGF$_2\alpha$-induced estrus in broodmares remains variable (2 to 15 days after treatment). Mares in diestrus with large follicles present ($\geq$35 mm in diameter) return to estrus and ovulate sooner than mares with smaller follicles present. In many such cases, behavioral estrus may not occur, may be partial, or may be abbreviated to 1 or 2 days. The incidence of "silent estrus" (ovulation without accompanying signs of estrus) after prostaglandin injection averages approximately 15% (see Table 3-5). Therefore, both estrus and ovulation can easily be missed if daily teasing and regular monitoring of follicular status are not initiated at the time PGF$_2\alpha$ is given.

Precise synchronization of estrus and ovulation in groups of mares is difficult because of incomplete sensitivity of the equine corpus luteum to PGF$_2\alpha$ administered before 6 days after ovulation, and administration after 9 days after ovulation does not significantly shorten the interovulatory interval. These phenomena prevent precise synchronization of ovulation in groups of mares with single or multiple injections of PGF$_2\alpha$. However, because of cost, availability, and ease of administration, synchronization schemes using PGF$_2\alpha$, either alone or in combination with other hormones, are commonplace. A routine protocol used for synchronizing estrus in a group of mares is to administer two intramuscular injections of PGF$_2\alpha$ 14 days apart. The rationale for the two-injection scheme is that more mares have corpora lutea that regress after the second injection, permitting a greater percentage of mares to return to estrus in a synchronous manner. In a group of randomly cyclic mares, approximately 50% have a corpus luteum 5 to 15 days old that is capable of responding to a single injection of PGF$_2\alpha$, but most of the group of randomly cyclic mares should have a corpus luteum capable of responding to the second injection of PGF$_2\alpha$ later. Typical responses to a two-injection scheme of PGF$_2\alpha$ are shown in Table 3-5.

Because prostaglandins, including cloprostenol (an analog), can produce side effects such as sweating and abdominal cramping, some practitioners recommend using smaller doses than listed on the product labels. The standard dose for PGF$_2\alpha$ (Lutalyse, Upjohn, Kalamazoo, MI) is 5 to 10 mg, and the standard dose for cloprostenol is 250 to 500 μg, injected intramuscularly. Nie and coworkers (2004) investigated the ability of lower doses of these drugs to effectively induce luteolysis and found 25 μg cloprostenol and 0.5 mg PGF$_2\alpha$ were generally luteolytic without producing side effects, with best results obtained with the microdose of cloprostenol. Luteolysis was more protracted with these lower doses of prostaglandins, but significant extension in the interovulatory interval did not occur compared with standard dose administration. Some practitioners commonly use these smaller doses of prostaglandins but repeat them in 24 hours to ensure luteolysis. Whether this is a necessary practice is unknown.

Progestogen administration, in the form of progesterone in oil (150 mg/d, IM) or altrenogest (0.044 mg/kg per day, PO), to artificially prolong the luteal phase of the estrous cycle has been used to synchronize the ensuing estrus in mares. Rationale for efficacy of progestogen therapy to synchronize estrus is based on progestogen inhibiting LH release from the anterior pituitary and thereby blocking ovulation. When administered for a long enough period of time to cyclic mares, corpora lutea regress but subsequent ovulation is blocked by the exogenous progestogen. When progestogen administration ceases, mares return to estrus and ovulate. Administration of progestogen for 14 to 15 days should be more effective than shorter periods of administration by allowing mares with fresh ovulations at the onset of treatment sufficient time for spontaneous luteal regression to occur. Interval to estrus is somewhat variable after cessation of progestogen administration but averages 4 to 7 days. Ovulation usually occurs, on average, 7 to 12 days after cessation of progestogen treatment. Because follicular development is not uniformly inhibited, even by relatively high doses of progestogen, follicles in a wide range of developmental stages exist after termination of treatment, resulting in highly variable intervals to ovulation among mares.

Control of follicular growth during the treatment period is requisite for achieving precise control of ovulation in the mare. Several findings in the last 30 years have led to development of more precise ovulation control in the mare. Daily administration of 10 mg **estradiol-17β** was found to suppress follicular growth. Subsequently, daily administration of progesterone (to artificially prolong the luteal phase) in combination with daily administration of estradiol (to suppress follicular growth) was hypothesized to provide for a more predictable interval to ovulation after cessation of steroid treatment. This hypothesis was confirmed in cyclic mares, postpartum mares, and maiden and barren mares that had been maintained under an artificially increased photoperiod for at least 60 days.

An additional problem contributing to variability in interval to ovulation has been the tendency for corpora lutea to persist (**persistent luteal function**) beyond cessation of progestogen treatment. This is the result of: (1) a number of mares ovulating after steroid treatment is initiated, with resulting corpora lutea continuing to produce progesterone after cessation of exogenous progestogen treatment, and (2) corpora lutea of some mares occasionally spontaneously persisting longer than the usual diestrous period, thereby remaining functional after progestogen treatment is discontinued. Administration of PGF$_2\alpha$ after cessation of progestogen treatment has therefore been recommended to ensure that remaining corpora lutea regress and treated mares return to estrus in a timely manner. With use of Loy's recommended protocol of 150 mg progesterone plus 10 mg estradiol-17β in oil injected daily for 10 consecutive days, combined with a single injection of PGF$_2\alpha$ on the last day of steroid treatment, followed by an ovulation-inducing drug when a follicle 35 mm or more in diameter was first detected, approximately 80% to 85% of mares ovulated 19 to 22 days after the first steroid injection on day 1 (ovulations typically range from 18 to 25 days after the last steroid injection; see Figure 3-5). Unfortunately, time-consuming daily injections of 150 mg progesterone and 10 mg estradiol-17β in oil are required, and no commercial preparation containing estradiol-17β is approved in the United States for veterinary use. Progesterone and estradiol combinations must currently be obtained from veterinary pharmaceutical compounding companies.

Pharmaceutical companies are pursuing implant technology that provides for sustained release of various compounds, including hormones, for prescribed periods of time. Such formulations have the advantage of only having to be administered once. Investigations have been performed with biodegradable microspheres containing progesterone and estradiol-17β. The microsphere preparations were formulated to release desired amounts of the hormones over a period of 12 to 14 days in mares. Field trials with these preparations were encouraging in that estrus and ovulation are more precisely controlled, and fertility in treated mares is normal.

HORMONAL THERAPY TO IMPROVE FERTILITY OF MARES EARLY IN THE POSTPARTUM PERIOD

The **first postpartum estrus,** commonly referred to as **foal heat,** is characterized by normal follicular development and ovulation within 20 days post partum. The onset of the foal heat occurs within 5 to 12 days after parturition in more than 90% of mares. In a study involving 470 Thoroughbred mares in central Kentucky, 43% had ovulated by day 9, 93% by day 15, and 97% by day 20 after parturition. The average interval from parturition to first ovulation was 10.2 ± 2.4 days. In a recent study of 93 Quarter Horse mares in southeast Texas, the day of first postpartum ovulation was 12.3 ± 2.9 days and was significantly influenced by month of foaling. Ovulations in June foaling mares occurred 3 days earlier than ovulations in March foaling mares. That study also revealed the day of ovulation was not influenced by age or parity of the mare.

Pregnancy rates achieved by breeding during foal heat are reported to be 10% to 20% lower than those obtained by first breeding at subsequent estrous periods. The decreased pregnancy rate associated with foal-heat breeding has been suggested to be from failure of the uterus, particularly the endometrium, to be completely restored and ready to support a developing embryo. In support of this hypothesis, Kentucky workers showed that the pregnancy rate from foal-heat breeding was higher in mares that ovulated after 10 days post partum compared with those that ovulated before this time. Because a 5-day interval after ovulation is required before the embryo enters the uterus, ovulation after day 10 post partum helps ensure that the histologic appearance of the endometrium has returned to normal, and fluid normally present within the uterine lumen during the first week or two post partum has been fully expelled, before embryo

entry. Also of interest is that, in the previously cited Kentucky study, foal-heat pregnancy rates were farm-dependent (i.e., some farms achieved pregnancy rates decidedly lower when mares were bred on the first postpartum estrus compared with mares bred on the second postpartum estrus, and no significant difference in pregnancy rates was found between these breedings at other farms). This emphasizes the need for the practitioner to use common sense in evaluating the practice of breeding on first versus second postpartum estrus, taking farm (management) practices and previous success rates on a given farm into consideration.

Attempts to improve pregnancy rates from breeding in the early postpartum period have been centered around either attempting to enhance the rate of uterine involution or delaying breeding until involution is more complete. To enhance fertility achieved on foal-heat breeding, several methods have been used in an attempt to speed uterine involution in normal foaling mares. Some of the methods tested include: repeated uterine lavage during the first week post partum; repeated administration of uterine ecbolics (e.g., prostaglandins, oxytocin, methylergonovine; to promote uterine contraction and evacuation) during the first 10 days post partum; and administration of steroid hormones (progestogen, progesterone, estradiol and progesterone plus estradiol) during the first few days to 2 weeks post partum. None of the methods tested has enhanced uterine involution rate (measured by gross uterine involution, histologic repair of the endometrium, or evacuation of uterine fluid) in normal foaling mares. Therefore, we believe that currently the best method to enhance fertility of mares in the early postpartum period is to delay breeding until histologic involution and expulsion of intrauterine fluid is complete.

The two methods currently used to postpone breeding in the postpartum period until normal pregnancy rates can be achieved are: 1, to delay the onset of the foal heat; or 2, to shorten the interval to the second postpartum estrus. Pregnancy rates achieved by breeding on foal heat appear to be higher in mares in which estrus is delayed with progestogen therapy. Altrenogest has been given daily for 8 or 15 days after foaling. Prostaglandin should be administered on the last day of treatment because progestogen therapy alone may not prevent ovulation from occurring even though estrus is suppressed. Daily treatment with a combination of progesterone and estradiol-17β for as few as 5 days has also been used to delay onset of the first postpartum estrus and ovulation. Treatment should commence as soon as practical on the day of foaling before gonadotropin surges responsible for follicular recruitment occur.

The major objection to the use of progestogen therapy for several consecutive days, beginning at the time of foaling, is that the treatment delays the onset of the first postpartum estrus to an extent that foaling intervals are not significantly reduced. If treatment of postparturient mares for 2 or 3 days after foaling would delay ovulation only until just after day 10 post partum, progestogen treatment might offer the best method for increasing pregnancy rate without significantly extending the parturition to breeding interval in early postparturient mares. Preliminary trials with 150 mg progesterone and 10 mg estradiol-17β for the first 2 days post partum have been encouraging in this respect, ensuring that no treated mares ovulate before day 10 post partum.

Administration of $PGF_2\alpha$ at 5 to 7 days after the first postpartum ovulation hastens onset of the second postpartum estrus, which normally does not occur until approximately 30 days post partum. Although this management technique is expected to increase pregnancy rate at the first breeding post partum, such is not always the case. In addition, when compared with breeding during the foal heat, the parturition to breeding interval is delayed approximately 2 weeks (i.e., approximately 1 week is saved compared with waiting and breeding on the second postpartum estrus). We believe the best method for using this technique is to monitor postparturient mares closely for ovulation and uterine fluid accumulation with transrectal palpation and ultrasonographic evaluation. Mares are bred on foal heat if they had no parturient or postparturient complications such as retained placenta, if it does not appear that they will ovulate before day 10 post partum, and little or no fluid remains in the uterus. If complications are associated with foaling, if ovulation occurs before day 10 post partum, or if significant fluid accumulation is present in the uterus, instead of breeding during the foal heat, the mare can be injected with $PGF_2\alpha$ 5 to 6 days after ovulation and bred on the subsequent induced estrus.

BIBLIOGRAPHY

Alexander SL, Irvine CHG: Control of the onset of the breeding season in the mare, its artificial regulation by progesterone treatment, *J Reprod Fertil* 44(Suppl):307-318, 1991.

Besognet B, Hansen BS, Daels PF: Induction of reproductive function in anestrous mares using a dopamine antagonist, *Theriogenology* 47:467-480, 1997.

Blanchard TL, Thompson JA, Brinsko SP, et al: Effects of breeding to ovulation interval and repeat service during the same estrus on pregnancy rates in Throughbred mares, *Proc 53rd Ann Mtg Am Assoc Equine Pract* 568-572, 2007.

Burns SJ, et al: Fertility of prostaglandin-induced oestrus compared to normal postpartum oestrus, *J Reprod Fertil* 27 (Suppl):245-250, 1979.

Card C, Green J: Comparison of pregnancy rates by week from stallion exposure and overall pregnancy rates in pasture-bred mares synchronized with CIDR and/or prostaglandin F2 alpha, *Proc 50th Ann Conv Am Assoc Equine Pract* 514-517, 2004.

Duchamp G, Daels PF: Combined effect of sulpiride and light treatment on the onset of cyclicity in anestrous mares [abstract], *Theriogenology* 58:599-602, 2002.

Fitzgerald BP, Schmidt MJ: Absence of an association between melatonin and reproductive activity in mares during the non-breeding season, *Biol Reprod* (Mono 1):425-434, 1995.

Ginther OJ: *Reproductive biology of the mare: basic and applied aspects,* ed 2, Cross Plains, WI, 1992, Equiservices, 158-161.

Jochle W, Trigg TE: Control of ovulation in the mare with Ovuplant: a short-release implant (STI) containing the GnRH analogue deslorelin acetate: studies from 1990-1994, *J Equine Vet Sci* 14: 632-644, 1994.

Kenney RM, et al: Noninfectious breeding problems in mares, *Vet Scope* 19:16-24, 1975.

Loy RG: Characteristics of postpartum reproduction in mares, *Vet Clin North Am Large Anim Pract* 2:345-358, 1980.

McCue PM, Warren RC, Appel RD, et al: Pregnancy rates following administration of GnRH to anestrous mares, *J Equine Vet Sci* 12:21-23, 1992.

McCue PM, Nickerson KC, Squires EL, et al: Effect of altrenogest on luteinizing hormone concentrations in mares during the transition period, *Proc 47th Ann Mtg Am Assoc Equine Pract* 249-251, 2001.

McCue PM, Hudson JJ, NBruemmer JE, et al: Efficacy of hCG at inducing ovulation: a new look at an old issue, *Proc 50th Ann Mtg Am Assoc Equine Pract* 510-513, 2004.

McCue PM, Magee C, Gee EK: Comparison of compounded deslorelin and hCG for induction of ovuation in mares, *J Equine Vet Sci* 27: 58-61, 2007.

McCue PM, LeBlanc MM, Squires EL: eFSH in clinical equine practice, *Theriogenology* 68:429-433, 2007.

Morehead JP, Blanchard TL: Clinical experience with deslorelin (Ovuplant) in a Kentucky Thoroughbred broodmare practice, *J Equine Vet Sci* 20:358-402, 2000.

Morehead JP, Colon JL, Blanchard TL: Clinical experience with native GnRH therapy to hasten follicular development and first ovulation of the breeding season, *J Equine Vet Sci* 21:54,81-88, 2001.

Nagy P, Guillame D, Daels PF: Seasonality in mares, *Anim Reprod Sci* 60/61:245-262, 2000.

Nickerson KC, McCue PM, Squires EL, et al: Comparison of two dosage regimens of the GnRH agonist deslorelin acetate on inducing ovulation in seasonally anestrous mares, Proceedings of Annual Symposium Equine Nutrition and Physiology Society, *J Equine Vet Sci* 18:121-124, 1998.

Nie GJ, Goodin AN, Braden TD, et al: How to reduce drug costs and side effects when using prostaglandins to short-cycle mares, *Proc 50th Ann Mtg Am Assoc Equine Pract* 396-398, 2004.

Niswender KD, McCue PM, Squires EL: Effect of purified equine follicle-stimulating hormone on follicular development and ovulation in transitional mares, *J Equine Vet Sci* 24:37-39, 2004.

Niswender KD, Roser JF, Boime I, et al: Induction of ovulation in the mare with recombinant equine LH, *Proc 52nd Ann Mtg Am Assoc Equine Pract* 387-388, 2006.

Palmer E, Draincourt MA, Ortavant R: Photoperiodic stimulation of the mare during winter anestrous. *J Reprod Fertil Suppl* 32:275-282, 1982.

Peres K, Fernandes C. Alvarenga M, et al: Effect of eFSH on ovarian cyclicity and embryo production of mares in spring transitional phase, *J Equine Vet Sci* 27:176-180, 2003.

Sharp DL, et al: Photoperiod. In McKinnon AO, Voss JL, editors: *Equine reproduction,* Philadelphia, 1993, Lea & Febiger, 179-185.

Squires EL, et al: Relationship of altrenogest to ovarian activity, hormone concentrations and fertility of mares, *J Anim Sci* 56:901-910, 1983.

Stich KL, Wendt KM, Blanchard TL, et al: Effects of a new injectable short-term release deslorelin in foal-heat mares, *Theriogenology* 62:831-836, 2004.

Taylor TB, et al: Control of ovulation in mares in the early breeding season with ovarian steroids and prostaglandin, *J Reprod Fertil* 32(Suppl):219-224, 1982.

Wendt KM, Stich KL, Blanchard TL: Effects of deslorelin administration in vulvar mucosa, with removal in 2 days, in foal-heat mares, *Proc 48th Ann Mtg Am Assoc Equine Pract* 61-64, 2002.

Breeding Soundness Examination of the Mare

CHAPTER 4

OBJECTIVES

While studying the information covered in this chapter, the reader should attempt to:
- Acquire a working understanding of the procedures used for performing a breeding soundness examination of the mare.
- Acquire a working understanding of how abnormalities of the genital tract may adversely affect fertility of the mare.

STUDY QUESTIONS

1. List information (history) that should be obtained to assess prior reproductive performance and to identify potential problems to be considered in a breeding soundness examination of a mare.
2. Describe procedures that are integral parts of the breeding soundness examination of the mare (e.g., assessment of vulvar conformation, vaginal speculum examination, procurement of specimens for uterine cytology, culture and biopsy).
3. List benefits of a properly taken and interpreted uterine cytology specimen.
4. List abnormalities that can be detected only with uterine biopsy.
5. List abnormalities that can be detected with intrauterine endoscopy.
6. Summarize the purposes for performing a breeding soundness examination of a mare.

HISTORY

A breeding soundness examination should begin with a gathering of all pertinent reproductive history regarding the mare. A thorough history may uncover information about a mare that may not otherwise be obtained. For instance, the following queries should be answered: How old is the mare? Has the mare been bred previously? If so, has she become pregnant and delivered any foals? How many foals? How long since she last foaled? Has she been bred each year? Has she been bred to fertile stallions with good breeding management procedures? Has she been bred to different stallions each year? Has she had any difficulties associated with foaling? Were any diagnoses of early pregnancy loss confirmed? Has she had any abortions or stillbirths? If so, at what gestational ages were pregnancies lost? Has the mare had any genital discharges? Has the mare previously been treated for genital infection? If so, what treatments were administered and when?

Mare age is important because, as a population, mares become less fertile with increasing age. A recent study involving Quarter Horse–type mares in good body condition revealed that for every year increase in age, the odds ratio for becoming pregnant on foal-heat breeding was 0.937 (i.e., approximately a 6% lower chance of becoming pregnant). In another study that investigated some of the factors affecting fertility in

Thoroughbreds bred in central Kentucky, once mares passed the age of 10 years, odds ratios for becoming pregnant during the season significantly declined (Table 4-1).

The status of the mare at the beginning of the year (i.e., *foaling mare,* mare that delivered a foal that year; *maiden mare,* mare that has not been bred in previous years; *barren mare,* mare bred the previous year that did not become pregnant; *not bred mare,* mare that the owner elected not to breed the previous year; or *aborted mare,* mare that became pregnant the previous year but lost the conceptus before a live foal could be born) can also be a significant predictor of expected fertility. A number of studies have identified maiden and foaling mares as the most fertile groups in broodmare bands; other groups of mares (particularly barren mares) are usually less likely to become pregnant and produce foals.

One should also collect information regarding the mare's estrous cycle. Mares are seasonal breeders with the peak of fertility corresponding to the longest days of the year. The mares typically have normal estrous cycles during the physiologic breeding season (spring and summer), then enter a state of reproductive quiescence in the late fall, as day length decreases. Mares that are reproductively normal generally enter into estrus (heat) every 18 to 24 days (approximately every 3 weeks) during the breeding season, with heats that typically last for a period of 4 to 7 days (see Chapter 2). Because of seasonal variations in the duration of estrus, a better indicator that the mare has regular estrous cycles is that the period between heats is 14 to 16 days. This interval remains relatively constant regardless of season. Whether or not the mare has normal estrous cycles and exhibits strong outward signs of heat (i.e., is sexually receptive) when exposed to a stallion during estrus should be noted. In addition, the method of teasing should be obtained because most mares fail to show strong signs of estrus unless teased by a stallion. Numerous mare owners believe otherwise, yet we have teased mares

with a stallion when the owners thought the mares were showing heat to a gelding or another mare, often finding the mares were not in estrus. In contrast, we have also teased mares thought by the owners to be out of heat when we suspected they actually were in heat (based on palpation findings) and usually found that the mares express behavioral estrus when presented to a stallion.

Shortened estrous cycles (e.g., less than 18 days) suggest the possibility of an underlying uterine infection (i.e., acute endometritis causing premature luteolysis). Lengthened estrous cycles in nonbred mares suggest the possibility of prolonged luteal function; in mares that have been bred, the possibility exists for early embryonic or fetal death. A less likely cause of irregular estrous cycles is endocrine dysfunction. If a mare has regular estrous cycles, the likelihood of endocrine dysfunction is low.

If possible, the examiner should collect previous breeding and medical records regarding the mare of interest and determine specifically whether the mare has had any reproductive or general medical problems that have necessitated treatment. A variety of ailments may reduce or abolish a mare's reproductive potential. A sample breeding soundness examination form for recording of history, examination findings, diagnosis, and treatment recommendations is provided in Figure 4-1.

GENERAL PHYSICAL EXAMINATION

Just because a mare is being examined for reproductive potential does not mean that her general body condition should be ignored. Texas workers, using a body condition scoring system of 1 to 9, found that mares with body condition scores of 5 or more had higher pregnancy rates and fewer cycles per pregnancy than mares with lower body condition scores. They also found that mares that entered the breeding season in high body condition, and were maintained in high body condition during the season, had earlier onset of regular estrous cycles and

TABLE 4-1				
Effects of Mare Age (Odds Ratios for Different Age Groups) on Pregnancy Outcome				
	Odds Ratio	**Lower CL**	**Upper CL**	**$P < 0.05$**
Mare age: 6-10 yr	0.89	0.63	1.20	NS
Mare age: 11-15 yr	0.66	0.45	0.92	S
Mare age: 16-20 yr	0.46	0.29	0.73	S
Mare age: >20 yr	0.33	0.13	0.66	S

CL, Confidence limit; *NS,* not significantly different from reference age group; *S,* significantly different ($P < 0.05$) from reference age group (mares ≤5 years of age).
Investigated with a stepwise multiple logistic regression model, adjusting for factors that significantly affected fertility during one season at a large Thoroughbred breeding farm in central Kentucky. Mares older than 10 years of age had significantly lower odds of becoming pregnant.

Mare Information:
Name:
Case #:
Age:
Breed:
Color:
Lip Tattoo #:
Registration #:
Markings / Brands:
Present Breeding Status:

Owner/Agent:
Address:

Telephone:
Fax:
Referring Veterinarian:
Address:

Telephone:
Fax:

History:

General Body Condition:

Genital Examination:
  Method(s) Used: ☐ Palpation   ☐ Ultrasound
● Anus/Perineum:
● Vulva:

● Clitoris:
● Vestibule:
● Vagina:
        ☐ Speculum examination:
        ☐ Digital examination:
● Cervix:
        ☐ Palpation per rectum:
        ☐ Speculum examination:
        ☐ Digital examination:
● Uterus:
        Right horn:
        Left horn:
        Body:
● Ovaries:
        Right:
        Left:
● Mammae:
● Other Findings:

Laboratory Tests:
☐ Endometrial culture:
☐ Endometrial biopsy:
        Category: Prognosis for supporting foal to term:
        Diagnosis:
☐ Endometrial cytology:
☐ Other tests performed:

Diagnosis/Recommendations:

Signature: Date:

Figure 4-1   Example of a breeding soundness examination form for the mare.

higher pregnancy rates and were less likely to lose pregnancies than were mares that entered the breeding season in poor body condition or that lost body condition during the breeding season.

Good general health also extends the longevity of broodmares and favors the ability of a mare to support a pregnancy to term and provide sufficient high-quality colostrum/milk for adequate foal development. All body systems (e.g., digestive, respiratory, urinary, cardiovascular, and nervous systems and special senses) should receive at least a cursory examination to prevent overlooking of conspicuous problems. Common laboratory tests (Coggin's test, urinalysis, blood analysis, and fecal egg counts) can be used in conjunction with a physical examination to assess the general health of a mare. Evaluation of conformation for defective traits that are potentially heritable is also prudent.

REPRODUCTIVE EXAMINATION

Restraint

With examination of a mare's reproductive tract, one must assess the mare's demeanor and ensure that she is properly restrained. Such precautions prevent or reduce undue injury to the mare or veterinarian during the examination process. Methods of restraint are the same as those discussed for palpation per rectum (see Chapter 1).

Examination of the External Genitalia

The first part of the reproductive examination involves a thorough inspection of the external genitalia. Conformation of the vulva, perineum, and anus is closely evaluated. To prepare the area for examination, the tail can be wrapped in a plastic sleeve, which is itself secured at the base of the tail with tape. The tail is then elevated by lifting it directly over the mare's rump to improve visualization of the external genitalia (Figure 4-2). Another useful method is to wrap the tail in a gauze bandage, pull the tail up to the side, and tie the gauze around the mare's neck. The disadvantage of this method is that exposure of the perineal area is reduced; however, it is useful for keeping the tail out of the way when a stock is not available.

The long axis of the vulva should be vertical, with the vulvar labia well apposed to produce an intact vulvar seal against contamination (see Figure 1-11). Any conformational abnormalities or vulvar discharge are noted. The perineum should be intact, and the anus should not be recessed (sunken) (see Figure 1-12) because this conformation predisposes the mare to excessive vulvar contamination during defecation. The labia of the vulva can be parted gently to document that the mare has an intact vestibulovaginal seal. If the vestibulovaginal seal is incompetent, parting the vulvar lips results in aspiration of air, heard as a sucking noise. This seal is also important to deter ascending uterine infection.

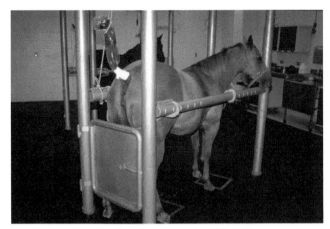

Figure 4-2 Mare placed in a stock with tail wrapped in a plastic sleeve and tied overhead in preparation for a breeding soundness examination.

Palpation per Rectum

With the arm protected with a plastic sleeve, a veterinarian can palpate the internal genital organs of the mare. With use of a systematic approach, the cervix, uterus, and ovaries are evaluated for normalcy. The uterus should be examined for evidence of pregnancy before more thorough palpation. If the mare is determined to be nonpregnant, the examination is continued. (Ultrasonographic evaluation is covered in Chapter 5.)

The ovaries of the mare are generally bean-shaped and range in size from that of a golf ball to a tennis ball (see Chapter 1). The ovulation fossa can be readily palpated in the normal ovary. Mares can have ovarian tumors develop that result in substantial increase in ovarian size and loss of the ovulation fossa (Figure 4-3). Ovarian size can also be markedly increased with hematoma formation (Figure 4-4), which occurs when excessive bleeding follows ovulation and formation of a corpus hemorrhagicum. The ovaries are examined for follicles (Figure 4-5) or corpora lutea (Figure 4-6),

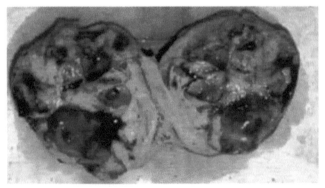

Figure 4-3 Surgically removed granulosa cell tumor of an ovary of a mare. The affected ovary was enlarged and firm, and the contralateral ovary was atrophied (small, inactive). The mare was behaviorally anestrous, with elevated circulating concentrations of inhibin and testosterone.

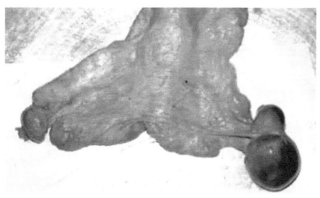

Figure 4-4 Ovarian hematoma from a mare. Mares affected with ovarian hematomas usually continue to have regular estrous cycles and do not have contralaterally atrophied ovaries. The enlarged ovary shrinks over time. Hormone assay results reveal no abnormalities in hormone concentrations.

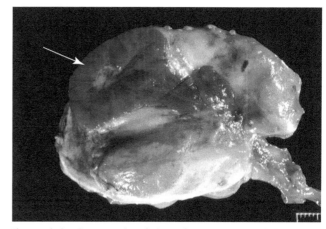

Figure 4-6 Cross-sectional view of mare ovary with functional corpus luteum *(arrow)* present. (Photo courtesy of Dr. John Edwards.)

findings that suggest that the mare is having normal estrous cycles. Occasionally, incidental parovarian cysts are detectable but seldom interfere with fertility. Cysts formed in the fossa region are thought to be peritoneal fragments that become embedded in the serosal surface of the ovary after ovulation. Other parovarian cysts are likely to be distended remnants of the embryonic mesonephric system or paramesonephric tubules or ducts and are located at the mesovarium near the ovary (Figure 4-7) or on the ovary (epoophoron). Very small (1 to 2 cm in diameter) hypoplastic ovaries are sometimes found bilaterally, in which case gonadal dysgenesis as a result of sex chromosome abnormalities should be suspected. If one ovary is enlarged and the other is small and inactive, a granulosa cell tumor involving the enlarged ovary should be suspected. Sometimes, one or both ovaries may be absent. If only one ovary is missing, it was likely removed previously because of an ovarian tumor. Some performance mares have both ovaries surgically removed in an attempt to eliminate objectionable behavior associ-

ated with estrus. If an ovariectomized mare is sold, the new owner may be unaware that the ovaries have been removed.

The uterus of the nonpregnant mare is T (or Y) shaped, consisting of two uterine horns and a singular uterine body (see Chapter 1). It is palpated in its entirety for size, symmetry between uterine horns, and evidence of luminal contents. Numerous uterine abnormalities can be detected via palpation per rectum and include atrophy of endometrial folds (Figure 4-8), localized atrophy of uterine musculature, large lymphatic cysts (Figure 4-9), uterine tumors (Figure 4-10), and presence of large quantities of purulent material or other abnormal fluid within the lumen of the uterus (Figure 4-11).

The cervix, a tubular structure that connects the uterus with the vagina, can be easily palpated per rectum. It is evaluated primarily to aid in estimating the stage of the estrous cycle; it is elongated and closed

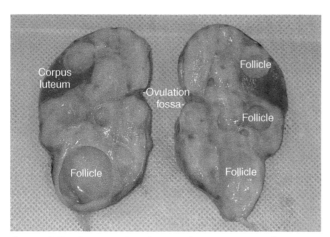

Figure 4-5 Cross-sectional view of mare ovary with various-sized follicles present.

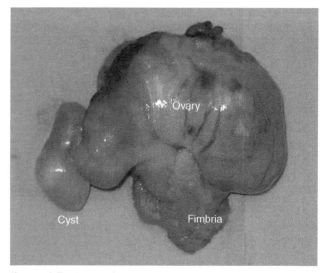

Figure 4-7 Parovarian cyst next to ovary from a mare. Such cysts are not uncommon and are not believed to interfere with fertility.

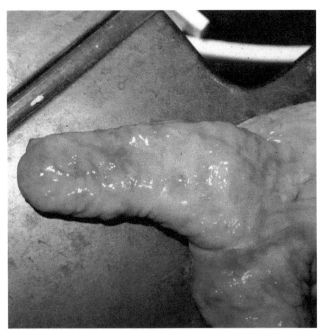

Figure 4-8 Uterus from mare with atrophied endometrial folds. The uterus has been turned inside out so that the endometrial surface is outermost.

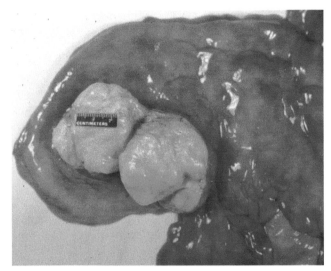

Figure 4-10 Uterine tumor (leiomyoma) near end of right horn of mare uterus; cut surface shown with endometrium outermost. On palpation per rectum, the tumor was firm and easily mistaken for the ovary, except that the tumor was contained within the uterus and the ovary was palpable just beyond the tip of the uterine horn.

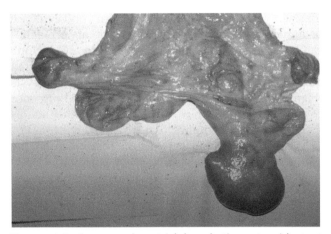

Figure 4-9 Large endometrial lymphatic cyst evident at base of uterine horn. The uterine wall was thin (atrophied) and a prominent sacculation was present at the base of one uterine horn during palpation per rectum.

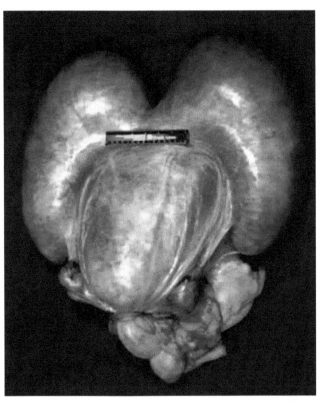

Figure 4-11 Uterine distention with purulent material from a mare with chronic pyometra.

when a mare is in diestrus (i.e., out of heat) and shortened and dilated when a mare is in heat (estrus). Most abnormalities of the cervix affect its lumen and cannot be readily identified via palpation per rectum. For this reason, the cervix is also evaluated with visual inspection and digital palpation per vaginum. For digital palpation, the index finger is inserted into the cervical lumen, the thumb is apposed on the outside of the protruding cervix, and the entire circumference of the cervix is palpated between the thumb and forefinger to determine whether muscle separations or lacerations are present (Figure 4-12). Luminal adhesions can also be detected by advancing the index finger along the entire length of the cervical lumen. In some cases, particularly

in older maiden mares, the cervix may be difficult to dilate. Such mares tend to accumulate fluid within the uterus because of insufficient ability of the cervix to properly dilate when in estrus.

One part of the internal reproductive tract that cannot be examined readily via palpation per rectum is the

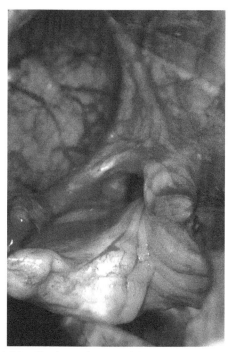

Figure 4-12 Pie-shaped cervical laceration evident during speculum examination of mare cervix.

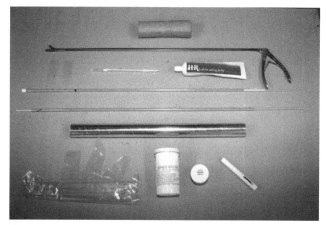

Figure 4-13 Equipment used for breeding soundness examination in the mare. *From top:* Gauze tail wrap; alligator-type uterine biopsy forceps for procuring endometrial biopsy; microscope slides for making of endometrial cytology preparation for staining; transport media to contain uterine swab during shipment to bacteriology laboratory; sterile, nonbactericidal/nonbacteriostatic lubricant; guarded and unguarded (i.e., no distal occlusion) culture instruments for taking uterine culture or cytology; disposable vaginal speculum; rectal sleeve; fixative vial and shipping container for transport of endometrial biopsy sample to reference laboratory; and light for illumination of vagina during viewing through speculum.

oviduct. The mare has two oviducts. These tiny tubes connect the uterine horns with their corresponding ovaries, serve as a sperm reservoir after breeding, are the site of fertilization, and transport fertilized oocytes to the uterus for continued development. Oviductal problems that interfere with fertility in mares are considered to be rare. However, this consensus may change as improved technology allows better assessment of oviductal function. Blockage of the oviducts by inspissated protein concretions (presumably from follicular fluid) has been reported as a potential cause of unexplained infertility in older broodmares. Perhaps one of the more promising methods for reestablishing oviductal patency (as opposed to attempting to mechanically flush the oviducts by accessing the fimbria for cannulation via flank laparotomy) is to drip 0.2 mg prostaglandin E_2 (PGE$_2$)-laced gel (Dinoprostin, Upjohn, Kalamazoo, MI) along the surface of the oviducts via a laparoscope. English workers reported this to be a favorable treatment for mares with unexplained infertility over 1 to 4 years. Examination of effluent from uterine flushings obtained 3 to 4 days after PGE$_2$ administration may potentially reveal the presence of these uterine concretions and confirm that oviductal patency has likely been reestablished.

VAGINAL SPECULUM EXAMINATION

After thorough cleansing of the vulva and surrounding areas to avoid contamination of the upper reproductive tract, a sterile disposable tubular vaginal speculum can be inserted into the vaginal cavity to allow examination of this area (Figures 4-13 and 4-14). A small amount of

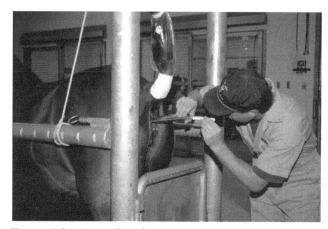

Figure 4-14 Procedure for viewing vagina and external os of cervix through a tubular vaginal speculum.

sterile lubricant is placed on the speculum before insertion, and a light is used to illuminate the vestibule and vagina through the speculum. The entire vestibule, vagina, and external cervical os can be viewed with this approach.

Alternatively, a reusable metal speculum (Caslick's or two-bladed speculum) (Figures 4-15 and 4-16) can be used for this purpose. An advantage of metal specula is that the vestibule and vulva can be further spread to provide better visualization. The two-bladed speculum also allows good visualization of the floor of the vestibule when the urethral opening needs further evaluation.

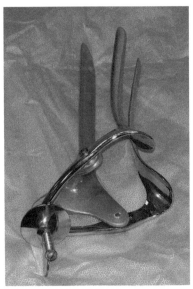

Figure 4-15 Three-bladed Caslick's speculum for vaginal examination.

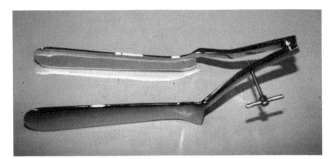

Figure 4-16 Two-bladed vaginal speculum for viewing vagina and vestibule.

Abnormalities that may be detected via vaginal speculum examination include persistent hymen (Figure 1-10), vaginitis/cervicitis, vaginal varicosities (Figure 4-17), adhesions (scarring of the cervical opening or vaginal vault), lacerations or tears of the posterior cervix (see Figure 4-12) or vaginal walls, and accumulation or purulent material or urine in the vaginal cavity (Figures 4-18 and 4-19).

UTERINE (ENDOMETRIAL) CULTURE

An endometrial (uterine) culture can yield valuable information regarding a mare's reproductive potential, provided it is properly obtained and interpreted in conjunction with other examination findings. The objective of an endometrial culture is to determine whether any microorganisms (i.e., bacteria or fungi) are present within the cavity of the uterus and are causing endometritis. An important point is that positive culture results alone, in the absence of signs of inflammation, do not indicate that the mare is infected. Unfortunately, contamination of the swab sample with microorganisms originating from the outside environment, perineum,

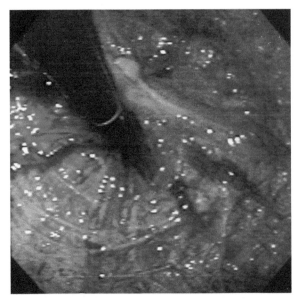

Figure 4-17 Vaginal varicosities on cranial aspect of vestibular fold and caudal vagina. The flexible endoscope was passed into the cranial vagina and turned to permit viewing of the back side of the vestibular fold. The mare had a history of recurrent episodes of hemorrhage from the vulva.

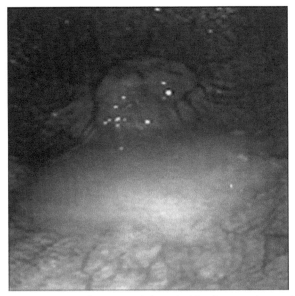

Figure 4-18 Purulent material pooled in the anterior vagina of a mare with endometritis.

vulva, vagina, or cervix is extremely easy to do. Such contamination often leads to the false impression that a mare has endometrial infection, particularly when endometrial cytology or biopsy is not performed in conjunction with the endometrial culture. Hence, it is essential to thoroughly cleanse and dry the mare's hindquarters and use a guarded swab and sterile equipment when swabbing the endometrium for bacteriologic culture (see Figure 4-13). To procure a swabbing for culture, one of two methods can be used. The first method involves carrying the guarded swab into the vagina with a sterile gloved hand. The index finger is

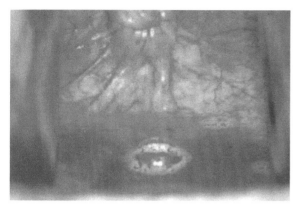

Figure 4-19 Urine and debris pooled in the anterior vagina of a mare with urovagina.

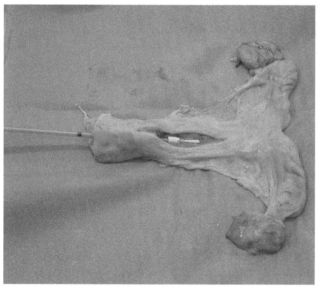

Figure 4-20 Method used for transcervical procurement of uterine swabbing for bacteriologic culture or cytologic analysis. The body of the uterus has been cut open to facilitate viewing of the extended swab.

placed in the cervical lumen, and the guarded swab is guided into the uterine lumen where the swab is then exposed (Figure 4-20). The swab should be retracted back into the guard before removing the swab from the uterus. For swabbing the endometrium through a speculum, a sterile vaginal speculum is passed into the cranial vagina to the cervical os. A light is used for illumination, and the sterile guarded swab is passed through the speculum and cervix into the uterine lumen where the swab is then exposed. Again, the swab should be retracted back into the guard before removing it from the uterus. Passing a uterine swab through an unrelaxed cervix of a mare can be difficult or impossible with the speculum technique; however, if the cervix is relaxed and moist (i.e., mare is in estrus), the technique works well.

New York workers reported that use of a small volume (60-mL) uterine flush with sterile phosphate buffered saline (PBS) solution infused through a 20F balloon catheter, with collection of as much effluent as possible, could lead to better recovery of bacteria than that achieved with simply sampling the endometrium with a guarded swab. The uterine effluent should be handled in an aseptic manner and put in a sterile tube for centrifugation, and the sediment should be used to inoculate the diagnostic culture medium. Although this technique requires more time to obtain the specimen for culture, the group reported better correlation with inflammatory changes detected on endometrial biopsy (i.e., more positive culture results in mares with endometritis) than was obtained from endometrial swabbing.

To further increase the chance that culture of the endometrial swabbing accurately reflects its microbial status, the culture swab must be handled correctly on transit to the laboratory for testing. We recommend use of transport media, such as Amie's charcoal or Stuart's medium, that maintain organism viability without encouraging contaminant overgrowth, particularly if much time-lapse will occur between obtaining the sample and inoculation of the culture medium. In addition, we recommend that culture results be obtained from direct inoculation on media rather than from broth culture, which likewise encourages overgrowth of contaminant bacteria. Finally, growth from direct inoculation of the plate should be quantified in some fashion because heavy growth at 24 or 48 hours of incubation is more likely to be significant than recovery of only a few colonies. Yeast or fungal organisms sometimes require longer incubation periods for sufficient growth to occur on the medium to allow identification. If practitioners prefer to perform their own cultures, 5% blood agar plates and MacConkey's agar can be inoculated with the uterine swabbing. Blood agar media incubated in aerobic conditions is adequate for recovery of most potential pathogens of the mare reproductive tract (the exception being the need for microaerophilic or anaerobic conditions for the mare with septic postparturient metritis). Antimicrobial susceptibility testing is also desirable to aid in selection of the proper drug for treatment of uterine infections. Antimicrobial susceptibility test discs and apparatus are available from several veterinary supply companies. We recommend the use of disks containing the antibiotics most commonly used for uterine infusions (e.g., penicillin, ampicillin, ticarcillin, timentin, gentamycin, amikacin, and polymyxin-B) to ensure selection of a suitable antimicrobial for the more common causes of endometritis in mares. Other antimicrobial discs are available as well.

To minimize misinterpretation of culture results, the findings should be compared with those of endometrial cytologic analysis or biopsy. Cytologic analysis or biopsy allows the detection of endometrial inflammation, a process that accompanies presence of microorganisms if the mare truly has infectious endometritis.

UTERINE (ENDOMETRIAL) CYTOLOGY

By using a swab (the same method described for obtaining a swabbing for culture) or other device, cells can be retrieved from the uterine cavity and endometrial surface for examination for the presence of an active inflammatory process that accompanies infectious endometritis. If a swab is used to collect material for cytology, it should immediately be gently rolled across the surface of a microscope slide; the material is allowed to air dry and then fixed and stained with a suitable stain such as Diff-Quik (Fisher Scientific, Pittsburgh, Pa.) If a loop or small scoop is used to collect a specimen for cytology, the fluid from the collection device should be gently tapped onto a microscope slide, smeared and allowed to air dry, and then stained in a similar manner. Stained cytology preparations are examined with a microscope for the presence of white blood cells (usually neutrophils), microorganisms, and healthy or unhealthy luminal epithelial cells. Normal endometrial cytologic preparations contain healthy-appearing sheets of, and individual, columnar epithelial cells with few or no white blood cells and no bacteria, fungi, or yeast organisms (Figure 4-21). Cytologic preparations from mares with acute or subacute endometritis contain increased numbers of white blood cells and unhealthy-appearing (degenerate) epithelial cells. A simple method of evaluating endometrial cytology is to examine at least five cellular fields with a 40× objective and obtain an average number of neutrophils (polymorphonuclear cells; PMNs) per high power field (hpf). A normal cytology sample should contain less than 1 PMN/hpf; 1 to 2 PMNs/hpf indicates mild inflammation, 3 to 4 PMNs/hpf indicates moderate inflammation, and 5 or more PMNs/hpf is indicative of severe inflammation.

Kentucky workers have proposed using a low-volume uterine flush for preparing samples for cytologic analysis (a modification of that described by New York workers previously). A Bivona (Bivona Inc, Gary, IN) uterine catheter (EUF 80) is passed aseptically into the uterus 10 to 12 cm beyond the cervix (i.e., into a uterine horn). The retention cuff is not inflated within the uterine lumen. Sixty mL of sterile physiologic saline solution is infused into the uterine lumen, and a hand is inserted into the rectum for massage of the fluid throughout the uterus for at least 30 seconds. The fluid is then collected via gravity flow while the tip of the horn is lifted per rectum. An aliquot of the mixed fluid is centrifuged for 10 minutes, and the supernatant is decanted. The remaining pellet is sampled with two sterile swabs (one used for inoculation of culture media and one used for cytologic preparation). For cytologic analysis, the swab is rolled across a microscope slide, which is then prepared as described previously. The investigators report that this technique is well correlated with inflammatory changes detected in endometrial biopsy and with recovery of pathogens on culture.

The value of uterine cytology is usually limited to documentation of an active (i.e., acute or subacute) inflammatory response, as neutrophils are a prominent luminal component of endometritis (Figure 4-22). In addition, staining of uterine cytology preparations remains the best way to demonstrate infection with yeast or fungi (Figure 4-23) because these organisms tend to proliferate in the uterine lumen and on the surface of the luminal epithelial cells. However, more subtle inflammatory changes of the endometrium, such a chronic endometritis, are usually not detectable with this approach. Nevertheless, uterine cytology can provide a gauge of the representativeness of uterine culture results, particularly when time is of the essence. For example, when a mare is presented for examination

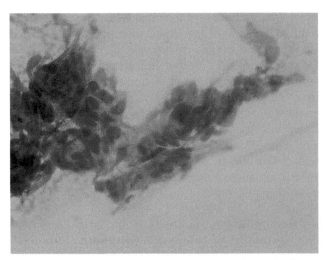

Figure 4-21 Cytologic preparation (Diff-Quik stain) of normal endometrial cells. Normal endometrial cytology includes healthy-appearing simple columnar epithelial cells, often in clumps, and few or no neutrophils.

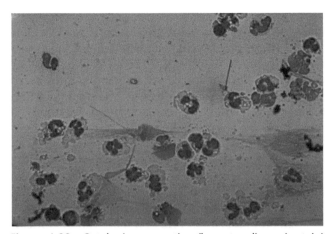

Figure 4-22 Cytologic preparation (hematoxylin-eosin stain) from a mare with an acute endometritis associated with *Streptococcus* infection. Cytologic preparations from mares with acute or subacute endometritis yield numerous neutrophils that are often degenerate and may contain phagocytosed bacteria along with many singular degenerate epithelial cells.

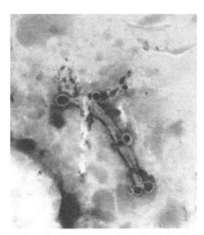

Figure 4-23 Cytologic preparation (Diff-Quik stain) from a mare with fungal endometritis revealing hyphae and encapsulated yeast spores.

early during estrus, if the uterine cytologic analysis and culture suggest that inflammation is not present, the mare can be bred during the same estrous period. Likewise, if evidence of only mild inflammation/infection exists, treating the uterus before and after breeding is sometimes an option (see Chapter 6). If the practitioner had to wait for endometrial biopsy results, breeding on that estrus would most likely have to be skipped (e.g., ovulation would be missed because of the lag in report time). In addition, if cytologic analysis was not performed and positive culture results were obtained because of contamination, the mare might not be bred on that cycle because of the erroneous belief that she needed treatment for a uterine infection that did not really exist.

Endometrial Biopsy

Provided that the gross physical condition of the mare and reproductive tract is within normal limits, evaluation of an endometrial biopsy is probably the single most important means of assessing the mare's potential as a broodmare. In other words, biopsy results can be categorized according to the prognosis for the mare to become pregnant and carry a foal to term:

  Category I: 80% to 100% chance
  Category IIA: 50% to 80% chance
  Category IIB: 10% to 50% chance
  Category III: Less than 10% chance

A biopsy can easily be taken from the endometrium by passing an appropriately designed instrument through the cervix and into the uterus for sample retrieval. The aseptic procedure is the same as that for procuring an endometrial swabbing for culture, except that the closed biopsy punch must be passed far enough into the uterus to ensure that a representative specimen of endometrium is obtained. Ideally, routine biopsy specimens should be obtained at the base of one of the uterine horns, where, after cessation of the mobility phase, early development of the embryo occurs. Endometrial specimens obtained too near the cervix have reduced

glandular density and shallow gland penetration into the lamina propria, which prevents accurate assessment of glandular normalcy or pathology. After the biopsy punch is inserted into the uterus, one hand is inserted into the rectum and the other hand holds the biopsy grip. With the hand in the rectum, the biopsy punch can be further guided to the base of one of the uterine horns. The biopsy jaws are opened, and the uterine wall is lifted (if the sample is to be procured from the ventral surface of the uterine horn) (Figure 4-24) or pressed (if the sample is to be procured from the dorsal surface of the uterine horn or body) (Figure 4-25) into the jaws which are then

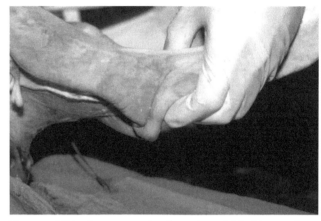

Figure 4-24 Procurement of endometrial biopsy from ventral surface of the uterus. The uterine wall is gently lifted with the fingers into the jaws of the biopsy punch and held in this position until the jaws are closed, thereby clipping off a portion of the endometrium.

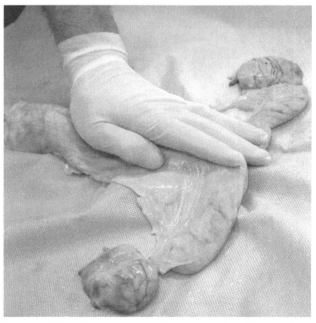

Figure 4-25 Procurement of endometrial biopsy from dorsal surface of the uterus. The uterine wall is gently pressed into the underlying jaws of the biopsy punch and held in this position until the jaws are closed, thereby clipping off a portion of the endometrium.

closed, thereby clipping off a portion of the endometrium. The biopsy punch is removed from the mare's reproductive tract, and the endometrial specimen is placed in a suitable fixative, such as Davidson's solution or 10% buffered formalin, and transported to a reference laboratory for interpretation. Bouin's solution was once the preferred fixative for endometrial biopsies; however, because of its volatile nature, more stringent regulations have made proper shipment and disposal of Bouin's solution problematic.

Many abnormalities that can adversely affect a mare's fertility can be detected only with microscopic evaluation of an endometrial biopsy. Examples include periglandular fibrosis, cystic glandular distention, lymphatic distention, and chronic inflammatory changes within the endometrium (Figures 4-26 to 4-32). Biopsy evaluation is also an excellent way to monitor patient response to therapy when uterine infections or other

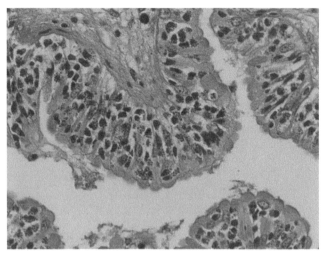

Figure 4-28 Transepithelial migration of eosinophils commonly occurs when pneumouterus is present.

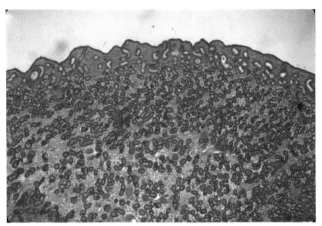

Figure 4-26 Normal active endometrium (category I: 80% or better chance of foaling). Glands are numerous, randomly dispersed, and active. Inflammatory cells are absent or infrequent in occurrence.

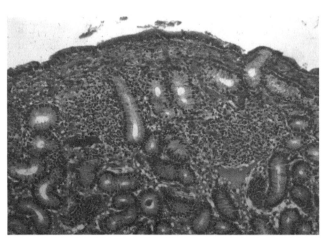

Figure 4-29 Chronic endometritis with lymphocyte infiltration into lamina propria (category IIA: 50% to 80% chance of foaling). This type of inflammation may not be detected with uterine cytology.

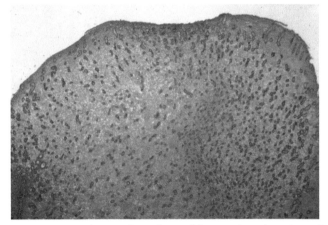

Figure 4-27 Seasonal endometrial atrophy. Atrophy of glands (shrunken, straight, and nontortuous) and luminal epithelium (flattened, cuboidal) are evident during seasonal atrophy. Fertility is likely to be reduced until seasonal atrophy is corrected.

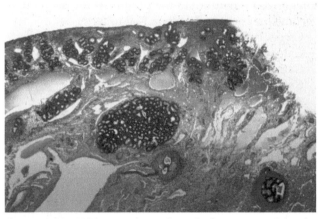

Figure 4-30 Widespread, moderately frequent periglandular fibrosis (category IIB: 10% to 50% chance of foaling). Clumped (nested) glands are distended and are surrounded by a few layers of connective tissue.

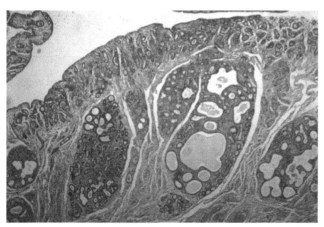

Figure 4-31 Widespread, frequent periglandular fibrosis (category III: less than 10% chance of foaling). Gland nesting (clumping) from fibrosis is so frequent that it affects almost all glands within the stratum spongiosum (deeper lamina propria).

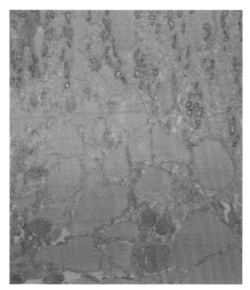

Figure 4-32 Widespread, frequent lymphatic lacunae (category IIB: 10% to 50% chance of foaling). Lymphatic vessels, particularly in core areas of the lamina propria, are distended with homogeneous eosinophilic fluid.

endometrial abnormalities are diagnosed and treated. Workers in the United Kingdom have shown that improved biopsy scores after treatment (i.e., pathologic changes detected in a previous endometrial biopsy have disappeared or are less severe) are more closely related to subsequent fertility of mares than a prognosis based simply on a single pretreatment biopsy.

OTHER DIAGNOSTIC AIDS

Additional diagnostic tests can be incorporated into a breeding soundness examination if more information is necessary to judge a mare's breeding potential. Two of the more commonly used procedures are transrectal ultrasonographic examination of the reproductive tract

and transcervical endoscopic examination of the uterine cavity. Ultrasound examinations use high-frequency sound waves to visualize reproductive structures (e.g., the ovaries and uterus, which are otherwise hidden from view) with a relatively noninvasive approach. It improves diagnostic capability for several reproductive abnormalities, including ovarian tumors or hematomas; uterine tumors, cysts, abscesses; and pathologic fluid accumulations within the uterine cavity.

Endoscopic examinations allow direct visualization of the uterine cavity. A specialized viewing instrument (disinfected endoscope or videoscope of sufficient length to fully visualize the entire uterus) is passed directly into the uterine cavity via the cervix. The uterus is insufflated with sufficient air or fluid to dilate the uterine cavity, and the endoscope is advanced to the internal bifurcation (Figure 4-33) and then to the end of a uterine horn (Figures 4-34 and 4-35). After one uterine

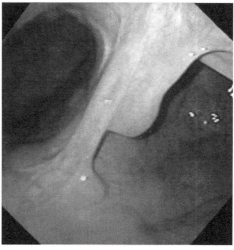

Figure 4-33 Endoscopic view of bifurcation of uterine horns. The uterus must be partially distended with air or fluid for visualization of the interior of the uterus.

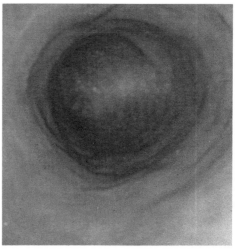

Figure 4-34 Endoscopic view of lumen of a uterine horn. Endometrial folds are not apparent as a result of distention of the uterine horn with air to facilitate visualization.

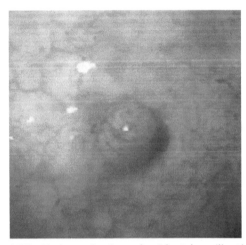

Figure 4-35 Endoscopic view of oviductal papilla, the location where the oviduct empties into the uterus.

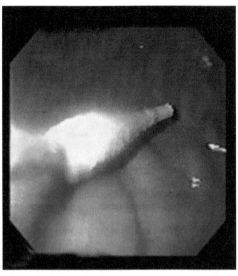

Figure 4-37 Endoscopic view of the tip of a Culturette inadvertently left in the uterus.

horn is viewed in its entirety, the endoscope is retracted and passed to the end of the other uterine horn in the same manner. The entire inner surface of the uterus can thus be viewed, permitting definitive diagnosis of abnormalities such as endometrial cysts (Figure 4-36), foreign bodies (e.g., cotton swabs that were broken off in the uterine cavity during a previous attempt at obtaining a uterine culture) (Figure 4-37), purulent luminal contents (Figure 4-38), transluminal adhesions (Figure 4-39), and other space-occupying lesions (Figure 4-40).

WRITTEN SUMMARY FOR CLIENT/OWNER

As with any type of soundness examination, a written report should be given to the client or owner that summarizes findings, including any definitive diagnosis, recommended treatment, and prognosis for future fertility. This document is also useful for review in determining response to treatments and in assessing breeding outcome.

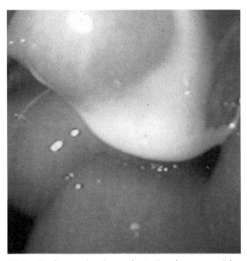

Figure 4-38 Endoscopic view of uterine lumen, with purulent material on luminal epithelium.

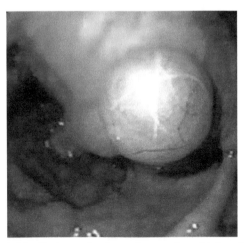

Figure 4-36 Endoscopic view of an endometrial cyst.

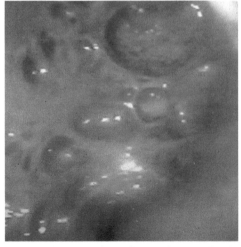

Figure 4-39 Endoscopic view of extensive transluminal adhesions occluding the uterine lumen.

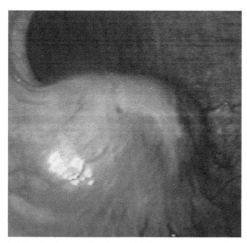

Figure 4-40 Endoscopic view of leiomyoma (uterine smooth muscle tumor) impinging on uterine lumen as a space-occupying mass.

BIBLIOGRAPHY

Allen WR, Wilsher S, Morris L, et al: Re-establishment of oviductal patency and fertility in infertile mares, Proc 9th Int Symp Equine Reprod, *Animal Reprod Sci* 94:242-243, 2006.

Baker B, Kenney RM: Systematic approach to diagnosis of the infertile or subfertile mare. In Morrow DA, editor: *Current therapy in theriogenology,* Philadelphia, 1980, Saunders Co, 721-736.

Ball BA, Shin SJ, Patten VH, et al: Use of a small volume uterine flush for microbiologic and cytologic examination of the mare's endometrium, *Theriogenology* 29:1269-1283, 1988.

Brook D: Uterine cytology. In McKinnon AO, Voss JL, editors: *Equine reproduction,* Philadelphia, 1993, Lea & Febiger, 246-254.

Henneke DR, Potter GD, Kreider JL: Body condition during pregnancy and lactation and reproductive efficiency of mares, *Theriogenology* 21:897-909, 1984.

Kenney RM: Cyclic and pathologic changes of the mare endometrium as detected by biopsy, with a note on early embryonic death, *JAVMA* 1978;172:241-262.

Kenney RM, Ganjam VK, Bergman RV: Non-infectious breeding problems in mares, *Vet Scope* 19:16-24, 1975.

Kenney RM, Doig PA: Equine endometrial biopsy. In Morrow DA, editor: *Current therapy in theriogenology,* ed 2, Philadelphia, 1986, Saunders, 723-729.

LeBlanc MM, Magsig J, Stromberg AJ: Use of a low-volume uterine flush for diagnosing endometritis in chronically infertile mares, *Theriogenology* 68:403-412, 2007.

Transrectal Ultrasonography in Broodmare Practice

CHAPTER 5

OBJECTIVES

While studying the information covered in this chapter, the reader should attempt to:
- Acquire a working understanding of the principles and equipment used for performing ultrasonographic examination on the mare reproductive tract.
- Acquire a working knowledge of the ultrasonographic appearance of the reproductive organs of the mare.
- Acquire a working understanding of the ultrasonographic appearance of the mare reproductive tract and conceptus during the estrous cycle and early pregnancy.
- Acquire a working understanding of the ultrasonographic appearance of ovarian and uterine abnormalities of the mare reproductive tract.

STUDY QUESTIONS

1. List the components and characteristics of an ultrasound machine suitable for use in examination of the mare reproductive tract.
2. Describe the technique for safely performing a transrectal ultrasonographic examination of the mare reproductive tract. Emphasize the importance of a systematic approach to ensure thorough scanning of the uterus of a mare for early pregnancy diagnosis.
3. Describe the ultrasonographic appearance of:
   a. The anestrous ovaries
   b. A preovulatory follicle
   c. An ovulatory follicle (within 24 hours after ovulation)
   d. The developing corpus luteum
   e. The mature corpus luteum
   f. The estrous uterus
   g. The diestrous uterus
   h. An anovulatory follicle
   i. An ovarian hematoma
   j. A granulosa cell tumor
   k. Uterine lymphatic cysts
   l. Intrauterine fluid accumulation associated with endometritis
4. Summarize the characteristic location and transrectal ultrasonographic appearance of the equine conceptus in the following periods of pregnancy:
   a. 12 to 14 days
   b. 17 to 18 days
   c. 20 to 21 days
   d. 28 to 30 days
   e. 34 to 36 days
   f. 38 to 40 days
   g. 45 to 50 days
   h. 60 to 65 days

In 1980, real-time ultrasonography was first reported as a potentially valuable diagnostic modality in the discipline of equine reproduction. Since this original report, applications of diagnostic ultrasonography in equine reproduction have expanded to the point that ultrasound has become a fundamental, indispensable tool for both veterinary clinicians and research scientists.

The two-dimensional grayscale image produced with **B-mode** (brightness-modality) **real-time** ultrasonography provides a detailed cinematographic view of the structure being studied. With this modality, the observer can actually visualize "hidden" reproductive organs and follow various reproductive events in a noninvasive manner, with no apparent adverse biologic effects incurred by the patient. More recently, color Doppler ultrasound has been used to assess blood flow in the uterus, ovary, and uterus of the mare. Transvaginal ultrasound has also been used for aspiration of oocytes from ovarian follicles, twin reduction, and deposition of embryos into the uterus. Although the technology behind real-time ultrasonography is quite complex, operation of the unit is relatively simple for the trained theriogenologist, requiring only a basic knowledge of ultrasound principles and ultrasonic anatomy of the reproductive tract.

INSTRUMENTATION

A B-mode real-time ultrasound system consists of a **transducer** that is connected by a long cord to a base unit containing a **display monitor** and **control panel** (Figure 5-1). The transducer transmits and receives **high-frequency sound waves** to produce images of soft tissues and organs on the display monitor. Tissues vary in echogenicity (i.e., the ability to propagate or reflect sound waves); therefore, the proportion of reflected sound waves is dependent on the innate characteristics of the tissues or fluids being examined. For instance, fluids readily propagate sound waves, whereas air and dense tissues reflect most or all sound waves. Reflected sound waves that are received by the transducer are then converted to electronic impulses and subsequently displayed on the monitor. The monitor consists of a two-dimensional array of closely aligned dots. The brightness of the dots is directly proportional to the amplitude of the echoes (or reflected sound waves). Hence, highly **echogenic** tissues (e.g., bone or connective tissue) appear *white* on the ultrasound monitor whereas nonechogenic **(anechoic)** fluids are *black*. A continuum of gray shades between white and black allows one to distinguish tissues of intermediate echogenicity. The control panel of the ultrasound unit allows the operator to adjust the quality of the image and label or measure structures of interest. Because air interrupts the transmission of ultrasound waves, when air is present within a viscus, bright echogenic lines or spots are seen on the monitor. When

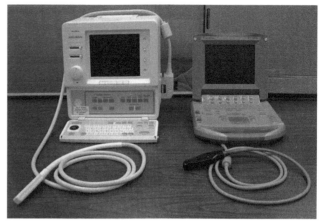

Figure 5-1 Two ultrasound systems for use in transrectal ultrasonographic examination of the mare. Shown on the *left* is a portable unit with a display monitor and fold-down control panel, 5-MHz transducer, and attached cord. Newer computer-based ultrasound machines (hand-held, battery-powered portable unit located on the *right*) use software that allows labeling and filing of images, with storage to internal or external devices that permit downloading to personal computers for editing, labeling, printing and publication. The stored images can also be accessed for viewing, enhancement, and sending as a viewable image over the Internet. Most portable ultrasound systems can be purchased with a number of different probes for varied uses.

sufficient blockage of ultrasound waves occurs, artifactual shadows or reverberations may be produced below the initially sound-impacted echogenic structure or tissue on the monitor. For example, dark shadows are visible on the monitor below sound-impacted bone, such as fetal ribs. Reverberation echoes are bright artifacts repeated at even intervals, but with lesser reverberation, because blocked sound waves are bounced back and forth between the probe and a gas-filled viscus. Artifacts not only interfere with the ability of the examiner to visualize surrounding tissue but may be falsely interpreted to be pathologic structures.

Linear-array 5-MHz transducers are amenable to most needs encountered in equine reproduction. The higher resolving power of 7.5-MHz transducers allows a more detailed study of structures, but the tissue-penetrating capacity of these transducers is more limited. Transducers with lower sound wave frequencies (e.g., 2.5 to 3.5 MHz) permit greater tissue penetration, so they may be more useful for evaluation of the uterus and its contents during advanced pregnancy; however, image resolution is reduced accordingly. Curvilinear transcutaneous probes available for thoracic or abdominal imaging can be useful for monitoring fetal viability (e.g., heartbeat, fetal activity), character and amount of amniotic or allantoic fluid, uteroplacental thickness, and separation of the placenta.

Color Doppler ultrasound is becoming available in less expensive, often portable, machines. This field of study could increase diagnostic information available to the theriogenologist. The basis for the technology is in the shift in ultrasound frequency of echoes from red blood cells in motion as they move toward or away from the transducer. This allows pictorial assessment of blood flow, which can be seen on the monitor in color-flow mode. Characterizing changing blood flow (perfusion) may be an important indicator of viability of transitional follicles, corpora lutea, and pregnancy, providing information that would otherwise not be available. Many of the portable Doppler ultrasound units use linear or curvilinear probes that are easily used within the rectum or vagina.

PROCEDURAL CONSIDERATIONS

Ultrasound evaluation of the mare's reproductive tract is generally performed with a transrectal approach. Usefulness of transcutaneous ultrasonography is limited to evaluation of the uterus and fetus during more advanced (3 to 4 months to term) pregnancy.

Precautions regarding mare restraint and reproductive examination per rectum are similar to those issued for palpation per rectum. Minimal but effective restraint of the mare greatly reduces the likelihood of equipment damage or injury to the mare or operator during the examination process. When examining the mare's reproductive tract via transrectal ultrasonography, the following steps should be taken:

1. All manure is removed from the rectum with a well-lubricated arm. Care is taken to avoid entry of air into the rectum during the manure-evacuation process because air effectively prevents transmittance of ultrasound waves into surrounding structures.
2. The internal genital organs are palpated in their entirety and in a systematic manner.
3. Palpation per rectum is followed by an ultrasonographic examination, with the transducer well shielded by the examiner's hand to avoid undue trauma to the wall of the rectum. A methodical approach should be used during the examination.
4. The transducer should be well lubricated and should have good contact with the rectal wall. Manure or air should not be interposed between the transducer and the tissue of interest.
5. If the mare resists excessively, the examination should be discontinued, or the mare should be sedated, given a tocolytic (e.g., Buscopan, Boehringer Ingelheim Pharmaceuticals, Ridgefield, Conn.), an infusion of intrarectal lidocaine, or epidural anesthetic, before continuing. If so treated, the mare's reproductive tract should be examined as soon as deemed prudent to prevent pneumorectum from developing as anal sphincter

relaxation occurs. Pneumorectum increases the risk of injury to the rectum during the examination and also interferes with transducer contact with the rectum, thereby reducing ultrasound image clarity.

For ultrasound examination of the mare reproductive tract per rectum, we prefer to advance the transducer over the cervix and body of the uterus until the bifurcation of the uterus is visualized (Figures 5-2 to 5-5). The transducer is slowly moved toward the tip of one uterine horn, with care taken to ensure the image of the uterine horn in cross section remains in the center of the monitor screen. As the transducer moves beyond the tip of the uterine horn, the ovary is scanned (Figure 5-6) in its entirety. The transducer is then moved slowly back down the uterine horn to the bifurcation, and the opposite uterine horn and ovary are scanned in a similar manner. After scanning the opposite ovary, the transducer is moved slowly back to the bifurcation and is rotated slightly in a back-and-forth motion across the uterine body and cervix as it is withdrawn from the rectum. This systematic scanning procedure ensures that the entire reproductive tract is examined twice, permitting accurate identification of the location of singleton or multiple pregnancies and uterine pathologic conditions, and provides confidence that no conceptus was overlooked during the examination process.

Transabdominal ultrasonography allows maximum visualization of the fetus and placenta, sometimes beginning as early as 60 to 80 days of gestation. Lower frequency (2.5 to 3.5 MHz) curvilinear transducers in various configurations are used for this

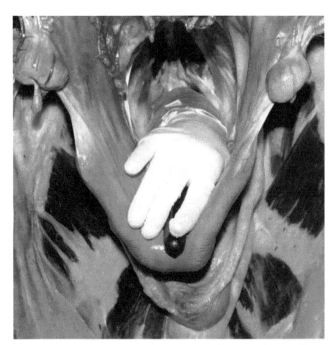

Figure 5-2 Examiner advancing the ultrasound transducer to the bifurcation of the uterus.

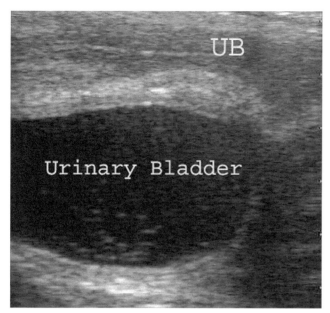

Figure 5-3   Transrectal ultrasound image of longitudinal section through the cervix and uterine body (UB) of a mare in diestrus. The white spectral reflection delineating the mucosal surface of the uterine lining is often visualized at this time.

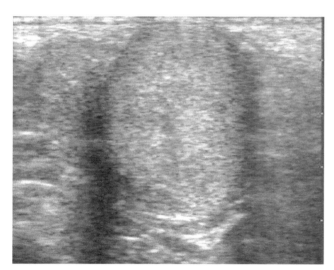

Figure 5-4   Transrectal ultrasound image of cross section through the base of a uterine horn.

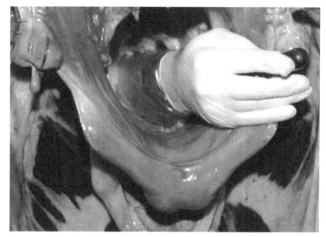

Figure 5-5   Examiner moving the ultrasound transducer to the tip of the uterine horn and ovary.

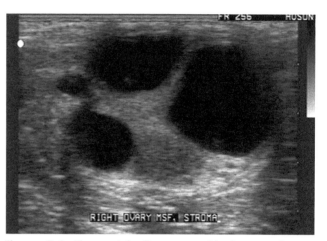

Figure 5-6   Transrectal ultrasonographic image of mare ovary containing anechoic (black) follicles.

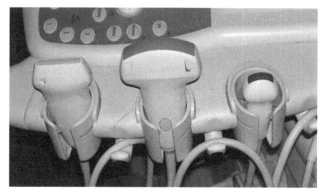

Figure 5-7   Three ultrasound probes available for transabdominal or transthoracic ultrasonographic examination. In general, lower frequency (2.5 to 3.5 MHz) curvilinear array probes are used for transcutaneous applications. A variety of size and configurations are available for different purposes. The low-frequency ultrasound waves emitted permit greater penetration into tissues, which is necessary to visualize structures deep within the abdomen.

purpose (Figure 5-7) and may allow assessment of the uterus in the inguinal area in some cases. In later gestation, maximal penetration into the ventral abdomen is necessary. Application of ultrasound gel or alcohol is helpful for improving contact between the transducer (ultrasound probe) and skin, allowing underlying structures to be more easily visualized. Because hair traps air, which interferes with sound wave propagation, it may be necessary to clip the hair closely, from the xiphoid-sternum to the udder, and on the lower flanks on either side of the midline, to improve transducer contact and thus image clarity.

For advanced pregnancy, the transducer is initially placed between the sternum and the mare's udder (Figure 5-8), followed by slow movement from side to side and cranial to caudal, until the fetus is located. Fluid within a viscus (especially the nongravid horn) is searched for to locate the uterus. Fetal structures (e.g., skull, foot, ribs) or membranes are often visualized, which aids in identification of the gravid uterus. Locating the fetal skull or thorax is helpful for orientation. Fetal heart rate, movement, amount and character of fluid (amniotic/allantoic), uteroplacental thickness, and evidence of separation between the uterus and placenta are typically evaluated by the examiner to determine normalcy (see Chapter 9). Examination for two fetuses is also possible if a question about twin status exists.

Per vagina ultrasonography has recently been used in horses for transvaginal aspiration of oocytes (follicular aspirations) and transvaginal aspiration or injection of the yolk sac or allantois of an early twin conceptus (see Figure 8-26). A common apparatus uses a stainless steel needle guide installed in an elongated plastic probe extension handle that accommodates a small curvilinear ultrasound probe in the tip (Figure 5-9). After sterilization and assembly, a 24-inch, 12- to 16-gauge, single- or double-port needle is inserted into the needle guide in the probe handle. The handle is used to insert the ultrasound probe into the cranial vagina; the operator uses the other hand in the rectum to position the structure of interest immediately next to the probe held in the vagina (Figure 5-10). Some ultrasound machines have software installed that delineates a dotted line on the ultrasound monitor and indicates where the needle will pass once inserted through the vaginal tissue. While the structure of interest (ovary with follicle, portion of uterine horn containing the twin conceptus) is held firmly against the ultrasound probe, the needle is

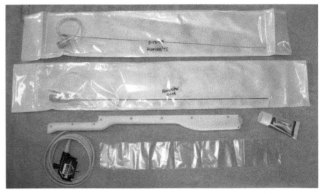

Figure 5-9 Handle and probe assembly used for transvaginal ultrasonographic applications. Autoclavable plastic handle is made to accommodate a small curvilinear 5.0-MHz probe and stainless steel needle guide. A 24-inch single-port needle, which is inserted through the needle guide, is shown.

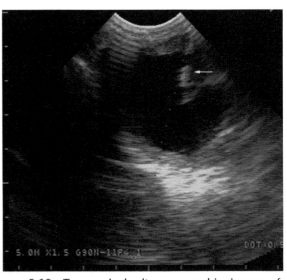

Figure 5-10 Transvaginal ultrasonographic image of an ovary positioned next to the intravaginal probe in preparation for aspiration of an oocyte from a follicle. The *dotted line* indicates the needle path for insertion. The *arrow* indicates echogenic needle tip.

forced through the cranial vagina, retroperitoneal fascia, and peritoneum into the structure of interest.

Diagnostic ultrasonography is used in the broodmare for (1) evaluation of ovarian activity, (2) detection and evaluation of pregnancy, and (3) diagnosis of pathologic changes in the reproductive tract. Although transrectal ultrasonography is emphasized in this chapter, transabdominal ultrasonographic images are shown in Chapter 9.

EXAMINATION OF THE OVARIES

The ovaries of the mare are easily visualized with transrectal ultrasonography. The connective-tissue stroma is uniformly echogenic (white). Follicles are fluid-filled

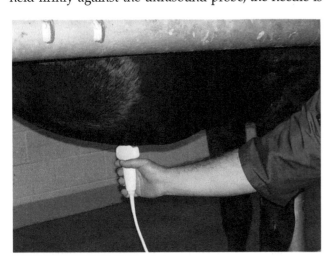

Figure 5-8 The examiner is performing a transabdominal ultrasonographic examination. The skin of the mare's abdomen was soaked with rubbing alcohol to improve contact with the ultrasound probe in preparation for the examination.

and, hence, represented as circular or irregularly shaped anechoic (black) images on the ultrasound monitor (see Figure 5-6). The ultrasonographic appearance of a corpus luteum is variable and ranges from a uniformly hyperechoic image (Figure 5-11) to a heterogeneous or mottled image, in which only a portion of the gland contains echogenic material (Figure 5-12). Because of the distinct border, many corpora lutea can be distinguished from the surrounding stroma throughout their life span.

Estimating the Stage of the Estrous Cycle by Ovarian Characteristics

Because of the ease with which follicles and corpora lutea can be detected with transrectal ultrasonography, this technique can be used to approximate the stage of the estrous cycle in mares. One can also distinguish those mares that exhibit reproductive cyclicity from those that are seasonally anestrous or are in transitional estrus.

The advent of high-quality real-time ultrasound imaging has permitted detailed study of follicular dynamics in mares throughout the estrous cycle. Mares tend to have either one or two follicular waves during the estrous cycle, with one follicular wave being the most common pattern. In either case, the ovulatory follicle becomes ultrasonically identifiable approximately 10 to 12 days before ovulation (see Chapter 2). Diestrous follicles (i.e., large follicles detected while a functional corpus luteum is present) sometimes become quite large (e.g., ≥35 mm in diameter), although the preovulatory follicle of estrus is generally the largest follicle of the estrous cycle.

Follicles destined to ovulate tend to grow rapidly (approximately 3 to 5 mm per day increase in mean diameter) beginning approximately 7 days before

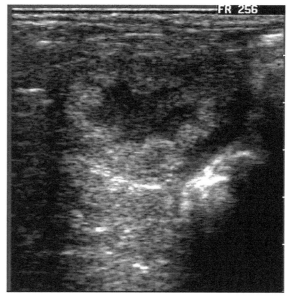

Figure 5-12 Ultrasonographic image of an atypical corpus luteum (2 days after ovulation) with hyperechoic periphery and mottled hypoechoic center.

ovulation, with corresponding atresia of other follicles within the same follicular wave. If a 5-MHz transducer is used for the examination, corpora lutea tend to be identifiable throughout their functional life span (generally about 13 to 14 days). Occasionally, the gland remains ultrasonically visible through the following ovulation. Unless a clear border is visible around the corpus luteum, differentiation between a corpus luteum (CL) and ovarian stroma may be difficult, as both are echogenic. "Mare-side" progesterone assays can be of help in such cases. If progesterone concentration in the blood is high (>2 ng/mL), a functional CL must be present. If progesterone concentration is low, the echogenic tissue in the ovary is more likely to be stroma or a regressed CL. When all of the ultrasonographic features of the ovarian structures are used in conjunction with echotexture of the uterus and palpable characteristics of the cervix, the stage of the estrous cycle can be predicted much more accurately than with palpation per rectum alone.

Ovarian inactivity (i.e., small ovaries with minimal or no follicular activity and no luteal structures) is typical of mares in seasonal **anestrus** (Figure 5-13). **Transitional estrus** has typically been characterized as protracted, sometimes irregular, estrous behavior with pronounced follicular activity (i.e., multiple follicles of varying size) in the absence of a detectable corpus luteum. However, English workers recently showed that as many as seven waves (average, three) of follicular growth with development of uterine edema can occur during transitional estrus before the first ovulation of the year finally occurs.

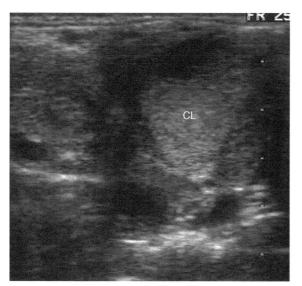

Figure 5-11 Ultrasonographic image of a mare ovary containing a hyperechoic corpus luteum (CL).

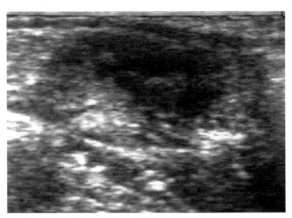

Figure 5-13 Ultrasonographic image of an anestrous ovary (typically 2 to 3 cm in diameter) containing few small follicles.

Prediction or Detection of Ovulation

With use of transrectal ultrasonography, the cross-sectional size and shape of follicles and the echogenicity of the follicular fluid can be used to aid in prediction of ovulation. The diameter of preovulatory follicles generally ranges from 40 to 50 mm. However, the size may be smaller, especially for double unilateral preovulatory follicles. Within 24 hours before ovulation, the shape of most, but not all, follicles tends to change from spherical to conical or pear shape, and the follicular wall may become "scalloped" or thickened in appearance (Figures 5-14 and 5-15). The apex of the conical follicle is located at the ovulation fossa. Occasionally,

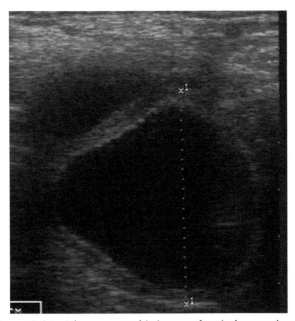

Figure 5-14 Ultrasonographic image of typical preovulatory follicle (within 1 day before ovulation). Note the thickened borders of the follicular wall, loss of round shape, and conical appearance near the center of the ovary (i.e., near the ovulation fossa).

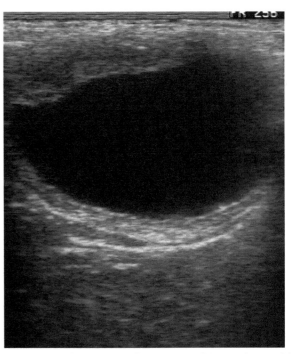

Figure 5-15 Ultrasonographic image of preovulatory follicle, 24 hours after administration of hCG to induce ovulation. The follicular borders are no longer round, and pronounced thickening of the ventral follicular wall (granulosa) is visible.

the echogenicity of the follicular fluid increases slightly just before ovulation.

Wisconsin workers recently performed frequent (up to hourly) ultrasonographic examinations of pre-ovulatory follicles until ovulation occurred. Characteristics they noted as typically occurring in the follicle before ovulation included serration of granulosa (irregular or notched appearance of the inner follicular wall); decreased turgidity (softening); loss of spherical shape; development of an apex, sometimes with a stigma (nipple); and appearance of hyperechoic spots within the antrum. They found that no single criterion approached 100% as a reliable predictor of impending ovulation when mares were examined at 12- to 24-hour intervals. The best single criterion for detecting impending ovulation was serration of the granulosa (present in 59% of ovulating follicles when the mare was examined twice daily). However, when hourly examinations were performed, serration of the granulosa and softening of the follicle occurred sometime between 1 and 8 hours immediately before ovulation in 100% of the ovulating follicles examined, and all but one of the criteria (development of hyperechoic spots, which occurred in only 50% of ovulating follicles) occurred in all follicles examined 1 hour before ovulation. Interestingly, although development of hyperechoic spots in the follicular antrum only occurred in 50% of ovulating follicles, when the spots did appear, the follicles ovulated within an hour or two. If mares were examined only once daily, the chance of detecting these criteria of impending ovulation was only about 1 in 3, which emphasizes the importance of use of all criteria available for predicting the best time to breed a mare.

At the time of ovulation, follicular fluid may be discharged either abruptly or gradually (i.e., within a 1-minute to 7-minute period). The echogenicity of the follicle changes from a predominantly anechoic appearance to a heterogeneous echotexture as the fluid is released, the blood clot organizes, and luteal development begins. The developing corpus luteum usually contains a small anechoic center that results from retained follicular fluid or blood or, alternatively, may retain variable echolucent areas within or surrounding the developing corpus luteum for several days. Infrequently, regressing follicles may collapse without subsequently forming a corpus luteum.

Ultrasonographic examination of a mare's ovaries during the periovulatory period ensures precise determination of the number, location, size, and shape of ovarian follicles. As opposed to palpation per rectum, ultrasonography can accurately detect multiple ovulations of adjacent follicles on a single ovary.

Diagnosis of Pathologic Conditions

Ultrasonography has been useful for diagnosis of various ovarian abnormalities.

Anovulation

Anovulation is considered a common and normal phenomenon during transitional estrus in the spring or fall; however, it occurs infrequently during the ovulatory season and is considered abnormal during that time. The cause of anovulation during the ovulatory season is not known. Although some anovulatory follicles simply seem to regress, they more commonly are considered to become hemorrhagic (i.e., **hemorrhagic follicle**) and are characterized ultrasonographically as large (sometimes 6-cm to 10-cm in diameter) hypoechoic follicular structures that gradually begin to show echogenic specks within the follicular antrum. They may have a highly echogenic rim, possibly associated with some luteinization of the follicular wall (Figure 5-16). Maximal size is usually reached during this apparent consolidation process. After the structure ceases growing, organization becomes apparent (sometimes with the appearance of fibrinous strands within the cavity; Figure 5-17), and the hemorrhagic follicle slowly decreases in size over a 3-week to 6-week period until it is no longer apparent.

Whether hemorrhagic follicles are more common in mares with normally appearing follicles that are treated with ovulation-inducing agents is unknown. In a discussion of these structures, Ginther (1992) suggested they may be associated with deficient estrogen production because uterine echotexture during the estrus in which they develop is often reduced or absent. He also stated that, in some instances, hemorrhagic follicles that

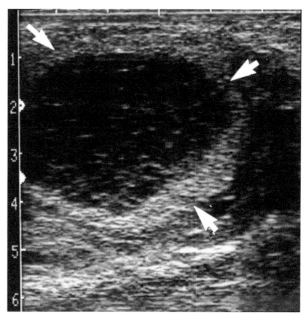

Figure 5-16 Ultrasonographic image of a hemorrhagic anovulatory follicle. Fluid in the follicle is slightly echogenic *(white speckling)* and the follicular wall *(arrows)* is greatly thickened.

occur during the breeding season are associated with prolonged interovulatory intervals and may be associated with low levels of progesterone production. Clinical experience suggests that once they have formed, they do not predictably respond to treatment with either human chorionic gonadotropin (hCG) or deslorelin by either ovulating or organizing into an ultrasonographically solid-appearing luteal structure. We have

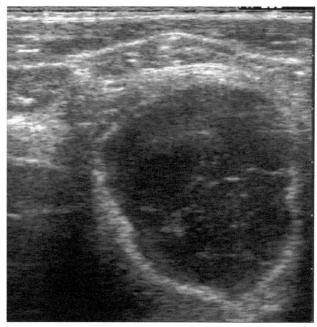

Figure 5-17 Ultrasonographic image of hemorrhagic follicle that has become more fibrinous in appearance.

also noted that in some mares that develop hemorrhagic follicles during the breeding season, the level of progesterone production while the structure is in the hyperechoic-flecked stage (as in Figure 5-16) is low, and simply administering prostaglandin-$F_2\alpha$ ($PGF_2\alpha$) after they develop is an unreliable method of inducing a return to estrus.

Colorado workers recently reviewed cases of hemorrhagic follicles that were detected in embryo transfer donors over several seasons. They found the rate of occurrence to be 4% to 8%, with a higher incidence in older mares. Return to estrus after development of a hemorrhagic follicle was delayed, with the interovulatory interval extended to 39 ± 15 days (sometimes exceeding 100 days). They also noted that mares with a hemorrhagic follicle tended to have an unpredictable, usually long, period of low progesterone secretion. However, once progesterone levels began to rise (>1 ng/mL), 70% of affected mares responded to injection of $PGF_2\alpha$ with return to estrus in 10 ± 6 days. Unfortunately, approximately one in three mares developed another hemorrhagic follicle on the next estrus. Further investigation of the cause is justified because the occurrence during the breeding season is frustrating to the practitioner, resulting in an unpredictable delay in the chance to get the mare rebred and pregnant.

Ovarian Hematoma

Ovulation tends to be a hemorrhagic event in the mare; hence, hematomas infrequently develop on the ovary, presumably at the time of ovulation (see Figure 4-4). Affected ovaries sometimes are quite large (e.g., 10 cm to 30 cm in diameter), although smaller hematomas are probably more common. When the ovary rapidly fills with blood and ovarian tissue becomes dwarfed in comparison, its ultrasonographic appearance is initially hypoechoic. As the blood clots, the echotexture first becomes fibrinous or honeycombed, and eventually mottled to heterogeneous in pattern (Figure 5-18). Regression of large ovarian hematomas occurs more slowly than that of anovulatory hemorrhagic follicles, sometimes requiring months for ovarian size and appearance to return to normal. However, mares almost invariably continue to have regular estrous cycles even though an ovarian hematoma is present.

The effects of ovarian hematomas on fertility are not well documented. Large ovarian hematomas tend to pull the uterus into a pendant position, which might interfere with sperm migration to the oviduct, or uterine motility (migration of the early conceptus) and thus maternal recognition of pregnancy, thereby causing embryonic death. Large ovarian hematomas might also occlude the ovulation fossa, resulting in interference with oocyte release or pick up by the associated fimbria, which results in failure of fertilization to occur. We have observed smaller ovarian hematomas (8 to 12 cm in diameter) in mares that became pregnant and

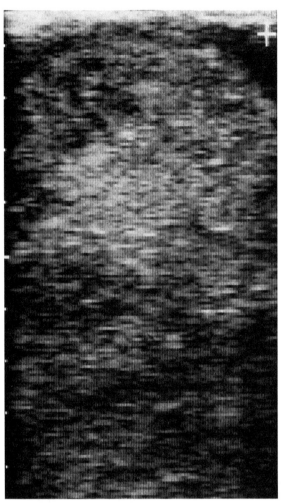

Figure 5-18 Ultrasonographic image of a large, well-organized ovarian hematoma. Hematomas typically appear with a mottled or spider web pattern. Corpora hemorrhagica and corpora lutea sometimes also have this ultrasonographic appearance, but they are not as large as ovarian hematomas and they become echogenic as a result of organization much sooner than ovarian hematomas.

maintained pregnancy to term. No treatment is generally necessary for ovarian hematomas. They should be differentiated from ovarian tumors, which usually do interfere with fertility.

Inactive Ovaries

Ovarian activity normally subsides as mares enter seasonal anestrus. Inactive ovaries are also observed in prepubertal fillies and sexually senescent mares during the breeding season. Ovarian inactivity of a pathologic nature primarily results from malnutrition or abnormalities that involve the sex chromosomes. Malnutrition leads to ovarian atrophy, whereas chromosomal abnormalities usually result in profound ovarian hypoplasia. Ovarian inactivity is characterized by small ($4 \times 3 \times 3$ cm or less) echodense stroma with few (very small) or no follicles visible with ultrasonographic imaging (Figure 5-19). Profound ovarian hypoplasia

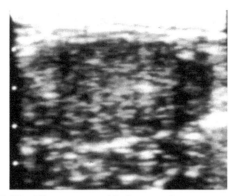

Figure 5-19 Ultrasonographic image of an anestrous ovary, devoid of developing follicles or corpora lutea.

(1 to 2 cm in diameter) from sex chromosome abnormalities can be confirmed with karyotyping studies. The most frequently identified sex chromosome abnormality associated with this condition is Turner's syndrome (63 X,O).

Ovarian Neoplasia

Ovarian neoplasia is rather common in mares, with granulosa-theca cell tumors (see Figure 4-3) and teratomas detected most frequently. The ultrasonographic appearance of granulosa cell tumors is quite variable, depending on structure and composition. They may be uniformly echogenic (if the tumor is solid), heterogeneous with a honeycomb appearance (if the tumor is multicystic) (Figures 5-20 and 5-21), or largely hypoechoic or anechoic (if the tumor consists primarily of a single fluid-filled cyst). Hypoechoic or anechoic granulosa cell tumors are usually quite large with a thick (up to 1 to 2 cm), echodense wall and are sometimes

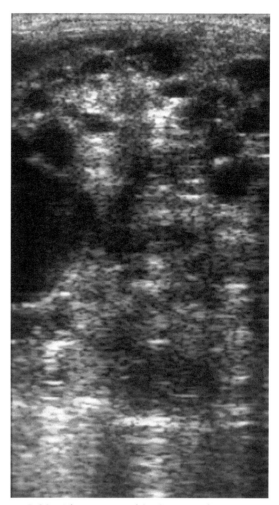

Figure 5-21 Ultrasonographic image of a more solid-appearing granulosa-theca cell tumor of a mare ovary.

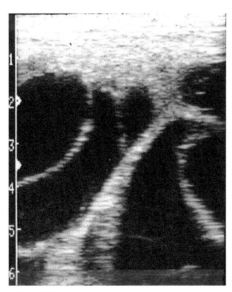

Figure 5-20 Ultrasonographic image of a multicystic granulosa-theca cell tumor of mare ovary that shows a honeycomb appearance. The tumor was too large to permit complete visualization with a 5-MHz probe.

stippled with echogenic material (probably clotted blood because the tumors are highly vascularized). Ultrasonographic characteristics are too inconsistent to enable definitive identification of granulosa cell tumors, but they may aid in narrowing the differential diagnosis when used in conjunction with other diagnostic measures (e.g., historical findings and evaluation of the contralateral ovary, which typically is atrophied and inactive; hormonal assay). The ultrasonographic characteristics of teratomas may mimic those of granulosa-thecal cell tumors, unless the tumor contains highly echogenic components such as cartilage, teeth, or bone (Figures 5-22 and 5-23). Demonstration of high inhibin or testosterone concentrations in hormonal assays from a mare with an enlarged, firm ovary and atrophy of the contralateral ovary confirms the diagnosis of granulosa-theca cell tumor. Although stallion-like behavior is the most demonstrable behavioral change associated with granulosa-theca cell tumors, note that many of these tumors do not secrete testosterone, and the most common behavioral change is anestrus from the suppressive effects of inhibin, which is elevated in most granulosa-theca cell tumors.

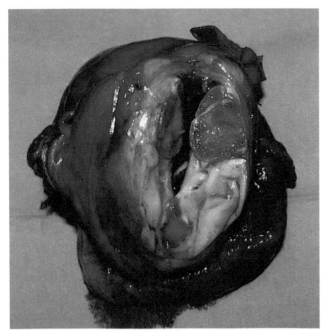

Figure 5-22 Ovarian teratoma of mare ovary. The tumor has been incised and fluid drained from the center of the ovary before photograph was taken. The mare had produced foals via both artificial insemination and embryo transfer but only when ovulating from the other ovary. Ultrasound examination demonstrated multicystic appearance with bright hyperechoic areas. Hair, cartilage, and bone were found within the ovarian stroma of the enlarged ovary.

Treatment of an ovarian tumor is surgical removal of the affected ovary. With secretory granulosa cell tumors, most, but not all, mares begin having regular estrous cycles during the next breeding season. Some mares need 2 years to begin having regular estrous cycles after surgical removal of a granulosa cell tumor; the rare mare never returns to ovarian cyclicity.

EVALUATION OF THE TUBULAR TRACT

Although the oviducts cannot be easily detected with a 5-MHz transrectal transducer, the remainder of the tubular tract can usually be imaged in its entirety. The exception is a uterus that is greatly enlarged as a result of (1) incomplete involution during the early postpartum period, (2) advanced pregnancy, or (3) pathologic conditions (e.g., pyometra, mucometra, large endometrial-lymphatic cysts, leiomyomas). In these instances, only a portion of the uterus can be viewed because of incomplete penetration of sound waves emanating from the transducer. With use of a linear-array transducer, the uterine horns are typically scanned in a transverse (cross-sectional) plane, and the uterine body and cervix are scanned in a longitudinal plane.

Estimating the Stage of the Estrous Cycle by Uterine Characteristics

Uterine echotexture can be used to differentiate diestrus (i.e., the luteal or progesterone-dominated phase of the estrous cycle) and estrus (i.e., the follicular or estrogen-dominated phase of the estrous cycle). The diestrous uterus is characterized by a relatively *homogeneous echotexture* (Figure 5-24). The uterine lumen and endometrial folds are less discernible during diestrus (approximately days 2 to 3 through days

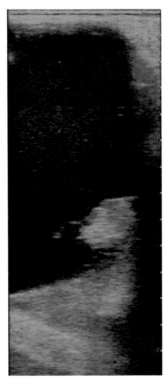

Figure 5-23 Ultrasonographic image of teratoma shown in Figure 5-22, before fluid was drained from the large central cystic cavity. Note the hyperechoic ventral areas suggestive of cartilaginous sheet or bone present within the tumor.

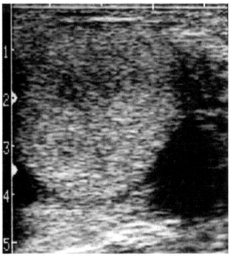

Figure 5-24 Ultrasound of cross section of a uterine horn of a mare in diestrus. The echotexture is homogeneous and nonedematous.

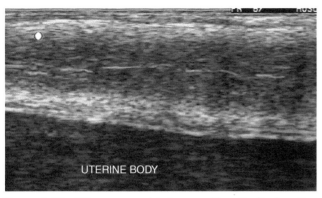

Figure 5-25 Ultrasonographic image of longitudinal section of uterine body of a mare in diestrus. The bright reflection *(white line)* evident along the center of the body identifies the endometrial surface.

14 to 16 after ovulation during the breeding season). A bright reflection (white line) often identifies the endometrial surface of the uterus viewed in longitudinal section during diestrus (Figure 5-25). During estrus, the endometrial folds become prominent and the uterus has a *heterogeneous appearance* (i.e., a mixture of hyperechoic and hypoechoic areas). This ultrasonographic pattern results from edema within the endometrium and, occasionally, free fluid within the uterine lumen. A characteristic "starfish" pattern may be evident in cross-sectional images of the uterine horns of mares in estrus (Figure 5-26). The degree of uterine heterogenicity (i.e., endometrial edema) tends to peak approximately 1 to 3 days before ovulation (when the appearance is that of a sliced tomato) and begins to decrease within a day preceding ovulation, and a homogeneous uterine echotexture typical of diestrus is restored within 1 to 3 days after ovulation. Endometrial edema scores are typically recorded as 0 (none),

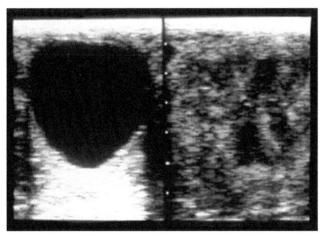

Figure 5-26 Ultrasonographic appearance of cross section of a uterine horn and an ovary containing a 45-mm diameter follicle of a mare in estrus. Note the edematous (hypoechoic) starfish-like appearance of the uterine horn cross-sectional image, which is the result of accumulation of fluid within the edematous endometrial folds.

1 (slight), 2 (moderate), and 3 (heavy). Changes from homogenous to heterogenous patterns (and vice versa) are more gradual during the fall months in mares that are still having regular estrous cycles.

The cervix of diestrus is well demarcated, hyperechoic, and contracted. During estrus, it becomes less distinct, relaxed, and loses some of its echogenicity. The cervical lumen is more likely to be visualized with ultrasound during estrus than during diestrus.

DIAGNOSIS AND EVALUATION OF PREGNANCY WITH TRANSRECTAL ULTRASONOGRAPHIC EXAMINATION

One of the first uses of diagnostic ultrasound in mares was early pregnancy detection. With a high-quality ultrasound unit equipped with a 5-MHz transrectal transducer, embryonic vesicles can be detected within the uterine lumen as early as 9 to 10 days after ovulation, when the vesicle is 3 to 4 mm in diameter and is found in the uterine body 60% of the time. Thereafter, an extensive mobility phase of the vesicle ensues, with the vesicle traversing the entire uterine lumen (both horns and body) several times per day.

Recent studies with color Doppler ultrasonography, performed by Wisconsin workers, revealed vascular perfusion increased in the uterine horn containing the migrating vesicle within 7 minutes after the vesicle entered that horn. The group also discovered an early endometrial vascular indicator of the future position of the embryo proper, which they described as a colored spot visible at the apposition of the endometrium and the wall of the embryonic pole, in the antimesometrial position (opposite from the mesometrial [broad ligament] attachment) (Figure 5-27). The spot was visible approximately 2 to 3 days before the embryo proper could be detected (which can be done 2 to 3 days earlier with color Doppler ultrasonography than with standard B-mode ultrasound (Figure 5-28) and was noted to become visible about ½ a day after fixation of the conceptus at the base of a uterine horn. With color Doppler ultrasonography, the embryonic heartbeat could also be detected as color flow signals within the embryo proper as early as day 22 of pregnancy.

With use of standard B-mode ultrasonography, the embryo proper is visible by days 20 to 21 after ovulation, and the heartbeat of the embryo is discernible ultrasonographically by days 24 to 26 after ovulation. The gender of the fetus can also sometimes be determined; the optimal time for gender determination is 60 to 70 days after ovulation. At this stage of gestation, the location of the *genital tubercle* can be used to aid in differentiating fetal gender. The genital tubercle is under the tail of the female fetus and just

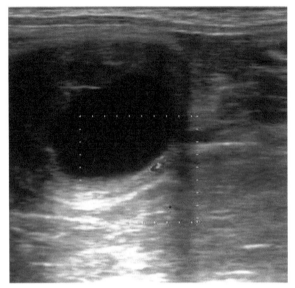

Figure 5-27 Color Doppler ultrasonographic image of early vascular indicator of the future position of the embryo proper. The colored spot within the endometrium close to the wall of the embryonic pole can be noted approximately ½ day after vesicle fixation at the flexure of a caudal segment (base) of the uterine horn and marks the site adjacent to where the embryo proper will eventually be situated within the embryonic vesicle.

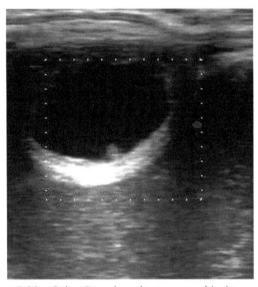

Figure 5-28 Color Doppler ultrasonographic image of a 22-day pregnancy showing color flow change (heartbeat) within the embryo proper. Note that the embryo is located opposite the encroaching (thickening) endometrium, which is thought to play a role in rotation of the embryonic vesicle so that final positioning of the embryo proper is ventral (opposite to the mesometrium, or antimesometrial).

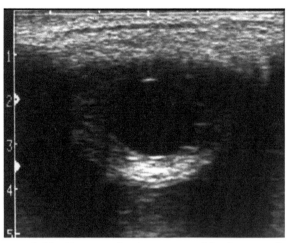

Figure 5-29 Transrectal ultrasonographic image of an equine pregnancy 12 days after ovulation. The pregnancy is located in a uterine horn in this case but can be located anywhere throughout the uterus during the prefixation stage, often being found in the body of the uterus.

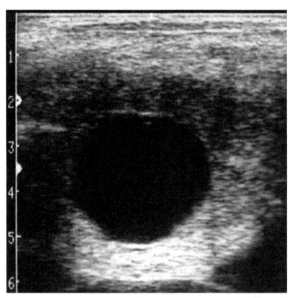

Figure 5-30 Transrectal ultrasonographic image of an equine pregnancy 16 days after ovulation. The pregnancy is located at the base of the uterine horn and is round.

behind the umbilical cord of the male fetus. Estimation of conceptus age during early pregnancy (i.e., days 10 to 50 after ovulation) can be made with the previous information in addition to:

▪ Size and shape of the embryonic vesicle (Figures 5-29 to 5-31).

▪ Location and fixation of the embryonic vesicle within the uterine lumen. The embryonic vesicle typically becomes fixed at the base of one uterine horn approximately 16 days after ovulation (see Figure 5-30).

▪ Percentage of the embryonic vesicle occupied by yolk versus allantoic fluid (e.g., the allantois occupies 25% of the vesicle at 25 to 26 days, 50% of the vesicle at 28 to 30 days, 75% of the vesicle at 34 to 36 days, and nearly 100% of the vesicle at 38 to 40 days; Figures 5-32 to 5-35).

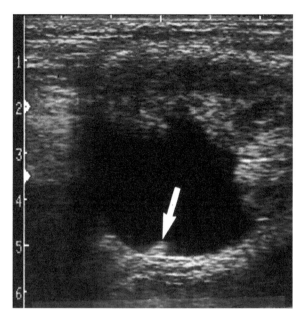

Figure 5-31 Transrectal ultrasonographic image of an equine pregnancy 21 days after ovulation. The pregnancy is located at the base of the uterine horn and is no longer round, gaining a triangular or guitar-pick shape from hypertrophy of the dorsal uterine wall. The embryo proper can be visualized at the base of this vesicle (arrow).

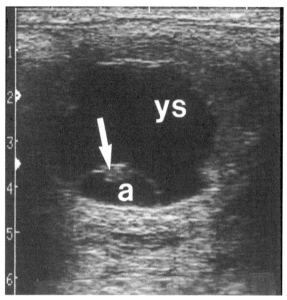

Figure 5-33 Transrectal ultrasonographic image of an equine pregnancy 26 days after ovulation. The embryo *(arrow)* and allantois *(a)* occupies the bottom portion of the vesicle, and the yolk sac *(ys)* occupies the top portion.

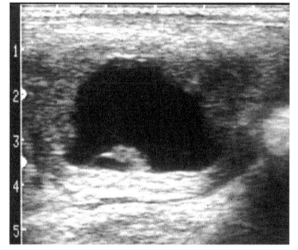

Figure 5-32 Transrectal ultrasonographic image of an equine pregnancy 22 days after ovulation. The embryo can be visualized at the bottom of the embryonic vesicle, and the allantois is beginning development.

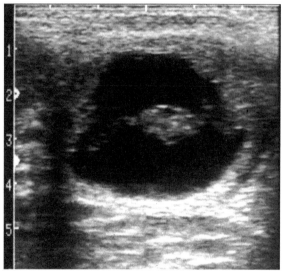

Figure 5-34 Transrectal ultrasonographic image of an equine pregnancy 28 days after ovulation. The embryo is positioned at the center of the vesicle, with the regressing yolk sac located above and the developing allantois located below.

- Location of the embryo (or fetus) within the vesicle (e.g., the embryo is located ventral in the vesicle at 21 days and rises to a dorsal position by 38 days, after which the membranes separating the yolk sac, dorsally and allantois, ventrally fuse to become the umbilical cord; the fetus then descends to a ventral position by 45 to 50 days; see Figures 5-32 to 5-37).

Current understanding of early pregnancy events in the mare (e.g., the role of conceptus mobility in maternal recognition of pregnancy, the incidence of twin pregnancy [both unicornual and bicornual], embryonic development, and natural mechanisms involved in twin elimination) has markedly improved as a result of transrectal ultrasonography. This new knowledge has led to advancements in breeding management and improved methods for manual reduction of twin pregnancies to singleton pregnancies. Better ways for assessing conceptus viability may now also be used.

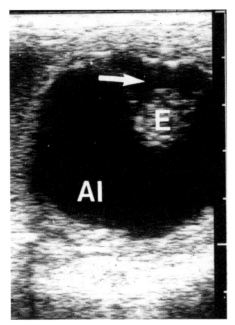

Figure 5-35 Transrectal ultrasonographic image of an equine pregnancy 36 days after ovulation. The embryo *(E)* is positioned near the top of the vesicle, and the yolk sac *(arrow)* is mostly resorbed. The allantois *(Al)* occupies the greatest portion of the vesicle at this time.

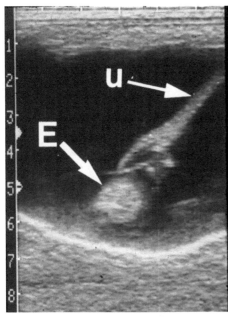

Figure 5-36 Transrectal ultrasonographic image of an equine pregnancy 47 days after ovulation. The embryo *(E)* is positioned near the bottom of the vesicle, and the umbilicus *(u)* is prominent.

DETERMINATION OF FETAL GENDER WITH TRANSRECTAL ULTRASONOGRAPHY

Transrectal ultrasonography has been increasingly used to determine fetal gender (fetal sexing) in the last 15 years. Considerable study and practice are needed to become proficient in this technique. The ability to

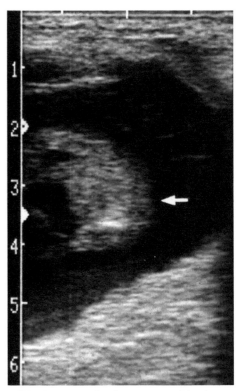

Figure 5-37 Transrectal ultrasonographic image of an equine pregnancy at 52 days after ovulation. A sagittal view of the fetus *(arrow)* can be visualized within the amnion. The head, neck, trunk, one forelimb, and two hind limbs can be seen.

determine fetal gender with this method is based on assessing the location of the **genital tubercle**, which is the embryonic structure that differentiates into either the **penis** (male) or **clitoris** (female). As differentiation progresses, associated structures (i.e., **prepuce** in the male, identifiable with gross inspection by day 77, and pendulous by day 115, of gestation; **vulvar lips** in the female, begin extending dorsally from the clitoris by 55 days gestation) develop sufficiently to lend additional echogenic patterns that aid in determining location of the genital tubercle. The location of the undifferentiated genital tubercle is between the hind limbs, midway between the anus and umbilicus. As fetal growth progresses, the genital tubercle becomes relatively closer to the umbilicus in males or anus in females. The ideal time for determining fetal gender with transrectal ultrasound has been determined to be between 60 and 70 days of gestation, when the genital tubercle location is sufficiently obvious to reduce the incidence of mistaken diagnoses (Figures 5-38 and 5-39). Determination of fetal gender is possible with transrectal ultrasonography beyond 70 days of gestation (Figure 5-40), but because of size and location of the enlarging pregnancy, proper imaging of the desired area of the fetus becomes increasingly difficult. However, other organs become sufficiently developed to aid in gender determination beyond 80 to 115 days of gestation (e.g., mammary buds, prepuce, and scrotum).

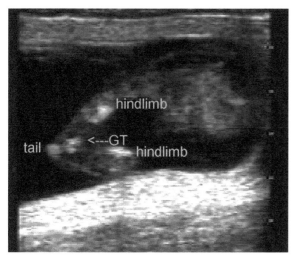

Figure 5-38 Transrectal ultrasonographic image of female 65-day-old filly fetus. The genital tubercle *(GT)* represents the clitoris and is located within the triangle formed by the coccygeal vertebrae of the tail and the long bones of the two hind limbs.

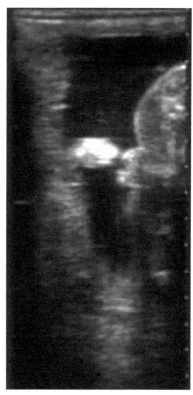

Figure 5-40 Transrectal ultrasonographic image of a female fetus 193 days after ovulation. The fetus lies on its side with the tail, labia, and buttocks visible *(from left to right)*.

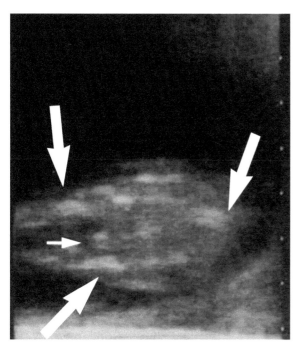

Figure 5-39 Transrectal ultrasonographic image of male fetus 65 days after breeding. The genital tubercle *(small arrow)* represents the prepuce/penis and is located between the hocks of the two hind limbs and the tail head *(large arrows)*.

DIAGNOSIS OF PATHOLOGIC UTERINE CONDITIONS WITH TRANSRECTAL ULTRASONOGRAPHY

Ultrasonography has been quite useful in the diagnosis of endometrial cysts and pathologic fluid accumulations within the uterine lumen. Other pathologic conditions (e.g., leiomyomas, abscesses, periuterine masses) may also be examined ultrasonically, but their prevalence is quite low.

Uterine Cysts

Uterine cysts that can be identified ultrasonically are generally of lymphatic origin and are more frequently located in the endometrium than other uterine layers. Lymphatic cysts range in size from microscopic to several centimeters in diameter, and cysts as small 2 to 5 mm can oftentimes be detected with a 5-MHz transducer. They can be unilocular or multilocular (Figures 5-41 and 5-42), with the larger cysts obviously protruding into the uterine lumen. The cysts are anechoic but can have hyperechoic trabeculae if they are multilocular. The prevalence rate of endometrial cysts in mares is fairly high (possibly ranging from 10% to 15% and up to 27%), with the cysts more common in mares older than 10 years. Although cysts may be located anywhere within the uterus, they may be predisposed to development in the ventral surfaces of the corpus cornual junctions.

The presence of endometrial cysts is important because (1) they can be mistaken for an embryonic vesicle during early pregnancy examinations; (2) they may increase pregnancy wastage, especially if sufficiently numerous or large enough to interfere with conceptus mobility (Figure 5-43) or placental-endometrial interaction; and (3) they are likely to represent evidence of an underlying problem such as lymphatic stasis. When an embryonic vesicle becomes fixed immediately adjacent to an endometrial cyst, orientation of the embryo may be altered from normal configuration (i.e., normally

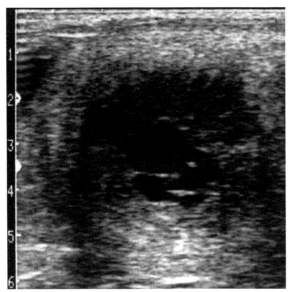

Figure 5-41 Ultrasonographic image of a multilocular uterine lymphatic cyst in the uterus of a mare.

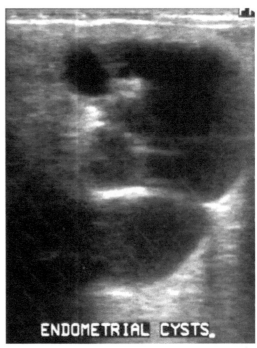

Figure 5-43 Ultrasonographic image of a large (5-cm diameter) uterine cyst at the base of a uterine horn in a mare. Such a large cyst may interfere with embryo mobility and result in failure to maintain pregnancy; it may also interfere with ability of the inseminate to reach the oviductal papillae or uterine flushing to remove an embryo.

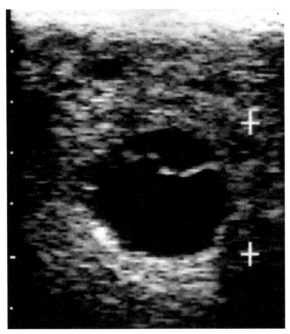

Figure 5-42 Ultrasonographic image of two-chambered lymphatic cyst in uterine horn of a mare. The structure mimics an equine pregnancy except that it is too small and an embryo proper is not present.

developing ventrally in the antimesometrial position), which may result in predisposition to early embryonic demise from reduction in contact of absorptive surfaces with normal glandular endometrial epithelium (i.e., endometrial cyst epithelium is devoid of endometrial glands).

Whether endometrial cysts have a depressant effect on fertility in the absence of other uterine pathology

remains controversial. Ginther (1986) suggested that single cysts and groups of small cysts do not adversely affect fertility. A subsequent Wisconsin study found a tendency for mares with more than 5 cysts or cysts larger than 1 cm in diameter to have lower 40-day pregnancy rates than mares with smaller or fewer cysts. Louisiana workers reported that in 215 Thoroughbred mares, number and size of cysts was unrelated to ability of mares to become pregnant or to maintain the pregnancy to term. We have certainly noted that some mares presented for examination because of failure either to become detectably pregnant or failure to maintain pregnancy have numerous endometrial cysts of varying size present without accompanying severe changes in endometrial biopsies that would otherwise account for pregnancy failure.

Until further research better characterizes potential adverse effects of endometrial cysts on fertility, we recommend that treatment of endometrial cysts is seldom necessary if (1) cysts are small (<2 to 3 cm in diameter) and infrequent (less than five located throughout the uterus) and they are not grouped together at the corpus-cornual junction, and (2) other potential causes of infertility have been eliminated. Although the relationship between lymphatic lacunae and endometrial cysts remains conjectural, if extensive pooling of lymphatic fluid in the endometrium is present (e.g., widespread, frequent medium to large lymphatic lacunae detected in endometrial biopsy samples), we believe the mare is a poor candidate for treatment (i.e., because cysts seem to be more likely to recur).

Uterine Intraluminal-Fluid Accumulations

A small amount of anechoic free fluid is sometimes detected within the uterine lumen of reproductively normal mares during estrus. It has generally been thought that if the fluid is of large volume (i.e., 1 to 3 cm or greater height of luminal distention) or echogenic character (Figures 5-44 and 5-45), it should be considered abnormal. However, even lesser accumulations of anechoic fluid during estrus, or particularly during the immediate postovulation period, could possibly adversely affect fertility. Wisconsin workers have shown that any free fluid within the uterine lumen during diestrus should be considered abnormal because it is associated with reduced pregnancy rates and increased embryonic losses. Such fluid accumulations are indicative of **endometritis** (perhaps identifying mares inefficient at mechanically evacuating the uterus; see Chapter 6) and should be treated accordingly. The degree of fluid echogenicity is related to the concentration of inflammatory cells and debris. Pyometra or mucometra can also be easily distinguished from advanced pregnancy with use of ultrasonography because of the lack of uniformly anechoic appearance and the failure to detect an embryo/fetus, umbilicus, or fetal membranes (Figure 5-46). The contents of the urinary bladder can sometimes be confused with uterine contents with use of transrectal ultrasonography, so distinguishing between the two organs is imperative when performing the examination (Figure 5-47).

Pneumouterus

Hyperechoic areas in the uterus may be an indication of pneumouterus (air in the uterus) (Figure 5-48). If the condition is unassociated with examination or treatment procedures that resulted in entry of air into the uterus, pneumovagina or cervical incompetency should be suspected. Treatment for pneumouterus from pneumovagina or cervical incompetency is surgical correction of the anatomic defect predisposing to the condition.

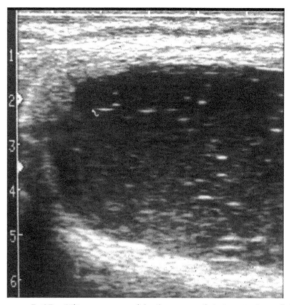

Figure 5-45 Ultrasonographic image of intrauterine fluid accumulation in a mare. Note the intermediate echogenicity of the fluid, suggesting the presence of inflammatory products and debris.

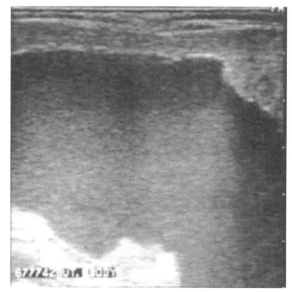

Figure 5-46 Ultrasonographic image of pyometra in a mare. Note the hyperechoic nature of the fluid. No fetus or fetal membranes were detected.

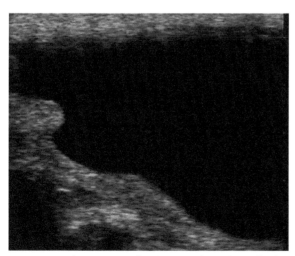

Figure 5-44 Ultrasonographic image of anechoic fluid present within the uterine lumen.

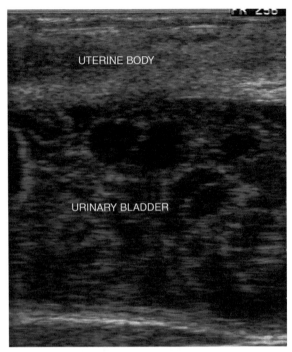

Figure 5-47 Contents of the urinary bladder can sometimes be confused with uterine contents during an ultrasonographic examination.

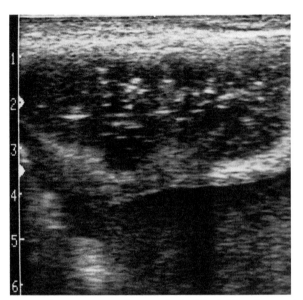

Figure 5-48 Numerous hyperechoic "flecks" in the uterine body can be indicative of pneumouterus (air within the uterus) and should be differentiated from pyometra.

BIBLIOGRAPHY

Adams GP, et al: Effect of uterine inflammation and ultrasonically-detected uterine pathology on fertility in the mare, *J Reprod Fertil* 35(Suppl):445-454, 1987.

Curran S, Ginther OJ: Ultrasonic diagnosis of equine fetal sex by location of the genital tubercle, *J Equine Vet Sci* 9:77-83, 1989.

Curran S: Fetal gender determination. In Rantanen NW, McKinnon AO, editor: *Equine diagnostic ultrasonography,* Baltimore, 1998, Williams & Wilkins, 165-169.

Eilts BE, et al: Prevalence of endometrial cysts and their effect on fertility, *Biol Reprod* 1(Mono):527-532, 1995.

Gastal EL, Gastal MO, Ginther OJ: Serrated granulosa and other discrete ultrasound indicators of impending ovulation in the mare, *J Equine Vet Sci* 26:67-73, 2005.

Ginther OJ: *Reproductive biology of the mare: basic and applied aspects,* ed 2, Cross Plains, WI, 1992, Equiservices, 173-230, 305-311, 392-396.

Ginther OJ: *Ultrasonic imaging and animal reproduction: color-Doppler ultrasonography,* Cross Plains, WI, 2007, Equiservices, 257.

Ginther OJ: *Ultrasonic imaging and reproductive events in the mare,* Cross Plains, WI, 1986, Equiservices, 370.

McGladdory A: Fetal ultrasonography. In, McKinnon AO, Voss JL, editors: *Equine reproduction,* Philadelphia, 1993, Lea & Febiger, 171-180.

McKinnon AO, Carnevale EM: Ultrasonography. In McKinnon AO, Voss JL, editors: *Equine reproduction,* Philadelphia, 1993, Lea & Febiger, 211-220.

McCue PM, Squires EL: Persistent anovulatory follicles in the mare, *Theriogenology* 58:541-543, 2002.

Silva LA, Gastal EL, Beg MA, et al: Changes in vascular perfusion of the endometrium in association with changes in location of the embryonic vesicle in mares, *Biol Reprod* 72:755-761, 2005.

Silva LA, Ginther OJ: An early vascular indicator of completed orientation of the embryo and the role of dorsal endometrial enchroachment in mares, *Biol Reprod* 74:337-343, 2006.

Endometritis

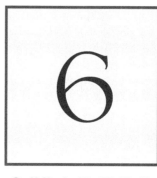

CHAPTER 6

OBJECTIVES

While studying the information covered in this chapter, the reader should:
- Acquire a working understanding of the mechanisms by which normal fertile mares are able to eliminate potentially pathogenic organisms from the genital tract.
- Understand the anatomic and physiologic deficiencies that contribute to establishment of uterine infections in the mare.
- Understand how persistent postmating endometritis differs from chronic infectious endometritis and identify methods used to reduce the incidence of embryonic loss associated with persistent postmating endometritis.
- Acquire a working understanding of rationales for selecting methods for treatment of genital infections in the mare.

STUDY QUESTIONS

1. Review the barriers to uterine infection in the mare.
2. Discuss potential roles for the following factors in eliminating microorganisms from the uterus of the mare:
   a. Immunoglobulins
   b. Neutrophil migration
   c. Opsonins
   d. Physical clearance mechanisms:
      (1) Secretions
      (2) Uterine tone and contractility
      (3) Lymphatic drainage
      (4) Transcervical drainage
3. Regarding mares considered susceptible to postmating endometritis, discuss how to recognize which mares might be affected and how to optimize management during estrus to enhance resolution of the postmating endometritis.
4. Regarding treatment of uterine infections in the mare, discuss the rationale for and procedures used in:
   a. Local antibiotic therapy
   b. Uterine lavage
   c. Administration of oxytocin or prostaglandins.
   d. Infusion of immunity enhancers (colostrum, plasma, or bacterial filtrates)
   e. Uterine curettage
   f. Hormonal therapy
5. List the most common locations for genital infections in the mare.
6. List the most common organisms associated with genital infections in the mare.
7. Discuss signs of and techniques for diagnosis of endometritis in the mare.
8. Discuss methods for prevention of genital infections in the mare.

TERMINOLOGY FOR GENITAL INFECTIONS

Most uterine infections in the mare involve only the endometrium (endometritis). Very few endometrial infections progress into deeper uterine tissues such as the myometrium (metritis). If infection progresses this deeply into the uterine wall, it can result in perimetritis and peritonitis and lead to septicemia and laminitis. The cervix can become involved (cervicitis), as can the vagina (vaginitis), usually as an extension of endometritis. Fortunately, infection of the oviducts (salpingitis) is rare because of the tight uterotubal junction in the mare. Even in the mare with a distended uterus from pyometra, the exudate rarely penetrates through the oviduct papilla to enter the oviduct.

ENDOMETRITIS

Endometritis has long been recognized as a major cause of reduced fertility in mares. Sources of uterine contamination that lead to development of endometritis include parturition, reproductive examination (even under strictly hygienic conditions), artificial insemination or natural mating, and self-contamination from conformational characteristics. Reproductively normal mares respond to uterine contamination with a transient inflammatory response that includes the activation of humoral or antibody-mediated defense mechanisms, recruitment of polymorphonuclear cells (PMNs) for bacterial phagocytosis, the release of prostaglandins, and increased uterine contractility to mechanically rid the uterus of luminal contents. These normal defense mechanisms render the reproductively normal mare resistant to persistent endometritis.

Mares that are not reproductively normal experience a breakdown in this natural defense mechanism and are considered to be susceptible to persistent endometritis. Some of the mechanisms proposed for development of persistent endometritis include insufficient opsonization of bacteria by PMNs within the uterine lumen and defective physical clearance of uterine contents. Defective physical clearance of uterine contents can result from dysfunctional uterine contractility, obstruction of physical clearance from failure of cervical relaxation, and conformational changes (e.g., pendulous uterus) that make physical removal of intrauterine contents more difficult. Persistent endometritis can be divided into two categories: persistent postmating endometritis and chronic infectious endometritis.

Persistent Postmating Endometritis

After mating or insemination, reproductively normal mares experience a transient inflammatory reaction within the uterus (in response to the presence of bacteria and sperm), which is quickly resolved (i.e., within 24 to 48 hours). This efficient clearance of the uterus after mating provides ample time for the intrauterine environment to return to normal, thus allowing for embryonic survival when the embryo enters the uterus 5 to 6 days after ovulation. In contrast, mares in which postmating endometritis fails to resolve within 48 to 72 hours are considered to have a persistent postmating endometritis. In a field fertility study that included more than 700 mare cycles, Zent et al. (1998) reported that 14% of Thoroughbred mares developed a persistent postmating endometritis. They noted that mares that accumulated a large amount of fluid after breeding tended to have lower pregnancy rates.

Management of Mares Susceptible to Persistent Postmating Endometritis

The key to enhancing fertility of mares susceptible to persistent postmating endometritis is to identify the mares before breeding and then to manage them in a manner to aid physical clearance of uterine contaminants during and immediately after the estrus of breeding. In general, mares susceptible to persistent postmating endometritis are pluriparous and older in age. However, older maiden mares may also be predisposed to this problem because of a tight cervix that fails to adequately relax during estrus, leading to retention of semen, bacteria, and inflammatory byproducts within the uterus. The result is a sustained inflammatory response that renders the environment incompatible with establishment of pregnancy.

Reproductively normal mares may accumulate a small volume of fluid within the uterus during estrus. Ultrasound examination of normal mares during estrus reveals evidence of edema within the endometrium with no fluid, or less than 1 to 2 cm in height of anechoic fluid within the lumen of the uterine horns or uterine body. One can often visualize the uterus contracting and moving fluid toward the cervix in such mares during transrectal ultrasonographic examination. In contrast, most mares that are susceptible to persistent postmating endometritis tend to accumulate larger than normal volumes of fluid within the uterus during estrus (>2 cm in luminal distention), and fluid may become hyperechoic in nature. These mares have been hypothesized to have deficient lymphatic drainage of endometrial edema, resulting in dramatic endometrial edema patterns when viewed using ultrasound. Poor uterine contractility not only impairs the lymphatic drainage but also results in failure of the uterus to evacuate contaminants. Note that uterine fluid during estrus is probably sterile unless the uterus has been contaminated. The contamination that results from breeding leads to infectious endometritis in the mare whose uterus fails to clear the bacterial contaminants. Texas workers have shown that the presence of estral uterine fluid more than 2 cm in height on ultrasound scans is a very good indicator of susceptibility to mating-induced endometritis, which allows practitioners to identify susceptible mares before breeding.

Prudent management of the mare susceptible to persistent postmating endometritis includes routine ultrasound examination during the estrus before insemination and treatment as needed with uterine ecbolics (i.e., oxytocin or prostaglandins) to stimulate uterine contractility and expel uterine contents. Uterine lavage before breeding may be indicated in those mares in which systemic treatment with ecbolics is unsuccessful in controlling intrauterine fluid accumulation. Lactated Ringer's solution has been shown to be a safe medium for uterine lavage immediately before breeding so long as most of the fluid is evacuated during the lavage procedure.

Minimizing uterine contamination and inflammation is also important. Problems encountered during breeding that contribute to increased contamination of the uterus include excessive trauma to the genital tract, improper hygiene during breeding, excessive breeding, and a large bacterial inoculant in the stallion ejaculate. Iatrogenic contamination during artificial insemination or during examination and treatment of the genital tract can also contribute to an overwhelming inoculum. A nonsterile reusable vaginal speculum used for vaginal or cervical examination is a common culprit. Insemination should be performed under strict hygienic conditions, and semen should first be mixed with a suitable extender that contains broad-spectrum antibiotics to control bacterial growth. Ideally, breeding should be done only once within 24 to 48 hours before ovulation. Mares that must be bred by natural service may benefit from infusion of 30 to 50 mL of prewarmed antibiotic-containing semen extender into the uterus immediately before mating.

Intrauterine infusion of antibiotics after breeding is a common practice in Thoroughbred mares. However, studies evaluating the efficacy of routine postbreeding antibiotic infusions are limited, and most of the published data indicate that either the practice is either of no benefit in improving pregnancy rates or that it can in fact be detrimental. Infusion of an antibiotic solution into the uterus of a mare may be counterproductive if the solution remains retained within the uterus.

Postbreeding uterine lavage as early as 4 hours after insemination/mating aids in removal of uterine contents yet apparently does not interfere with sperm colonization of the oviducts. Therefore, we believe the safest practice is for uterine lavage or infusion to be accompanied by the use of ecbolics to promote clearance of the fluid from the uterus.

Unfortunately, the ideal interval for ecbolic administration after the uterus is infused remains unstudied. The practitioner is faced with the knowledge that administration of an ecbolic too soon after infusion could result in expulsion of the antibiotic before it may exert its beneficial effects on resident bacteria. When endometrial concentrations of various antimicrobials infused into the uterine lumen of cows and mares were evaluated, results suggested relatively rapid penetration of the few drugs studied. Therefore, until further research is done, we offer the following recommendations:

1. If uterine lavage results in complete evacuation of uterine contents, antimicrobial infusion can immediately follow the lavage. If ecbolic administration is desired, the ecbolic can be administered 4 to 8 hours later. Hopefully, this allows sufficient time for beneficial effects of the antimicrobial drug to be exerted before being expelled from the uterus.

2. If uterine lavage is accompanied or followed immediately by ecbolic administration, sufficient time should be allowed for uterine contractility to diminish before the antimicrobial infusion. Because oxytocin administered intravenously commonly results in increased uterine contractility for 20 to 50 minutes, the antimicrobial infusion could be performed as soon as 1 hour after lavage and ecbolic administration. Because the prostaglandin analog cloprostenol has been reported to result in 2 to 4 hours of sustained uterine contractions, antimicrobial infusion should be delayed by at least this interval of time.

3. If oxytocin is administered intravenously immediately before uterine lavage and if uterine lavage requires 20 to 30 minutes to complete, the antimicrobial could be infused immediately after lavage when uterine contractility from oxytocin administration should be diminishing.

Mares susceptible to persistent endometritis should be reevaluated daily after breeding via transrectal ultrasound examination until ovulation is confirmed. Uterine lavage and treatment with ecbolics may be indicated daily (or perhaps twice daily) to rid the uterus of fluid. Oxytocin administration for ecbolic effects has been shown to be safe for 2 or perhaps 3 days after ovulation. However, research has shown that administration of prostaglandins during the early postovulatory period (0 to 3 days) lowers corpus luteum (CL) production of progesterone during the ensuing diestrus, albeit for only 6 to 7 days. Because this process may contribute to CL demise, thus causing early embryonic death, the use of prostaglandins for their ecbolic effect is not recommended after ovulation has occurred. The use of oxytocin and prostaglandins during estrus and after ovulation is further discussed later in this chapter.

Chronic Endometritis

Infectious agents are capable of causing disease if the mare has a defective uterine clearance mechanism or the reproductive system is overwhelmed by a large or repeated inoculum. A common underlying problem associated with genital infection in the mare is pneumovagina, which can lead to pneumouterus. The presence of these conditions implies aspiration of air and debris into the genital tract. When these conditions exist, one or more of the three physical barriers to contamination of the uterus has been disrupted: the vulvar seal, the vestibulovaginal sphincter, or the cervix. Continuing insult, coupled with the inability to overcome infection, results in chronic endometritis. Long-standing, more severe disease shows significant infiltration of the endometrium with lymphocytes and plasma cells, confirming the chronicity of the infection. Plasmacytic infiltration implies the continuing presence of antigen, and therefore, the prognosis is guarded.

Causes of Infectious Endometritis

Numerous agents of infectious endometritis in the mare have been identified and include bacteria (both aerobic and anaerobic), fungi, and yeasts. The role of mycoplasmas, chlamydiae, and viruses is thought to be relatively insignificant, but few studies have focused on identifying these organisms as the cause of genital infections in the mare.

Diagnosis of Endometritis

Treatment of genital infections in the mare should always be preceded by a proper diagnosis. Mares are sometimes treated empirically without first pursuing a diagnosis to justify treatment, and far too often, mares are treated based on a positive culture alone, even when no evidence of inflammation is found. To substantiate a diagnosis of endometritis, signs of inflammation (e.g., the presence of fluid in the uterus or genital discharges, particularly from the uterus) should be present. Endometritis is easily confirmed with uterine cytologic analysis or biopsy. Ideally, cytology should accompany every uterine culture. Recovery of the offending organism on culture and determination of its in vitro sensitivity to antimicrobial agents allow selection of a suitable drug for treatment. The earlier the diagnosis is made, the less likely significant damage to the endometrium will occur. For this reason, mares found to be barren during fall pregnancy rechecks should be examined and treated as soon as possible.

Criteria for genital infections are presented next, followed by guidelines for various diagnostic modalities.

External Signs of Infection
These signs are rarely seen with low-grade endometritis.
- Matting of tail hairs from chronic discharge may be present.
- Occasional exudate is seen at the ventral commissure of the vulva.
- Obvious exudate is seen at the vulva with an open cervix pyometra or metritis.

Findings on Examination per Rectum
- Fluid accumulation in the uterine lumen is indicated by an enlarged uterus. An echogenic character to the fluid often indicates the presence of purulent material. Extensive fluid accumulation in diestrus, even when it is anechoic, has also been correlated with endometritis. However, the presence of small amounts of anechoic intrauterine fluid during estrus has been documented even in the absence of endometritis. A small volume of anechoic intrauterine fluid during estrus (<2 cm of intraluminal distention) is often seen in reproductively normal mares. Excessive intrauterine fluid during estrus (>2 cm) suggests poor uterine clearance mechanisms and is associated with an increased susceptibility to persistent mating-induced endometritis.
- Massage of the uterus or vagina per rectum may express contents through a dilated cervix or vagina as vulvar discharge.
- A slight thickening of the uterine wall may be detected in some mares with acute endometritis, but poor tone of the uterus is not a reliable indicator of endometritis.

Findings on Vaginal Speculum Examination
Findings may include:
- Presence of inflammation indicated by reddening or increased vascularity.
- Presence of discharge through the cervix.
- Presence of urine pooled in the anterior vagina.
- Presence of debris (such as manure) in the anterior vagina.

Endometrial (Uterine) Swabbing for Culture
- Avoid contamination of the swab. Use a guarded culture instrument (i.e., a distal occlusion should be present on the swab container that prevents exposure of the swab until it is placed within the uterus), and properly clean the hindquarters of the mare. One can pass the culture instrument through a speculum to obtain a swabbing; however, with this technique, passing the instrument through the cervix of maiden mares or mares not in estrus may be difficult.
- Perform culture when appropriate. Culture is best done in early estrus when the cervix is relaxed and the uterus is more resistant to infection, but uterine swabs can be cultured during any stage of the cycle. However, the cervix must be dilated manually to swab the uterus during diestrus.
- Avoid interpretive error. Isolation of bacteria alone is not evidence of endometritis. Compare the results of the culture with the presence of signs of inflammation on cytology (or particularly on biopsy) to determine the significance of results. Even when guarded uterine culture swabs are used, disagreement between culture and cytology or biopsy findings is possible. This disagreement means that positive culture results can be obtained from mares without endometritis and negative culture results can be obtained from mares with endometritis.

Bacterial Endometritis

The following four organisms (listed in decreasing order of frequency) are responsible for most confirmed cases (80%) of endometritis in the mare:

- *Streptococcus zooepidemicus*
- *Escherichia coli* (also *Enterobacter* spp.)
- *Pseudomonas aeruginosa*
- *Klebsiella pneumoniae*

α-Hemolytic streptococci, *Staphylococcus* spp., and other bacteria may be recovered but are commonly regarded as contaminants unless accompanied by significant signs of inflammation.

Another organism less commonly linked to endometritis in the United States is *Taylorella equigenitalis*, a microaerophilic gram-negative coccobacillus believed to have originated in Thoroughbreds in France and Ireland. *T. equigenitalis* is the cause of contagious equine metritis (CEM). This organism is venereally transmitted to mares at breeding by stallions, which serve as lesionless carriers of the organism. Some mares develop a copious gray vaginal discharge within 2 to 10 days after breeding, whereas other mares may show no clinical signs except shortened diestrous periods. Some mares recover spontaneously; others remain chronic carriers. Codes of practice have been developed to control spread of this disease, which must be reported to federal authorities if discovered.

Yeast and Fungal Endometritis

Candida spp., *Aspergillus* spp., and *Mucor* spp. are the most common yeast and fungal organisms seen. These organisms are more likely to be detected in cytologic specimens than in biopsy preparations. Yeast and fungal infections are usually superficial, in which case they often readily respond to treatment; however, they may also result in chronic deep endometritis that responds poorly to treatment. Some mares with chronic yeast infections have copious fluid accumulations with a thin mucus-like discharge.

Endometrial Cytologic Analysis

Endometrial cytologic analysis, although it does not provide as definitive a diagnosis of endometritis as that obtained with biopsy, does provide an immediate indicator of acute endometrial inflammation. A suitable sample for cytologic analysis can be obtained from uterine swabbing or with various custom-made cell accumulation devices. Guarded instruments must be used for collection of samples to ensure that inflammatory cells collected are from the uterus (endometrium). A uterine flushing can also be obtained for culture, and following centrifugation, cells are harvested for the cytologic specimen. LeBlanc et al. (2007) reported that low-volume flush with 60 mL of saline solution was more sensitive in detecting chronic endometritis from *E. coli* than was the use of a uterine swab.

Usually the prepared slide is air dried, fixed, and stained. Diff-Quik (Fisher Scientific, Pittsburgh, PA) is a commonly used stain for air-dried specimens. New methylene blue is a commonly used stain for cover-slipped wet mounts. The slide is observed under a microscope for the presence and condition of epithelial cells, bacteria, yeast or fungi, and inflammatory cells. The presence of a significant number of neutrophils, which may be degenerate and may contain phagocytized bacteria or yeast, indicates an acute inflammation (see Chapter 4 for more detailed information).

Endometrial Biopsy

An endometrial biopsy sample is obtained with a stainless steel uterine biopsy punch. The biopsy sample can provide information on various types of endometrial pathologic conditions, including acute or chronic endometritis. Biopsy is considered to be the definitive test for endometritis. In some cases, special stains can be used to identify the types of pathologic organisms involved. Proper interpretation of the endometrial biopsy findings enables the practitioner to suggest types of treatment that may be beneficial in an individual mare (see Chapter 4 for more detailed information).

TREATMENT OF GENITAL INFECTIONS

For successful treatment of genital infections, any underlying problems that contribute to reinfection must be eliminated. Problems that necessitate surgical correction include pneumovagina, urovagina, cervical lacerations, perineal lacerations, and rectovaginal fistulas. Retained placenta or delayed uterine involution should be treated early in the postpartum period to overcome uterine contamination. Finally, poor management practices, such as unhygienic breeding or examination, or excessive breeding, should be corrected to minimize contamination of the genital tract.

The organism that is causing the infection must be identified and eliminated. A number of techniques are commonly used by veterinarians to eliminate uterine infections, including the following.

Uterine Lavage

Uterine lavage is an important therapeutic tool for treatment of uterine infections. Reasons for uterine lavage include (1) removal of microbes, nonfunctional neutrophils, and other substances (e.g., proteolytic enzymes) that are likely to interfere with the function of potentially useful neutrophils or antibiotics; (2) stimulation of uterine contractility to aid in the physical clearance of uterine contents; and (3) recruitment of fresh neutrophils and possibly opsonins (through mechanical irritation of the endometrium) to combat infectious agents.

Typically, the uterus is lavaged with gravity-driven instillation and removal of 1 to 2 L of warmed (42°C to 45°C) solution through a large-bore (e.g., 8 mm inside diameter) catheter with a balloon cuff to facilitate retention in the uterus (the balloon is distended with air after passage beyond the cervix) (Figures 6-1 to 6-3).

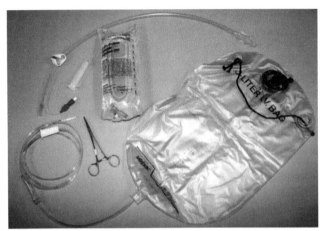

Figure 6-1 Equipment used to perform uterine lavage. A modified Foley catheter with balloon cuff, a syringe for filling the cuff with air, lavage fluid, a lavage bag to contain fluid with attached tubing and connector, and forceps for controlling the flow of fluid through the catheter are shown.

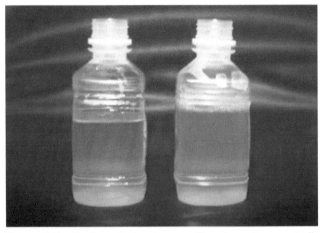

Figure 6-3 During uterine lavage, the uterus is repeatedly filled with 250 mL to 1 L of sterile saline solution and drained. Lavage is generally continued until resulting effluent is clear. The bottle on the *left* contains the initial cloudy effluent obtained from a mare with subacute endometritis. The bottle on the *right* contains clear effluent obtained at the end of the lavage procedure.

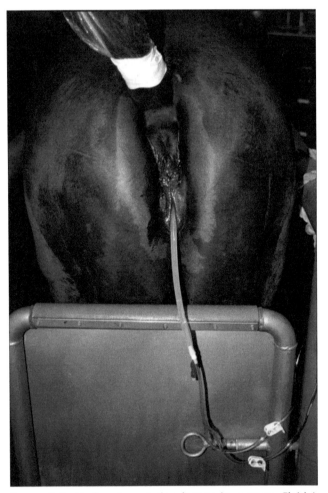

Figure 6-2 Performing uterine lavage in a mare. Fluid is instilled into the uterus by gravity flow; return effluent is caught for examination of character.

Older pluriparous mares may need larger volumes to fully distend the uterus. The procedure is oftentimes combined with uterine massage per rectum to further stimulate uterine contraction and more thoroughly distribute the solution within the uterine lumen. This process is generally repeated sequentially until the effluent is clear or nonturbid and should be performed for several consecutive days until the effluent of the first flush of the day is normal in appearance.

Isotonic saline solution or other balanced salt solutions such as lactated Ringer's solution is generally preferred for uterine lavage. Dilute povidone-iodine solutions can also been used. A suitable lavage solution can be made by mixing 10 mL of Betadine Veterinary (5% povidone-iodine, Purdue Pharma, Stamford, Conn.) or 5 mL of Betadine (10% povidone-iodine) solution in 1 L of sterile saline or lactated Ringer's solution. Studies involving other species (e.g., human, rat, dog, or rabbit) indicate a dose-dependent inhibition of neutrophil migration in vitro at povidone-iodine concentrations greater than 0.05%. Work specific to the horse revealed no depressive effect of povidone-iodine on directional or random migration of neutrophils in vitro at concentrations of 0.02% or less but a complete inhibition of neutrophil motility at povidone-iodine concentrations of 0.2% or more. Differences noted in neutrophil sensitivity between the two investigations may have been the result of greater resistance of horse neutrophils to damage or simply of differences in experimental design (e.g., methods of in vitro motility analysis). An interesting observation is that normal cellular morphology of horse neutrophils was maintained at higher povidone-iodine concentrations than those observed in other species, suggesting enhanced resistance of horse neutrophils to the cytotoxic effects of povidone-iodine

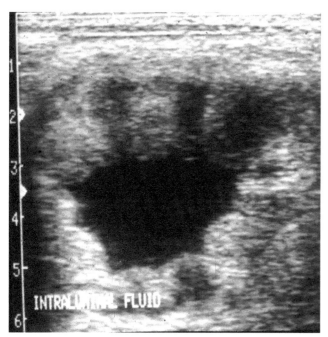

Figure 6-4 Ultrasonographic image of intrauterine fluid accumulation in a mare.

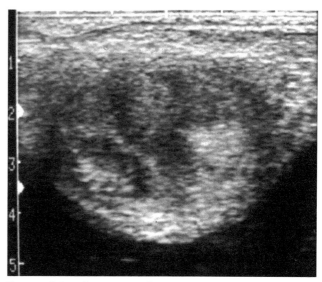

Figure 6-5 Ultrasonographic image of the uterine horn shown in Figure 6-4 30 minutes after intravenous administration of 20 units of oxytocin. Fluid retention was not ultrasonographically detectable anywhere within the uterus at this time, indicating that evacuation of fluid from the uterus had been achieved.

solution. Because the inhibition of neutrophil motility was associated with detectable cytotoxic effects (i.e., cellular pyknosis and lysis), it is probable that phagocytic activity is rendered nonfunctional at similar povidone-iodine concentrations.

Administration of Ecbolics

Because some mares susceptible to endometritis have been found to be unable to physically expel uterine contents through the cervix and to have impaired lymphatic drainage from the uterus, administration of uterine ecbolics (stimulate myometrial contraction) such as oxytocin (with or without concurrent uterine lavage) has been proposed as an adjunctive treatment for endometritis (Figures 6-4 and 6-5). Oxytocin (20 units intravenously, or 20 to 40 units intramuscularly) is the most commonly used uterine ecbolic in equine practice, and it is often combined with uterine lavage to treat endometritis. Whether administration of oxytocin via the intramuscular route is superior to intravenous administration is not known, but intramuscular administration has been shown to prolong the duration of uterine contractions in other species. Some practitioners administer oxytocin several times on a given day. Information on the ability of the equine uterus to respond repeatedly to routinely administered doses of oxytocin or the importance of the dose of oxytocin used to the type of uterine contractions generated (i.e., spasmodic versus peristaltic) is lacking. However, Florida workers have suggested that administration of more than 20 units of oxytocin intravenously or administration more often than once every 4 to 6 hours induces spasmodic uterine contractions that are likely to be unproductive in eliminating uterine fluid. Treatment

with oxytocin should be repeated for 1 to 2 days if uterine lavage effluent remains cloudy or intrauterine fluid accumulation remains evident on ultrasound examination. Texas workers showed that once-daily injection of oxytocin (20 units intravenously) during estrus had no detrimental effect on fertility, provided that treatment was postponed until 4 hours after breeding on the same day that a mare was bred. Oxytocin treatment near the time of breeding is currently discouraged because it has been shown recently by Texas workers to potentially decrease fertility, perhaps because semen is expelled from the uterus before adequate numbers of sperm access the oviduct. Treatment more than 2 to 3 days after ovulation is also generally discouraged.

Intramuscular administration of 250 μg of cloprostenol (Estrumate, Intervet/Shering-Plough Animal Health, Whitehouse Station, N.J.), a prostaglandin analog, has been advocated by Florida workers to aid in evacuation of uterine contents in mares being treated for endometritis. The analog results in a longer duration of induced uterine contractions (2 to 4 hours) compared with oxytocin administration (30 minutes to 1 hour). Cloprostenol (or prostaglandin-$F_2\alpha$) should not be administered to mares after ovulation has occurred. Several studies have shown that administration of prostaglandins on the day of ovulation or 1 to 2 days after ovulation lowered serum progesterone concentrations during the ensuing diestrus. Pregnancy rates were 50% lower in the mares receiving prostaglandin on the day of and 1 day after ovulation than in mares receiving oxytocin or saline solution control. If intrauterine uterine fluid continues to accumulate in the postovulatory period, uterine lavage or oxytocin administration is the preferred treatment. Cloprostenol is not approved for use in horses in the United States, but it is in some other countries. Side effects are reportedly minimal, although we have noted sweating and abdominal cramping (colic) in some mares after treatment with this product; these effects appear to be dose-dependent.

Antimicrobial Therapy

Some commonly used antimicrobial drugs and dosages for treatment of uterine infection in mares are provided in Table 6-1. The antibiotic chosen should be selected based on the susceptibility pattern obtained from culture. Distribution patterns of several antibiotics in reproductive tissues of the mare have been studied after intrauterine infusion. With standard infusion doses, endometrial and uterine lumen levels of most antibiotics (penicillin, ampicillin, chloramphenicol, gentamicin, amikacin, etc) remain at or above bacteriostatic/bacteriocidal concentrations for at least 24 hours. In contrast, higher doses and administration more often (two to four times daily) is usually necessary to achieve the same levels in the endometrium and uterine lumen after systemic administration of these same antibiotics. Therefore, most veterinary practitioners prefer to administer antibiotics with once-daily intrauterine infusion. In general, we recommend once-daily infusion for 3 days for treatment of slight endometritis (as judged from endometrial biopsy), for 5 days for treatment of moderate endometritis, and for 7 days for treatment of severe endometritis. To enhance efficacy, particularly if aminoglycosides are used, uterine lavage to remove organic material and particulate matter should be done before infusion. This procedure is thought to help avoid inactivation of the antibiotic infused.

Some antibiotics have a very acidic or alkalotic pH, which can be quite irritating to the endometrium if they are not buffered to a more neutral pH before infusion. Gentamicin and amikacin have an acidic pH, but when buffered with sodium bicarbonate, they can be infused with minimal irritation to the endometrium. In contrast, enrofloxacin has a basic pH. Unfortunately, when buffered to a more neutral pH, enrofloxacin has been reported to be less effective for bacterial killing, and infusion of unbuffered enrofloxacin may be very irritating to the genital tract. If the susceptibility patterns of bacterial infection suggest the use of enrofloxacin, systemic treatment is recommended. Pennsylvania workers found oral administration of 5 mg/kg enrofloxacin twice daily resulted in endometrial levels of enrofloxacin that were above the minimum inhibitory concentration of many bacteria that can cause endometritis.

One consideration for antibiotic selection is the antibiotic-neutrophil interaction in microbial killing. Some antibiotics (e.g., polymyxin B, tetracycline) are readily capable of penetrating phagocytes and thus may cause enhanced intracellular killing of microbes. Other antibiotics (e.g., penicillins, streptomycin, and gentamicin) pass into phagocytes only with difficulty.

Once intracellular access is attained, these antibiotics may augment bacterial killing. However, ingested bacteria can also be protected from the action of extracellular antibiotics, allowing some bacteria to actually continue multiplication within neutrophils.

Many studies have been conducted to evaluate the effect of various antibiotics on specific aspects of neutrophil function (e.g., chemotaxis, phagocytic activity, oxidative metabolism). Several antibiotics have been incriminated as damaging to neutrophil chemotaxis (e.g., tetracyclines, gentamicin, or amikacin), phagocytosis (e.g., tetracyclines or polymyxin B) or oxidative metabolism (e.g., tetracyclines or polymyxin B) in other species. However, conflicting reports make data interpretation difficult. One investigation specific to the horse revealed that gentamicin or amikacin significantly reduced in vitro phagocytic activity of neutrophils, whereas phagocytosis was unchanged in the presence of penicillin or ticarcillin.

During the breeding season, many mares are treated concurrently during the same estrus cycle in which they are bred. Such treatments most commonly involve intrauterine infusion of antibiotic (with or without prior uterine lavage) either early in the estrus cycle before breeding or late in the estrus cycle after breeding, often after ovulation is confirmed. Infusion of antimicrobials on the day of breeding (i.e., before breeding) should probably not be done because many antimicrobials have spermicidal properties when present in high concentrations. In some instances, practitioners lavage or infuse the uterus after a mare is bred. It is critical that any intrauterine treatment not be done less than 4 hours after breeding so that oviductal colonization with sperm is not disturbed. In addition, we do not recommend intrauterine treatment for more than 2 to 3 days after ovulation because of concerns of causing sufficient endogenous prostaglandin release to impair corpus luteum function.

Intrauterine Infusion of Disinfectant

Although intrauterine infusion of disinfectants is widely practiced, precautions should be taken when a disinfectant is chosen and used. Some disinfectants are quite irritating to tissues, including Lugol's iodine and chlorhexidine, particularly when they are not sufficiently diluted. Severe irritation from inadequate dilution has resulted, in some cases, in the formation of transluminal adhesions of the tubular tract. Intrauterine deposition of disinfectants has also been shown to kill neutrophils, possibly interfering with an important cellular immune defense mechanism.

Infusion of 500 mL of a 0.2% povidone-iodine solution induces a marked inflammatory response by the endometrium, which generally subsides within 7 days after treatment. This povidone-iodine concentration has been used successfully as a uterine treatment in mares with endometritis, when infused during the estrus before the cycle in which the mare is bred. Higher iodine concentrations are generally not recommended.

TABLE 6-1

Guidelines for the Administration of Some Commonly Used Intrauterine Drugs

Drug	Dose	Comments
Penicillin (Na⁺ or K⁺ salt)	5 million U	Very effective for streptococci; economical and commonly used.
Gentamicin sulfate	500-1000 mg	Highly effective; generally nonirritating when mixed with an equal volume of $NaHCO_3$ and diluted in saline solution.
Ticarcillin	1-3 g	Use for *Pseudomonas*; do not use for *Klebsiella*.
Timentin	3-6 g	Broad-spectrum activity against many gram-positive and gram-negative bacteria; contains ticarcillin and clavulanic acid to protect ticarcillin against degradation by β-lactamase enzyme–producing bacteria.
Amikacin sulfate	1-2 g	Use for *Pseudomonas*, *Klebsiella*, and persistent gram-negative organisms; mixed with equal volume of $NaHCO_3$ and diluted in saline solution.
Ceftiofur sodium	1 g	Third-generation cephalosporin; has been used empirically once daily either intramuscularly or via intrauterine infusion; broad-spectrum effectiveness against gram-positive and gram-negative bacteria.
Cefazolin sodium	1 g	First-generation cephalosporin; has been used empirically once daily intramuscularly for 2 to 3 weeks; broad-spectrum effectiveness against gram-positive and gram-negative bacteria.
Kanamycin sulfate	1 g	Toxic to sperm. Do not use close to breeding.
Polymyxin B	1 million U	Use for gram-negative bacteria, particularly *Pseudomonas*.
Neomycin sulfate	3-4 g	Use for sensitive *E. coli*; can be irritating; routine postbreeding use of oral preparations containing neomycin mixed with other antimicrobials has lowered pregnancy rates in mares.
Chloramphenicol	2-3 g	Can be very irritating, especially in the oral form.
Nitrofurazones	50-60 mL	Effectiveness is highly questionable.
Povidone-iodine	5 mL of stock Betadine solution/L of lavage solution	If solutions are too concentrated, severe endometritis may result or neutrophil function may be impaired. In vitro bactericidal activity is maintained at concentrations as low as 0.01% to 0.005%; indicated for lavage of uteri with nonspecific inflammation or fungal/yeast infections.
Nystatin	500,000 U	Used primarily for yeast (e.g., *Candida albicans*) in the growing phase; dilute in 100 to 250 mL sterile water; makes an insoluble suspension that must be vigorously mixed immediately before infusion.
Amphotericin B	200 mg	Used for infections with *Aspergillus*, *Candida*, *Histoplasma*, or *Mucor*; dilute in 100 to 250 mL sterile water; makes a relatively insoluble suspension.
Clotrimazole	700 mg	Used for yeast infections *(Candida* spp.); available as cream, tablets, or suppositories; preferable treatment is with tablets crushed and mixed with 40 mL sterile water; generally infused after uterine lavage.
Miconazole	200 mg	Is most efficacious for yeast infections *(Candida* spp.) but has been used by some practitioners for resistant fungal infections in mares by infusing once daily for up to 10 days; dilute in 40 to 60 mL sterile saline solution before infusion.
Fluconazole	100 mg	Synthetic triazole antifungal agent; proposed as infusion for treatment of fungal or *Candida* endometritis once daily for 5 to 10 days; adjust pH to 7 if necessary, as pH varies from 4 to 8.
Vinegar	2% (v/v) 20 mL/L of saline solution	Used empirically as an adjunct for treating yeast endometritis; 1-L uterine lavage; efficacy not critically tested.

Continued

TABLE 6-1

Guidelines for the Administration of Some Commonly Used Intrauterine Drugs—cont'd

Drug	Dose	Comments
Dimethyl sulfoxide	Dilute to 5% of stock solution; infuse 50-100 mL	Used as penetrating agent to carry drugs; effectiveness and safety unknown.
EDTA-Tris	1.2 g NaEDTA + 6.05 g Tris/L of H_2O; 250 mL	Titrate to pH 8.0 with glacial acetic acid. Infuse antibiotic 3 hours later. EDTA theoretically binds Ca^{2+} in bacterial cell walls, making cell wall permeable and thus more susceptible to antibiotic; use confined to persistent gram–negative infections such as from *Pseudomonas*.
Mannose	50 g/L of saline solution	In vitro study showed that mannose decreased adhesion of *E. coli*, *P. aeruginosa, and S. zooepidemicus* to equine endometrial cells in culture; proposed as a therapy in uterine lavage; bacteria bind to the sugar and are removed in lavage effluent; not critically tested in naturally infected mares.

Because no controlled studies have shown superior efficacy of disinfectants over antibiotics or antifungal agents when instilled into the uterus, we tend to avoid their use except in certain instances. For example, when lavage of the postpartum uterus must be performed in a field setting where large volumes of sterile solution are not available, a tamed iodine solution (such as povidone-iodine) can be prepared by mixing 30 to 40 mL of Betadine Veterinary solution with 1 gal of clean warm tap water to which 34 g of NaCl is added. Similar dilutions of "tamed" iodine solutions (mixed in sterile saline solution) are also sometimes used to treat yeast or fungal infections of the uterus of the mare.

Intrauterine Infusion of Plasma

Intrauterine plasma infusion, combined with uterine lavage, is one approach for treatment of chronic infectious endometritis because of the neutrophil-enhancing properties of serum and the reported success of this treatment combination. Only heparin or citrate should be used as an anticoagulant during the plasma collection process because ethylenediamine tetraacetic acid (EDTA) inactivates complement, the principal opsonin in serum. Autologous plasma is often recommended for intrauterine infusions because transmission of infectious agents or immunologic incompatibilities is possible when heterologous plasma is used. However, use of heterologous plasma is commonplace. The plasma is generally infused in 50-mL to 100-mL aliquots once daily for 4 to 5 days. Suitable plasma can be stored for later use for 100 days if frozen at –20°C. Aminoglycosides are believed to interfere with plasma function, whereas penicillin and ticarcillin do not.

Two studies found no improvement in infectious endometritis after intrauterine plasma infusions, but the therapeutic protocol in each study was different from that originally proposed by Florida workers. In contrast, in an Australian study involving 1341 breeding cycles in 905 Thoroughbred mares, lactating and barren mares treated with intrauterine antibiotics and autologous plasma once 12 to 36 hours after breeding had better pregnancy rates than similar mares either not treated or treated only with antibiotics. More studies are needed to definitively verify or reject intrauterine plasma infusion, in conjunction with uterine lavage or other therapies, as an important therapeutic strategy.

Uterine Curettage

Benefits have been reported from mechanical curettage of uteri in mares with persistent endometritis. Improvement is thought to be gained by inducement of acute inflammation, with attendant movement of neutrophils and serum-derived opsonins into the uterine lumen. Infusion of strongly irritating solutions has been advocated as a method of uterine curettage (e.g., termed chemical curettage). Chemical curettage is accomplished by infusing irritating solutions (e.g., strong disinfectant solutions, diluted kerosene, or magnesium sulfate solution) that cause endometrial necrosis. The irritant is held within the uterus for 5 to 10 minutes followed by a lactated Ringer's solution lavage and emollient medication of the vagina for protection against scalding. Daily or every other day lavage for a few days may decrease the chances of intrauterine adhesion formation. Direct comparisons between mechanical and chemical methods of inducing uterine inflammation have not been made. Overzealous curettage, be it by mechanical or chemical means, can incite excessive tissue damage and permanent infertility. The practitioner is cautioned that more controlled experimentation with the technique of mechanical or chemical curettage is needed to justify its appropriateness as a treatment modality for any form of endometrial pathologic changes, including endometritis.

Colostrum Infusions

Infusion of equine colostrum, an abundant source of immunoglobulins, has been reported as a successful treatment for infectious endometritis in mares. Although not critically studied, its efficacy remains questionable because the uteri of mares susceptible to endometritis apparently do not have a quantitative deficiency of immunoglobulins. Continued studies are needed to more completely understand the effects of the uterine environment on biologic activity of immunoglobulins. As with plasma, heterologous colostrum is a potential means of disease transmission or cause of immunologic complications. Aseptic collection and storage of colostrum are essential to avoid iatrogenic induction or propagation of infection. One of the authors examined breeding records from one farm in which colostrum infusions were often administered after breeding and found significantly lower pregnancy rates in the colostrum-treated mares.

Hormonal Therapy

Existing studies indicate that mares under estrogen influence are more capable of eliminating uterine infections than mares under progesterone influence. Improved microbial clearance in estrous mares may be the result of enhancements in migrational capacity of neutrophils, neutrophil phagocytic or microbicidal ability, uterine physical clearance mechanisms, or a combination thereof. Given the potential advantages of an estrous over a diestrous state to eliminate uterine infections, a logical approach to treatment includes increasing the percentage of time that a mare is in physiologic estrus. This effect can be achieved in the cyclic mare by administering an exogenous prostaglandin 5 to 6 days after ovulation to reduce the length of diestrus.

Advantages of exogenous estrogen for treatment of endometritis in cyclic mares have not been shown. Diestrus (i.e., progesterone influence) may mask any beneficial effects exerted by exogenous estrogen therapy. Many commercially available estrogens are esterified, resulting in heightened potency and prolonged (and unpredictable) duration of action; hence, complications may arise from their use. When estrogen therapy is contemplated by the practitioner, small doses (e.g., 0.5 to 1.0 mg of estradiol cypionate or 5 to 10 mg of estradiol-17β) should be used. Estrogens are not currently approved for use in horses.

Locally Applied Prostaglandin E

Some mares that tend to repeatedly accumulate fluid within the uterus seem to have insufficient relaxation of the cervix during estrus. This problem is particularly prevalent in older maiden mares. Because cervical relaxation is necessary to allow expulsion of uterine contents, we have tried local application of either 2 mg of prostaglandin E2 (Sigma Aldrich, St. Louis, Mo.), mixed in 2 to 4 mL of lubricating jelly and deposited in the cervical canal and external cervical os, or 200 µg to 1 mg of misoprostol (prostaglandin E1 analog) tablets (Cytotec, G.D. Searle and Co, Omaha, Neb.) softened in a small volume of sterile saline solution or lubricating jelly and inserted into the external cervical os once daily. Use of these compounds appears to result in cervical softening and dilation that facilitates uterine drainage in such mares. Further investigation on use of prostaglandin E in mares is warranted.

Use of Immunomodulators

Some products have been used empirically in an attempt to stimulate immunity to overcome uterine infection. Such treatments remain unstudied and of questionable efficacy. Products that have been used include the following:

- Levamisole given once daily (1 mg/lb) for 3 days, then stopped for 4 days, and then repeated for three to four series of treatments. Severe anaphylaxis and colic are potential side effects, so this treatment should be used with caution.
- Mebendazole (Telmin Pitman-Moore Inc, Washington Crossing, N.J.) given once daily (1 mg/lb) for 3 days, then stopped for 4 days, and then repeated for three to four series of treatments. Apparently, side effects are unlikely with this treatment, although we have no personal experience with it.
- An immunostimulant made from the bacterium *Propionibacterium acnes* (EqStim, Neogen Corporation, Lexington, Ky.) was reported to be efficacious when injected intravenously (4 mL/454 kg body weight) on days 1, 2, and 7 after diagnosis of endometritis. A subsequent field trial also claimed benefit.

The US Department of Agriculture (USDA) has recently approved an emulsified product derived from the cell wall of *Mycobacterium phlei* (Settle, Bioniche Animal Health, Athens, Ga.) for the treatment of endometritis caused by *S. zooepidemicus*. This product purportedly modulates the endometrial immune response, reduces bacterial contamination of the uterus, and improves pregnancy rates when compared with placebo treatment. The product can be administered intravenously or as a uterine infusion and can be used as a stand-alone therapy or in conjunction with other therapeutic modalities such as antibiotics or uterine lavage. However, critical studies involving adequate numbers of mares and suitable controls have not been performed.

Recently, the use of corticosteroids to reduce the inflammatory response of mares susceptible to persistent mating induced endometritis has been investigated. In one study, a single dose of prednisolone acetate (0.1 mg/kg) concomitant with the administration of human chorionic gonadotropin (hCG) resulted in a significant increase in pregnancy rate over that in susceptible mares not receiving corticosteroids (64.5% versus 0.0%, respectively). In another study, administration of dexamethasone (50 mg, intravenously) at the time of insemination was reported to reduce the inflammatory response and improve pregnancy rates.

PREVENTION OF GENITAL INFECTION

Prevention is of paramount importance for controlling genital infections of mares. Prevention techniques are varied but involve common sense. Too often the veterinarian is relied on to overcome less than optimal breeding hygiene and management through the use of antibiotics. Whether natural cover or artificial insemination is used, instituting the use of minimal contamination techniques and limiting the number of breedings per cycle will minimize the potential for uterine contamination. Conditions such as pneumovagina or urovagina should be controlled with corrective surgery. Proper hygiene during parturition, breeding, and genital examination is critical. Artificial insemination with a suitable antibiotic-containing semen extender or infusion of 30 to 50 mL of antibiotic-containing extender into the uterus of the mare immediately before natural cover can be of benefit in preventing infection of the genital tract.

BIBLIOGRAPHY

Asbury AC: Bacterial endometritis. In Robinson NE, editor: *Current therapy in equine medicine,* Philadelphia, 1983. Saunders.

Ball BA, Shin SJ, Patten VH, et al: Use of a small volume uterine flush for microbiologic and cytologic examination of the mare's endometrium, *Theriogenology* 29:1269-1283, 1988.

Brendemuehl JP: Influence of cloprostenol, PGF$_2\alpha$ and oxytocin administered in the immediate postovulatory period on corpora luteal formation and function in the mare, *Proc Equine Symp Soc Theriogenol* 267, 2000.

Bucca S, Carli A, Buckley T, et al: The use of dexamethasone administered to mares at breeding time in the modulation of persistent mating induced endometritis, *Theriogenology* 70:1093-1100, 2008.

Evans MJ, Hamer JM, Gason LM, et al: Factors affecting uterine clearance of inoculated materials in mares, *J Reprod Fertil* 35(Suppl): 327-334, 1987.

Giguere S, Sweeney RW, Belanger M: Pharmacokinetics of enrofloxacin in adult horses and concentration of the drug in serum, body fluids, and endometrial tissues after repeated intragastrically administered doses, *Am J Vet Res* 57:1025-1030, 1996.

Gunthle LM, McCue PM, Farquhar VJ, et al: Effect of prostaglandin administration postovulation on corpus luteum formation in the mare, *Proc Equine Symp Society Theriogenol* 139, 2000.

Hughes JP, Loy RG: Investigations on the effect of intrauterine inoculations of *Streptococcus zooepidemicus* in the mare, *Proc Am Assoc Equine Pract* 15:289-292, 1969.

LeBlanc MM: Recurrent endometritis: is oxytocin the answer? *Proc Am Assoc Equine Pract* 40:17-18, 1994.

LeBlanc MM, Magsig J, Stromberg AJ: Use of a low volume uterine flush for diagnosing endometritis in chronically infertile mares, *Theriogenology* 68:403-412, 2007.

Liu IKM: Uterine defense mechanisms in the mare. In Van Camp SD, editor: *The veterinary clinics of North America: equine practice,* vol 4, Philadelphia, 1988, Saunders.

Neely DP: Evaluation and therapy of genital disease in the mare. In Neely DP, Liu IMK, Hillman RB, editors: *Equine reproduction,* Nutley, NH, 1983, Veterinary Learning Systems.

Papa FO, Dell'aqua JA Jr, Alvarenga MA, et al: Use of corticosteroid therapy on the modulation of uterine inflammatory response in mares after artificial insemination with frozen semen, *Pferdeheilkunde* 24:79-82, 2008.

Pascoe DR: Effect of adding autologous plasma to an intrauterine antibiotic therapy after breeding on pregnancy rates in mares, *Biol Reprod Monogr* 1:532-543, 1995.

Peterson FB, McFeely RA, David JSE: Studies on the pathogenesis of endometritis in the mare, *Proc Am Assoc Equine Pract* 15:279-287, 1969.

Rohrbach BW, Sheerin PC, Cantrell CK, et al: Effect of adjunctive treatment with intravenously administered *Propionibacterium* acnes on reproductive performance in mares with persistent endometritis, *J Am Vet Med Assoc* 231:107-113, 2007.

Scott MA, Liu IKM, Overstreet JW: Sperm transport to the oviducts: abnormalities and their clinical implications, *Proc Am Assoc Equine Pract* 41:1-2, 1995.

Troedsson MHT: Uterine clearance and resistance to persistent endometritis in the mare, *Theriogenology* 52:461-471, 1999.

Troedsson MHT, Liu IKM, Thurmond M: Function of uterine- and blood-derived polymorphonuclear neutrophils in mares susceptible and resistant to chronic uterine infection: phagocytosis and chemotaxis, *Biol Reprod* 49:507-514, 1993.

Watson ED: Uterine defense mechanisms in mares resistant and susceptible to persistent endometritis: a review, *Equine Vet J* 20: 397-400, 1988.

Zent WA, Troedsson MHT, Xue J-L: Postbreeding uterine fluid accumulation in a normal population of Thoroughbred mares: a field study, *Proc Am Assoc Equine Pract* 44:64-65, 1998.

Pregnancy: Physiology and Diagnosis

7

CHAPTER

Objectives

While studying the information covered in this chapter, the reader should attempt to:
- Acquire a working understanding of the physiologic events of pregnancy in the mare.
- Acquire a working knowledge of the procedures used to diagnose pregnancy in the mare.

Study Questions

1. Discuss the following physiologic events of pregnancy in the mare:
   a. Entrance of embryo into the uterus
   b. Conceptus mobility throughout the uterus
   c. Embryonic vesicle fixation
   d. Maternal recognition of pregnancy
   e. Endometrial cup formation
   f. Supplementary corpus luteum (CL) formation
   g. Placentation
2. Describe the hormonal events of pregnancy in the mare, paying particular attention to source and timing of progesterone production (i.e., primary CL of pregnancy, supplementary CL of pregnancy, placental progestogen production). Also include in your description the concentrations of estrogen and equine chorionic gonadotropin in the blood stream of the mare.

3. Discuss methods of pregnancy detection at various stages of gestation in the mare. Include advantages and disadvantages of each method.
   a. Behavioral assessment
   b. Progesterone assays
   c. Vaginal speculum examination
   d. Palpation per rectum
   e. Transrectal ultrasound examination
   f. Equine chorionic gonadotropin (eCG) detection
   g. Serum estrone sulfate detection
   h. Urinary estrone sulfate detection

EARLY EVENTS OF PREGNANCY

Maternal endocrine status during the first 14 days of pregnancy is similar to that of the nonpregnant mare in diestrus. If the mare is not pregnant, the endometrium releases prostaglandin-$F_2\alpha$ ($PGF_2\alpha$) on approximately days 14 to 15 after ovulation, which causes regression of the corpus luteum and permits the mare to return to estrus. If the mare is pregnant, the corpus luteum does not undergo lysis on days 14 to 15 but persists and continues to secrete progesterone, which is responsible for pregnancy maintenance. The process whereby luteolysis is prevented by the presence of the conceptus is referred to as **maternal recognition of pregnancy.**

The embryo enters the uterine lumen approximately 6 days after ovulation. The early equine conceptus has been shown to be endocrinologically active, with the young embryo expressing enzymes for synthesis of prostaglandins E and F (PGE and PGF, respectively). The signal for activating this prostaglandin synthesis is still unknown. Idaho workers showed that the morula and early blastocyst secrete prostaglandin E (PGE), which plays a role in transport of the embryo from the oviduct into the uterus. Later in development, the early embryo secretes PGF, which is thought to stimulate myometrial contractions.

Unlike embryos of other domestic species, which typically remain in the uterine horn ipsilateral to the ovulatory ovary and elongate to facilitate maternal recognition of pregnancy, the equine **embryonic vesicle** remains spherical and is quite *mobile* after its descent into the uterus, migrating through both uterine horns and the uterine body several times each day. Mobility is maximal on day 11 or 12 and is maintained to approximately day 16. Movement of the embryonic vesicle is passive, dependent on uterine contractions that propel it through the uterine lumen. However, experiments have shown that simulated conceptuses move more slowly through the uterus than do viable conceptuses, which indicates that the embryo itself provides an active stimulus to uterine mobility.

Movement throughout the uterus is thought to be important for the conceptus to *"signal"* the dam that pregnancy has occurred (because of the small trophoblastic surface of the equine conceptus compared with that of other species), thereby preventing luteolysis. The factor involved in maternal recognition of pregnancy has not been identified in the equine, but in vitro studies have shown that the conceptus secretes a low–molecular weight ($\leq$10 kDa) protein that inhibits $PGF_2\alpha$ production by the endometrium.

Another unique feature of the equine embryo, described by Canadian workers, is the formation of a polysaccharide-rich *capsule* that forms between the trophectoderm and zona pellucida of the embryo within 48 hours of entering the uterus. The capsule continues to grow along with the embryonic vesicle until about day 18 and thereafter disappears by day 23 of pregnancy. The capsule is postulated to protect the conceptus from mechanical damage when it is propelled throughout the uterus during the mobility phase and may also be involved in protecting the conceptus from being recognized as immunologically foreign to the dam. The capsule undergoes rapid changes in protein composition at the time the conceptus becomes fixed within the uterus.

The corpus luteum, called the **primary corpus luteum (CL) of pregnancy**, can be visibly identified in the ovary for up to 180 to 220 days. The primary CL regresses at approximately the same stage of gestation as the supplementary corpora lutea. *The critical time for maternal recognition of pregnancy, to prevent luteolysis of the primary CL and subsequent loss of the pregnancy, is thought to be 14 to 16 days after ovulation in the mare.* Suppression of mobility of the conceptus through the uterus during days 10 to 16, or conditions that prevent the conceptus from migrating throughout the uterus (e.g., blocked uterine horn), will interfere with maternal recognition of pregnancy, resulting in failure to prevent endometrial production and release of $PGF_2\alpha$, and the mare returns to estrus in spite of conceiving.

The embryonic vesicle becomes stationary by approximately day 16 after ovulation. This process is referred to as **fixation** and is apparently largely the result of restriction of the enlarging conceptus at the base of one uterine horn. The process of embryonic vesicle fixation should not be confused with the process of fetal-maternal attachment. Soon after the time of fixation, the cross-sectional shape of the embryonic vesicle typically changes from circular to *triangular;* this change in shape is identified by transrectal ultrasonographic examination. The change in vesicle shape is the result of thickening *(hypertrophy)* of the dorsal uterine wall (see Figures 5-30 and 5-31). The encroachment of the dorsal aspect of the endometrium onto the vesicle is thought to play a role in orienting the embryo proper to a ventral 6 o'clock position, opposite the mesometrial attachment (antimesometrial).

When the reproductive tract is under progesterone influence from the primary CL of pregnancy and estrogen influence from the developing conceptus (estrogen is produced by day 12), the uterus begins to develop a characteristic shape with marked **tone** that becomes readily apparent on palpation per rectum by day 16 to 18 after ovulation (Figure 7-1). Examination via palpation per rectum usually reveals suggestive, but not definitive, evidence of early pregnancy at this point because the conceptus may not yet be readily palpable. The conceptus does not begin attaching to the endometrium until

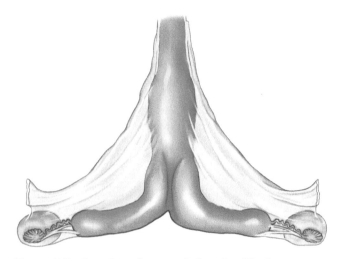

Figure 7-1 Drawing of uterus during day 18 of pregnancy. The cervix is elongated and firmly closed. The uterine horns are palpably turgid, making the bifurcation between the two uterine horns prominent on palpation per rectum.

day 40 to 45 of gestation, so the increased tone of early pregnancy is thought to help keep the embryo and developing membranes in close apposition with the endometrium during this time period to maximize nutrient transfer. The advent of ultrasonography has allowed considerable progress in pregnancy diagnostics in the mare because this technique enables detection of embryonic vesicles in the uterus as early as 9 to 10 days after ovulation. Pregnancy can typically be confirmed via palpation per rectum by most examiners at 25 to 35 days of gestation.

The process of **fetal-maternal attachment** is gradual. The vascularized trophoblast is closely associated with the uterine epithelium by day 25. Beginning interdigitation of **trophoblastic microvilli** and uterine epithelium has been described as occurring by days 38 to 40. Fetal **macrovilli** (which become the **microcotyledons** and are distinct from microvilli) begin appearing by day 45 as rudimentary structures and gradually develop until full placental attachment occurs in the form of well-developed **microplacentome**s (microcotyledons with maternal microcaruncles) by day 150 (Figure 7-2).

ENDOMETRIAL CUP FORMATION

A unique feature of the equine placenta is the development of endometrial cups early in gestation. On about day 25 of gestation, a specialized annular band of the **trophoblast** undergoes cellular changes to form the **chorionic girdle** at the junction of the developing allantois and regressing yolk sac. These trophoblastic cells of the chorionic girdle invade the adjacent uterine epithelium on approximately day 38 of gestation, migrating into the underlying lamina propria to develop into the prominent decidua-like cells of the **endometrial cups.** The endometrial cups are identified as a circular or horseshoe arrangement of pale irregular outgrowths on the luminal surface of the gravid uterine horn (Figure 7-3). They attain maximal size at about day 70 of gestation and then begin to undergo degeneration and eventually are completely sloughed by approximately day 130 of gestation. The endometrial cups secrete a hormone known as **equine chorionic gonadotropin (eCG),** previously termed pregnant mare serum gonadotropin *(PMSG).* Equine chorionic gonadotropin is first detectable in maternal blood on days 35 to 42, rapidly increasing in concentration to peak levels on days 55 to 65; then concentrations decline slowly to low or nondetectable levels by days 100 to 150. This hormone is believed to assist in the formation of supplementary corpora lutea and is thought to also be a necessary stimulus for maintenance of the primary CL during approximately days 35 to 120. Progesterone output from the primary CL actually increases during days 35 to 40, before acquisition of significant progesterone production by the supplementary corpora lutea. Equine chorionic gonadotropin is also thought to play an important immunoregulatory role during pregnancy.

Endometrial cup formation is an important consideration in the management of early embryonic loss. If pregnancy loss occurs before the formation of the endometrial

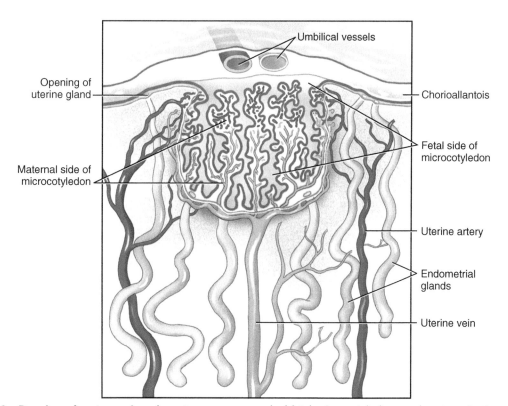

Figure 7-2 Drawing of mature microplacentomes composed of fetal microcotyledons and maternal microcaruncles.

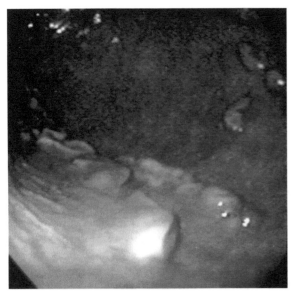

Figure 7-3   Endoscopic view of endometrial cups present in uterus after pregnancy termination at day 70 of gestation.

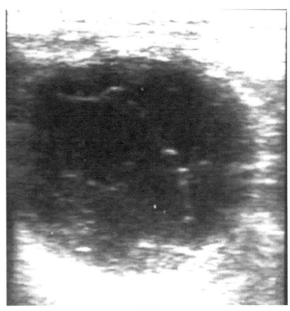

Figure 7-4   Anovulatory follicle in a mare that aborted between 70 and 75 days gestation. Multiple PGF$_2\alpha$ injections were given to regress corpora lutea and bring the mare into estrus for rebreeding, but ovulation failed. (Courtesy Dr. James Morehead, Lexington, Ky., 2001.)

cups (days 36 to 40), the mare returns to estrus within a short period of time (less than 1 month). Because only the primary CL is present, a single injection of PGF$_2\alpha$ promotes CL regression and return to estrus. *If pregnancy loss occurs after endometrial cup formation, eCG production continues and the mare may not return to estrus for 3 months, when the endometrial cups degenerate, thereby allowing supplementary corpora lutea to regress.* In addition, a mare that loses a conceptus after days 36 to 40 of gestation remains positive for pregnancy according to eCG detection tests (e.g., Equi-Chek, Endocrine Technologies Inc, Newark, Calif.) for up to 3 months although the mare is no longer pregnant, because these tests assay for presence of circulating blood levels of eCG, not pregnancy itself. *Of additional importance, repeated PGF$_2\alpha$ injections may cause a mare that has aborted after 40 days of gestation to return to estrus by inducing regression of supplementary corpora lutea, but the estrus is seldom fertile as long as endometrial cups remain.* Another aggravating problem when attempting to rebreed a mare that has endometrial cups remaining after abortion, even when the mare has been induced to return to estrus with repeated PGF$_2\alpha$ injections, is the tendency for follicles to fail to ovulate. Such mares have also been noted to ovulate smaller-than-normal follicles, luteinize follicles that do not ovulate, or form structures similar in appearance to hemorrhagic anovulatory follicles (Figure 7-4).

DEVELOPMENT OF SUPPLEMENTARY CORPORA LUTEA

Through the control of the pituitary gland and endometrial cups, the ovaries begin to develop **supplementary corpora lutea** about day 40 of gestation. In response to increasing eCG levels, progesterone production increases from resulting **secondary corpora lutea** (which arise from ovulations over days 40 to 70) and **accessory corpora lutea** (which arise from luteinization of existing follicles over days 40 to 150). The secondary corpora lutea and accessory corpora lutea together are referred to as supplementary corpora lutea (Figure 7-5). The additional progesterone produced by supplementary corpora lutea contributes to that produced by the primary corpus luteum in supporting the fetus during the first 5 months of pregnancy. *All corpora lutea degenerate*

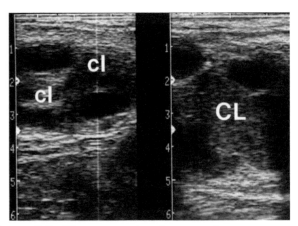

Figure 7-5   Ultrasonograph of ovary of pregnant mare (at 65 days of gestation) depicting primary corpus luteum *(CL)* of pregnancy on right ovary and supplementary corpora lutea *(cl)* on left ovary.

by days 150 to 200 of gestation; by then, the placenta has assumed the sole role of progestin secretion (and thus, pregnancy maintenance) until parturition.

In rare instances, mares may not develop supplementary corpora lutea. This phenomenon has been described as one potential cause of abortion in mares before 100 to 150 days of gestation. During the transition from pregnancy dependence on ovarian progesterone to placental progestin, the mare may experience increased susceptibility to abortion from adverse environmental influences. Abortion may occur during this time span (days 70 to 150 of gestation) from stress-related causes such as unaccustomed exercise, transport, inclement weather, or maternal illness.

PROGESTIN PRODUCTION BY THE FETOPLACENTAL UNIT

The fetoplacental unit synthesizes and secretes high levels of **progestins** (primarily 5α-pregnanes) into the maternal circulation during mid to late pregnancy. These progestins first appear in the maternal circulation between days 30 and 60 and increase gradually through day 300 of gestation. Fetoplacental progestin production is sufficient to maintain pregnancy in mares in mid- to late gestation. Studies involving ovariectomy during different gestational stages have led to the conclusion that an ovarian source of progesterone is requisite for maintaining pregnancy in some mares as late as day 70 but is not essential beyond days 100 to 140 of gestation. Indeed, many ovariectomized mares maintain pregnancy in the absence of exogenously administered progesterone from day 100 to term. A summary of hormonal and reproductive changes that occur during pregnancy in the mare is provided in Figure 7-6.

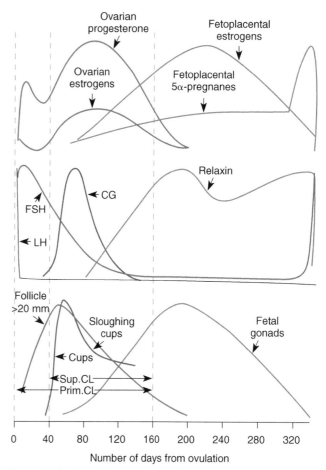

Figure 7-6 Graphic summary of hormonal and reproductive changes that occur during equine pregnancy. *CG*, Chorionic gonadotropin; *FSH*, Follicle-stimulating hormone; *LH*, luteinizing hormone; Prim. CL, primary corpus luteum; Sup. CL, supplementary corpora lutea. (Modified from Ginther OJ: *Reproductive biology of the mare: basic and applied aspects,* ed 2, Cross Plains, WI, 1992, Equiservices.)

SUMMARY OF METHODS OF PREGNANCY DIAGNOSIS

Several methods of pregnancy detection are available to the veterinarian. The type of diagnostic aid used is dependent on equipment availability, clinician expertise, and stage of pregnancy. Some methods of pregnancy diagnosis currently used are outlined.

Behavioral Assessment

Monitor sexual behavior of the mare by daily teasing with a stallion. A mare that is not pregnant should demonstrate behavioral estrus approximately 16 to 20 days after ovulation. Failure of the mare to return to estrus is suggestive evidence of pregnancy.

False-positive and false-negative results are likely to occur. Some pregnant mares exhibit behavioral estrus. Persistent luteal function and early embryonic death (after day 14 of gestation) may result in uninterrupted signs of diestrus in a nonpregnant mare.

This is a nonspecific indicator of pregnancy.

Serum/Milk Progesterone Assay

Progesterone assay is performed 18 to 20 days after ovulation. A high progesterone level implies the presence of a functional CL, thereby suggesting pregnancy.

False-positive results can result from a persistent luteal function (spontaneous, or from early embryonic death after maternal recognition of pregnancy has occurred that prevents CL regression).

This is a nonspecific indicator of pregnancy.

Vaginal Speculum Examination

Vaginal speculum examination is performed 18 to 21 days after ovulation, usually in conjunction with examination of the reproductive tract per rectum. Speculum examination is not indicated unless per rectum examination is equivocal. The presence of a dry, pale, tightly closed cervix with the external os protruding into the center of the cranial vagina is suggestive of pregnancy.

This is a nonspecific indicator of pregnancy; it simply indicates the presence of elevated progesterone secreted by a functional corpus luteum.

Palpation of the Reproductive Tract per Rectum

Until the advent of the use of transrectal ultrasonography, palpation of the reproductive tract per rectum was the most common and rapid pregnancy detection method used. It can be used to detect pregnancy at most any stage of gestation after 18 to 20 days.

Detection of Early Pregnancy at 18 to 21 Days After Ovulation (Figure 7-1)

During this time period, an increased **tone** and **tubularity** of the uterine horns is noted. The increased tone makes the external bifurcation between the two uterine horns noticeable as a prominent **cleft** or indentation. *Ovarian follicular activity is usually quite pronounced, and the cervix is elongated, firm, and tightly closed.* The cervix is so prominent that it feels much like a pencil per rectum, being longer than is usual for a mare in diestrus. If the mare were not pregnant, she should be approaching ovulation at this time and have a flaccid uterus and cervix. Therefore, a tonic uterus and an elongated tight cervix in the presence of significant follicular development (e.g., 30-mm to 35-mm follicles) 18 to 21 days after breeding are indicative of pregnancy. In mares with a small uterus, such as maiden mares, a small swelling about the size of a ping pong ball may occasionally be detected at the base of a uterine horn. However, because false-positive and false-negative results may occur with early embryonic death or a persistent luteal function, transrectal ultrasonographic examination is often required to confirm pregnancy at this stage.

Detection of Pregnancy at 25 to 30 Days After Ovulation (Figure 7-7)

The prominent uterine tone and tubularity, elongated cervix, and pronounced follicular activity noted at 18 to 21 days gestation are still present. In addition, a resilient spherical or ovoid *bulge (approximately the size of a golf ball or hens egg)* can often be noted on the anteroventral aspect of the uterine horn near the external bifurcation. The ventral surface of the uterine horns must be gently picked up in the fingers because the bulge of early pregnancy is easy to miss if only the dorsal surface of the uterine horns is palpated. The uterine wall over the well-circumscribed bulge is thin, with less tone than the adjacent uterine wall, feeling much like a balloon filled with water.

Detection of Pregnancy at 35 to 40 Days After Ovulation (Figure 7-8)

Palpation per rectum of the mare 35 to 40 days pregnant reveals the previous findings, plus a resilient spherical to ovoid bulge of *tennis ball to baseball size* at the base of one uterine horn.

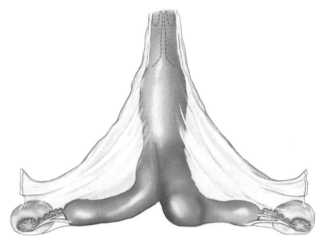

Figure 7-7 Drawing of appearance of uterus of mare at 25 to 30 days of gestation. The pronounced uterine tone and tubularity typical of early pregnancy remain, along with the palpably elongated cervix. A resilient spherical or ovoid bulge approximately the size of a golf ball or hen egg is often palpable at the base of one uterine horn.

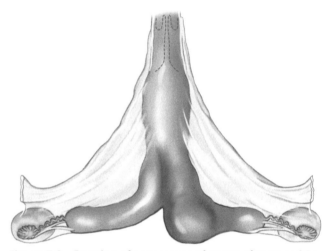

Figure 7-8 Drawing of appearance of uterus of mare at 35 to 40 days of gestation. The pronounced uterine tone and tubularity typical of early pregnancy remain, along with the palpably elongated cervix. A resilient spherical or ovoid bulge approximately the size of a tennis ball or baseball is present at the base of one uterine horn.

Detection of Pregnancy at 45 to 50 Days After Ovulation (Figure 7-9)

Palpation per rectum of the mare 45 to 50 days pregnant reveals the previous findings, plus a resilient spherical to ovoid bulge approximately the size of a *softball* that fills the palm and fingers of the hand. The ventral uterine wall typically feels thin and more fluid-filled than earlier in pregnancy.

Detection of Pregnancy at 60 to 65 Days After Ovulation (Figure 7-10)

While the cervix remains quite elongated and firm, the progressive filling of the uterus as pregnancy advances tends to feel less tonic than earlier in pregnancy. In

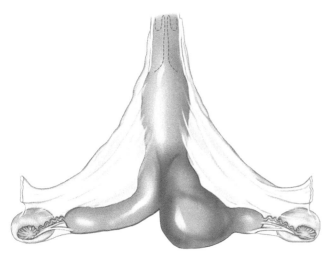

Figure 7-9 Drawing of appearance of uterus of mare at 45 to 50 days of gestation. The elongated cervix and increased uterine tone remain. A resilient spherical or ovoid bulge approximately the size of a softball or grapefruit is present at the base of one uterine horn.

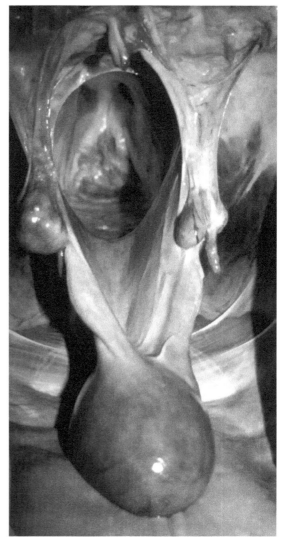

Figure 7-10 Appearance of uterus of mare at 60 to 65 days of gestation. The rectum and abdominal viscera have been removed. The elongated cervix remains readily palpable per rectum, and the bulge at the base of one uterine horn has moved into the body of the uterus and is the size of a cantaloupe or small football.

addition, the pregnancy is *beginning to expand into the uterine body*, and the uterus begins to descend into the ventral abdomen as pregnancy progresses. The uterine bulge tends to lose some of its earlier resiliency. The uterine bulge is approximately the size of a *cantaloupe or small football.*

Detection of Pregnancy 100 to 120 Days After Ovulation (Figure 7-11)

The pregnancy continues its expansion into the uterine body and is easier to detect here than in the uterine horn. The pregnancy is easily felt more dorsally than before, with the bulge being *volleyball to basketball sized.* Ballottement of the fetus within the uterus is possible, but is more difficult at this stage of pregnancy than it is in the cow. Because of the increased size and more cranioventral location of the uterus, this can be the most difficult stage of gestation to detect pregnancy via transrectal palpation. *It is quite easy to mistake a full urinary bladder for a pregnant uterus at this stage, so the examiner must take care to ensure that the fluid being felt is within the uterus.* Tracing the fluid-filled organ back to the cervix confirms it is the uterus and not the urinary bladder. If the cervix is not located, the examination must be repeated, with even more care taken to search for anatomic markers of the reproductive tract, including the ovaries.

Detection of Pregnancy at 150 to 210 Days After Ovulation

As pregnancy progresses and the uterus enlarges, the heavy uterine contents pull the suspending broad ligaments and ovaries into a more medioventral position.

Uterine descent into the ventral abdomen is complete at 150 to 210 days of gestation, and the pregnant uterus is too large to be encompassed with the outreached arm. The fetus is located in the ventral abdomen but may usually be detected with ballottement.

Detection of Pregnancy at 240 Days of Gestation to Term

The enlarging uterus begins to expand upward with most fetal growth occurring during this period. As the fetus enlarges markedly, proportionately less fluid is present in the uterus, making the hard fetus easy to feel. Although the position and approximate size of the fetus can usually be detected, a precise estimation of the gestational age of the fetus is quite difficult.

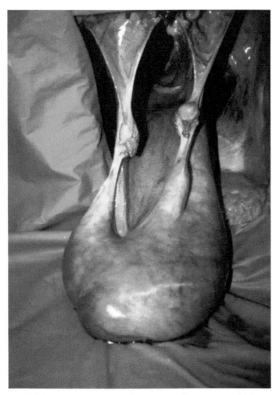

Figure 7-11 Appearance of uterus of mare at 100 to 120 days of gestation. The rectum and abdominal viscera have been removed. The elongated cervix remains readily palpable per rectum, and the bulge in the uterus typically is the size of a volleyball or basketball.

DETECTION OF PREGNANCY WITH ULTRASOUND EXAMINATION

Major advantages of transrectal ultrasound for pregnancy detection in the mare are:

- Earliest positive detection of pregnancy, with the embryonic vesicle visible as early as day 9 or 10 of gestation. The accuracy of vesicle detection approaches 99% by 15 days of gestation.
- Embryonic vesicle and embryo growth charts are available (and sometimes programmed into the ultrasound software) that permit more accurate determination of embryo/fetal age.
- Permits early detection of twin pregnancy, allowing methods of intervention to be pursued earlier and with greater success.
- Permits assessment of early embryonic loss by comparing expected development based on ovulation or breeding dates against expected values.
- Permits assessment of embryonic and fetal viability (i.e., heartbeat, movement, expected development for age).
- Permits fetal sexing at approximately days 60 to 70 of gestation.

Transrectal ultrasonography does have its limitations. It cannot replace palpation per rectum; indeed, to effectively use ultrasound, the veterinarian must first be an accomplished palpator. The equipment is expensive, so some clients find the charges for ultrasound pregnancy diagnosis to be prohibitive. Interpretive errors are also possible. Finally, the fetus is often difficult to visualize with transrectal ultrasound between 3 to 5 or 6 months of gestation because of the progressive enlargement of the gravid uterus moving it beyond the reach of the examiner. Transabdominal ultrasonography with a 2.5-MHz to 3.5-MHz curvilinear or sector probe is often helpful in assessing fetal viability during this period of mid-term gestation, and during late-term gestation.

Refer to Chapter 5 for a discussion of characteristics of early pregnancy that are detectable with transrectal ultrasonographic examination.

EQUINE CHORIONIC GONADOTROPIN DETECTION

Recall that eCG is produced by endometrial cups in the pregnant mare uterus beginning on days 36 to 40 of gestation. The period of detection of eCG in mare serum is limited to days 40 to 120 of gestation.

To test for presence of eCG, serum either can be submitted to a reference laboratory for testing or can be analyzed with a commercially available "mare-side" kit. However, false-positive reactions are possible. If a pregnancy is lost after days 36 to 40 of gestation, when endometrial cups are already functional, a false-positive result occurs (i.e., eCG is present in spite of pregnancy loss).

False-negative reactions occur if serum is evaluated before days 36 to 40 of gestation, when concentrations of eCG in the mare's serum may be too low to detect, or after day 120 of gestation, when concentrations have declined after endometrial cup regression. In addition, false-negative results are common (81%) in mares carrying mule fetuses.

ESTROGEN DETECTION IN BLOOD OR URINE

The developing conceptus has a remarkable estrogen-producing capability as early as day 12 of pregnancy. Concentrations of estrogens in the blood and urine parallel each other. By day 60 to 100 of pregnancy, estrogen concentrations in blood or urine exceed those noted during estrus. Because the estrogens are secreted primarily by the fetoplacental unit, the assay for estrogens has been advocated as a noninvasive means for assessing fetal viability during pregnancy. Concentration of estrogens in feces has even been reported for pregnancy diagnosis in feral horses. Blood serum or plasma can be submitted to a reference laboratory for measurement of estrogen concentration. Circulating estrogen concentration peaks at days 180 to 240 of gestation, then slowly declines until parturition. Estrone sulfate levels drop rapidly with fetal death or abortion, and estrogen tests have been advocated for diagnosing pregnancy and fetal viability or stress from 60 to 80 days of gestation through term. However, estrone sulfate levels have not been found to be useful for detecting early placentitis. We have noted that in some pregnant mares, equivocal or negative test results (estrone sulfate concentrations below that expected for pregnant mares) at 60 to 70 days of gestation became positive (estrone sulfate concentrations consistent with viable pregnancy) at 80 days of gestation. Premature elevations in estrone sulfate levels have been observed with twin conceptuses, whereas donkeys and miniature mares have been noted to lag in the elevation of estrone sulfate levels.

BIBLIOGRAPHY

Aurich C, Budik S: Expression of enzymes involved in the synthesis of prostaglandins in early equine embryos. *Proceeding of a workshop on maternal recognition of pregnancy in the mare III*, Monograph series no. 16, Barbados, West Indies, 2004, Havemeyer Foundation, 31-32.

Bergfeldt DR, Adams GP, Pierson RA: Pregnancy. In Rantanen NW, McKinnon AO, editors: *Equine diagnostic ultrasonography*, Baltimore, 1998, Williams & Wilkins, 125-140.

Ginther OJ: *Reproductive biology of the mare: basic and applied aspects*, ed 2, Cross Plains, WI, 1992, Equiservices, 642.

McKinnon AO: Diagnosis of pregnancy. In McKinnon AO, Voss JL, editors: *Equine reproduction*, Philadelphia, 1993, Lea & Febiger, 501-508.

Neely DP: Equine gestation. In Neely DP, Liu IMK, Hillman RB, editors: *Equine reproduction*, Nutley, NY, 1983, Veterinary Learning Systems Co, 40-55.

Quinn BA, Hayes MA, Waelchli RO, et al: Major proteins in the embryonic capsule, and in yolk-sac and uterine fluids, during the second to fourth weeks of pregnancy in the mare. *Proceeding of a workshop on maternal recognition of pregnancy in the mare III*, Monograph series no. 16, Barbados, West Indies, 2004, Havemeyer Foundation, 47-49.

Silva LA, Ginther OJ: An early endometrial vascular indicator of completed orientation of the embryo and the role of dorsal endometrial encroachment in mares, *Biol Reprod* 74:337-343, 2006.

Stout TAE, Rambags BPB, van Tol HTA, et al: Low molecular weight proteins secreted by the early equine conceptus, *Proceeding of a workshop on maternal recognition of pregnancy in the mare III*, Monograph series no. 16, Barbados, West Indies, 2004, Havemeyer Foundation, 50-52.

Pregnancy Loss

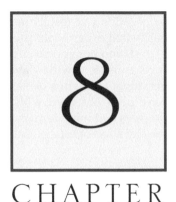

CHAPTER 8

OBJECTIVES

While studying the information covered in this chapter, the reader should attempt to:
- Acquire an understanding of the factors that contribute to pregnancy loss in the equine embryonic, fetal, natal, and neonatal periods.
- Acquire a working knowledge of the signs of placental and fetal infection.
- Acquire a working knowledge of procedures to be followed to maximize the chance of diagnosing the cause of an abortion.
- Acquire a working knowledge of the more common gestational abnormalities in the mare, including management of each condition.

STUDY QUESTIONS

1. Give the length of the embryonic, fetal, and neonatal periods of the horse.
2. List signs of embryonic loss in the mare, and discuss methods that can be used to confirm it.
3. Discuss management options for embryonic death in the mare.
4. List the causes of placental dysfunction in the mare.
5. List the more common infectious and noninfectious causes of abortion in the mare.
6. Explain why most aborted fetuses submitted for examination are 6 to 11 months of gestational age.
7. Explain how placentitis results in abortion.
8. Identify the routes of placental and fetal invasion by microorganisms.
9. Design a thorough diagnostic approach to an abortion problem on a broodmare farm.
10. Describe the more common gestational abnormalities in the mare, and discuss methods of diagnosis, treatment, and probable outcomes for each.

In a review of publications of pregnancy losses in horses, Ginther (1992) suggests an average expected loss rate of 18% when pregnancy diagnosis is done at 20 days after ovulation. He also notes that the loss rate per day should be expected to remain steady until approximately 60 days of gestation, after which loss rate per day should decline. Other reviewers have reported that equine pregnancy loss occurs with greater frequency early in pregnancy than later. Bain reported that, of pregnancies that were lost, 55% occurred by day 39 of gestation and 75% by day 49. Most authors agree that the rate

of pregnancy loss apparently diminishes after day 60 to 75 of gestation. In a recent 5-year review of breeding records from a Quarter Horse–type herd, Texas workers reported an 11.0% pregnancy loss rate (79 of 715), with 42% of the losses occurring by 42 days of gestation. A similar proportion of losses occurred with the fall pregnancy examination (2 to 5 months of gestation), with 17% of losses occurring later (>5 months) in gestation (Figure 8-1). Within individual mares with early loss of pregnancy, subsequent pregnancy loss is reportedly not different from that in the rest of the mare population

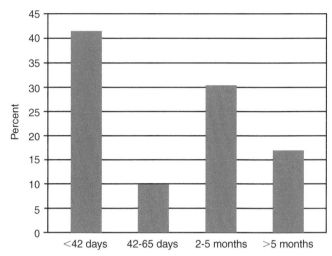

Figure 8-1 Distribution of pregnancy losses over a 5-year period in a Quarter Horse–type herd in southeast Texas. Overall pregnancy loss rate was 11.0% (79 of 715). Stillbirths and neonatal deaths are not included.

(i.e., pregnancy loss is no more likely to recur than in mares without previous pregnancy loss). In spite of this report, some mares seem to be predisposed to recurring pregnancy losses. In addition, pregnancy loss rates tend to gradually increase in broodmares older than 12 to 15 years of age. Thus, a widely held belief is that aged barren mares not only are less likely to become pregnant than maiden or foaling mares but are also more likely to lose the pregnancy.

Many genetic, maternal, and environmental factors can contribute to pregnancy loss during critical periods of development. These periods include the **embryonic period** (conception through organogenesis), the **fetal period** (completion of organogenesis through end of gestation), the **natal period** (birth), and the **neonatal period** (first 28 days of life). The susceptibility of the embryo to injurious agents varies with the stage of development. Cattle and sheep embryos less than 14 days of age (period of preattachment) are resistant to teratogens but susceptible to genetic mutations and chromosomal abnormalities. During the rest of the embryonic period, the embryo is highly susceptible to teratogens until this susceptibility begins to decrease as the various organ systems develop. The **embryonic period** in the equine includes *the period from conception to 40 days of gestation* (according to review by Ginther, 1992).

Limitations in accurate determination that conception has occurred prevent accurate assessment of the incidence of **embryonic death** in most animals. For the equine, the rate of pregnancy loss between days 15 and 50 after ovulation has been reported to be 10% to 15%. These estimates are based on losses that occur after early pregnancy diagnosis with transrectal ultrasonography. Estimates of earlier pregnancy loss (i.e., before ultrasonographic detection is possible at 10 to 14 days after ovulation) are more difficult to assess but have

been obtained from flushing uteri on different days (7 to 10 days after ovulation) and comparing actual embryo recovery rates at those times with known fertilization rates obtained in other populations of mares (by determining whether ova are cleaved in the oviducts). Nonrecovered oocytes or embryos, a problem with any recovery methodology, add a measure of inaccuracy to such estimates.

Estimates for embryonic death rates in the equine vary from 5% to 24% and average 20% for conception to day 40 of gestation in some groups of fertile mares. Because fertilization rates are generally quite high in both fertile and subfertile mares (exceeding 80% to 90%), a significant cause of subfertility may be early embryonic death. New York researchers reported the incidence of embryonic death before day 14 of gestation to be 7 to 8 times as frequent for aged subfertile mares as for young fertile mares. Other investigators have found that older mares are more likely to produce defective oocytes that presumably, when fertilized, are more susceptible to embryonic death.

The nonviable embryo is resorbed or expelled from the uterus and is therefore seldom observed. If embryonic death occurs before maternal recognition of pregnancy, affected mares return to estrus at the usual time expected if the mares had failed to conceive (i.e., interestrus interval of 3 weeks). In such cases, early embryonic death goes unsuspected. When interestrus intervals are prolonged (e.g., beyond 24 to 25 days), embryonic death with delayed return to estrus can be suspected.

CAUSES OF EMBRYONIC DEATH

Possible causes of embryonic death include infectious agents, chromosomal abnormalities, teratogenic agents, immunologic reactions, genetic abnormalities, local oviductal or uterine disturbances, nutritional factors (particularly deficient dietary energy or protein intake), and temperature stress. Ball (1993) divides potential factors that contribute to embryonic mortality into three general areas: (1) maternal; (2) external; and (3) embryonic.

Maternal Factors

- Endocrine: Low progesterone production from *failure of maternal recognition of pregnancy, primary luteal deficiency,* or *uterine-induced luteolysis* caused by endometrial irritation (e.g., endometritis).
- Oviductal environment: Reduced levels of embryotrophic factors, elevated levels of embryotoxic factors, improper timing of oviductal transport; *salpingitis.*
- Uterine environment: Commonly including *endometritis* and *periglandular fibrosis;* intraluminal fluid accumulation (often from endometritis) during early pregnancy; endometrial cysts when embryonic vesicle fixation occurs at cyst location.

- Age: Increased embryonic death rates as mares age; attributed in part to age-related degeneration of the uterus and oocyte quality.
- Lactation: If nutritional demands result in *declining body condition; delayed uterine involution* or *persistent endometritis.*
- Age-related anatomic changes in the genital tract (such as those that lead to pneumovagina, urovagina, or a pendant uterus that drains poorly and accumulates fluid) can contribute to infection that compromises the fetal-placental unit, thereby leading to pregnancy loss.

External Factors

- Stress: Hypothesized to decrease progesterone production, which may result in pregnancy loss.
- Inadequate nutrition: Particularly when mares lose body condition in late gestation or early lactation.
- Ingestion of toxins or infectious agents: Particularly those that have a predilection for the developing fetus. Consumption of Eastern tent caterpillars has been linked in mares in central Kentucky to a reproductive loss syndrome termed mare reproductive loss syndrome (MRLS).

Embryonic Factors

- Small size, morphologic defects.
- Embryos from aged subfertile mares have reduced survival rates when transferred to uteri of normal recipient mares.
- Chromosomal abnormalities: From *gamete aging* or other causes.

DIAGNOSIS OF EMBRYONIC DEATH

In a thorough discussion of ultrasonographically detectable signs of impending embryonic loss, Newcombe (2000) suggests the following criteria for predicting its occurrence:

Small-for-Age Embryonic Vesicles

Embryonic vesicles are sometimes visible as early as days 10 to 11 after ovulation, at a diameter of 3 to 4 mm. Vesicle size (diameter, top to bottom) typically increases 3 to 4 mm in diameter each day until day 16, plateaus during days 17 to 25, and resumes increasing in diameter by 1.8 mm/day by day 28 (Ginther, 1986). Whenever the diameter of the vesicle (through 30 days) is retarded in development by more than 1 to 2 days, particularly when undersized on more than one examination, embryonic viability should be questioned (Figure 8-2). Colorado workers recently found that the percentage of examinations during which the vesicle was found to be undersized was significantly higher for abnormal conceptuses (44.4%) than for normal conceptuses (<1%). Some veterinary ultrasound machines are programmed with gestation tables that permit the practitioner to

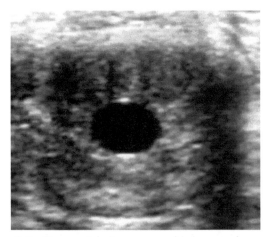

Figure 8-2 Transrectal ultrasonographic image of an embryonic vesicle 16 days after ovulation. The vesicle was smaller than expected (only approximately 1 cm in diameter) for gestational age, and the pregnancy was lost by day 21.

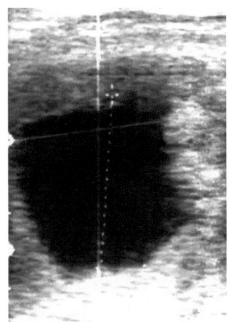

Figure 8-3 Transrectal ultrasonographic image of a small-for-gestational-age embryonic vesicle on day 32 after ovulation. The vesicle had been normal sized on days 14 and 16 after ovulation, but no embryo was visualized on days 27 or 32. The conceptus was no longer detectable by day 36.

estimate gestational age based on ultrasonographic measurements, which is useful for determining whether conceptuses are small for gestational age.

Anembryonic Vesicles

On occasion, vesicles fail to develop an embryo (Figure 8-3). Such vesicles often are first noted to be small for gestational age when detected early in pregnancy before the embryo is visible with ultrasound (typically by days 20 to 21). If an embryo is not visible by days 24 to 26, embryonic viability should be questioned. Colorado workers have found the incidence of anembryonic vesicles to be 4.4%.

Retarded Development of the Embryo

Normal progression in embryo development, as outlined in Chapter 5, should be apparent during examination for pregnancy. With use of B-mode ultrasonography, the embryo proper is typically apparent by 21 days and the embryonic heartbeat by 24 to 25 days. The allantois should occupy approximately half of the vesicle by 28 to 30 days and most of the vesicle (with the embryo having migrated dorsally within the vesicle) by 33 to 36 days; it should migrate to the ventrum of the allantois by 48 to 50 days. The embryo should also increase in size and development during this time. When development is retarded, heart beat is lost, allantoic shrinkage occurs, or separation of membranes from the endometrium occurs (Figure 8-4), impending pregnancy loss should be suspected.

Abnormalities of Embryo Location and Orientation

Ginther (2007) postulates there are three potential contributors to final orientation of the equine vesicle with the embryo ending up located in the ventral (antimesometrial) position within the uterine horn. Those contributors are (1) differences in tensile strength between two-celled and three-celled layers of the vesicle (i.e., two layers without interposed mesoderm on one side, with three layers including mesoderm [from which embryo develops] on the other side); (2) differential dorsal thickening of the endometrium (encroachment) at the site of fixation; and (3) massaging action of uterine contractions. Ginther notes that the vesicle "rolls" during migration through the uterine lumen before fixation so that orientation of the vesicle before fixation is variable. Immediately after fixation, the previous factors are involved in orienting the embryonic vesicle so that the embryo finally appears in the 6 o'clock position (antimesometrial) within the uterine horn. As

pregnancy progresses, the embryo moves dorsally to the 12 o'clock position (mesometrial) within the vesicle during allantoic development and then migrates ventrally as the umbilicus lengthens (back to the antimesometrial position).

Although many singleton pregnancies (beyond 21 days of gestation) have been noted to be in an altered orientation within the uterine horn, variations from the usual have not been proved to be prone to embryonic death. When unilateral twins are present, and one conceptus is spontaneously reduced, it is not uncommon for the eventual orientation of the embryo of the surviving conceptus to be altered. Altered orientation of the embryo also commonly results from development of a conceptus adjacent to an endometrial cyst (Figure 8-5). In these two conditions, the normal mechanism of dorsal endometrial thickening (encroachment) and the massaging action of uterine contractions may be interfered with in some manner by the adjacent twin or cyst.

The embryonic vesicle almost invariably becomes fixed and develops at the flexure (base) of one of the uterine horns. Rarely, the embryonic vesicle develops within the body of the uterus (*body pregnancy*) instead of at the base of one of the uterine horns. Body pregnancies are thought to be prone to failure even though early development appears normal.

Development Adjacent to Endometrial Cysts

The influence of endometrial cysts on fertility is discussed in Chapter 5. Although whether endometrial cysts affect fertility independent of mare age (from age-related changes in the endometrium that are often present in addition to cysts) remains controversial, when the embryonic vesicle develops adjacent to a cyst, an increased likelihood of pregnancy failure may be found.

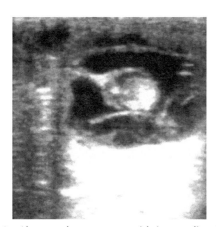

Figure 8-4 Abnormal pregnancy with impending loss is evident in this transrectal ultrasonographic image of a conceptus on day 38 after ovulation. An embryonic heartbeat was not present, and the chorioallantois had separated from the endometrium.

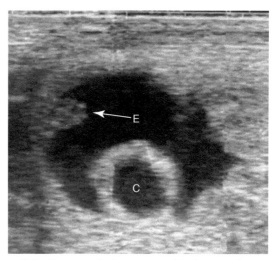

Figure 8-5 Transrectal ultrasonographic image of a 21-day-old conceptus developing over an endometrial cyst. The embryo *(E)* is located in a more dorsal position than typical as a result of disorientation of the conceptus *(C)*.

Certainly many such pregnancies continue to develop normally, with viable foals being delivered at term, so the size of the cyst and early orientation of the embryo in relation to the cyst may be important (Figure 8-6). Newcombe (2000) hypothesized that when the embryo begins development adjacent to the uterine wall, it is likely to develop normally, whereas if it begins development directly adjacent to a cyst, nutrient deprivation is more likely to occur and can result in pregnancy loss, similar to the deprivation hypothesis for spontaneous twin reduction proposed by Ginther (1992).

DEVELOPMENT OF UTERINE EDEMA DURING EARLY PREGNANCY

On occasion, a mare in early pregnancy (14 to 17 days after ovulation) has development of pronounced uterine edema, sometimes associated with behavioral estrus. Assay of progesterone concentration sometimes reveals a low concentration consistent with estrus. Some such pregnancies can be salvaged with immediate administration of progesterone or progestogen, which should be continued until either another ovulation occurs and forms a functional corpus luteum or progesterone supplementation is no longer deemed necessary to support the pregnancy (usually by 100 to 150 days of gestation). Newcombe (2000) suggests that conceptuses in such mares are more likely to be abnormal, particularly when embryonic vesicles are smaller than expected at 12 to 14 days after ovulation; thus, they are more likely to fail even though progesterone supplementation is

implemented. An additional cause to be considered is developing endometritis (Figure 8-7), which can precipitate endometrial prostaglandin-$F_2\alpha$ ($PGF_2\alpha$) release. Close monitoring of embryonic development is warranted in such progesterone-supplemented mares.

MANAGEMENT OF MARES WITH SIGNS OF ABNORMAL EMBRYONIC DEVELOPMENT

With the exception of progesterone and progestogen supplementation of mares developing uterine edema during early pregnancy, the most prudent management of mares with signs of abnormal embryonic development is serial reexaminations at intervals of 1 to 3 days. Colorado workers suggest that if an embryo and heartbeat cannot be identified with ultrasound by day 25 (Figure 8-8), monitoring through day 30 is indicated. If a viable embryo with an evident heartbeat does not become apparent by this time, $PGF_2\alpha$ should be administered to induce luteal regression and return to estrus for rebreeding. Newcombe (2000) also suggests that manual crushing of the conceptus at the time of induced luteolysis, immediately followed by uterine lavage to remove any remaining embryonic debris, might improve chances of conception when such mares are immediately rebred. We have noted that cloudy fluid accumulates in the uterus of some mares after the conceptus is manually crushed, so performing uterine lavage after the crush procedure is recommended. Treatment for more than 1 day may be necessary.

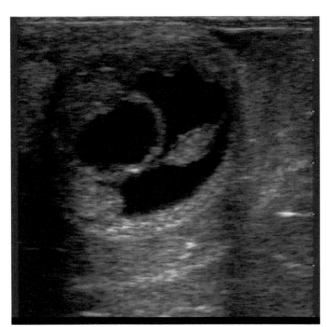

Figure 8-6 Transrectal ultrasonographic image of an embryonic vesicle developing adjacent to an endometrial cyst 28 days after ovulation. This pregnancy was maintained to term.

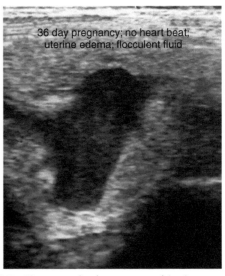

Figure 8-7 Transrectal ultrasonographic image obtained during a pregnancy recheck on day 36 after ovulation. An embryo with heartbeat was no longer detectable, and endometrial edema had developed. The remaining fluid had a flocculent character.

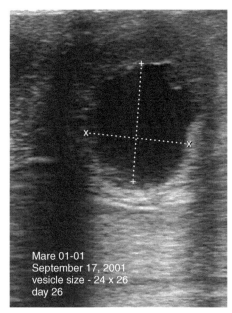

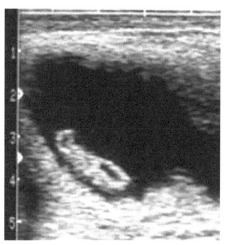

Figure 8-9 Transrectal ultrasonographic image from exam performed on day 42 after ovulation. The embryo is dead, with no heartbeat or activity. Ballottement of the uterus caused the dead fetus to float up and down.

Figure 8-8 Transrectal ultrasonographic image of an anembryonic vesicle on day 26 after ovulation. The pregnancy should be reexamined at 30 days after ovulation, and if no embryo is visible at that time, PGF$_2\alpha$ should be administered to induce return of the mare to estrus before the formation of endometrial cups.

PREGNANCY LOSS BEYOND THE EMBRYONIC PERIOD

Early fetal death (i.e., abortion early in gestation), or pregnancy loss beyond 40 days gestation, usually occurs with no premonitory signs. The expelled fetus and membranes may be found in stall bedding or on pasture but frequently go unnoticed. Ultrasound examination during the period of early fetal death (before expulsion) may reveal intact membranes and fetal fluids of normal echogenicity but a dead fetus (no heartbeat, inactive) (Figure 8-9). In other cases, fetal fluids become more hyperechoic (flocculent or "fuzzy") in appearance, suggesting the presence of debris or purulent material (Figure 8-10).

Most commonly, early fetal death is idiopathic and of sporadic incidence. Although no specific pathogens that restrict their attack to the early fetus have been identified, the agents involved in mare reproductive loss syndrome (MRLS) were first thought to have a predilection for pregnancy during the early fetal period. Texas and Kentucky workers showed that the increased fetal losses occurred without a concurrent increase in embryonic losses, despite that many mares carrying embryos (<40 days of gestation) were exposed on the same farms during the outbreak. University of Kentucky workers identified Eastern tent caterpillar involvement in MRLS, which presented as a multifaceted clinical syndrome with pericarditis and unilateral uveitis in adult horses, birth of weak foals, and early (40 to 150 days gestation) fetal loss. However, most susceptible

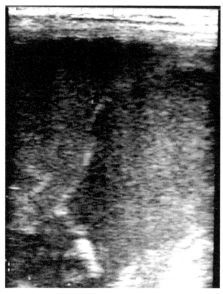

Figure 8-10 Transrectal ultrasonographic image of "cloudy" (increasingly echogenic) fetal fluids obtained when rechecking a pregnancy of a Thoroughbred mare in the first trimester of gestation during an MRLS outbreak. With repositioning of the probe, fetal thorax and other remnants could be visualized. (Courtesy Dr. James Morehead, Equine Medical Associates, PSC, Lexington, Ky.)

pregnancies were in this early stage of gestation when the outbreak occurred. Later, less severe outbreaks with signs consistent with MRLS (abortion with amnionitis or funiculitis) involved fetuses of later gestational age. Outbreaks of abortion (early or late fetal loss) of similar presentation have been described elsewhere in the United States and in other countries.

When embryonic death (<35 to 40 days) occurs during the breeding season, there is a good chance the affected mare will return to a fertile estrus and thus become pregnant again before the breeding season ends. Regardless of the cause of early fetal death, if endometrial cups are present, the affected mare can rarely be successfully rebred with establishment of another pregnancy during the same breeding season (Figure 8-11). For this reason, early fetal death usually results in failure to produce a foal for another year.

Fetal susceptibility to teratogens decreases with increasing age, except for those structures that differentiate later (e.g., cerebellum, palate, and urogenital system). Regarding infection, the extent of fetal damage that occurs likewise depends on fetal age at the time of infection and degree of fetal immunocompetence, virulence of the infectious agent, and extent of placental lesions and degree of placental dysfunction.

Although the exact level of function necessary to support fetal life and development is difficult to define, a critical level of placental function is deemed necessary to support the developing embryo and fetus to term. Therefore, **placental dysfunction** is a common cause of pregnancy loss. Possible causes of placental dysfunction include acute or chronic *placentitis, hypoxia* resulting from alterations in perfusion ratios between uterine and placental blood flow (as occurs with uterine torsion), a *defective placenta* (e.g., as occurs in hydrallantois), *inadequate placental attachment, edema of the placenta,* local immunologic reactions in the placenta, and *maternal disease or malnutrition.* Placental dysfunction may result in a malformed fetus, fetal death, mummification, abortion, fetal growth retardation (Figure 8-12), prematurity, full-term stillbirth, and neonatal weakness and death.

Low birth weights in neonates are often attributed to placental dysfunction caused by infection with

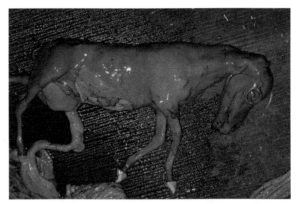

Figure 8-12 Intrauterine growth retardation (undersized for gestational age) was apparent in this aborted autolytic equine fetus.

microorganisms. Signs in the neonate (such as neonatal weakness and septicemia) that may occur as a result of fetal infection in utero are usually encountered in the first week of life, particularly within the first 24 hours.

Abortion is the termination of pregnancy before the conceptus is capable of extrauterine life. Causes of abortion can be *infectious* or *noninfectious.* The overall rate of abortion reported in the horse population varies from 5% to 15%, but "abortion storms" (outbreaks) have been reported in populations of susceptible pregnant broodmares exposed to reproductive pathogens (e.g., Equine herpesvirus [EHV-1], *Equine viral arteritis* [EVA], MRLS) (Figure 8-13). Observed abortions after 4 months of gestation usually account for a small fraction of equine pregnancy wastage; however, abortions before 4 months of gestation are rarely observed because fetal and placental tissues are relatively small and often overlooked in bedding or on pasture and genital discharges are usually scant after abortion at this early stage. Therefore, most aborted fetuses examined are 6 to 11 months of gestational age. Most equine abortions are the result of placental dysfunction.

Abortions may be acute or chronic in nature. **Acute abortions** occur with no premonitory signs, such as with Equine herpesvirus (EHV-1) abortion; **chronic abortions** follow premonitory signs, such as occurs with twin, mycotic, and most bacterial abortions. The fetus usually dies in utero, but some may be delivered alive yet nonviable. With all abortions, the placenta, fetus, and fluids should be regarded as *potentially infective* to other pregnant mares until EHV-1, leptospirosis, and *Salmonella abortus-equi* have been eliminated as causes. The percentage of equine abortions in which an etiologic cause is determined has been reported to be approximately 60%.

Placentitis is the lesion most common to causes of infectious abortion. For a discussion of the diagnosis and treatment of placentitis, refer to Chapter 9. In **acute placentitis,** hyperemia and hemorrhage lead to

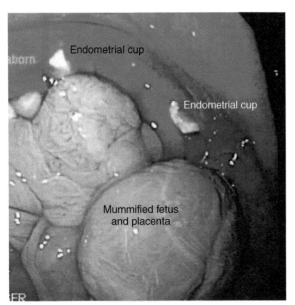

Figure 8-11 Endoscopic view of early fetal death with presence of endometrial cups and mummified fetus and fetal membranes. Mummification of the dead fetus is an uncommon occurrence; the dead fetus and membranes are usually expelled from the tubular tract.

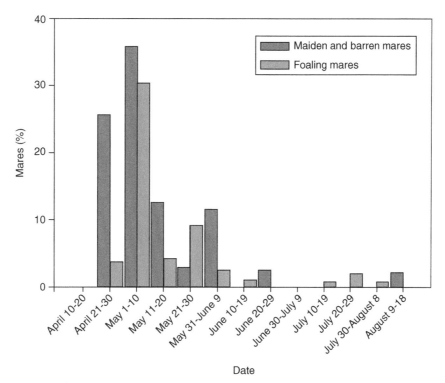

Date

Figure 8-13 Distribution of early fetal losses during 10-day periods in a population of pregnant Thoroughbred mares on four farms in Kentucky during spring 2001. In this population of 288 pregnant mares, 90% of the losses occurred between April 27 and June 26, with the median date of losses being May 7. The syndrome (abortion storm) was later defined as mare reproductive loss syndrome (MRLS) and was found to be related to exposure to an unusually high population of Eastern tent caterpillars. University of Kentucky workers estimated more than 30% of the Thoroughbred foal crop was lost. (Modified from Morehead JP, Blanchard TL, Thompson JA, et al: Evaluation of early fetal losses on four equine farms in central Kentucky: 73 cases, *J Amer Vet Med Assoc* 220:1828-1830, 2002.)

degeneration and necrosis that extends from the chorionic villi to the surrounding chorioallantois. Organisms and toxins then invade and kill the fetus. In **chronic placentitis,** infection extending through the placenta leads to edema and thickening of the chorioallantois, causing gradual separation of affected chorionic villi. As the edema progresses, the affected chorioallantois changes color from bright red to yellow, and even to a leathery brown (Figures 8-14 and 8-15). Few diseases have been implicated as affecting the amnion, but amnionitis (Figure 8-16) and

funiculitis (inflammation of cord portion of placenta) were implicated as components of abortions from MRLS that were seen in some cases.

Placental invasion by microorganisms can occur hematogenously (e.g., leptospirosis), by extension from the uterus, or more commonly by ascending from the vagina (e.g., streptococci, fungi) (see Figure 8-14). When

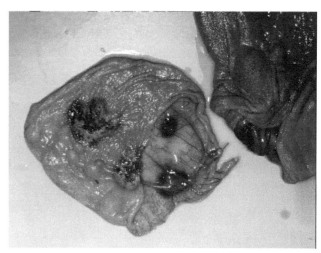

Figure 8-14 Thickened yellow-brown areas of chronic placentitis. An ascending pattern of placentitis is apparent.

Figure 8-15 Section of placenta illustrating focal necrotic placentitis typical of fungal infection.

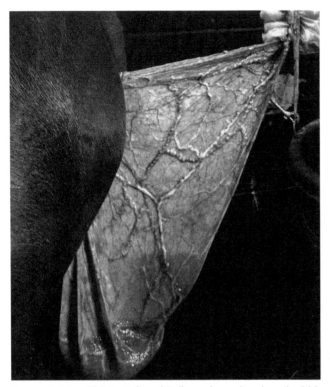

Figure 8-16 Thickened and inflamed amnion (amnionitis), with engorged vessels, from a Thoroughbred mare aborting a 270-day-old fetus during MRLS outbreak. (Courtesy Dr. James Morehead, Equine Medical Associates, PSC, Lexington, Ky.)

more discernible. Abortion of fetuses at 8 to 11 months of gestation is likely to be accompanied by apparent placental lesions (if the placenta was involved) and evident fetal lesions (because the fetus is becoming progressively more immunocompetent, permitting inflammatory reactions to occur). Full-term fetal deaths occur with **stillbirth** (i.e., birth of a term, full-sized fetus that is dead although it was alive in utero). Stillbirths occur commonly with dystocia, asphyxia, or sometimes with EHV-1 infection (Figures 8-18 and 8-19). **Dysmature fetuses** (small and underdeveloped for gestational age) are also often delivered as stillborn or as weak emaciated neonates (Figure 8-20).

Gross signs suggestive of intrauterine infection of the fetus include:
- Incomplete development of the fetus
- Fetal edema
- Fibrin stands or sheets in serous cavities of the abortus
- Necrotic foci in the abortus liver and other organs.
- Variable degrees of fetal autolysis

Microscopic lesions associated with intrauterine infection are found most commonly in the placenta and in fetal liver, lung, and intestine. Although fetal liver is one of the most commonly affected organs, because it undergoes autolysis quickly, the fetal lung is often more likely to yield identifiable lesions.

microorganisms *invade the fetus*, the organisms may invade *directly* (via the umbilical vein) or *indirectly* (via the amniotic fluid through fetal inhalation or ingestion or by invasion through the skin).

Dennis (1981) explains that aborted fetuses may be broadly divided into three groups: (1) those with no evidence of infection; (2) those with evidence of infection; and (3) those that are too autolytic to evaluate. Lesions detected in aborted fetuses are associated with the time of fetal death. Fetuses aborted at 4 to 6 months of gestation are usually autolytic (Figure 8-17), often from bacterial septicemia. Fetuses aborted at 6 to 8 months of gestation are usually less autolytic, and placental lesions are

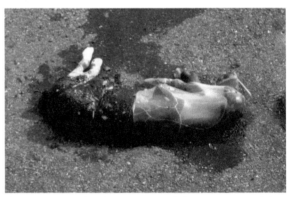

Figure 8-18 Fresh stillborn fetus delivered encased in placenta. Viral isolation procedures yielded EHV-1.

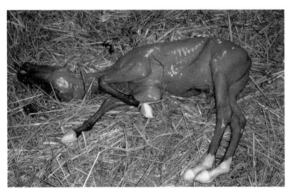

Figure 8-17 Autolytic 270-day-old fetus from mare in Figure 8-16. (Courtesy Dr. James Morehead, Equine Medical Associates, PSC, Lexington, Ky.)

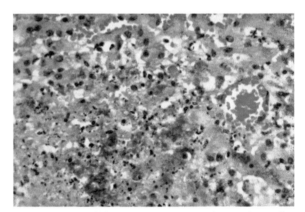

Figure 8-19 Focal hepatic necrosis in fetus aborted as a result of EHV-1 infection.

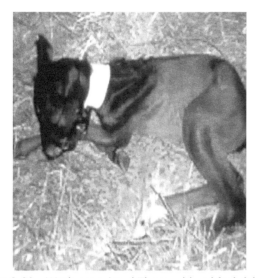

Figure 8-20 Weak, emaciated Thoroughbred foal delivered at 343 days of gestation. The foal was euthanized 7 days later because of toxemia and renal failure. The dam had begun premature udder development and lactation at 9 months of gestation, and placental separation was confirmed with transabdominal ultrasound examination. Treatment of the pregnant mare included administration of broad-spectrum antimicrobials for 3 weeks and an oral progestogen (Regumate) daily through term. Fetal heart rate remained within normal limits through birth. At delivery, the chorion of the placenta was covered with a thick tenacious brown exudate and had extensive villus atrophy and a chronic necrotizing placentitis caused by a gram-positive branching bacillus. (Courtesy Dr. D. Konkle, Equine Medical Associates, PSC, Lexington, Ky.)

Diagnosis of Abortions

Each abortion should be regarded as infective to other in-contact pregnant mares until proven otherwise. When more than one pregnant mare is present on the premises, an abortion should be treated as a potential herd problem. Because the gross placental and fetal findings with most causes of infectious abortion are similar and nonspecific, practitioners require laboratory assistance for diagnosis. The quality of laboratory assistance depends primarily on the practitioner. Laboratory assistance typically involves serologic, microbiologic, and histopathologic procedures.

A **complete history** should be submitted with specimens sent to a diagnostic laboratory and should include:
- Reproductive history of the mare
- Stage of pregnancy at which abortion occurred
- Other pregnant animals involved (i.e., an abortion outbreak) or in contact with (exposed to) the mare aborting
- Clinical signs observed before and after abortion
- Herd or group history: Vaccinations, diseases, closed or open herd, other animals transported to and from competition events or shows, and so on
- Housing and environment of the dam.
- Sources of feed and water.

Specimens submitted to the diagnostic laboratory should be collected and sent as promptly as possible to avoid development of autolytic changes that interfere with diagnosis. The best specimen to submit is the *aborted fetus and placenta.* This should be placed in a leak-proof plastic bag or container and should be transported *chilled* (not frozen) to the laboratory. If submitting the entire fetus and placenta is not practical, a field postmortem examination should be performed and the following samples should be submitted to the diagnostic laboratory in separate labeled containers:

1. Intact *stomach and contents.* Tie off the esophagus and duodenum.
2. *Liver*
3. *Lung*
4. *Kidney*
5. *Spleen*
6. *Adrenal glands*
7. *Placenta.* Submit as much as possible. Although isolation of an infectious agent from the placenta does not establish pathogenicity, with histologic involvement, diagnosis can sometimes be made directly from the placenta for mycotic abortions (see Figure 8-10) and occasional bacterial abortions (e.g., *Nocardia*).
8. *Uterine fluid*

Although less desirable, instead of submitting the fetus or tissue samples for bacteriologic examination, swabs can be taken from abdominal and thoracic fluids, stomach contents, liver, lung, spleen, and cardiac blood. With a badly decomposed fetus, brain contents can be collected aseptically for bacteriologic examination. Uterine swabbings can also be taken from the aborting dam for culture.

Items 2 to 7 should also be submitted in 10% buffered neutral **formalin** for histology.

Fetal serum (if possible) and peritoneal fluid can be submitted for **serologic examination**. *Paired serum samples* should be submitted from the dam. Collect acute and convalescent (i.e., at the time of abortion and approximately 2 to 3 weeks later) serum samples from the dam and submit as paired samples to the diagnostic laboratory. A rising or falling serum titer for a given infectious agent after abortion provides circumstantial evidence for it as the causative agent. However, a rising titer is often not seen if the abortion follows infection by a few weeks or more. In some cases, a very high titer may be found that is suggestive of a cause (e.g., *Leptospira*). Interpretation of serologic data is most reliable when microbiologic, histologic, and cytologic findings are also taken into consideration.

Noninfectious causes of abortion also exist for the mare. The most common noninfectious cause of abortion is twinning (see next section "Gestational Abnormalities"). Other noninfectious causes of abortion include fescue toxicosis, congenital anomalies, uterine body pregnancy, maternal stress and malnutrition, and possible hormonal abnormalities.

A summary of the more common causes of equine abortion, including recommendations regarding prevention, is presented in Table 8-1.

TABLE 8-1

Diagnostic Summary of Some Common Abortion-Causing Diseases of Horses

Disease	Etiology	Clinical Signs	Placental Lesions
Equine rhinopneumonitis (EHV-1)	Equine herpesvirus 1 Incubation up to 4 mo; abortions 1 to 4 mo after respiratory outbreak in weanlings	Primarily a respiratory disease but also causes late abortions (>5 mo), stillbirths, or weak infected foals (septicemia, viremia); can produce abortion storms (1% to 90%) Respiratory disease and abortions rarely seen concurrently Occasionally seen with neurologic form of disease	None apart from some edema Chorioallantois usually separates from endometrium; thus, fetus usually expelled fresh and often *within* the intact fetal membranes Usually no retained fetal membranes
Equine streptococcal abortion	*Streptococcus zooepidemicus*	Sporadic abortion often <200 days but can occur at any stage	*Chronic placentitis:* May show ascending pattern
Nocardioform placentitis abortion	Unclassified gram-positive filamentous branching bacteria	Sporadic abortions, usually in late gestation (8 to 11 mo) with extensive placental involvement; usually accompanied with impending signs of abortion, such as premature lactation	Focally extensive placentitis evident predominantly in the portions of the placenta that occupy the base of the uterine horns or cranial uterine body
Other bacterial abortions	*Escherichia coli, Pseudomonas aeruginosa*	Sporadic abortions often >200 days but can occur at any stage	*Chronic placentitis:* May show ascending pattern
Equine mycotic abortion	*Aspergillus fumigatus, Allescheria boydii, Mucor* spp.; primarily ascending infection	Sporadic abortions, usually at 5 to 11 mo of gestation (most around 10 mo)	*Chronic placentitis:* Chorion is extensively involved; edematous and necrotic, with adherent viscous exudate; typical plaques are round with necrotic centers Amniotic lesions in only 10% of cases; necrotic plaques
Leptospirosis	*Leptospira interrogans;* serotypes: *pomona, canicola, autumnalis*	Mild disease in horses except for periodic ophthalmia (moon blindness) Abortion is rare; occasionally follows mild illness by 1 to 3 wk Late abortions >6 mo	Not specific

Fetal Lesions	Laboratory Diagnosis	Other
Fresh: Little or no autolysis; mild icterus, hydrothorax, hydroperitoneum; multifocal hepatic necrosis (1-mm to 2-mm diameter foci); pulmonary edema or congestion Histopathologic findings: Necrotic foci in liver with eosinophilic *intranuclear inclusions* in surrounding hepatocytes Inclusions may also be in bronchiolar and alveolar epithelium, spleen, and adrenal cortex	Histopathologic findings: *Pathognomonic intranuclear inclusions* Fluorescence antibody test (FAT): fetal liver, lung, thymus Viral isolation Serology: Not a definitive test (just indicates exposure to virus); rising complement fixation (CF) titer in paired sera may aid in diagnosis	Presumptive diagnosis with fresh fetus and gross lesions Vaccine does not guarantee protection against abortion but should reduce the incidence of EHV-1 abortion in a herd Until more is known about vaccine protection, avoid switching types or brands of vaccine during pregnancy Management: Isolation of weanlings and yearlings, aborting mares; separation of pregnant mares; closed herd
Septic fetus, variable degrees of autolysis; congestion, yellow-red dirty discoloration of tissues Excessive fluid in pleural and peritoneal cavities, scattered petechiae	Culture: Placenta, fetus, uterine discharge Organism readily isolated Direct smear of placental surface: Gram-positive cocci Histopathologic findings: Gram-positive cocci and low-grade inflammation	Most common cause of bacterial abortion No vaccine; prevent ascending infection
Fetus may be small for gestational age and emaciated; may be expelled alive	*Culture:* Placenta, fetus, uterine discharge; demonstration of organism in placental lesions; bacteria grow slowly on blood agar	No effective treatment developed as yet because disease is incompletely understood Has become most commonly identified cause of placentitis in central Kentucky in recent years
No specific lesions; septic fetus, variable degrees of autolysis	Culture: Placenta, fetus, uterine discharge; organism readily isolated Direct smear of placental surface; gram-negative rods Histopathologic findings: Gram-negative rods and low-grade inflammation	*E. coli* second most common bacterial cause of abortion No vaccine; prevent ascending infection
Fetus small for gestational age and emaciated (as with any chronic placental dysfunction); may be expelled alive; rare lesions, occasional 1-mm to 3-mm gray-white nodules in lungs (2% of cases); skin lesions quite rare	*Culture:* Placenta, fetus (lung, liver); *hyphae* in chronic placental lesions and fetal stomach contents	May account for 5% to 30% of all infectious abortions No vaccine; prevent ascending infection
Usually autolytic	*Culture:* Leptospires in fetal fluid or blood; laboratory animal inoculation; darkfield or phase-contrast microscopy FAT Serology-paired sera	Leptospirosis endemic in horses (i.e., in some studies, 50% of horses have titer of 1:400 to 1:800) No vaccine prepared for the equine; protection afforded by cattle vaccines questionable

Continued

TABLE 8-1

Diagnostic Summary of Some Common Abortion-Causing Diseases of Horses—cont'd

Disease	Etiology	Clinical Signs	Placental Lesions
Equine infectious anemia (EIA)	Retrovirus	Abortions usually last half of gestation; low incidence rate	Not specific
Protozoal abortion (piroplasmosis)	*Babesia caballi* or *Thelaria equi* (formerly *Babesia equi*)	Some severely stressed mares abort Mares may have pronounced icterus or hemoglobinuria	Not specific
Equine viral arteritis (EVA)	Togavirus	Rare outbreaks of severe systemic and respiratory disease with abortion as a complication; abort within 1 to 14 days of onset of clinical signs in these cases; however, abortions reported to occur with only mild or no visible illness of mares No retained fetal membranes	Autolytic
Twinning	Placental insufficiency 65% to 70% of twins are aborted or stillbirths	Most abort by 8 to 11 mo of gestation, but can occur at any stage Abortion often follows premature mammary development	Contacting surfaces of twin placentas are devoid of chorionic villi
Uterine body pregnancy	Placental insufficiency	Majority abort by 8 to 11 mo of gestation, but can occur at any stage	Placenta fails to extend fully into uterine horns (short placental horns noted during examination of expelled fetal membranes)

GESTATIONAL ABNORMALITIES

The more common gestational abnormalities in the mare include twinning, premature placental separation, uterine torsion, hydrallantois, and ruptured prepubic tendon. Pathologic prolonged gestation is a rare condition in the mare and is usually related to fescue toxicosis. Fetal mummification, with the exception of a mummified twin, is a rare occurrence.

Twinning is an undesirable condition in the mare. If twins are not reduced to a singleton at an early stage of gestation, the usual outcome is late-term abortion (Figures 8-21 and 8-22). Few twins are carried to term and survive. Complications that can arise with late-term abortion of twins, or delivery of twins at term, include dystocia, retained placenta, delayed uterine involution and metritis, and of course, death of one or both twins. Although confirmation of monozygotic twins was recently described by Texas workers, it is still believed that most twins arise from double ovulations; thus, most twins are believed to be dizygotic. As one would suspect,

the incidence of twin conceptions varies with breed and is more common in those breeds with a higher incidence of multiple ovulations (e.g., Thoroughbreds have the highest incidence rate of multiple ovulations at approximately 15% to 25%). English workers have raised concern that the now routine method of manually reducing

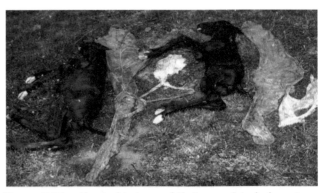

Figure 8-21   Aborted twins and their associated placentas.

Fetal Lesions	Laboratory Diagnosis	Other
Not specific	Isolate virus	No vaccine; no effective treatment
	Agar gel immunodiffusion test: mare sera (100% of horses have titer by 45 days after infection)	
Excessive fluid in pleural and peritoneal cavities	FAT: Fetal red blood cells (RBCs) of foal or dam	Primarily limited to Florida
Mild icterus sometimes	CF test: Mare sera	
Autolytic	FAT: Fetal tissues	Can be transmitted venereally via infected semen
No specific gross lesions	Viral isolation (culture of aborted fetus)	Infection is endemic in Standardbred horses
	Serology (virus neutralization test): Antibodies develop 1 to 2 wk after infection and persist for years	Vaccine available but generally requires approval of state and federal authorities (i.e., live virus vaccine); mares bred to known shedding stallions should be vaccinated before breeding
	Clinical findings in aborting mares	
Retarded growth	Placenta (lack of chorionic villi on portion of chorion that contacts placenta of twin)	Most common cause of equine abortion (20% to 30% of all diagnosed abortions)
Often have mummification of one of the twin fetuses	Twin fetuses, sometimes mummies	
Retarded growth	Short-horned placenta	Uncommon occurrence

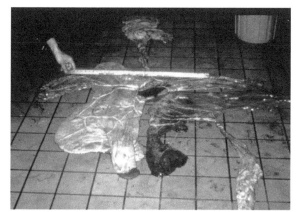

Figure 8-22 The placentas from this set of aborted twins occupied approximately equal portions of the uterus.

twins to a singleton pregnancy, which has been highly successful, may be increasing the prevalence of double-ovulating twin-producing mares in the population (i.e., because of a possible genetic component that controls multiple ovulations, producing more foals from multiple ovulating mares might result in raising more fillies that end up producing multiple ovulations when they enter the broodmare population).

Multiple ovulations may be *synchronous* (occurring within 1 day of each other) or *asynchronous* (occurring more than 1 day apart). Synchronous ovulations (when more than one oocyte is fertilized) often produce twin conceptuses similar in size when examined with ultrasound; asynchronous ovulations produce twin conceptuses that can vary in size by several millimeters. Once twin conceptuses are present within the uterus, they migrate throughout both uterine horns and the uterine body (Figure 8-23) just as singleton conceptuses do. When the conceptuses become fixed in the same uterine horn at 16 to 17 days of gestation, they are referred

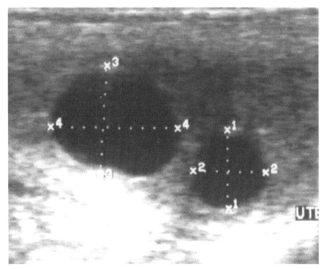

Figure 8-23 Transrectal ultrasonographic image of twin conceptuses located within the body of the uterus on day 15 after ovulation.

to as *unilateral* (or unicornual) twins. If instead, each twin conceptus becomes fixed in a different uterine horn, they are referred to as *bilateral* (or bicornual) twins. Mares are able to spontaneously reduce unilateral twins to a singleton pregnancy with a high degree of efficiency (i.e., 75% of unilateral twins at 16 to 17 days of gestation are reduced to a singleton pregnancy by 40 days of gestation). However, mares with bilateral twin pregnancy, or with unilateral twin pregnancy beyond 40 days of gestation, are likely to abort both twins late in gestation when placental contact with the uterus becomes insufficient to maintain fetal life. In some cases, one twin dies and becomes mummified, allowing the other twin to continue to develop and be maintained to term. The area of adjacent placental contact is avillous, as contact with the uterus is prevented (Figure 8-24).

Diagnosis of twins is best made via transectal ultrasound examination at 14 to 15 days after ovulation, before fixation occurs. Performing the examination at this time reduces the chances of missing the smaller twin if the twins arose from asynchronous ovulations (because one twin is 1 to 2 days smaller in size, and thus more difficult to detect, than the other twin) yet permits the diagnosis to be made before fixation when the twin conceptuses might become fixed in one uterine horn. With unilateral twin fixation, it is extremely difficult to manually crush one twin without damaging the other. If twins are diagnosed, and are not yet fixed, they are more easily separated and one twin can be crushed (per rectum) (Figure 8-25). It remains controversial whether crushing of the smaller conceptus improves the probability that the remaining conceptus will survive to term, but most practitioners follow this practice. It is logical that the healthiest embryo, at least if synchronous ovulations occurred, is the larger one. With experience, success rates approximate 90% (i.e., 90% of singleton pregnancies carried to term) when one twin is manually reduced during the mobility phase of gestation. Mares that lose both pregnancies usually return to a fertile estrus within 2 weeks. The same technique Manual crushing can be applied for perhaps 1 to 2 weeks longer, with good success rates expected if bilateral fixation of twins has taken place. Highest success rates are achieved with twin reduction by crushing when it is attempted at less than 30 days of gestation. However, manual crushing of one twin becomes progressively less successful (i.e., both twins are lost) the longer the twins are allowed to survive before intervention. If both pregnancies are lost after endometrial cup formation (approximately days 36 to 40 of gestation), the mare usually does not return to fertile estrus until endometrial cups and supplementary corpora lutea spontaneously regress (e.g., approximately 3 months later), depending on the gestational age at the time of pregnancy loss. Even if supplementary corpora lutea are induced to regress with daily injections of

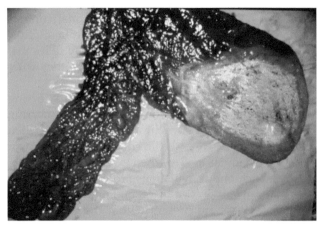

Figure 8-24 Avillous area of placenta where a mummified twin prevented contact of placenta with endometrium, thereby yielding an area devoid of villi.

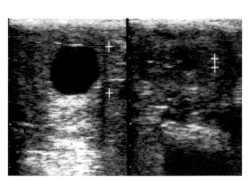

Figure 8-25 Ultrasonographic appearance of viable and nonviable twin conceptuses. The photograph was taken immediately after the conceptus on the right was manually crushed. A small amount of fluid remained in the luminal area where the conceptus was crushed.

prostaglandin-$F_2\alpha$, the induced estrus often will not result in the establishment of pregnancy while endometrial cups remain. More problematic is the tendency for developing follicles to become hemorrhagic or to luteinize rather than ovulate as long as endometrial cups remain active. The failure to ovulate precludes establishment of pregnancy. So, if twins are not spontaneously or manually reduced to a singleton pregnancy before 35 days of gestation, prostaglandin is usually administered (a single injection is sufficient to induce abortion before endometrial cup stimulation of supplementary corpora lutea formation) to ensure the mare returns to a fertile estrus in time to be rebred during the same breeding season.

Other methods of twin reduction to a singleton pregnancy that have been used with limited success include: aspiration of vesicle (allantoic) fluid through a needle inserted into the uterus per vagina (*transvaginal aspiration*) (Figure 8-26); injection of the allantoic space or fetal heart (again, through a needle inserted into the uterus per vagina) with a toxic substance such as colchicine, potassium chloride solution, or procaine penicillin G; or fetal cardiac puncture later in gestation, beyond 100 days, through a needle inserted into the uterus via transabdominal ultrasound–guided needle injection. Kentucky workers recently described a technique that they have had success with when reducing a twin of 60 to 90 days of gestation. The mare is given flunixin meglumine (1 mg/kg intravenously [IV]) and detomidine HCl (10 to 20 mg IV) before the procedure

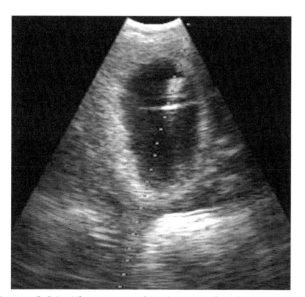

Figure 8-26 Ultrasonographic image of twin conceptus being reduced with ultrasound–guided transvaginal needle aspiration of allantoic fluid. The *dotted line* represents the direction the needle is expected to travel. A needle with an echogenic tip is used to facilitate visualization *(bright spot)* during the puncture procedure. When the needle is placed within the allantoic space, fluid is aspirated until the chorioallantois collapses. Some practitioners claim better results with injection of 2 to 3 mL of procaine penicillin G instead of aspiration of fluid.

is performed. With a rectal tocolytic (e.g., 60 to 120 mg Buscopan or 30 to 60 mg propantheline bromide, IV), the head of the smaller fetus is located with transrectal ultrasound examination. The transducer is removed from the rectum, and the hand is used to isolate the fetal head. The fetal head is stabilized between the thumb and forefinger, and the head is bent from side to side until ligaments are freed (making movement of the head easy). The thumb is then placed at the base of the head and pushed forward and dorsal until dislocation is achieved. The separation allows placement of the thumb and forefinger between the cervical vertebrae and the head. The procedure has also used in twin pregnancies by performing the procedure though a flank laparotomy or through a colpotomy. After surgery, regardless of technique, the mare is treated with Regumate (0.88 mg/kg, orally [PO]), along with parenteral antibiotics if surgical laparotomy was used. If treatment is successful, fetal heartbeat may take up to 40 days to cease, but the dead fetus and its membranes mummify and the other fetus continues to term.

To *induce abortion of twins* if they are detected between 40 and 110 days of gestation, multiple injections of prostaglandin-$F_2\alpha$ (once daily for 4 to 5 days) usually induce abortion of both conceptuses. For pregnancies that do not respond to multiple injections of prostaglandin (typically those beyond 110 to 150 days of gestation), the fetal membranes can be punctured transcervically and a toxic substance (such as dilute tamed-iodine solution) infused into the allantoic space. Infusion of dexamethasone has also been reported to be successful. Reexamination at intervals of 1 to 2 days is required to ensure that fetal death and expulsion of the fetuses and fetal membranes have occurred. Recently, South African workers have proposed the use of prostaglandin E2 (PGE_2) for elective abortion in mares 100 to 300 days of gestation. They instilled 0.5 to 1.5 mg PGE_2 into the cervical canal, followed in 2 hours by manual dilation of the cervix sufficient to allow the hand to be passed into the uterus. The fetus and fetal membranes were then extracted with no complications.

Body Pregnancy

Infrequently, the conceptus becomes fixed in the uterine body during early pregnancy *(body pregnancy)* as opposed to fixation in the flexure (base of either uterine horn). Further growth of the conceptus continues, but abortion usually follows later in gestation because of placental insufficiency. Placental insufficiency results from failure of the placenta to expand sufficiently into the two uterine horns. If a body pregnancy is detected after the period of embryonic mobility (i.e., after day 16 to 17 of gestation), the mare should be given a single injection of $PGF_2\alpha$ (or an analog) before day 35 of pregnancy to ensure early return to estrus and rebreeding. Caution should be exercised as body pregnancy is uncommon, and development of the pregnancy at the corpus corneal junction (just cranial to the uterine body–which may appear to be a body pregnancy on cursory examination) will most likely proceed to term.

Premature Placental Separation

Premature placental separation occurs most commonly during birth. The chorion separates from the endometrium without the fused chorioallantois rupturing and releasing allantoic fluid. Because gas exchange is impaired, the separation causes fetal hypoxia/anoxia that can contribute to weakness and dysmaturity ("dummy foal") or even stillbirth. The condition is diagnosed by visualizing the reddish, velvet-like surface of the chorion bulging between the vulvar labia during birth (Figure 8-27). The chorioallantois should be manually ruptured or incised to allow the fetus to be delivered without the placenta being forced along with it. The fetus may already be compromised, so fetal delivery should be accomplished as soon as possible once the membranes are ruptured and allantoic fluid is released. Resuscitative procedures may be necessary, including administration of oxygen, to save the foal's life (see Chapter 11).

Premature placental separation sometimes also occurs in mid to late gestation with placentitis, death of a fetal twin, or impending abortion. The mare may begin to *lactate prematurely* in such cases. When fetal membrane separation during gestation is suspected, a thorough examination of the reproductive tract, including assessment of fetal well being, should be performed (see Chapter 9). If abortion is imminent, assistance can be provided to ensure the mare delivers the abortus without dystocia. If the cervix is closed and the fetus is alive, therapy with progestogen (altrenogest or progesterone) or flunixin meglumine should be instituted. Pentoxyphylline (7.5 to10 mg/kg, every 8 to 12 hours PO or IV) may provide added benefit to improve malleability of red blood cells and thus potentially improve circulation through the intact placenta. Some practitioners have used clenbuterol (Ventipulmin Syrup, Boehringer Ingelheim, Ridgefield, Conn.) to prevent uterine contractions and thereby reduce placental separation and impending abortion. If concern about concurrent placentitis exists, systemic antimicrobial therapy can be added to the treatment regime. Treatment for 1 to 2 weeks is indicated, if abortion does not occur in the meantime. In some cases in which a fetal twin has died, the twin may mummify and be delivered at term with the other fetus.

Uterine Torsion

Uterine torsion occurs occasionally in pregnant mares, usually during mid to late term (5 to 9 months of gestation). Although it can occur in term mares, it is much less common at this time. The cause is speculative, sometimes thought to develop when a mare takes a sudden fall. The direction of the uterine twist can be either clockwise or counterclockwise (when viewed from the rear). Torsions of less than 180 degrees seldom cause a problem. Torsions greater than 180 degrees are painful and create a low-grade, persistent colic that is nonresponsive to analgesics (although some short-term relief may occur, abdominal pain returns). If the torsion restricts blood flow sufficiently, the uterus can become congested, friable, or even necrotic if left unattended. Unattended uterine torsions may lead to uterine rupture with loss of the fetus into the abdominal cavity. Alterations in blood flow from uterine torsion place the fetus at risk of hypoxia; if fetal death occurs, abortion follows in a few days to a week or more even if the torsion was corrected. In some cases in which uterine torsion is corrected and the fetus is alive when the mare is discharged from the hospital, abortion occurs 1 or 2 weeks later.

Uterine torsion is diagnosed by palpation of the genital tract per rectum. The direction of the twist is determined by following the broad ligaments to their respective ovaries; that is, a clockwise torsion presents with the left broad ligament passing over the top of the uterus (and down if the torsion is greater than 180 degrees) to the right, and the right broad ligament passes underneath the uterus toward the left. The broad ligament passing over the top of the uterus is easier to locate than the ligament passing underneath the uterus. Because most uterine torsions in the mare do not involve the cervix or vagina, only rarely can the diagnosis of a uterine torsion be confirmed via palpation per vaginum (i.e., finding that the cranial vaginal vault is narrowed and twisted). Treatment of preterm uterine torsion involves one of three methods: (1) anesthetizing the mare and placing a board low in the flank to aid in maintaining pressure on the uterus while the mare is rolled in the direction of the torsion until it is corrected (in essence, the uterus and fetus are held in place while the mare is rotated around them) (Figure 8-28); (2) performing a standing flank laparotomy, reaching under the uterus and lifting the fetus and uterus up and over into the

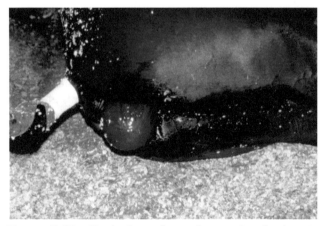

Figure 8-27 Chorionic surface of unruptured placenta presented beyond vulva as a result of premature placental separation.

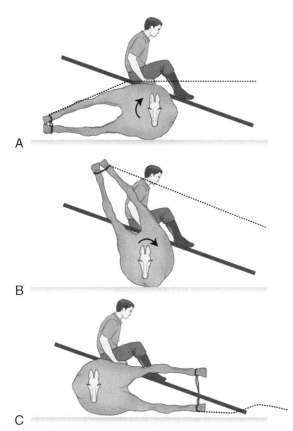

Figure 8-28 Illustration of rolling technique used to correct uterine torsion in a preterm mare. **A,** The position of the mare, fetus, and plank before rolling; the direction of rolling is indicated *(arrow)*. **B,** Uterine and fetal position are maintained by applying weight on the plank during rotation; the direction is indicated *(arrow)*. **C,** The positions after a reduction of 180% of uterine torsion. The procedure is repeated until the full extent of torsion has been corrected.

torsion until it is corrected; and (3) performing a midventral laparotomy and either correcting the torsion through the incision or performing a Cesarean section and then correcting the torsion. In all cases in which the fetus is not removed at the time of correction, the mare is at risk of abortion if severe fetal distress has occurred. Rolling the mare works best for torsions that occur earlier in gestation and is less likely to be successful in near-term or full-term uterine torsions. If the torsion is greater than 180 degrees, the mare most likely will have to be rolled more than once. The position of the uterus and broad ligaments is checked by an examiner per rectum, and the mare remains under general anesthesia. If further rolling is necessary, the mare should be gently rolled over her feet, and the procedure begun again. This ensures the mare is never rolled in the wrong direction. Once torsion is fully corrected, the mare is allowed to recover from anesthesia and is assisted in standing. Once the mare is standing in a stable position, the position of the uterus and broad ligaments should be checked per rectum one final time to ensure no torsion of the uterus remains.

Hydrallantois and Hydramnios

Hydrallantois is an uncommon condition that is thought to develop as a result of placental dysfunction (Figure 8-29). Excess allantoic fluid accumulates (as many as 100 to 200 L or more), usually in mid to late gestation, overfilling the uterus. The placenta is sometimes quite edematous (Figure 8-30), as placental dysfunction is thought to play a role in the disease. The condition generally develops over a period of a few weeks, and the mare is noted to have developed an extremely enlarged abdomen, predisposing the mare to rupture of the prepubic tendon. Hydrallantois is diagnosed by palpating (per rectum) the extremely enlarged, fluid-filled uterus. The uterus is sometimes so distended with fluid that it is elevated to or above the level of the floor of the pelvis and little else, including the fetus, can be palpated. *Hydramnios* has been reported in the mare but is thought to be a rare occurrence. Uterine distention with hydramnios is reportedly less dramatic and may not develop as quickly. Reimer (1997) reports that transabdominal ultrasound

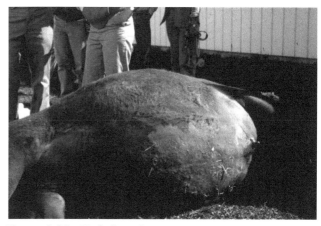

Figure 8-29 Hydrallantois apparent in a recumbent mare. The abdomen is greatly distended from accumulation of excessive fetal fluids in the uterus.

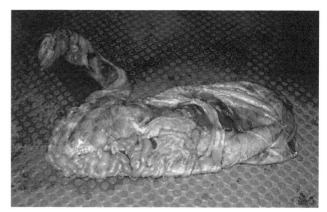

Figure 8-30 Extreme edema evident in placenta, with engorged lymphatics, from a mare with hydramnios.

examination may aid in diagnosis when excess accumulation of allantoic or amniotic fluid is unequivocally found. In a series of nine cases, Reimer reported three in which fetal death had already occurred at the time of ultrasonographic diagnosis.

Because the fetus is usually severely compromised, the treatment consists of inducing parturition to deliver the fetus and expel the fetal fluids from the uterus. Frazer (2000) reports that approximately 50% of fetuses are born alive, with euthanasia of a living fetus indicated as a result of nonviability. If the mare is judged to be in such poor condition that she may enter shock as a result of the sudden loss of the tremendous volume of fluid, pretreatment with intravenous fluids and corticosteroids may be beneficial. The cervix should be manually dilated and the fetal membranes punctured to allow allantoic fluid to escape slowly for a period of time (perhaps a half hour or more). If so desired, the cervix can be treated with prostaglandin E1 (PGE_1) (Cytotec, G.D. Searle and Co, Omaha, Neb.), 500 to 1000 μg mixed with sterile lubricating jelly and placed in the cervical canal). Use of prostaglandin E has been reported to hasten softening of the cervix and improve its ability to dilate when the mare is induced with oxytocin 6 to 24 hours later. Frazer (2000) suggests that siphoning of fluid through a catheter placed transcervically into the allantoic space may be necessary in some cases to gradually evacuate some of the excess fluid. If labor does not begin spontaneously, oxytocin can be administered. Texas workers usually administer oxytocin in 5- to 20-unit injections (intramuscularly [IM] or IV) given at 15-minute intervals; Frazer (2000) suggests administering oxytocin in an intravenous drip at the rate of 1 unit per minute. Assistance should be given in fetal delivery, and the mare should be encouraged to lie quietly for as long as possible before rising after giving birth. Abdominal support wraps may be necessary for a period of time until abdominal muscle tone returns. The mare's condition should be monitored closely thereafter until danger of retained placenta, metritis, and laminitis is past. Uterine involution is delayed, and rebreeding on foal heat should be discouraged. Anecdotal reports suggest that although fertility may be reduced during the season of occurrence, fertility in ensuing seasons is normal and the condition is unlikely to recur.

Ruptured Prepubic Tendon

A ruptured prepubic tendon sometimes occurs in aged mares with hydrallantois or in those carrying a large fetus or twins. A thickened, edematous plaque develops ventrally extending from the udder to the xiphoid, sometimes before rupture of the tendon. Rupture of the prepubic tendon results in loss of ventral abdominal support to the pelvis, so a typical sawhorse stance develops wherein the pelvis is tipped cranially and the feet are extended fore and aft. Support for the udder is lost, and it becomes swollen and congested (Figure 8-31). The

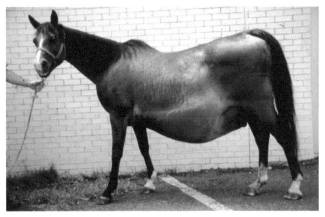

Figure 8-31   Mare with sawhorse stance typical of ruptured prepubic tendon from loss of ventral abdominal support, tipped pelvis, and elevated tail head. The udder is also swollen and congested.

affected mare is reluctant to move, and her condition rapidly deteriorates. Palpation per rectum reveals the abdominal floor falling away from the brim of the pelvis. If rupture has not occurred, and the objective is to save the mare, induction of parturition is indicated. Assistance with fetal delivery is likely to be necessary because the mare will probably have a weakened abdominal press. If the objective is to save the foal, and the expected foaling date is near, sometimes support wraps and nursing care permit the mare to maintain the foal until induced parturition can be performed at a time when foal survival is more likely. If the mare's life is spared, she should not be rebred if partial disruption of the prepubic tendon occurred because it is likely to recur during the next gestation. A similar condition, managed in a similar manner, is *abdominal wall rupture* or *herniation*. However, with minor herniation, delivery of the fetus is often possible and the hernia can sometimes be repaired surgically after the foal is weaned. The mare can then be rebred to carry a foal to term without recurrence of the hernia.

Prolonged Gestation

In the mare, prolonged gestation (>340 days) seldom results in birth of an oversize fetus that contributes to dystocia as occurs in the cow. Numerous reports exist of mares undergoing gestation lengths of 1 year or more that deliver foals of normal size and viability. The causes of prolonged gestation are not known in the mare, but Vandeplassche hypothesized that arrest of embryonic/fetal development sometimes occurs during early pregnancy. The arrested development has been postulated to sometimes last for 3 to 5 weeks, resulting in a corresponding delay in interval to birth. Placental insufficiency is also likely to play a role in prolonged gestation. The foals born from these prolonged gestations are normal but may be small for gestational age. Another factor contributing to gestations longer than the expected 340 days is season.

Mares that conceive early in the breeding season (February and March) tend to carry the fetus longer than mares that conceive in late April and May. Regardless of the cause, induction of parturition should not be attempted unless cardinal signs of fetal maturity and impending parturition are present. Currently, adequate udder development and, most important, the presence of good quality colostrum of high calcium content constitute the best indicator that the fetus is mature and the mare is ready to deliver a live-foal (see Chapter 9).

Pathologic prolonged gestation can occur in mares grazing *Acremonium*-contaminated fescue grass **(fescue toxicosis).** The placenta is typically thickened, partly because of an increase in connective tissue, and stillbirth with the foal still encased in the fetal membranes may occur. Udder development is minimal *(agalactia)* in affected mares, presumably as a result of ergot alkaloids present in infested fescue acting as dopamine receptor agonists. Missouri workers recently showed that pony mares affected with fescue toxicosis had low circulating levels of relaxin, which were associated with placental disease and agalactia. Pennsylvania workers went further, documenting low circulating relaxin levels in mares with other forms of placental disease or insufficiency.

Prevention of the condition is best accomplished with pasture management to control infestation by the fungus, supplemental feeding of nonfescue hay, and rotation of pregnant mares to a noncontaminated pasture for the last 3 months of gestation. Drugs that have been used to stimulate prolactin production and overcome agalactia have included thyrotropin-releasing hormone (TRH) (2.0 mg, subcutaneously [SQ], twice daily), reserpine (0.5 to 2.0 mg, IM, once every 2 days), and perphenazine (0.3 to 0.5 mg/kg, PO, twice daily). Missouri workers reported treatment with a long-acting D2-dopamine receptor antagonist (fluphenazine deconate, 25 mg, IM) 2 to 3 weeks before expected parturition increased circulating relaxin levels and decreased the incidence of fescue toxicosis–related problems in pony mares and their foals. Perhaps the most success has been gained by administering a dopamine-D2 receptor antagonist, sulpiride or domperidone. South Carolina workers have shown that domperidone (Equidone, Dechra Veterinary Products, Overland Park, Kan.) (1.1 mg/kg, PO, once daily) before foaling was helpful for treating gravid mares grazing *Acremonium*-contaminated fescue pastures in reducing the incidence of dystocia,

stillbirth, placental retention, and agalactia. Beginning treatment 10 to 15 days before expected foaling gave better results than initiating treatment later, but treatment near or after foaling still appeared to reduce the incidence and severity of agalactia.

BIBLIOGRAPHY

Bain AM: Foetal losses during, pregnancy in the thoroughbred mare: A record of 2, 562 pregnancies, *New Zealand Vet J* 17:155-158, 1969.

Ball BA: Embryonic death in mares. In McKinnon AO, Voss JL, editors: *Equine reproduction,* Philadelphia, 1993, Lea & Febiger, 517-531.

Cross DL, Anas K, Bridges WC, et al: Clinical effects of domperidone on fescue toxicosis in pregnant mares, *Proc Ann Mtg Am Assoc Equine Pract* 45:203-209, 1999.

Dennis SM: Pregnancy wastage in domestic animals, *Comp Cont Educ Prac Vet* 3:S62-S70, 1981.

Frazer G: Hydrops, ruptures and torsions, *Proc Soc Therio* 2000, 33-38.

Ginther OJ: *Ultrasonic imaging and reproductive events in the mare,* Cross Plains, WI, 1986, Equiservices, 195-223, 253-285.

Ginther OJ: *Reproductive biology of the mare: basic and applied aspects,* ed 2, Cross Plains, WI, 1992, Equiservices, 546-560.

Ginther OJ: *Ultrasonic imaging and animal reproduction: color-Doppler ultrasongraphy,* Book 4, Cross Plains, WI, 2007, 156-176.

McCue PM: Lactation. In McKinnon AO, Voss JL, editors: *Equine reproduction,* Philadelphia, 1993, Lea & Febiger, 588-595.

Morehead JP, Blanchard TL, Thompson JA, et al: Evaluation of early fetal losses on four equine farms in central Kentucky: 73 cases (2001), *J Am Vet Med Assoc* 220:1828-1830, 2002.

Newcombe JR: Embryonic loss and abnormalities of early pregnancy, *Equine Vet Educ* April:115-131, 2000.

Redmund LM, Cross DL, Trickland JR, et al: Efficacy of domperidone and sulpiride as treatments for fescue toxicosis in horses, *Am J Vet Res* 55:722-729, 1994.

Reimer JM: Use of transcutaneous ultrasonography in complicated latter -middle to late gestation pregnancies in the mare: 122 cases, *Proc Am Assoc Eq Pract* 43:259-261, 1997.

Ryan P, Bennet-Wimbush K, Loch W, et al: Effects of fescue toxicosis and fluphenazine on relaxin concentrations in pregnant pony mares, *Proc Ann Mtg Am Assoc Equine Pract* 44:60-61, 1998.

Ryan P, Vaala W, Bagnell C: Evidence that equine relaxin is a good indicator of placental insufficiency in the mare, *Proc Ann Mtg Am Assoc Equine Pract* 44:62-63, 1998.

Taylor TS, Blanchard TL, Varner DD, et al: Management of dystocia in mares: uterine torsion and cesarean section, *Comp Cont Educ Prac Vet* 11:1265-1273, 1989.

Vandeplassche M: Obstetrician's view of the physiology of equine parturition and dystocia, *Equine Vet J* 12(2):45-49, 1980.

Vanderwall DK, Squires EL, Brinsko SP, et al: Diagnosis and management of abnormal embryonic development characterized by formation of an embryonic vesicle without an embryo proper in mares, *J Am Vet Med Assoc* 217:58-63, 2000.

Wolfsdorf KE, Rodgerson D, Holder R: How to manually reduce twins between 60 and 120 days gestation using cranio-cervical dislocation, *Proc 51st Ann Mtg Am Assoc Equine Pract* 2005, 284-287.

Management of the Pregnant Mare

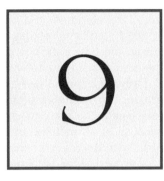

CHAPTER

9

OBJECTIVES

While studying the information covered in this chapter, the reader should attempt to:
- Acquire a working understanding of procedures used to manage the pregnant and parturient mare.
- Acquire a working understanding of procedures used to monitor fetal viability during gestation.
- Acquire a working knowledge of the rationale and procedures for monitoring the mare for readiness for birth.
- Acquire a working understanding of the birth process, including the three stages of labor.
- Acquire a working knowledge of the events that occur in the early postpartum period in the healthy foaling mare.

STUDY QUESTIONS

1. Identify the average duration of gestation in the mare and discuss effects of season on gestation length.
2. Outline differences in nutritional needs for mares during early and late gestation and during lactation.
3. Outline a preventive healthcare program for pregnant mares on a broodmare farm.
4. Describe examination findings that indicate fetal well-being is at risk.
5. Describe the desirable characteristics of a foaling area or stall.
6. List changes that occur in the mammary gland and its secretions that are useful in prediction of readiness for parturition in the mare.
7. Describe the progression of events that occur during the three stages of parturition in the mare.
8. Outline methods for induction of parturition in the mare.
9. Explain the economic pressure to breed mares on foal heat.
10. Describe the progression of events that occur during uterine involution and return to pregravid condition in the healthy foaling mare.

Mares should be managed attentively during pregnancy to help ensure the birth of a strong healthy foal with no injury incurred by the dam. Maintaining the mare in good health, being familiar with the signs of impending parturition, and preparing a foaling environment conducive to mare and foal health increase the likelihood of a healthy foal. Although managerial programs are usually adapted to meet special needs of individual mares or owners, certain strategies and methodologies are universally applicable. This chapter discusses routine care of the pregnant mare, methods for monitoring fetal viability, preparation of the mare for foaling, and the physiologic events of parturition to provide background for managing the term mare and birth process.

LENGTH OF GESTATION

Average duration of gestation in the equine is 335 to 342 days. Occasionally, viable term foals can be born as early as 305 days of gestation, but foals born before

320 days of gestational age are typically premature and nonviable. Some authors define abortion as the expulsion of the fetus before day 300 of gestation and use the term **prematurity** to designate birth of an underdeveloped foal between days 300 and 320 of gestation. The reader should recognize that use of these precise days for definition purposes can be misleading because gestation length is so variable in the equine. Certainly, foals delivered at more than 320 days of gestation can fit other criteria used to describe prematurity. **Dysmaturity**, on the other hand, designates birth of a full-term but immature and often undersized foal.

The duration of gestation is sometimes exceedingly long, 360 days or more, with no untoward effects on the fetus or mare (i.e., the fetus is not oversized and is viable, and no increased risk of dystocia exists). These long gestational periods have been hypothesized to result from the ability of the equine conceptus to undergo a period of arrested development during the first 2 months of gestation and then reinitiate growth and development.

Seasonal effects on the duration of equine gestation are found, with mares due to foal in late winter and early spring carrying their foals approximately 5 to 10 days longer than mares that foal later in the breeding season (late spring or summer). This seasonal effect can partially negate efforts made to get mares pregnant early in the breeding season (February 15 or soon thereafter) and can be circumvented by exposing pregnant mares to artificial lighting regimens (beginning December 1) identical to those used to initiate early ovulatory estrus in nonpregnant mares. Exposure of pregnant mares to artificial lighting systems can reduce gestation length by an average of 10 days.

Other factors that may influence gestational length in mares include gender of the foal (males are carried slightly longer), maternal nutrition, and environmental stresses. Ingested toxins (e.g., ergot alkaloids in contaminated fescue grass or hay) may lengthen the duration of gestation.

PREVENTIVE HEALTHCARE

Vaccination of the Pregnant Mare

Preventive health measures recommended for pregnant mares include regular immunization for common infectious diseases. Immunization of the pregnant mare serves two purposes: protection of the dam (and gestating fetus) and eventual protection of the newborn foal. Two viruses—equine herpesvirus 1 (EHV-1) and equine arteritis virus (the agent of equine viral arteritis [EVA]—are of special concern to the pregnant mare because they can cause abortion or birth of infected live but severely compromised foals. Many infectious organisms can infect foals, which are compromised in the ability to develop a high level of their own immunity early in life. Immunoglobulins produced in response to vaccine antigens are

too large for diffusion across the placental barrier; nevertheless, the antibodies should be concentrated in colostrum and thus are made available to the newborn foal at the time of nursing (i.e., before "gut closure," generally by 24 hours of age). If protection of the foal is of foremost concern, booster vaccines should be administered approximately 4 to 6 weeks before the projected foaling date to optimize concentration of colostral immunoglobulins to be passively transferred to the foal.

Protection of newborn animals through maternal immunization has been widely practiced by the veterinary profession for many years (Box 9-1). Although the rationale for vaccination of the pregnant dam to enhance concentration of specific immunoglobulins in colostrum is well understood, documentation of efficacy for this practice for many specific vaccines so used is often lacking. Potential problems associated with vaccination of the pregnant dam include the following: (1) the pregnant dam may not respond as well to immunization (humoral response may be downregulated during gestation), which could lessen the desirable immune response of the dam to vaccine antigens administered during pregnancy; (2) administration of numerous different vaccines, even when given as multivalent products, at the same time might lessen the dam's ability to respond favorably to specific antigens (i.e., vaccine interference). Thus, some authors recommend administering no more than four vaccine antigens at one time and waiting for 2 to 4 weeks before other vaccine antigens are administered; and (3) passively acquired immunoglobulins can interfere with the growing neonate's ability to respond favorably to primary immunization against certain pathogens (e.g., influenza).

Routine vaccination with inactivated vaccines directed at many antigens is accepted as safe for the pregnant mare. Adverse impacts on pregnancy have not been shown for modified live intranasally administered strangles or influenza vaccines or for the modified live EHV-1 vaccine. The recombinant West Nile virus (WNV)

BOX 9-1

Prefoaling Vaccinations

8 months of gestation	Rotavirus
9 months of gestation	Rotavirus
10 months of gestation	Rotavirus
	Equine influenza
	Eastern and Western equine encephalitis
	West Nile virus
	Strangles (*Streptococcus equi*)
	Botulism

Note: When 10-month prefoaling vaccinations are given during a time when other vaccines are scheduled, be careful not to double-vaccinate.

vaccine is also thought to be safe for pregnancy. However, *modified live virus Venezuelan Equine Encephalitis (VEE) vaccines and live anthrax spore vaccines should not be used in pregnant mares.*

Selection of vaccines for immunization of pregnant mares should depend on many factors, including expected exposure to the disease, economic constraints, and vaccine efficacy and safety. Immunization programs should be tailored to meet needs of individual mares or owner needs (e.g., management practices that increase exposure to infectious disease) and disease control measures used on farms where mares reside. Also, parenterally administered vaccines are generally best for use in the prepartum period because intranasally administered vaccines are less effective for stimulating high levels of immunoglobulin G (IgG), the immunoglobulin that is transferred in high concentrations into colostrum. For a more thorough discussion of vaccinations for broodmares (and foals), including potential benefits, problems, and risks, the reader is referred to Wilson (2005) and the AAEP website (www.aaep.org/vaccination_guidelines/htm).

Although not exhaustive, some specific considerations regarding vaccination of pregnant dams follow.

Equine Herpesvirus Abortion

Equine herpesvirus type 1 **(EHV-1)** is the herpesvirus associated with abortion. The virus has also been associated with perinatal foal death; rhinopneumonitis in foals, growing horses, and some adult horses; and encephalomyelitis in adult horses. The virus is distinct from EHV-4, which is the major cause of rhinopneumonitis in foals and is only rarely isolated from equine abortions.

EHV-1 infection is acquired via inhalation, with the virus attaching to, penetrating, and replicating in upper airway mucosal epithelial cells. If local immunity fails to overcome infection, the virus breaches the basement membrane to invade the lamina propria of the respiratory mucosa and infects T lymphocytes and endothelial cells. The resulting viremia disseminates virus throughout the body. Abortion is the result of ischemia consequent to vasculitis of uterine vessels that disrupt the uteroplacental barrier. Lymphocytes resident within the endometrium are also thought to potentially transfer virus directly to uterine endothelium and result in abortion. This latter mechanism has been proposed to explain abortion of single mares in a group and abortions that occur many weeks or months after viremia.

Viral latency also occurs with EHV-1 infection, with periodic reactivation of latent virus resulting in asymptomatic shedding from the respiratory tract that may result in infection of in-contact horses. If local immunity has waned, reinfection and viremia can recur, again placing the fetus at risk. Although vaccinations do not eliminate preexisting latent EHV-1 infections, if they stimulate sufficient local immunity to prevent shedding, transmission of virus to other in-contact animals may be prevented.

Vaccination timing and efficacy against EHV-1 abortion remains controversial. Pneumabort-K +1b (Wyeth Animal Health, Guelph, Ontario) is a killed-virus preparation approved for use to protect against EHV-1 abortions in mares, with administration recommended during the fifth, seventh, and ninth months of gestation. Nonpregnant mares that may come in contact with pregnant mares should have vaccine administered at the same time as pregnant mares. Rhinomune (Pfizer, Animal Health, New York, NY) is an attenuated live virus preparation approved for use in preventing respiratory disease caused by EHV-1. Although the product label makes no claim for provision of protection against abortion, it does state that no adverse reactions have been reported in pregnant mares vaccinated with this product and further recommends vaccination of pregnant mares after the second month of gestation and at 3-month intervals thereafter. Prestige II with Havlogen (Intervet/Schering-Plough Animal Health, Whitehouse Station, N.J.) is a killed-virus preparation that contains EHV-1, EHV-4, and equine influenza subtypes A1 and A2; the product label makes no claims concerning provision of protection against abortion. Prodigy (Intervet/Schering-Plough Animal Health, Whitehouse Station, N.J.) is a killed-virus preparation of EHV-1 labeled for the prevention of abortion. Vaccination with this product is recommended at the fifth, seventh and ninth months of gestation. Recommendations for frequency of administration of booster vaccines, although they vary with the product used, are notably at frequent intervals because herpesviruses typically do not stimulate long-lasting immune protection (even immunity from natural infection wanes in 3 to 6 months). Although the efficacy of vaccination in the face of an abortion outbreak from rhinopneumonitis is unknown, Pneumabort-K +1b is labeled for this use.

Research regarding changing administration between vaccine types or brands during gestation is lacking. Some practitioners believe that switching vaccines during pregnancy leads to vaccine breaks in which EHV-1 abortion is more likely to occur. Until this phenomenon is studied, we caution against changing products during pregnancy in gestating mares.

Prevention and control of EHV-1 abortion cannot rely solely on a vaccination program because vaccination provides limited protection against viral shedding and the disease and properly vaccinated mares occasionally abort. One should use unerring management procedures in concert with a vaccination protocol to reduce mare exposure to the virus. Pregnant mares should be separated from the rest of the farm population. Permanent resident mares should not be allowed contact with transient boarders that normally reside elsewhere. Stress should be minimized to reduce the risk of activation of EHV-1 virus that may already be present in the mare. Mares that have aborted as a result of EHV-1 should be isolated from the rest of the herd. In addition, all mares that have been in contact with aborting mares should be segregated from those not yet exposed to the virus, and booster vaccines may be administered to in-contact mares in an attempt to stimulate immunity. Strict hygienic measures should be instituted to minimize spread of infection to the rest of the mares on the premises.

When facilities are limited for separating at-risk from nonexposed mares, the practitioner can perform polymerase chain reaction (PCR) testing on nasopharyngeal washes and whole blood samples collected from incoming mares. Procedures for nasopharyngeal washes are described by Conboy (2005). Submitting these samples to a diagnostic laboratory that can perform PCR testing for EHV-1 (e.g., University of Kentucky Livestock Disease Diagnostic Center, Lexington, Ky.) results in timely reporting of results, which can be used as a screening measure for either keeping animals isolated or allowing them to be moved into different locales on a farm. Animals with positive results on PCR testing of nasopharyngeal washes should at least be considered to have been exposed to the virus (but may not be actively infected, nor shedding the virus), and those with positive results in blood should be considered to be viremic and therefore likely to be shedding the virus. Some practitioners require maiden mares arriving at a breeding farm to be PCR negative for EHV-1 before they are allowed to mix with other mares at the farm or before they are allowed to be sent to a stud farm for breeding. Such a screening protocol may prove to be valuable in controlling an outbreak of EHV-1 respiratory or neurologic disease (although the test does not specifically identify the variant that causes neurologic disease).

Tetanus (Clostridium tetani)

Tetanus toxoid administration should be mandatory in all vaccination programs because of the incidence and life-threatening consequences of the disease for the dam and foal. The initial series of injections in unvaccinated horses consists of a two-dose series, with the second dose given 4 to 6 weeks after the first. For the pregnant broodmare, booster vaccines are given 4 to 6 weeks before the date of expected foaling to provide passive protection from colostrum intake by the newborn foal.

Encephalomyelitis (Sleeping Sickness)

This insect-transmitted neurologic disease is caused by viruses of the *Togaviridae* family, of which **Eastern**, **Western**, and **Venezuelan encephalomyelitis** viruses are most pathogenic. Horses in endemic areas should be immunized with a suitable inactivated-virus vaccine before the mosquito season each year, which corresponds to the foaling season. In areas where mosquito resurgence occurs in late summer or fall, a second annual dose should be given in late summer, just as for the inactivated WNV

vaccine. Pregnant mares are routinely administered a booster vaccination 4 to 6 weeks before the date of expected foaling in an attempt to provide passive protection to the newborn foal from colostrum intake.

West Nile Virus

This insect-transmitted neurologic disease is also caused by a virus transmitted mainly by mosquitoes, and outbreaks have occurred throughout the United States and worldwide. Three vaccines are currently available for horses: (1) an inactivated vaccine that requires an initial two-dose primary immunization series; (2) a recombinant canarypox vaccine that requires an initial two-dose primary vaccination series; and (3) a flavivirus chimera vaccine that requires only a single dose for primary immunization. Revaccination in late summer before mosquito population resurgence has been recommended for both the inactivated and the recombinant products. All products are thought to be safe for vaccination of the pregnant mare, but recommendations have been to provide the primary course of vaccination to previously unvaccinated mares while they are nonpregnant. However, a recent Texas study revealed no adverse effects when the inactivated vaccine was administered to previously nonimmunized pregnant mares at all stages of gestation. Pregnant mares are routinely administered a booster vaccination 4 to 6 weeks before the date of expected foaling in an attempt to provide passive protection from colostrum intake by the newborn foal.

Rabies

The risk of rabies is widespread across the United States. Because of the associated mortality and public health risks, immunization against this disease should be recommended for all horses. A single dose is recommended for primary immunization. Pregnant mares can be administered a booster vaccination 4 to 6 weeks before foaling in an attempt to provide passive protection from colostrum intake by the newborn foal. However, because of the relatively long duration of immunity, some authors recommend the vaccine be given after foaling but before breeding to reduce the number of prepartum vaccines given to a mare.

Rotavirus Diarrhea

Rotavirus is considered to be the most common infectious cause of diarrhea in foals, and farm outbreaks can affect a large proportion of the foals on a farm and become endemic. Foals of very young age are susceptible to adverse effects of rotavirus infection, which causes a profuse watery diarrhea. One of the better ways to provide protection to newborn foals is to vaccinate pregnant broodmares. A three-dose series (1 month apart) of vaccine administration is recommended, with the first dose given at 8 months of gestation. Thus, the last dose is given approximately 1 month before foaling to optimize colostral immunoglobulin concentration.

Immunization against other infectious diseases is sometimes desirable, depending on local risk factors such as endemic diseases, housing in contact with horses of other ages, and contact with outside (nonresident) horses at risk of contracting transmissible infectious diseases such as **influenza, strangles, botulism, anthrax,** and **Potomac horse fever**. Product labels should be examined because some products (e.g., FluAvert IN, Intervet/Schering-Plough Animal Health, Whitehouse Station, NJ, and anthrax vaccine) caution against use in pregnant mares.

Protection against **equine viral arteritis** (EVA) may be necessary in some instances. Special precautions are needed for use of vaccine, and state and federal authorities may need to be contacted for approval of its use and guidelines for its administration. EVA vaccine (Arvac, [Guelph, Ontario] a modified live virus vaccine) was previously thought to be unsafe for administration to pregnant mares, but recent outbreaks of the disease in Quarter Horse populations throughout the Midwestern United States prompted its widespread use in pregnant mares, with no published adverse effects on fertility or already established pregnancies. Because of potential export restrictions, all horses to be vaccinated should first have seronegative status documented. Recommendations are for mares recently vaccinated to be kept segregated from other seronegative horses for a minimum of 2 to 3 weeks to prevent in-contact seronegative horses from seroconverting.

Dental Care and Parasite Control

Regular **dental examination** and **floating** enables proper grazing and chewing of feeds, which helps maintain body condition and prevent digestive upsets. The frequency of dentistry necessary depends on each individual mare's dental conformation and wear but generally should be at 6- to 12-month intervals The goal of dental management is to ensure an ideal functional masticatory unit with regular filing and burring or cutting of teeth that are too long to balance the chewing surfaces from side to side and front to back. Sources of chewing discomfort should be identified and corrected.

Parasite control is second only to good nutrition in proper management. Discussion of the varied anthelmintics and programs for their use is beyond the scope of this chapter. However, three common methods of parasite control used for broodmares are (1) strategic dosing based on egg reappearance period (ERP); (2) regularly scheduled use of anthelmintics, performed at intervals (usually 2 or 3 months), with different chemical classes of dewormers in a rotating fashion in an attempt to avoid development of parasite resistance to products; and (3) continuous deworming, (e.g., daily feeding of Strongid C or Strongid C2X, Pfizer Animal Health New York, N.Y.). Any method should include twice-yearly (fall and spring)

deworming with a product that removes bots (with use of a macrolytic lactone such as ivermectin or moxidectin) and tapeworms (with praziquantel). Deworming medications are generally considered safe for use during pregnancy unless otherwise indicated on the product label. A variety of dewormers are approved for use during pregnancy, including ivermectin, pyrantel pamoate, and pyrantel tartrate. Thiabendazole, fenbendazole, and piperazine have been used regularly throughout pregnancy with no known untoward effects. Cambendazole should not be used during the first 3 months of pregnancy. Always read the precautions on the package insert of anthelmintics before administering to pregnant mares.

Administration of ivermectin to the broodmare on the day of foaling is common practice to minimize the parasitic load of *Strongyloides westeri*. The infective larvae of this parasite are transmitted to the foal via nursing beginning about 4 days after birth.

Any deworming program should be suited to the individual requirements of a farm or stable, with evaluation of program success by examination of feces at regular intervals to monitor parasitic egg levels (eggs per gram [epg]). Sound pasture management (e.g., low stocking density, regular pasture rotation, and pasture harrowing) should be used in concert with deworming protocols to establish an effective antiparasitic program. An example of one health program, including a deworming schedule, for broodmares is presented in Box 9-2.

Nutritional Considerations

Proper nutritional support of the broodmare improves fertility and promotes normal growth and vigor of the developing fetus. The reader is referred to a review of nutrient requirements for gestating and lactating mares for a thorough discussion of feeding guidelines (Hintz, 1993). Pregnant mares should be kept in good **body condition** (body score of 6 to 7, based on a scoring system of 1 to 9). Best pregnancy rates are achieved in mares of good to fat condition. and fertility of thin mares is improved if they are gaining weight at the time of breeding. Because late gestation and early lactation place enormous metabolic demands on the mare and most are rebred within 1 month after foaling, broodmares should be in a positive energy balance at the time of parturition. However, mares should not be obese because obesity has been reported to be associated with birth of weak undersized foals. Specific nutrient requirements for gestating mares are available from the National Research Council (NRC) (1989). In general, three different feeding programs—energy, protein, and minerals—are necessary for pregnant mares, with dietary requirements dictated by lactational status and stage of gestation. Digestible energy (DE) requirements for mares during the first 8 months of gestation are the same as for maintenance and gradually increase during

---

Box 9-2

Example of a Herd Health Program for Pregnant Mares Used on a Thoroughbred Farm in Kentucky

January	Deworming (rotational)
	Equine rhinopneumonitis vaccine
	Equine influenza vaccine
	Streptococcus equi vaccine
	Botulism vaccine (if never received before, administer three doses in January, February, and March)
February	Rabies vaccine (before breeding)
March	Deworming (rotational)
	Equine rhinopneumonitis vaccine
	Eastern and Western equine encephalomyelitis vaccine
	Tetanus toxoid
	West Nile virus vaccine
April	
May	Deworming (rotational)
	Equine rhinopneumonitis vaccine
June	*Streptococcus equi* vaccine
July	Deworming with praziquantel and ivermectin
	Equine rhinopneumonitis vaccine
	Equine influenza vaccine
August	Eastern and Western equine encephalitis vaccine
	West Nile virus vaccine
September	Deworming
	Equine rhinopneumonitis vaccine
October	
November	Deworming with praziquantel and ivermectin
	Equine rhinopneumonitis vaccine
December	

July and November dewormings include a product effective against bots and tapeworms.

Note: To simplify scheduling of rhinopneumonitis vaccination, the vaccine is administered to every broodmare on the farm at 2-month intervals. Vaccination for equine influenza and *Streptococcus equi* (strangles) is twice yearly due to a summer-fall pregnant mare sales season. Because of mosquito resurgence, which typically occurs in the fall in this locale, a second late summer vaccination against sleeping sickness and West Nile virus is performed.

---

late gestation over the maintenance requirement (1.11, 1.13 and 1.20 times maintenance requirements for 9, 10, and 11 months of gestation, respectively). The additional maternal nutrition needed during the last 3 months of gestation is indicated because 60% to 65% of fetal growth occurs during this period. Because the growing fetus increasingly takes up abdominal space during this time, feeding of some grain and good-quality hay high in DE is necessary (perhaps as much as 0.5 to 1.0 kg grain and 1 to 1.5 kg hay per 100 kg of body weight). Initial body condition is important for optimizing fetal growth and mare lactation, so constant monitoring of body condition should be done to ensure dietary energy requirements are met.

Regarding dietary crude protein (CP) requirements, mares in late gestation need 44 g of CP per megacalorie (mcal) of DE. A rule of thumb is to provide 9% to 10% of the total ration (on a dry matter basis) as CP during the last 3 months gestation, as opposed to 7% to 8% CP in the total ration during the first 8 months of gestation (Hintz, 1993). Alfalfa hay is a good source of protein for pregnant and lactating mares.

The primary minerals to be concerned with in pregnant mare rations are calcium and phosphorus. The NRC recommends calcium (in g/d) in the total ration be fed at a rate of 1.90 × mcal DE, or approximately 0.2% and 0.4% of total rations for maintenance (first 8 months gestation) and late gestation (last 3 months), respectively. Calcium should be added to the grain mixture, rather than feeding free choice in a salt-mineral mix, to avoid osteochondrosis of the fetus. Because legume hays are rich in calcium, feeding of alfalfa may preclude the need for calcium supplementation in the diet, whereas if grass hay is fed, the need for calcium supplementation may reach 0.6% of the grain mixture. Phosphorus content of the ration should be scrutinized closely so that mares in late gestation are fed a diet containing 0.3% phosphorus. However, phosphorus content should not exceed calcium content in the ration (Hintz, 1993). Recommendations for feeding of other minerals, including zinc, copper, manganese, iodine, and selenium, and for feeding of vitamins are discussed in the NRC guidelines. Finally, mares should be offered fresh clean water and salt ad libitum.

During the first 1 to 12 weeks of lactation, mares of light breeds produce milk equivalent to 3% of their body weight per day. Milk production is reduced to 2% of mare body weight per day later in lactation (i.e., 13 to 24 weeks). Lactation results in more nutrient drain on the mare than occurs during late gestation. Milk yield is markedly influenced by both water and feed consumption by the mare. The protein and energy content of milk are markedly reduced by 12 hours post partum and thereafter gradually decrease over the remainder of the lactation period. During the first 12 weeks of lactation, mares need approximately 70% more energy than for maintenance. This need is reduced to a 48% increase over maintenance in late lactation. Dietary protein requirement is nearly 120% over maintenance during early lactation and is reduced to 60% over maintenance during late lactation. Calcium and phosphorus requirements are similar for pregnant and lactating mares (Hintz, 1993).

Monitoring Fetal Viability

Illness or injury of the pregnant mare can predispose to fetal stress and abortion. Some pregnant mares have genital discharge or precocious udder development with premature lactation that alerts the owner or manager to the possibility of abortion or premature delivery. Rarely, a mare may have an overly large abdomen develop, worrying the owner that twins or hydrops of the fetal membranes may be present. In such instances, examination of the mare's physical condition, uterine status, and viability of the fetus is indicated.

The origin of genital discharge can usually be determined via vaginal speculum examination. This examination must be performed in an aseptic and expedient manner to avoid contaminating the vagina and cervix. Scanty mucopurulent discharges are most commonly the result of inflammation of the vulva or vestibulum, often from inadequate vulvar lip apposition (which can be corrected with Caslick's surgery) (see Chapter 15). Purulent or brownish bloody discharge through a relaxed cervix should alert the practitioner to the

probability of an impending abortion, and fetal viability should be assessed after the discharge is swabbed for microbial culture. Occasional older mares have development of urovagina from conformational changes associated with the enlarging pregnancy. Urovagina, uncontrollable by improving body condition and exercise, may necessitate reconstructive surgery to prevent infection from ascending through an inflamed cervix (see Chapter 15). Rarely, bloody discharge (sometimes with clots of blood) occurs in aged pregnant mares as a result of hemorrhage from prolapsed subepithelial veins in the vulva or vagina (sometimes referred to as vaginal hemorrhoids) (Figure 9-1). Bleeding from one of these vessels most often occurs on the cranial surface of the vestibular ring, which can be difficult to visualize without the use of a flexible endoscope. In most cases, treatment is not necessary because bleeding is minor and usually stops within a few days. Periodic application of over–the-counter hemorrhoidal cream is sometimes helpful in controlling hemorrhage. If bleeding is excessive or persistent, cauterization of affected vessels is usually effective in stopping bleeding, as is ligation.

To assess fetal viability during early gestation, transrectal ultrasonography can be performed to detect fetal movement, umbilical blood flow, and fetal heartbeat (Figure 9-2). The use of transrectal ultrasonography to assess these criteria is limited in advanced gestations by the examiner's inability to image the fetus. In advanced gestation, the fetus can be palpated per rectum to detect fetal movement, although the lack of fetal movement is no guarantee of fetal death. Transrectal

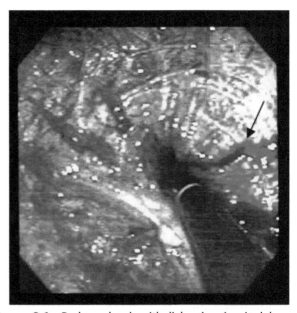

Figure 9-1 Prolapsed subepithelial veins (vaginal hemorrhoids) beneath vaginal mucosa visualized through an endoscope. The endoscope has been turned 180 degrees to visualize the cranial surface of the vestibular ring. The *arrow* points to a bleeding vessel.

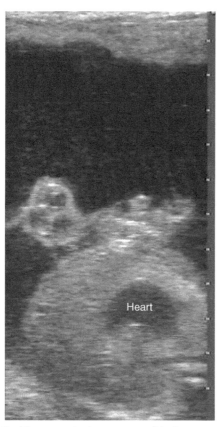

Figure 9-2 Transrectal ultrasonographic image of fetus at 3 months after breeding. Fetal movement and heartbeat were readily apparent. The distended heart is noted.

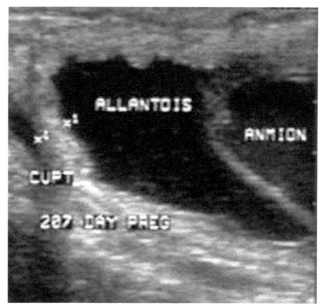

Figure 9-3 Transrectal ultrasonographic image obtained during assessment of uterine-placental thickness (combined uteroplacental thickness [CUPT] measured between cursors) in a mare at 207 days of gestation. The allantoic fluid (allantois) and amnionic fluid (amnion) are visible.

ultrasonography can also be used to assess the combined thickness of the uterus and placenta (CTUP) for detecting placental thickening, sometimes with separation and fluid accumulation between the endometrium and allantochorion. This technique is performed by placing the probe 1 to 2 inches cranial to the cervix and then rotating the probe laterally until the middle uterine artery is visualized. The CTUP is measured between the anterior wall of the middle uterine artery (caudal uterine wall) and the caudal margin of the allantoic fluid (Figure 9-3). Because of undulations in the uterine wall, measurements should be taken in at least three separate locations and the measurements averaged to provide a more accurate determination of the CTUP. Minnesota and California workers suggest that when combined thickness of the uterine wall and allantochorion exceeds 8 mm between 271 and 300 days of gestation, 10 mm between 301 and 330 days, and more than 12 mm after 330 days, the abnormal thickening is indicative of placental failure and pending abortion from ascending placentitis.

Transcutaneous ultrasonography, with 2.5-MHz to 5-MHz curvilinear probes, is a good method for evaluating the fetus, uterine fluids, uterus, and placenta of mares in mid to late gestation. Pennsylvania workers suggest use of a depth setting of 27.5 to 30 cm for scanning the ventral abdomen. Doppler ultrasonography

or M-mode echocardiography is especially useful for assessment of fetal cardiac rhythm. Reimer (1997) described abnormal pregnancies identifiable during transcutaneous ultrasonography, including visible anomalies of the fetus (omphalocele, fetal ascites), excessive echogenic retroplacental fluid accumulations resulting in placental separation (Figure 9-4), thickening of the placenta from placentitis (Figure 9-5), hydrallantois, hydramnios, compromised twin pregnancies missed on earlier transrectal ultrasound examinations (one or both dead), and fetal death. Determination of fetal heart beat and cardiac rate is also useful for evaluation of fetal health during late gestation. Florida and Pennsylvania workers determined that reduced fetal movement, combined with failure of the fetal cardiac rhythm to substantially increase in response to fetal movements, can be indicative of fetal hypoxic stress. Florida workers suggest that normal late-gestation equine fetuses should have a baseline heart rate of 60 to 92 beats per minute, accelerating by 25 to 40 beats per minute in the approximately 30-second period accompanying vigorous fetal movement. They also suggest monitoring fetal cardiac rhythm for periods of up to 10 minutes to evaluate fetal cardiac response during movement. Persistent bradycardia or tachycardia, particularly on more than one examination separated by a few hours, has been associated with poor fetal outcome in studies by several different groups.

Unfortunately, even with improved capability for monitoring fetal viability in the equine, methods for treatment that improve outcome remain limited. For example, in the mare with precocious udder

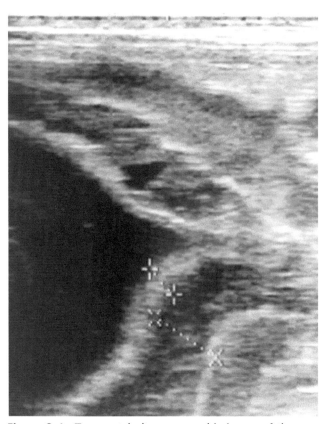

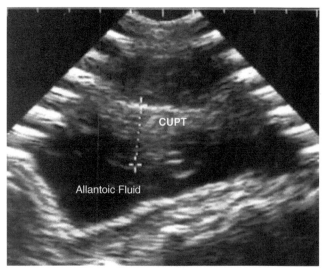

Figure 9-5 Transabdominal ultrasonographic image obtained during assessment of fetal well-being in a mare with premature udder development and lactation 4 weeks before her due date. Combined uteroplacental thickness *(CUPT)* was excessive (2 cm), and placental thickening and separation were apparent cranial to the cervix (Figure 9-4). Despite treatment with broad-spectrum antimicrobials, altrenogest, and flunixin meglumine, the foal was delivered 3 days later (red bag delivery). Extensive chronic placentitis was evident throughout the placenta, which occupied more than 5 gallons and weighed more than 20 lb. (Courtesy Dr. Jorge Colon, Lexington, Ky.)

Figure 9-4 Transrectal ultrasonographic image of the caudal uterine body/cervix obtained during assessment of fetal well-being at 9 months gestation. Premature udder development and cervical relaxation were apparent, and impending abortion caused by placental separation/placentitis was suspected. Fetal heart rate was normal. +—+ represents chorioallantois; X—X represents an area of separation between the chorioallantois and endometrium. (Courtesy Dr. Jorge Colon, Lexington, Ky.)

development and premature lactation, in which premature separation of the placenta or placentitis is suspected or confirmed yet the fetus remains alive, treatment typically consists of administration of uterine tocolytics and progestogens, antiprostaglandins, and broad-spectrum antimicrobials. Progesterone levels (P_4) are normally low in mid to late gestation and then rise dramatically within 1 week before parturition. A premature rise in P_4 levels at less than 310 days of gestation is indicative of fetal stress. Unfortunately, because of the amount of variation in P_4 levels within and amongst mares, comparison of a single sample with normal reference values may not be very informative. Florida and Kentucky workers reported that a minimum of three samples taken at 48- to 72-hour intervals was necessary to show a change in plasma progestin levels. With this method, these workers determined that a 50% change in progestin levels (higher or lower) from baseline indicated fetal stress.

Although its use remains controversial, supplementation of at-risk mares with estrogens is gaining favor among some practitioners. The rationale is based on the hormonal profile of pregnant mares and a clinical trial in which mares suspected of having placentitis and treated with estrogens but no progestins had a higher delivery rate of live foals (35 of 50, 70%) than in similar at-risk mares that did not receive estrogens or progestins (4 of 20, 20%) (Douglas, 2004). Both groups of mares had similar hormonal profiles between 106 and 280 days of gestation, with elevated progestin levels (~20 ng/mL) and low levels of estrogens (~600 pg/mL) In healthy pregnant mares, total progestin levels remain relatively low (typically between 4 and 10 ng/mL) from 100 to 300 days of gestation, whereas total estrogen levels exceed 1000 pg/mL from 150 to 310 days of gestation. Monitoring of both total estrogen and progestin in mid-term to late-term at-risk mares appears to provide additional information for the diagnosis of placentitis.

When evidence of placentitis exists, monitoring of fetal viability at regular intervals until parturition occurs is indicated, with the clinician being prepared to provide intensive care to a potentially dysmature foal. No doubt occasions exist in which monitoring of fetal viability enables the clinician to better make a decision regarding whether to induce parturition, taking into account increasing fetal risk versus capability of sustaining extrauterine life. In the case of detection of a dead fetus, twins (Figure 9-6), a prominent fetal abnormality, or hydrallantois, transcutaneous ultrasonographic examination of the uterus and its contents improves the clinician's ability to make a proper diagnosis and justify induction of abortion or parturition.

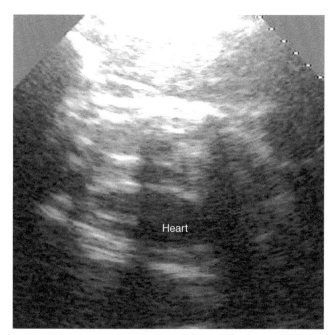

Figure 9-6 Transabdominal ultrasonographic image obtained during assessment of fetal well-being during advanced gestation. The mare had precocious udder development, and impending abortion was suspected. Twin fetuses were detected, with one dead (no heart beat) at the time of examination. The fetal thorax is visualized in this image (note *shadows* cast by ribs), with the anechoic structure being the heart.

MONITORING AND PREPARING THE MARE FOR PARTURITION

Approximately 4 to 6 weeks before the date of expected foaling, the mare should be moved to a location that is clean and dry and provides protection against inclement weather. Pasture is suitable if it is well drained and not overstocked and sheds or trees are available in rainy cold seasons. In cold climates, well-ventilated barns with clean, freshly bedded stalls are commonly used for housing mares overnight and in inclement weather. Moving a mare to the area of foaling 4 to 6 weeks before her due date serves a variety of purposes. It allows the mares to become acclimated to the foaling premises and handling procedures. During this time period, the mares are exposed to organisms indigenous to the foaling area, thus providing them with the opportunity to develop antibodies to organisms that may be infectious. The antibodies are then transferred to the foal through the colostrum. Moving to such a location also avails the near-term mare to closer, more frequent observation. Because the mare is accessible, it is also an opportune time to immunize with appropriate vaccines.

Before foaling, the mare's udder (and ideally the underside of the mare where the foal might attempt to nurse) should be cleansed; if the mare has had the vulva sutured, it should be opened to prevent vulvar tearing at parturition. For indoor foaling, the mare should be placed in a large (14 by 14–ft), recently cleansed, well-bedded, and ventilated stall. When weather permits, the mare can be turned out for exercise in a small paddock or pasture during the day. During observation, particularly at night, care should be taken to avoid disturbing the mare.

Throughout the last month before foaling, the mare should be examined frequently for physical changes that indicate nearness of delivery. Physical changes that occur as parturition nears include development of vulvar laxity and edema, scanty vulvar discharges, relaxation of pelvic ligaments, udder enlargement, and a change in the amount and character of mammary secretion. The most reliable indicator of impending parturition is a remarkable change in udder size and secretion. Mammary gland growth becomes quite apparent in the last month of gestation, particularly in the last 2 weeks. Filling of teats and changes in mammary secretion occur nearer to parturition. The udder typically becomes engorged within the last few days before foaling. The accumulation of waxy secretion on teat ends (Figure 9-7), from early colostrum formation, usually occurs 1 to 4 days before foaling but sometimes as early as 2 weeks before parturition or not at all. Occasionally, milk leaks from teats of pluriparous mares for several days to weeks before foaling, resulting in loss of colostrum. When this occurs, as much of the colostrum as possible should be harvested and stored frozen until the mare foals, or an alternative source of colostrum should be identified.

Monitoring of milk secretions is a valuable tool for predicting nearness of parturition. As parturition

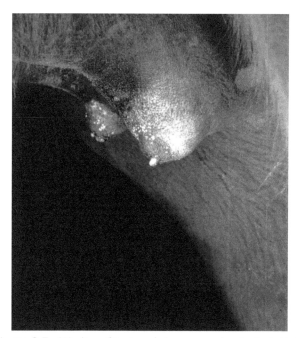

Figure 9-7 Waxing of teat ends in a mare due to foal. Note that the udder is well developed and the teats are full. Waxing of the teat ends usually occurs 1 to 4 days before foaling.

approaches, secretions change from thin straw-colored fluid to one that is milky white. Eventually, a thick viscous fluid that is yellow to orange in color becomes apparent as colostrum formation occurs. Good-quality colostrum should contain more than 60 g IgG/L. Although not all mares produce yellow viscous colostrum, a recent French study confirmed that yellow colostrum had significantly higher IgG concentration than white colostrum, and viscous colostrum also appeared to contain more IgG than liquid colostrum.

Changing electrolyte content of prefoaling udder secretions is related to fetal maturity and viability and thus readiness for birth. The ion concentration (particularly calcium and magnesium) of prefoaling udder secretion increases, especially in the last 2 to 4 days before parturition. Concentrations of Na^+ and K^+ in mammary secretions can also be used as an indicator of approaching parturition. The concentration of Na^+ is higher than that of K^+ in mammary secretions until 48 hours before parturition, when there is an inversion of the Na^+/K^+ ratio and K^+ concentrations exceed Na^+ concentrations (Ousey et al., 1984).

A number of methods can be used to measure calcium content in prefoaling udder secretions and require only a small sample be collected once or twice daily to monitor changes. With atomic absorption spectrophotometry, when calcium concentrations exceeded 10 μmol/L, 92% of mares (10 of 11) foaled spontaneously within 1 to 6 days (Peaker et al., 1979). The Predict-A-Foal Test Mare Foaling Predictor Kit (Animal Health Care Products, Vernon, Calif.) measures both calcium and magnesium concentrations (Figure 9-8). When one of five indicator squares changes color with this test, the mare has less than 1% chance of foaling within the next 12 hours. When four of five indicator squares change color, the mare has a more than 80% chance of foaling within the next 12 hours. A colorimetric test kit (FoalWatch test kit available

from CHEMetrics Inc, Calverton, Va.) has been adapted to measure calcium carbonate concentrations in prefoaling udder secretions of mares (Ley et al., 1998). After diluting 1.5 mL of udder secretion with 9 mL of distilled water, Ley and colleagues used concentrations of calcium carbonate less than 200 ppm in the diluted sample as an indicator that most mares (99% probability) would not foal within 24 hours; the predictive value that a mare would foal within 72 hours was 97% when secretions from mares with calcium carbonate concentrations exceeded 200 ppm. Most mares with colostrum testing results of 300 to 500 ppm of $CaCO_3$ foaled within a short period of time. Whenever possible, secretions should be obtained and measured in the evening, because calcium concentrations in term mares can be low in the morning and rise dramatically by the same evening as the mare approaches parturition.

Neonatal Isoerythrolysis Screening

In an effort to prevent neonatal isoerythrolysis (NI) in the newborn foal, veterinarians may use a screening test for the presence of the alloantibody in at-risk mares. The test is sometimes run on all mares on the farm or, more commonly, is run on those known to have produced a foal with NI in the past and on older pluriparous mares that are more likely to have become exposed to a factor that produces alloantibody (e.g., from delivering a foal; as a result of placentitis during pregnancy). Serum is obtained from the mare 2 weeks before foaling and is tested by a blood typing laboratory for the presence of alloantibody. The detection of alloantibodies in this fashion does not confirm that NI is impending, because the blood type of the foal is not known, but most practitioners muzzle the foal from a "positive" mare and feed it substitute colostrum. The muzzle can be left on for 24 to 36 hours (i.e., until gut closure occurs so that the foal cannot absorb these antibodies from the affected mare's colostrum). Alternatively, the mare can be milked at frequent intervals and, after a suitable period of time, a colostral sample from the mare plus an ethylenediamine tetraacetic acid (EDTA) anticoagulated blood sample from the foal is submitted to a laboratory for the JFA test (jaundiced foal agglutination test). Once the foal's red blood cells (RBCs) no longer agglutinate in the presence of the mare's colostrum, the muzzle can be removed from the foal and it can be allowed to nurse the mare thereafter. If an NI screening test has been performed on a mare but the mare has not foaled within 2 weeks of the test, the test should be performed again.

STAGES OF PARTURITION

Parturition, although it is a continuous process, has arbitrarily been divided into three stages for descriptive purposes. In mares, the **first stage of parturition** (or preparatory stage) usually requires 30 minutes to 4 hours. Shorter and less obvious signs may occur in

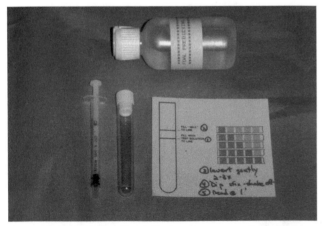

Figure 9-8 The Predict-A-Foal test uses an indicator test strip with succeeding squares changing color as calcium and magnesium contents increase in prefoaling udder secretions and the mare nears spontaneous parturition.

pluriparous mares. During the first stage, mares are restless and exhibit signs similar to that of colic (e.g., the mare may look back toward her flank, raise and switch her tail, urinate small quantities frequently, perspire, and lie down and get up frequently) (Figure 9-9). This period is associated with uterine contractions of increasing intensity and frequency and cervical dilation. Also during this stage, the cranial portion of the foal *rotates from a dorsopubic, through dorsoilial, and eventually to a dorsosacral position*. The uterine contractions eventually push the foal's forefeet and muzzle with the surrounding chorioallantoic membrane into the dilating cervix.

Once the determination has been made that the mare is in the first stage of labor, the tail should be wrapped and the perineal area scrubbed and dried. Late in this stage, the mare will lie down, roll from side to side, and stand up again (Figure 9-10). This activity may be very important in helping the fetus to reposition itself. As the fetus and fetal fluids (contained within the placenta) are forced against the cervix, cervical dilation progresses until the *chorioallantois* ruptures and several gallons of **allantoic fluid** escape from the genital tract (i.e., the "water breaks") (Figure 9-11). If the chorioallantois does not rupture and the velvety-red surface of the chorioallantois is presented at the vulva (red bag delivery; see Figure 8-27), it should be immediately ruptured because this indicates that the placenta is separating from the endometrium (i.e., **premature placental separation**) and fetal oxygenation will be impaired.

Once the chorioallantois ruptures, the **second stage of parturition** ensues, cervical dilation progresses, and the fetus passes into the birth canal. Fetal passage into the pelvic inlet elicits abdominal contractions and release of oxytocin from the neurohypophysis (posterior pituitary gland); these effects reinforce existing uterine contractions. The mare usually lies on her side

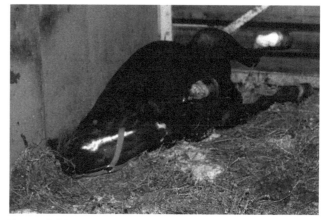

Figure 9-10 Pony mare in the first stage of labor. Regardless of the size of stall used for foaling, a mare may get cast in a corner when rolling during this stage of labor. If the mare gets caught in a corner, she should be pulled away from the corners so she may rise again or so she does not attempt to deliver the foal against a wall or into a corner where delivery is impeded.

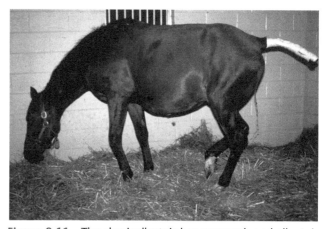

Figure 9-11 The chorioallantois has ruptured, and allantoic fluid escapes from the birth canal. The fluid may initially be released in a slow, almost undetectable stream or in a prominent stream that is obvious. This point marks entry into the second stage of labor.

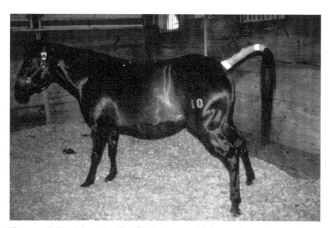

Figure 9-9 Mare in the first stage of labor. The tail has been wrapped and the perineal area and udder have been cleansed. The mare was sweating, stretching, lifting her tail, and urinating small quantities at periodic intervals.

and periodically strains forcefully during this active labor. The repeated abdominal press assists in fetal expulsion. Within 5 minutes after rupture of the chorioallantoic membrane, the **amnion** (the white, glistening membrane) is forced between the vulvar lips (Figure 9-12). As delivery progresses, first one forefoot and then the other become visible, with the soles of the hooves directed downward. The nose follows, with the head resting on the forelimbs at the fetlock or carpal level (Figure 9-13). It is not uncommon for the mare to rise when the forefeet are just being presented at the vulva and then turn around and lie down again a few moments to minutes later and resume active straining. The most forceful contractions occur when the head and shoulders pass through the mare's pelvis (Figure 9-14). The amnion usually ruptures at this point. If necessary,

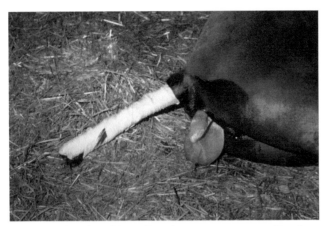

Figure 9-12   The white, glistening structure protruding from the vulva is the amnion, which contains the amniotic fluid. One foot is detectable within the amniotic cavity.

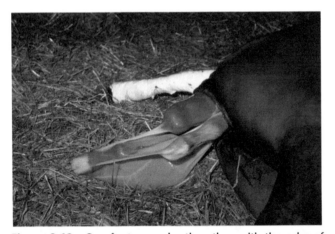

Figure 9-13   One foot precedes the other, with the soles of the feet directed downward, as the second stage of labor progresses. The muzzle of the foal is positioned at the carpus level. Because the amnion may remain intact at this point in delivery, some practitioners prefer to quietly enter the stall and remove the amnion from covering the foal's head to prevent suffocation.

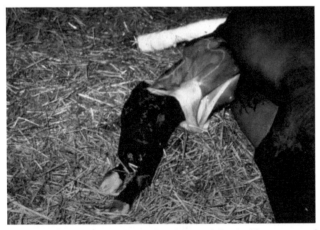

Figure 9-14   The head and shoulders of the foal have passed through the mare's pelvis. The amnion has been ruptured. The level of the shoulders represents the greatest cross-sectional diameter of the foal.

assistance can be provided at this time by gently pulling on the foal's forelimbs in synchrony with the mare's abdominal press (Figure 9-15). Once the foal's hips pass through the maternal pelvis, the mare usually rests for 15 or 20 minutes (Figure 9-16). If the foal has ruptured the amnion and cleared the fetal membranes, is breathing normally, and is able to struggle to a sternal position, the foal and the mare need not be disturbed. Letting the umbilical cord remain attached during this time may result in return of blood from the placenta into the newborn (Figure 9-17). If the mare is disturbed, she may rise and rupture the cord prematurely. In most circumstances, it is acceptable to let the cord break naturally when the mare stands or the foal attempts to rise. If manual separation is deemed necessary, the cord should be grasped with one hand on each side of the intended break point (e.g., the predetermined break site

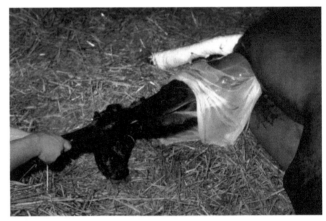

Figure 9-15   If traction must be applied during the dam's abdominal press, one foreleg should be pulled slightly in front of the other to ensure that one shoulder precedes the other during the foal's passage through the maternal pelvis, thereby reducing the effective diameter of the fetus at its shoulders.

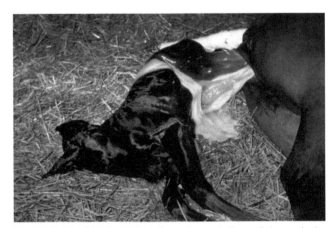

Figure 9-16   The foal's hips have been delivered through the maternal pelvis, and the foal's hind limbs remain within the vagina. The exhausted mare usually rests for a period of time before rising.

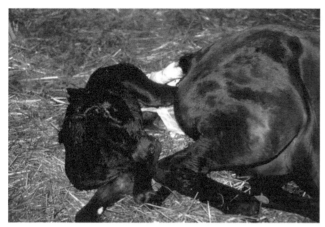

Figure 9-17 When possible, the umbilical cord should be left intact for a few minutes to ensure maximal blood flow from the placenta to the circulation of the newborn foal.

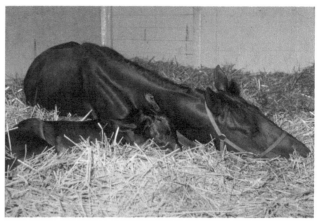

Figure 9-18 Once the umbilical cord has been detached, the foal can be moved toward the mare's head. This procedure can aid in relaxing the mare and can also facilitate the bonding procedure between the mare and the foal.

is seen on the umbilical cord as a pale strictured area 1 to 2 inches from the foal's abdomen; see Figure 11-11). The thumb and forefingers are used to twist and pull the cord apart. Caution should be used to avoid placing undue tension on the cord attachment to the abdominal wall, and the cord should not be cut, because this action may result in excessive hemorrhage or a patent urachus. The umbilical stump should be observed for hemorrhage, urine leakage, or swelling before being disinfected with 0.5% chlorhexidine (Nolvasan solution 2%, Fort Dodge Laboratories). California workers showed chlorhexidine to be superior to 1% or 2% tamed iodine, or 7% tincture of iodine, in reducing bacterial numbers without inducing tissue destruction of the foal navel. The *navel should be disinfected* several times during the first few days of life. An *enema* can also be given at this time to aid in prevention of meconial impaction. If the mare has not risen by this time, the foal can be moved near to the mare's head. This may reduce the likelihood of the mare stepping on the foal when rising (Figure 9-18). Unnecessary disturbances should be avoided, to allow dam-foal interaction during the early postpartum period and to permit the development of a strong bond between them. Guidelines for evaluation of the foal during the first 72 hours of life, including confirmation of sufficient transfer of immunoglobulins through ingestion of colostrum, are reviewed in Chapter 11.

Normally, second stage labor is explosive and short-lived; *delivery of the fetus usually occurs within 20 to 30 minutes*. If delivery is taking longer than this amount of time, or if progression of delivery ceases, fetal position and posture should be assessed immediately (i.e., to ensure **dystocia** is not a problem). The most common impediments to delivery are abnormalities in fetal posture, which must be corrected to facilitate delivery of a viable foal.

Stage 3 of parturition encompasses expulsion of the fetal membranes and uterine involution. Once the mare rises, or in the period immediately after birth when the mare is resting, the placenta can be tied to itself (Figure 9-19) so it hangs just above the hocks to avoid being stepped on until it is passed. The *placenta is typically expelled within 30 minutes to 3 hours* after foaling. If the placenta is not passed by this time, treatment may be necessary to hasten its expulsion and avoid uterine trauma and infection.

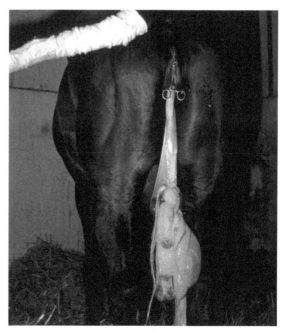

Figure 9-19 The placenta can be tied to itself so it hangs at the level of the hocks when the mare stands. This prevents the mare from stepping on the placenta until it is passed. The labia of the vulva can be temporarily apposed with towel clamps to minimize aspiration of air into the vagina when the mare rises after parturition.

To prevent undue aspiration of air into the vagina when the mare attempts to stand, temporary application of towel clamps has been advocated to appose vulvar labia. We do not find this procedure to be necessary except in some cases of dystocia when swelling and abrasion of tissues have occurred or when vulvar conformation is so poor that aspiration of air and feces is to be avoided. Care should be taken not to incorporate placental tissue in the towel clamps if they are applied, and clamps should be removed as soon as deemed possible. If conformational faults contribute to severe pneumovagina, suturing of the dorsal vulvar lips (see Chapter 15) can be done at this time.

INDUCED PARTURITION

Induction of parturition has been used in the mare for management of high-risk pregnancies, research, teaching, and convenience. Several drugs have been used to induce parturition in the mare. Regardless of which agent is used to induce parturition, the mare and the fetus must be ready for birth. Gestation should be at least 335 days in length. Adequate pelvic ligament and cervical relaxation should be apparent, and udder development and good quality colostrum should be present (refer to guidelines given earlier to determine readiness for birth). Although parturition can be induced in mares with a nonrelaxed cervix (providing other signs of readiness for birth are apparent), the first stage of labor is prolonged. Texas workers have shown that the prolonged first stage of labor is associated with an increased incidence of birth hypoxia and neonatal maladjustment. In a subsequent study, the Texas workers showed that placement of 2 mg prostaglandin E_2, (PGE_2) (Sigma Aldrich, St. Louis, Mo.) in the external cervical os 4 to 6 hours before inducing parturition resulted in softening of the cervix and a shorter interval to delivery, which should decrease the chances of birth hypoxia and neonatal maladjustment syndrome. Others have recommended 200 to 1000 μg of PGE_1 (Cytotec, G. D. Searle and Co, Omaha, NE.) can be used for promoting cervical softening before induction. Whenever parturition is induced, if delivery is not progressive or is delayed once labor begins, prompt examination for dystocia is indicated

Oxytocin is generally considered to be the drug of choice for inducing parturition in the mare. The drug has a rapid effect and usually results in delivery within 15 to 90 minutes after oxytocin administration is begun. The patterns of induction are consistent and seem to have little untoward effect on the term foal. Various methods of oxytocin administration have been used to induce parturition, including (1) injection of 40 to 120 units (intramuscularly); (2) injection of 2.5 to 20 units (intravenously, intramuscularly, or subcutaneously) at 15- to 20-minute intervals until the second stage of labor ensues; and (3) intravenous drip of 60 to 120 units in 1 L saline solution at a rate of 1 unit/min until the second stage of labor ensues. The uterus of the term mare is very sensitive to the effects of oxytocin, and the response is dose-dependent. Doses exceeding 40 units given as a bolus are unnecessary and can result in premature placental separation, malpositions, or malpostures from the rapid and forceful contractions that are induced.

When mares are near the time of spontaneous delivery, very low doses of oxytocin are capable of inducing parturition. Some practitioners have proposed that administration of a single daily microdose of oxytocin in the evening results in a response in only those mares ready for delivery. Those mares that do not respond can continue to be treated once daily until either they respond or deliver their foal spontaneously. Use of oxytocin in this manner can result in most foals being born at a predictable time when personnel are available for assistance if needed. Italian workers used this protocol for half of the mares on one Standardbred farm. Of the 148 mares that met criteria for readiness to deliver (e.g., >335 days of gestation, >200 ppm calcium concentration in udder secretions), intramuscular administration of 3.5 units of oxytocin once in the evening between the hours of 18:00 and 20:00 resulted in foaling 69% of mares within 2 hours of oxytocin administration on the first, second, or third evening of treatment (51% foaled the first night, 14% foaled the second night, and 3% foaled the third night). The remainder of the mares foaled either more than 2 hours after oxytocin administration or spontaneously at a time unrelated to oxytocin administration. Only two treated mares experienced dystocia.

Both natural and synthetic prostaglandins have also been used successfully for inducing parturition in the mare; however, the prostaglandin analogs are generally thought to produce more predictable responses with less risk to the foal. Fluprostenol (250 μg, intramuscularly) has been reported to induce parturition only in those mares in which the fetus is mature and capable of extrauterine life. However, this is not always the case because some premature foals have been delivered after administration of fluprostenol. In addition, the induction-parturition interval is more variable (1 to 6 hours) with fluprostenol than with oxytocin. Fenprostalene (0.5 to 1.0 mg, subcutaneously; in 2 hours, either repeat fenprostalene injection or initiate oxytocin administration) has also been used successfully to induce parturition in mares. When the two-injection scheme of fenprostalene was used, most mares delivered their foals within 2 to 4 hours after the first fenprostalene injection. When 2.5 units oxytocin was administered intravenously at 15- to 20-minute intervals beginning 2 hours after the initial fenprostalene injection, mares delivered foals within 2 to 3 hours. However, neither fenprostalene nor fluprostenol is currently available in the United States.

Unlike in cattle, corticosteroids generally are not effective for inducing parturition in the mare. However, based on work in women, administration of corticosteroids to mares with high-risk pregnancies is sometimes performed several days before induction of parturition in an effort to enhance fetal lung maturation. Preliminary studies by workers in England showed that daily administration of 100 mg of dexamethasone on days 315 to 317 of gestation hastened fetal maturation. Fully mature foals were born at 322 days of gestation. This treatment certainly warrants further investigation in the horse.

THE POSTPARTUM PERIOD

Breeding on the First Postpartum Estrus

For optimal economic return in broodmares, management personnel must strive to maximize the number of foals produced per dam lifetime. The major constraint to achieving this goal in the mare is the relatively long gestation period, which averages 340 days and permits only 25 days from parturition to conception to produce foals at yearly intervals. The pregnancy rate achieved by breeding during the first postpartum estrus (foal heat) is often lower (e.g., 10% to 20% lower) than that achieved by breeding on subsequent estrus periods (see Chapter 3 discussion of fertility in the early postpartum period). However, failure to establish pregnancy by foal-heat breeding results in an 18-day drift toward a later conception and a corresponding delay in the foaling date the following year. Registry-derived time constraints that are placed on equine breeding seasons often result in barrenness in late-foaling mares. Failure to produce foals on a yearly basis culminates in irretrievable economic loss because of expenses for feed and housing, transportation, animal care, and nonproductive breeding fees.

Uterine Involution

The decreased pregnancy rate associated with foal-heat breeding has been suggested to result from failure of the uterus, particularly the endometrium, to be completely restored to a pregravid state and therefore ready to support a developing embryo. Although a paucity of information is available on uterine involution and its relationship to fertility in the mare, changes that occur during the involution process have been studied. Vaginal exudate progressively decreases through the first postpartum ovulation, and the amount of fluid detected via ultrasound in the uterine lumen decreases until it is nondetectable by day 15 post partum. Uterine horns return to pregravid size by day 32 post partum, whereas involution of the endometrium occurs more rapidly. Resorption of microcaruncles is essentially complete by day 7 post partum, and the overlying luminal epithelium is intact by days 4 to 7 post partum. Endometrial gland dilation is absent by day 4 post partum, and glandular activity increases, as indicated by taller epithelial cells with increased mitotic activity, through day 12 post partum. The *endometrium usually has a normal pregravid histologic appearance by day 14 post partum.* This is probably the reason for increased pregnancy rates in mares that ovulate after 10 days post partum when bred on foal heat because embryo entry into the uterus occurs 5 to 6 days after ovulation when intrauterine fluid is absent and the endometrium is restored. For a review of hormonal treatments to delay breeding of postpartum mares until uterine involution has taken place, refer to Chapter 3.

Factors responsible for uterine involution are not well understood. Uterine contractility probably plays an important role in rapidly reducing the postparturient uterus to its pregravid state. Concurrent with this decrease in uterine size, a significant amount of lochial fluid is discharged from the uterine lumen. The histologic character of the endometrium correspondingly reverts to a condition more conducive to embryonic support.

Examination of the Postpartum Mare

Routine examination of the postpartum reproductive tract of the mare is done when pathologic conditions are suspected and to provide information on which to base a decision to breed a mare on the first postpartum estrus. Procedures used for these purposes include inspection of the vulva and perineum, palpation of the genital tract per rectum, transrectal ultrasound examination of the genital tract, and examination of the vagina and cervix digitally or through a speculum. Knowledge of characteristics of normal involution is necessary to accurately assess the status of the reproductive tract. The following listing is of events that occur in the progression of uterine involution and return to ovarian cyclicity in the postpartum mare.

- **Placental passage:** Normally within 3 to 4 hours after delivery of the foal.
- **Twelve to 24 hours post partum:** Marked decrease in uterine size; uterine discharge evident. Most uterine fluid is eliminated by 24 to 48 hours post partum.
- **Three to 5 days post partum:** Usual time of thorough postpartum examination. Both uterine horns are palpable per rectum, the gravid horn is more enlarged than nongravid horn, vulvar discharge ceases, blood-tinged discharge is noted at external cervical os, and the external cervical os is hyperemic.
- **Five to 15 days post partum:** Onset of first postpartum estrus (foal heat). The microcaruncles of the endometrium are no longer evident by day 7, the endometrium has a normal nonpregnant histologic appearance by day 14, the myometrium is still enlarged, the gravid horn is still more enlarged than the nongravid horn, the external cervical os may still be hyperemic, and the cervix

does not close from the time of parturition until after foal-heat ovulation occurs.

▪ **Foal heat (first postpartum estrus):** Onset at 4 to 14 days. A slight decrease in pregnancy rates achieved by breeding on the first postpartum estrus may be seen. The main advantage to breeding on foal heat over breeding on later postpartum estrus periods is a reduction in the interval from parturition to conception (25.3 versus 43.8 days open).

▪ **First postpartum ovulation:** Forty-three percent of mares ovulate by day 9, 93% of mares ovulate by day 15, and 97% of mares ovulate by day 20. Mares that ovulate after day 10 post partum are reputed to have normal pregnancy rates (i.e., the same as mares that are bred for the first time on the second or later postpartum heats).

▪ **Twenty-five to 32 days post partum:** Onset of second postpartum estrus. The uterine horns have returned to pregravid size.

BIBLIOGRAPHY

American Association of Equine Practitioners: *Guidelines for vaccination of horses,* 2008, available at www.aaep.org/vaccination_guidelines.htm. Accessed November 18, 2009.

Adams-Brendemuehl C: Fetal assesment. In Koterba AM, Drummond WH, Kosch PC, editors: *Equine neonatology,* Philadelphia, 1990, Lea & Febiger, 16-33.

Conboy HS: Preventing contagious equine diseases, *Proc 51st Ann Mtg Am Assoc Equine Pract* 439-445, 2005.

Douglas RH: Endocrine diagnostics in the broodmare: what you need to know about progestins and estrogens, *Proc Soc Theriogenology* 106-115, 2004.

Hintz HF: Nutrition of the broodmare. In McKinnon AO, Voss JL, editors: *Equine reproduction,* Philadelphia, 1993, Lea & Febiger, 631-639.

Ley WB, Parker NA, Bowen JM, et al: How we induce the normal mare to foal, *Proc 44th Ann Mtg Am Assoc Equine Pract* 194-197, 1998.

Loy RC: Characteristics of postpartum reproduction in mares, *Vet Clin N Am Large Anim Prac* 2:345-358, 1980.

McClure JJ: Diseases of the immune system. In Kobluk CN, Amers TR, Geor RJ, editors: *The horse: diseases and clinical management,* Philadelphia, 1995, Saunders, 1051-1063.

National Research Council: *Nutrient requirements of horses,* Washington, DC, 1989, National Academy of Sciences, National Research Council.

Ousey JC, Dudan F, Rossdale PD: Preliminary studies of mammary secretions in the mare to assess foetal readiness for birth, *Equine Vet J* 16:259-263, 1984.

Ousey J, Delcaux M, Rossdale P: Evaluation of three test strips for measuring electrolytes in mare's prepartum mammary secretions and for predicting parturition, *Equine Vet J* 21:196-200, 1989.

Ousey JC, Kölling M, Allen WR: The effects of maternal dexamethasone treatment on gestation length and foal maturation in thoroughbred mares, *Proceed 9th Int Symposium Equine Reprod Animal Reprod Sci* 94:436-438, 2006.

Peaker M, Rossdale PD, Forwyth IA, et al: Changes in mammary development and the composition of secretion during late pregnancy in the mare, *J Reprod Fert* 27(Suppl):555-561, 1979.

Reef VB, Vaala WE, Worth LT, et al: Transcutaneous ultrasonographic assessment of fetal well-being during late gestation: a preliminary report on the development of an equine biophysical profile, *Proc 42nd Ann Mtg Am Assoc Equine Pract* 152-153, 1996.

Reimer JM: Use of transcutaneous ultrasonography in complicated latter-middle to late gestation pegnancies in the mare: 122 cases, *Proc 43rd Ann Mtg Am Assoc Equine Pract* 259-261, 1997.

Roberts SJ: *Veterinary obstetrics and genital diseases, theriogenology,* ed 3, Woodstock, VT, 1986, SJ Roberts 277-352.

Rossdale PD, Ricketts SW: *Equine stud farm medicine,* ed 2, Philadelphia, 1980, Lea & Febiger, 220-276.

Slater R: Immunologic control of viral and bacterial pathogens, *Proc 46th Ann Mtg Am Assoc Equine Pract* 10-20, 2000.

Troedsson MHT, Renaudin CD, Zent WW, et al: Transrectal ultrasonography of the placenta in normal mares and mares with pending abortion: a field study, *Proc 43rd Ann Mtg Am Assoc Equine Pract* 256-258, 1997.

Villani M, Romano G: Induction or parturition with daily low-dose oxytocin injections in pregnant mares at term: clinical applications and limitations, *Reprod Dom Anim* 43:481-483, 2008.

Wilson WD: Strategies for vaccinating mares, foals, and weanlings, *Proc 51st Ann Mtg Am Assoc Equine Pract* 421-438, 2005.

Dystocia and Postparturient Disease

10

CHAPTER

OBJECTIVES

While studying the information covered in this chapter, the reader should attempt to:
- Acquire a working understanding of maternal and fetal contributions to dystocia and those factors that contribute to postparturient abnormalities in the mare.
- Acquire a working knowledge of procedures used to diagnose and relieve dystocia in the mare.
- Acquire a working knowledge of procedures used to diagnose and methodologies used to treat abnormalities of the postparturient period in the mare.

STUDY QUESTIONS

1. List equipment necessary to correct dystocia in the mare.
2. Describe procedures used to diagnose the cause of dystocia in the mare.
3. Define the following terms:
   a. Dystocia
   b. Fetal presentation
   c. Fetal position
   d. Fetal posture
   e. Mutation
   f. Repulsion
   g. Delivery via traction
4. Describe the more common obstetric procedures used to correct dystocia in the mare via mutation and delivery via traction.

5. Describe proper treatment of the following postparturient abnormalities in the mare:
   a. Retained placenta
   b. Metritis
   c. Laminitis
   d. Uterine prolapse
   e. Invagination of the uterine horn
   f. Uterine rupture
   g. Ruptured uterine or ovarian artery
   h. Other postparturient hemorrhages

Dystocia and postparturient disease are uncommon in the mare; however, when they do occur, they may carry a guarded prognosis for life or future fertility in affected mares. Prompt, sound clinical management of dystocia, retained placenta, and other postparturient disorders can preserve the breeding potential of valuable mares.

DYSTOCIA

For better recognition of dystocia, the processes and events of normal delivery must be well understood. Refer to Chapter 9 for a review of normal progression through the three stages of parturition. If either the first or the second stage of parturition is prolonged or not

131

progressing, dystocia is possible. Prompt veterinary examination is indicated to preserve the life of the foal and mare and to prevent injury to the mare's reproductive tract.

Obstetric Equipment and Lubricant

High-quality, clean (preferably sterile) obstetric equipment and lubricant should be readily available. Equipment should include, at a minimum, lubricant, obstetric chains or straps, obstetric handles, a bucket, cotton or paper towels, tail wrap, and disinfectant soap (Figure 10-1). For the special equipment needed to perform a fetotomy, the reader is referred to the monograph by Bierschwal and de Bois (1972).

When minimal obstetric manipulations are necessary, the authors sometimes apply a small amount of polyethylene polymer powder (J-Lube, Jorgensen Laboratories Loveland, CO) to the birth canal of the mare. The powder adheres to mucosal membranes, which provides excellent short-term lubrication for extracting the fetus. Note, however, that this product should be avoided if any chance of uterine rupture exists or if a cesarean section may be needed because even small amounts of J-lube contamination of the peritoneum can be fatal (Frazer et al., 2004). Liquid lubricants (e.g., carboxymethylcellulose solution) provide good protection to the fetus and genital tract and can be pumped into the uterine lumen and around the fetus through a sterile stomach tube. Lubricant solution can be sterilized in gallon containers before use, or 0.5 to 1 tablespoon of chlorhexidine solution can be mixed with each gallon of lubricant as a disinfectant. This amount of disinfectant does not seem to irritate the genital tract. Pumping lubricant into the uterine lumen provides some uterine distention that facilitates manipulation of the fetus. For fetotomy, petroleum jelly can be applied

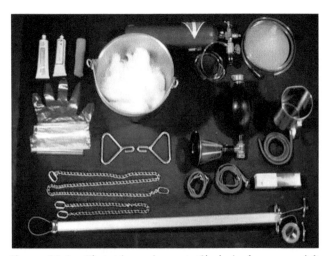

Figure 10-1 Obstetric equipment. *Clockwise from upper left:* Tubes of sterile lubricant, clean bucket containing cotton, oxygen bottle, administration set, enema bucket and tube, Ambu bag, obstetric straps, nasal catheter, fetatome, obstetric chains and handles, and obstetric gloves.

to the fetus and birth canal for extra protection against physical injury during the procedure.

Examination of the Mare

If possible, the mare should be standing for the initial examination. The examination is done in a clean environment with good footing for the mare and the veterinarian. The tail is wrapped and tied to the side, and the perineal area and rump are thoroughly scrubbed with an antiseptic soap and dried. If straining is a problem, the initial examination is made while the mare is being slowly walked. When necessary, a local anesthetic can be injected into the caudal epidural space to control straining. After the hair over the site of injection (usually coccygeal vertebrae 1 and 2, Cy1-Cy2) is clipped, the skin is scrubbed and disinfected. Lidocaine (1.0 to 1.25 mL of 2% lidocaine per 100 kg of body weight) can then be administered in the caudal epidural space to provide perineal analgesia and control straining. We prefer to use a combination of xylazine (35 mg/500 kg of body weight), Carbocaine-V (Pharmacia & Upjohn Co, New York, NY) (2.6 mL of 2% mepivacaine hydrochloride/500 kg of body weight), and sterile 0.9% NaCl solution (sufficient quantity [qs] to 7.0 to 8.0 mL/500 kg of body weight) for epidural anesthesia. The rationale for use of this combination is that perineal analgesia is optimized while the risk of hind limb ataxia associated with higher doses of local anesthetics is reduced. Note that because 30 minutes may be required for full anesthetic effect, valuable time can be lost if an epidural is used when a live fetus is present, which can result in the delivery of a compromised foal or stillborn fetus. In some cases, general anesthesia (xylazine, 1.0 mg/kg, intravenously [IV], followed by ketamine, 2 mg/kg, IV) may be necessary to facilitate obstetric procedures.

The hands and arms of the veterinarian are scrubbed with a disinfectant soap and then rinsed before entry into the birth canal. Sterile plastic sleeves can also be worn. The fetus is thoroughly examined to assess presentation, position, and posture and for the presence of any congenital abnormalities, such as contracted tendons, that might contribute to dystocia. An attempt is made to determine whether the fetus is alive with stimulation of reflex movements or with detection of a heartbeat or umbilical pulse if either the fetal thorax or umbilicus is within reach. Evidence of trauma that may indicate a previous attempt to deliver or allude to the duration of dystocia is noted.

For descriptive purposes, the reader should be familiar with terms used to describe the fetus at the time of its entrance into the birth canal or pelvis. **Presentation** refers to the relationship of the spinal axis of the fetus to that of the dam (*longitudinal* or *transverse*) and the portion of the fetus entering the pelvic cavity (head, *anterior* or *cranial;* or tail, *posterior* or *caudal*) in longitudinal presentations or ventral or dorsal in transverse presentations. **Position** refers to the relationship of the dorsum of the fetus in longitudinal presentation or the head in transverse presentation to the quadrants of the maternal pelvis (sacrum, right ilium, left ilium, or pubis). **Posture** refers to the relationship of the fetal extremities (head, neck, and limbs) to the body of the fetus; they may be flexed, extended, or retained beneath or above the fetus. The normal presentation, position, and posture of the equine fetus during parturition are anterior-longitudinal, dorsosacral, and with the head, neck, and forelimbs extended, respectively. Fetal postural abnormalities are the most common cause of dystocia in the mare. Equine fetuses are predisposed to postural abnormalities because of the long fetal extremities. Structural abnormalities of the fetus, such as hydrocephalus, may also result in dystocia. Caudal and particularly transverse fetal presentations are associated with a greatly increased incidence of fetal malformations (particularly contractures) that contribute to dystocia. Fetal death or severe compromise prevents the fetus from taking an active part in positioning for delivery, thereby contributing to dystocia.

Accurate assessments of fetal presentation, position, and posture; the presence of fetal abnormalities; whether the fetus is alive; the condition of the genital tract; and the general condition of the mare are necessary to formulate a plan for delivery. Unless structural abnormalities of the fetus are present, mutation and delivery via traction are often possible. If dystocia is prolonged, the birth canal and uterus may become contracted, edematous, and devoid of fetal fluids, necessitating the choice of an alternate route of delivery.

Delivery via Mutation and Traction

Mutation refers to manipulation of the fetus to return it to normal presentation, position, and posture for facilitation of delivery. It is helpful to first repel the fetus from the maternal pelvis into the abdominal cavity (where more space is available for repositioning and correction of fetal malposture). Additional room can sometimes be gained by pumping 1 or 2 gal of warm liquid lubricant into the uterine lumen and around the fetus. To avoid uterine rupture, obstetric manipulations must not be overly vigorous. Repulsion is not attempted if the uterus is devoid of fetal fluids, dry, and contracted; an alternative form of delivery (cesarean section) is chosen. General anesthesia and elevation of the hindquarters of the mare often result in sufficient gravitational repulsion and elimination of straining to permit mutation and delivery of the fetus.

In countries in which injectable clenbuterol (Ventipulmin Solution, Boehringer-Ingelheim, Burlington, Ontario) is available, slow intravenous administration of 0.17 to 0.35 mg/454 kg of body weight induces uterine relaxation sufficient to permit safer repulsion and repositioning of the fetus. Although this drug is antagonistic to the effects of prostaglandin-$F_2\alpha$ (PGF$_2\alpha$)

and oxytocin, its use apparently does not result in an increased incidence of uterine prolapse or retained placenta. Clamping the dorsal vulvar labia for 6 to 8 hours after correction of dystocia with this drug may, however, be indicated to reduce the chance of prolapse. More recently, practitioners have started using Buscopan (N-butylscopolammonium bromide, Boehringer-Ingelheim Pharmaceuticals, Ridgefield, CT) to relax the uterus and facilitate obstetric procedures.

Correction of Malposture

Regardless of presentation, the limbs of a full-term fetus must be extended to permit passage through the birth canal. To correct **carpal** or **hock flexion**, the flexed carpus or hock is repelled out of the pelvis while traction is applied to the foot until it is fully extended. Traction can either be applied entirely by hand or be assisted by first placing an obstetric chain or strap around the pastern and having an assistant pull on it while the other hand simultaneously repels the proximal portion of the limb. If adequate room is available, this procedure can sometimes be accomplished by introducing both arms into the birth canal. One hand should be cupped over the foot as it is brought outward to prevent uterine rupture when traction is applied on the distal end of a flexed limb.

Anterior presentations with deviations of the head and neck commonly lead to dystocia in mares. For correction of lateral or ventral head posture, the fetus is repelled and the jaw or muzzle of the foal is grasped and pulled toward the pelvic inlet. To gain more room for this procedure, one forelimb can first be placed in carpal flexion after a chain is placed around the pastern. The chain is helpful for correcting the carpal flexion after the head is replaced in the pelvic inlet. Securing a snare around the lower jaw may correct alignment of the head and neck, provided minimal traction is applied. Alternatively, a loop of obstetric chain can be secured to the head by placing it through the mouth and over the poll. Again, minimal traction should be applied and care should be taken to prevent damage to the uterus from incisors through a gaping mouth created with this technique.

When the fetus is presented normally (i.e., anterior longitudinal presentation, dorsosacral position, with the forelimbs, head, and neck extended), delivery can proceed. If the fetus is presented posteriorly, delivery can proceed after the hind limbs are extended. Traction straps or chains can be placed around the fetal pasterns, with the eye of the straps on the dorsal (extensor) aspect of the limbs. Placement of two loops on each limb, with the first encircling the distal cannon bone (immediately above the fetlock) and the second encircling the pastern (Figure 10-2), helps prevent damage to the distal limb when forceful traction is applied. Traction is gradual and smooth, applied only during the

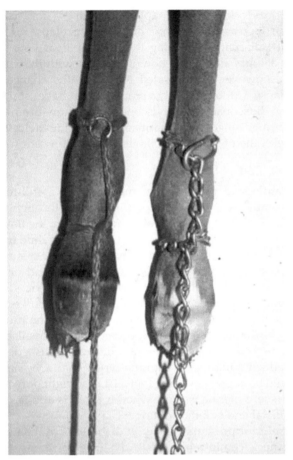

Figure 10-2 Obstetric strap and chain, each placed with two loops on the forelimb, with the first loop encircling the distal cannon bone above the fetlock and the second loop encircling the pastern.

dam's abdominal press. With anterior-longitudinal presentation, traction is applied such that one forelimb precedes the other until the shoulders travel through the birth canal.

Any impediments to delivery are corrected promptly to allow delivery to continue because the umbilicus may be compressed, thus restricting blood supply to the fetus. In posterior presentations, rupture or impaction of the umbilicus quickly leads to fetal anoxia, so delivery must be accomplished quickly to avoid fetal asphyxia.

If the fetus is in posterior presentation with bilateral hip flexion (**breech presentation**) or **transverse presentation**, the chances of delivery of a viable foal after dystocia are greatly reduced. The casual observer is frequently unaware that the mare is in labor in these cases because abdominal straining is often weak. More detailed procedures for mutation and delivery via traction are reviewed by Roberts (1986).

If the dystocia cannot be corrected within 10 to 15 minutes via fetal manipulations with the mare standing, anesthetization of the mare may increase the chance of a successful delivery. After induction of anesthesia, the mare is positioned in dorsal recumbency and the hindquarters are elevated with a hoist until the long axis of the mare is at a 30-degree angle to the floor or ground. If the mare is anesthetized in the field, placement of the mare in a head-down position on an incline often works as well. This procedure eliminates abdominal straining and increases the intraabdominal space for easier manipulation of the fetus.

If the fetus is dead and cannot be delivered via mutation and traction, an alternative method of delivery must be chosen. **Fetotomy** may provide a more satisfactory alternative than cesarean section in such cases. When fetotomy is correctly performed, major abdominal surgery is avoided, which results in a shorter recovery time for the mare and less aftercare than with cesarean section. The most common indication for fetotomy is to remove the head and neck of a dead fetus when manual correction of lateral or ventral head deviation is difficult. However, fetotomy should be avoided, if possible, in mares with protracted involution and fetal emphysema (because room to manipulate the fetus and fetatome is severely constrained), or if more than partial dismemberment (one or two cuts) of the fetus is necessary, to avoid the potential for severe damage to the genital tract.

Cesarean section is indicated if attempts to deliver a foal per vagina jeopardize the foal or mare or are apt to impair the mare's subsequent fertility. Such situations include certain types of malpresentation; emphysematous fetuses; deformed fetuses; certain types of uterine torsion; and abnormalities of the dam's pelvis, cervix, or vagina. Extremely large foals or small dams might also necessitate cesarean section for correction of dystocia. Refer to citations in the Bibliography for discussion of equipment, procedures, and techniques for performing percutaneous fetotomy and cesarean section.

Uterine Torsion

Uterine torsion occurs uncommonly in mares; however, it does account for a significant percentage of serious equine dystocias. Uterine torsion occurs more commonly in preterm mares (5 to 8 months of gestation) than in term mares. Preterm mares with uterine torsion exhibit signs of intermittent, unresponsive colic. The condition is diagnosed by determining displacement of the tense broad ligaments via palpation per rectum. Identification of the ovaries is helpful in determining that "twisted" structures are indeed the uterus and broad ligaments. Diagnostic methods are the same for preterm and term uterine torsion. The reader is referred to Chapter 8 for discussion of diagnosis and treatment of uterine torsion in preterm mares. Uterine torsion very rarely occurs at term with the cervix dilated. If the cervix is open, correction of the torsion may be possible in a standing mare by grasping the fetus ventrolaterally with the arm resting on the pelvic floor and then rocking the fetus to impart momentum until it can be lifted upward and rotated into (opposite to) the direction of the uterine twist. If this method is successful, the fetus and uterus rotate into the normal position, and the fetus can be delivered as soon as the cervix becomes fully dilated.

In many cases of uterine torsion, correction must be accomplished surgically. Surgical methods for correction of uterine torsion are described in citations in the Bibliography.

POSTPARTURIENT ABNORMALITIES

Retained Placenta

The fetal membranes are usually expelled 30 minutes to 3 hours after parturition. The placenta is considered to be retained if it is not expelled within 3 hours after birth of the foal. The percentage of postparturient mares with retained fetal membranes is reported to range from 2% to 17% but may be as high as 54% in draft breeds.

The probability of retained placenta increases after dystocia, probably as a result of trauma to the uterus and myometrial exhaustion. Disturbance of the normal uterine contractions at parturition also might make retained placenta more likely. Retention is particularly likely if severe placentitis was present. Placental retention is more common in the nongravid uterine horn (Figure 10-3), perhaps because of a progressive increase in the degree of placental folding and attachment from the gravid horn to the nongravid horn. Partial placental retention is also more likely to occur in the nongravid uterine horn than in the gravid horn because the chorioallantoic membrane is thinner, resulting in easier tearing.

Disturbed uterine contractions may result from fetomaternal endocrine dysfunction, inadequate release of oxytocin, or inadequate response of the myometrium to oxytocin. The role of oxytocin in placental expulsion is attested to by prompt placental expulsion after oxytocin-induced parturition and by the failure of some mares with retained placenta to exhibit the characteristic abdominal discomfort typically associated with uterine contraction and placental expulsion in the early postpartum period.

A variable portion of the placenta may be exposed through the vulvar opening. Occasionally, the veterinarian is alerted to the possibility of retained placenta when no placenta is found after foaling. Aseptic intrauterine examination may reveal the presence of the placenta within the uterine cavity. Alternatively, part of the placenta may remain in the uterus and continue to initiate mild straining or colic after most of the placenta has been removed. For this reason, the expelled fetal membranes should be examined to ensure that they are complete and that no portion remains in the uterus. Retention of portions of the placenta other than just the tip in the previously nongravid horn is also possible, so thorough examination of both surfaces of the expelled chorioallantois is necessary to detect less obvious missing portions. For facilitation of examination, the chorioallantois can be filled with water (Figure 10-4). If the expelled placenta has been damaged (by trampling or other means), determination of whether remnants remain in the uterus may be impossible from inspection of the placenta alone.

Sequelae of retained placenta range from none (particularly if mares are well managed and promptly treated) to the development of metritis, septicemia or toxemia, laminitis, and death. Uterine involution is often delayed even if mares do not have these sequelae develop. Retained placenta with serious sequelae is reportedly more common in draft horses than in Thoroughbreds or Standardbreds, and mares with retained

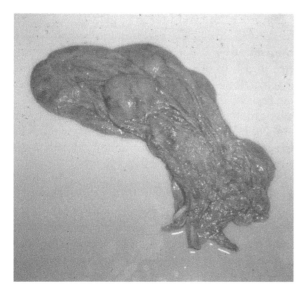

Figure 10-3 Tip of the placental horn typically retained in the uterus.

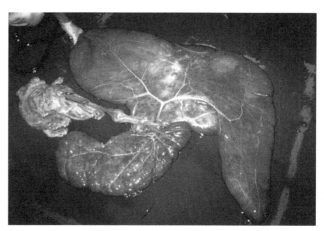

Figure 10-4 Expelled placenta is filled with water for examination.

placenta after dystocia have a greater risk for the development of toxic metritis and laminitis. Severe toxic metritis and laminitis after dystocia are believed to result from delayed uterine involution, increased autolysis of the placenta, and severe bacterial infection. In mares with toxic metritis after dystocia and retained placenta, the uterine wall becomes thin and friable or even necrotic. Absorption of bacteria and bacterial toxins probably follows loss of endometrial integrity and precipitates the peripheral vascular changes that lead to laminitis.

Various treatments for retained placenta in mares have been advocated. Manual removal was the probably the first method used to treat a retained placenta; although it is still widely practiced in some areas, we do not recommend it because of the potential for damage to the endometrium. Oxytocin therapy (alone or in conjunction with other treatments) is the most common and apparently the most beneficial form of management. Recommended doses range from 20 to 60 U (smaller doses are given intravenously, whereas larger doses are given subcutaneously or intramuscularly), and dosing can be repeated every 4 to 6 hours if the placenta is not passed. We prefer to inject 20 U intramuscularly to promote more physiologic (peristaltic-like) uterine contractions. Clinical signs of abdominal discomfort occur within a few minutes of injection and are usually followed by straining. Discomfort is more pronounced with large doses and might result from intense and perhaps spasmodic uterine contractions. A more physiologic, less intense response occurs during slow intravenous infusion of 30 to 60 U of oxytocin in 1 or 2 L of normal saline solution over a 30-minute to 60-minute period. Occasionally, uterine prolapse can occur after oxytocin administration, so care should be taken to observe for this potential complication. If not expelled shortly after injection of oxytocin, the placenta sometimes is expelled 1 or 2 hours later. The placenta can sometimes be extracted with gentle traction applied to the portion protruding from the patient's vulva. Mares that have undergone severe dystocia or that have aborted are less likely to respond. If the chorioallantois is intact, distention of the chorioallantoic cavity with 9 to 12 L of warm, sterile water or saline solution is an effective treatment for retained placenta (Figure 10-5). The opening of the chorioallantois is closed to contain the fluid. Stretch receptors are activated when the chorioallantois and uterus are distended, followed by endogenous release of oxytocin and separation of the chorionic villi from the endometrial crypts. Escaping fluid is forced back into the retained portion of the placenta until separation is complete and the placenta is expelled (usually 5 to 30 minutes). This treatment protocol can be used in conjunction with exogenous oxytocin therapy.

Other treatments that can be combined with oxytocin therapy include administration of systemic and

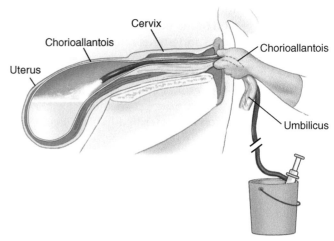

Figure 10-5   Distention of chorioallantoic cavity with fluid to promote expulsion of placenta.

local antibiotics, uterine lavage, exercise, and prophylactic measures to prevent laminitis (e.g., systemic administration of cyclooxygenase inhibitors or application of footpads). Whether intrauterine treatment should be continued after the fetal membranes have passed is a topic of controversy; use of such treatment is particularly questionable if contamination of the reproductive tract was minimal and placental passage after treatment was prompt.

The rationale for uterine lavage in mares that are at risk of metritis is that removal of debris and bacteria from the uterus reduces contamination and creates a less favorable environment for bacterial growth. Purulent material and cellular debris which may bind to and inactivate many antibiotics, are also removed with uterine lavage. After disinfection of the perineal and vulvar areas, a sterilized or disinfected nasogastric tube is passed into the uterus. The hand is cupped around the end of the tube to prevent the uterus and any remaining placenta from being siphoned into its end (Figure 10-6). The uterus is gently lavaged with warm (40°C to 42°C) physiologic saline solution (administered via a sterile or disinfected stomach pump) in 3-L to 6-L flushes until the effluent is relatively clear. If necessary, uterine lavage can be repeated on successive days until the initial effluent is free of purulent material and tissue debris. Oxytocin therapy (10 to 20 U, every 6 hours, intramuscularly [IM]), which stimulates uterine contractions that last 20 to 50 minutes, helps expel uterine contents.

If there is concern that the mare might develop septic or toxic metritis and laminitis, systemic and intrauterine antimicrobial therapy is indicated. Intrauterine antimicrobial agents are administered after evacuation of lavage fluid. Because antimicrobial agents infused into the uterus seldom reach acceptable levels anywhere except in the uterine lumen and endometrium, relatively high antibiotic doses are administered systemically to prevent or control the development of

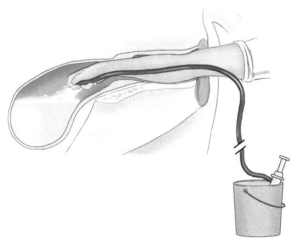

Figure 10-6 Technique used for lavage of the uterus of the postpartum mare. The hand should be cupped around the end of the tube to avoid injury to the uterus from the siphoning action.

septicemia from uterine infection that might involve tissue deeper than the endometrium. The agents chosen should be compatible and should have broadspectrum activity, because a wide variety of organisms have been recovered from the postpartum uterus. The antimicrobial regimen must be effective against anaerobic bacteria and endotoxin-producing organisms. Administration of gentamicin (6.6 mg/kg, every 24 hours, IV) and penicillin (22,000 to 44,000 U Na$^+$ or K$^+$ penicillin, every 6 hours, IV or IM; or 22,000 U procaine penicillin every 12 hours, IM) can be used for this purpose.

If evidence of toxemia is found (e.g., neutropenia with toxic neutrophils in the peripheral circulation, elevated heart and respiratory rates, altered mucous membrane perfusion, or other circulatory disturbance), cyclooxygenase inhibitors such as flunixin meglumine should be administered. Cyclooxygenase inhibitors attenuate or prevent the circulatory disturbances associated with experimentally induced endotoxemia. Flunixin meglumine therapy is continued until there is no more danger of endotoxemia. The agent is usually given intravenously at a reduced dosage (0.025 mg/kg three times daily) to avoid potential adverse side effects. Administration of polymyxin-B (1000 to 6000 U/kg, every 6 hours, slowly IV) may be added to the systemic antimicrobial regimen in an attempt to overcome endotoxemia. Pentoxyphylline (7.5 to 10 mg/kg, every 8 to 12 hours, by mouth [PO] or IV) may provide added benefit to improve malleability of the red blood cells (RBCs) and thus potentially improve circulation in vasculature of the foot.

Acute laminitis is a medical emergency, and treatment should commence as soon as possible. Many therapeutic regimens have been recommended for the treatment of laminitis. Refer to current equine medicine textbooks for discussion of various treatments for laminitis. Certainly, padding of the foot (frog) and restriction of movement are indicated if lameness or other signs of laminitis are present.

Uterine Prolapse

The uterus of the mare rarely prolapses. **Uterine prolapse** is more likely to occur immediately after parturition but sometimes occurs several days later. Conditions that cause strong tenesmus (e.g., vaginal trauma) combined with uterine atony predispose a mare to uterine prolapse.

One or both uterine horns may be prolapsed, or the uterine body may comprise the major portion of the exposed uterus. Uterine prolapse may be complicated by rupture of internal uterine vessels, shock, or incarceration and ischemia of viscera, leading to death. In addition, damage to the prolapsed contaminated uterus predisposes the mare to development of tetanus and metritis.

Treatment of uterine prolapse is first focused on control of straining, via either administration of sedatives, caudal epidural anesthesia, or general anesthesia. In mares kept standing, the uterus is lifted to the pelvic level in an attempt to restore circulation, reduce congestion, and decrease traction on ovarian and uterine ligaments that causes pain and straining (Figure 10-7). The uterus is gently cleaned with a disinfectant soap if it is grossly contaminated, and any placenta that remains loosely attached is carefully removed to better allow uterine replacement. Bleeding vessels should be clamped and ligated. Uterine tears should be sutured, with serosal surfaces brought into contact. If the urinary bladder is distended, catheterization may be necessary before uterine replacement. Application of petroleum

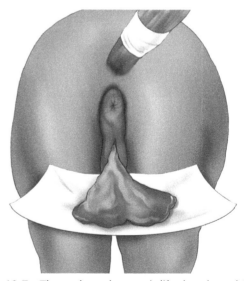

Figure 10-7 The prolapsed uterus is lifted to the pelvic level to restore circulation and reduce edema in preparation for replacement.

jelly to the endometrial surface protects against lacerations during massage and replacement. Placing the uterus inside two or three plastic garbage bags has been advocated to reduce the risk of puncturing or lacerating it during replacement (Figure 10-8). The garbage bags are removed as the uterus is pushed inside the vagina. Replacing the ventral aspect of the uterus allows gravity to help pull the remainder of the uterus over the pelvic brim and can greatly facilitate replacement. To avoid reprolapse, the uterus must be completely replaced. Gently filling the uterus with warm water or saline solution may help to ensure complete replacement of uterine horns. Excess fluid is then siphoned off through a stomach tube. Small doses (10 to 20 U) of oxytocin are administered in an attempt to stimulate uterine contractions and maintain uterine tone, and intrauterine antibiotics are given to control infection. Intravenous administration of 500 mL calcium gluconate solution, mixed in 5 L lactated Ringer's solution (LRS), may raise calcium levels when low, which improve uterine muscular contractions. Placing the mare in cross ties for 1 or 2 days (to keep her standing) has been advocated to reduce the chance of recurrence. Suturing the vulva prevents pneumovagina and speeds resolution of vaginal irritation, which might stimulate further straining. Broad-spectrum antibiotics are administered systemically to control infection. Tetanus prophylaxis is needed. Other treatment is the same as that described for metritis.

Invagination of Uterine Horn

An **invaginated uterine horn** is suspected when a postparturient mare has mild colic that is unresponsive to analgesics. The invagination is sometimes associated with a placenta that remains attached to the tip of the uterine horn, being partially inverted as a result of traction. Palpation per rectum may reveal a short, blunted uterine horn and tense mesovarium (Figure 10-9). Intrauterine examination typically reveals the dome-shaped, inverted tip of the horn projecting into the uterine lumen. The placenta may be incarcerated in the intussuscepted horn. Rarely, with advanced invaginations, a reddish-black discharge is associated with necrosis of the inverted uterus.

Treatment involves replacement of the uterine horn to its normal position, which may necessitate manual removal of the placenta. The mare is sedated to control straining. For digital separation of the placenta, it is carefully twisted at the vulvar opening while an attempt is made simultaneously to manually separate the chorion from the endometrium. The major portion of the placenta that protrudes from the vagina has to be severed if manual separation cannot be accomplished safely. This reduces the weight pulling on the tip of the uterine horn, permitting it to return to its normal position. The invaginated portion of the uterine horn is gently kneaded inward to its normal position. If the examiner's arms are too short to reach or fully correct the invagination, a clean bottle can be inserted into the affected horn and used to gently push against the invaginated horn to aid in its reduction. Infusion of 1 to 2 gal of warm, sterile water or balanced salt solution has also been used to facilitate complete replacement of the inverted uterine horn. Aftercare is the same as that described for metritis. If a portion of the placenta was left within the uterus, daily uterine lavage and intrauterine treatment are necessary until the retained portion is expelled.

Uterine Rupture

Rupture of the uterus occurs predominantly during the second stage of labor. The cause of the rupture is usually unknown, or it may result from dystocia. In rare

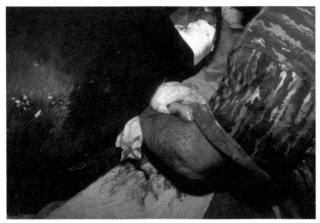

Figure 10-8 The prolapsed uterus is replaced after first covering the endometrium with petroleum jelly and then placing it inside clean plastic bags. The bags are removed as the uterus is pushed inside the vagina. This technique, described by Dr. Wendell Cooper, has been advocated to reduce the chances of lacerating the friable endometrium of the prolapsed uterus. The uterus should be completely replaced in its normal position to reduce the chance of reprolapse.

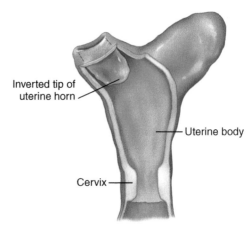

Figure 10-9 An invaginated uterine horn. Palpation per rectum reveals a short, blunted uterine horn and tense mesovarium.

instances, the fetus may be found free in the abdominal cavity, particularly if uterine torsion was present. Many ruptures occur during fetal manipulation to correct dystocia (Figure 10-10). The uterus may also rupture during overly vigorous treatment in the postparturient period (e.g., during uterine lavage).

A number of uterine ruptures are detected in mares after seemingly normal deliveries, usually in the tip of the previously gravid uterine horn. Wisconsin researchers used radiography to monitor fetal changes in position during delivery and showed that the caudal portion of the fetus completed its rotation to a dorsosacral position as the fetal abdomen passed through the birth canal. The hind limbs to the level of the fetlocks remained encased in the gravid horn during this rotation, and straightening of the hind limbs was a forceful process when the fetal stifles engaged the pelvic inlet. Perhaps this forceful extension of the hind limbs explains the occasional uterine rupture in the end of the gravid horn of mares with seemingly uneventful deliveries. When rupture of the tip of the gravid horn occurs, close examination of the expelled placenta may reveal a corresponding rupture in this area of the placenta.

Hemorrhagic vaginal discharge may be present after uterine rupture. Acutely, hemorrhage (and pain) from the torn uterine wall may result in signs of circulatory shock, including pale mucous membranes, elevated heart and respiratory rate, sweating, and extremities that are cold to the touch. Unless the hemorrhage is severe, a large decrease in the packed cell volume is

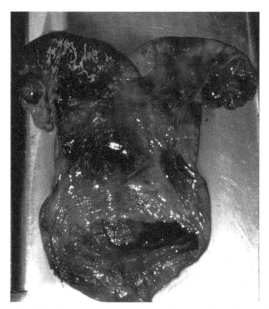

Figure 10-10 Transverse uterine rupture in the uterine body that was discovered after dystocia was relieved. Note that a rupture in the tip of the previously gravid uterine horn is also present.

seldom seen at this time. If the uterine rupture remains undiagnosed and untreated, the mare gradually develops signs of colic, or rapidly becomes depressed and febrile (within 24 hours). Although exsanguination is uncommon, blood loss may be sufficient to result in anemia and pale mucous membranes within 12 to 24 hours. Elevated white blood cell counts with degenerative left shifts from peritonitis eventually develop.

Dorsal uterine tears can sometimes be identified per rectum. Signs of discomfort may be elicited during palpation of the rupture. Careful palpation of the internal surface of the uterus per vagina is more likely to result in identification of a rupture. However, the large size of the postpartum uterus makes evaluation of the entire uterus impossible. Abdominocentesis provides evidence for intraabdominal hemorrhage, even with some partial-thickness tears when diapedesis and peritoneal contamination occur. An undetected, full-thickness uterine tear culminates in septic degenerative peritonitis, which can be confirmed with abdominocentesis. Although slight elevations in peritoneal fluid values may be observed, total protein (TP) levels should be less than 25 g/L and white blood cell (WBC) counts should less than 5000/μL in normal postpartum mares. Cloudy to serosanguinous peritoneal fluid, TP levels more than 30 g/L, and WBC counts more than 15,000/μL are indicative of a potentially life-threatening situation (Frazer, 2003). On occasion, viscera may herniate through the uterine rent and be found within the uterine cavity, in the vagina, or protruding from the vulvar opening.

Immediate treatment for hemorrhagic shock or dehydration is instituted. The best treatment for saving both the life and the breeding potential of the mare is laparotomy and surgical repair of the uterine rupture. This is best accomplished with a ventral midline approach with the mare under general anesthesia. After uterine closure, the abdominal cavity is lavaged to reduce contamination. If the mare's general condition makes her a poor candidate for anesthesia, conservative treatment is used, consisting of administration of 1 to 3 mg of ergonovine maleate intramuscularly every 2 to 4 hours (to contract smooth muscle in the uterus and uterine vessels), systemic administration of broad-spectrum antibiotics and flunixin meglumine, and intravenous replacement of fluids and electrolytes. Abdominal lavage can be performed to reduce contamination. Conservative treatment is most likely to be successful with small, dorsally located uterine tears, but the risk of development of fatal peritonitis is great. After either primary closure of the uterine tear or conservative treatment, the uterus should be massaged per rectum at 3- to 5-day intervals to break down adhesions that may form. Tetanus prophylaxis and additional treatments to prevent laminitis are also indicated.

Internal Hemorrhage

Rupture of the utero-ovarian or uterine artery, within the broad ligament, sometimes occurs at parturition or shortly thereafter. Rarely, the artery ruptures before parturition. External iliac artery rupture occurs less often. Right utero-ovarian, middle uterine, or the vaginal branch of the uterine artery rupture occurs more commonly than left artery rupture. Age-related (i.e., associated with mare age >10 years of age) degenerative changes in vessel walls, including aneurysms, predispose the mare to vascular rupture. Vascular rupture may also occur with uterine prolapse or torsion.

The affected mare may show signs of severe, unrelenting colic, with profuse sweating and evidence of hemorrhagic shock (pale mucous membranes, low packed cell volume, increased pulse and respiratory rate, sweating with cold extremities, weakness, and prostration). Alternatively, the mare may fail to show signs of pain, with hemorrhage controlled within the broad ligament. A hematoma, usually 20 to 30 cm in diameter, may be detected in the broad ligament of the uterus during routine prebreeding examination of mares in which hemorrhage has been restricted to this area.

Treatment of severe hemorrhage associated with rupture of uterine or iliac arteries is often unsuccessful. The mare should be confined in a darkened stall to prevent activity and excitement. The added excitement associated with possible therapeutic methods such as blood transfusion and the administration of drugs may raise the mare's blood pressure enough to exacerbate bleeding, causing the broad ligament to burst and death to occur. Analgesics, such as flunixin meglumine (0.5 to 1.0 mg/kg intravenously) and butorphanol tartrate (0.02 to 0.04 mg/kg intravenously) may be administered to control the pain associated with distention of the broad ligament. Corticosteroids can be administered to combat shock. Rupture of the broad ligament with intraabdominal hemorrhage usually leads to rapid extravasation and death. Intraabdominal hemorrhage can be confirmed with abdominocentesis.

Some mares with evidence of intraabdominal hemorrhage have survived after treatment for hemorrhagic shock. The mare's circulatory status should be evaluated to determine whether whole blood transfusion or plasma expansion therapy is necessary. Changes in laboratory parameters (e.g., a packed cell volume < 15%, a hemoglobin concentration <5 mg/dL, and a plasma protein concentration <4 mg/dL) are indicative of marked blood loss and deficient oxygen-carrying capacity. If these changes are seen, transfusion should be considered. The clinician should remember that when marked quantities of whole blood are lost, laboratory values supporting the need for transfusion often lag behind clinical signs of hypovolemic blood loss. Therefore, when clinical signs of hypovolemic blood loss (e.g., tachycardia, weak pulse, pale mucous membranes, weakness, and depression) are present, whole blood transfusion should be strongly considered. Guidelines for collection of blood from a suitable donor and for administration of blood to the affected mare are discussed in textbooks.

Administration of naloxone hydrochloride has been advocated for treatment of rupture of the uterine or utero-ovarian artery in mares. Endogenous opioids may be released during hemorrhagic shock, and naloxone, a narcotic antagonist, should block their effects. The rationale for this theory is predicated on the finding that the administration of naloxone attenuated some of the cardiovascular responses associated with experimentally induced shock in horses. Thus, naloxone has been proposed to have potential therapeutic value for shock treatment. Apparently, naloxone antagonizes the actions of endogenous opioids mobilized by pain or stress and is involved in the regulation of blood pressure by the central nervous system. The naloxone (8 to 20 mg) is administered intravenously to the mare that has already been placed in a darkened, quiet stall. Whether this treatment is superior to simply placing the mare in the same type of quiet environment, with or without the administration of other drugs, is not known.

An antifibrinolytic drug, aminocaproic acid, has also been used to control hemorrhage (e.g., with ruptured uterine arteries or incision sites of cesarean sections). This drug inhibits factors that promote clot lysis, thereby reducing secondary hemorrhage.

We do not generally recommend that the foal be separated from the mare unless it is necessary to protect the foal from inadvertent injury by the colicky mare. If removal of the foal from the dam is necessary, steps should be taken to ensure that the foal's nutrient and passive immunity needs are met.

Hematomas that remain contained within the broad ligament regress gradually over a few weeks. Some hematomas may remain palpable as firm uterine enlargements for several months or occasionally longer. Such uterine hematomas may be detected per rectum during prebreeding examination of mares in which no postpartum problems were suspected. Ultrasonographically, the consolidating hematoma will appear more echolucent than the rest of the uterus, with echodensities dispersed throughout the clot (Figures 10-11 and 10-12). The hematoma becomes palpably more firm and progressively more echodense as fibrous tissue organizes. If the hematoma is exceedingly large, deposition of extensive scar tissue around the reproductive tract may end the mare's reproductive career.

Some investigators suggest an increased likelihood of recurrence of vascular rupture, with fatal

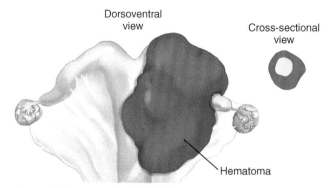

Figure 10-11 Drawing of uterine hematoma discovered during postpartum examination of the uterus of a mare, illustrating the extent of the surrounding hematoma.

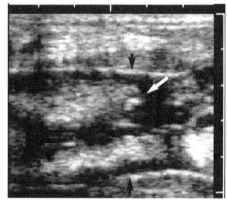

Figure 10-12 Transrectal ultrasonographic appearance of the hematoma depicted in Figure 10-11: margins of the uterine wall *(black arrows);* clotting blood becoming echogenic *(white arrow).*

hemorrhage at the subsequent parturition. However, a number of practitioners from large breeding farms report that affected mares are generally fertile once the hematomas regress and affected mares that are rebred usually deliver subsequent foals without recurrence of hemorrhage.

Other Postparturient Hemorrhages

Hemorrhagic vulvar discharge may originate from lacerations in the birth canal or from internal uterine trauma. Forceful, premature removal of fetal membranes may induce intrauterine hemorrhage. Hemorrhage may be profuse if a large blood vessel in the cervix, vagina, or vulva is ruptured. Alternatively, hemorrhage may be extravaginal (resulting in perivaginal hematoma) or intraperitoneal if the ruptured blood vessel is located within the abdomen. The mare may become anemic but usually survives.

Slight hemorrhage does not necessitate treatment. Profuse hemorrhage originating from blood vessels

identified per vagina can often be clamped and ligated. If bleeding vessels cannot be identified, 1 to 3 mg of ergonovine maleate is injected intramuscularly to stimulate contraction of uterine and arterial muscles in an effort to control the hemorrhage. Oxytocin (20 to 40 U) can be administered intramuscularly to stimulate uterine contractions but does not cause contraction of muscular elements in the vasculature. If intrauterine or intravaginal hemorrhage cannot be controlled, packing the uterus or vagina with long strips of cotton sheets lubricated with petroleum jelly may be beneficial. The sheets should be removed 1 to 2 days later. Sequential measurements of red blood cell count, packed cell volume, and plasma protein concentration should be obtained to monitor blood loss. Supportive therapy, including use of broad-spectrum antibiotics to control infection and perhaps whole blood transfusion, is administered as necessary. Lacerations in the vagina should be sutured if possible. Repair of cervical lacerations must be delayed until uterine involution is complete. Vaginal stenosis may result from intrapelvic or perivaginal bleeding (Figure 10-13). Organized blood clots beneath or around the cervix may interfere with normal cervical function. Perivulvar hematomas often become abscessed, necessitating surgical drainage (Figure 10-14).

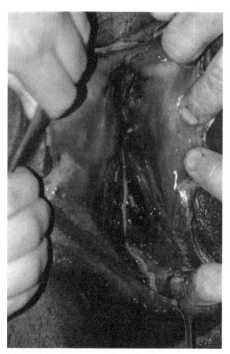

Figure 10-13 Vestibular and vaginal tearing and bruising, with superficial necrosis seen as discolored mucosa, in a postpartum mare.

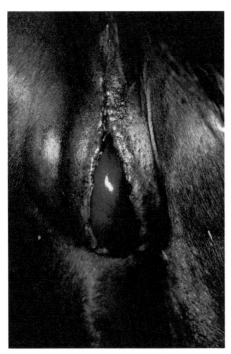

Figure 10-14 Perivulvar hematoma present in a postpartum mare. Abscesses of the organizing hematoma sometimes form.

BIBLIOGRAPHY

Bierschwal CJ, de Bois CHW: *The technique of fetotomy in large animals,* Bonner Springs, KS, 1972, VM Publishing.

Frazer GS: Postpartum complications in the mare: part 1:conditions affecting the uterus, *Equine Vet Edu* 5(Feb):45-54, 2003.

Frazer GS, Beard WL, Abrahamsen E, et al: Systemic effects of peritoneal instillation of a polyethylene polymer based obstetrical lubricant in horses, *Proc Soc Theriogenol* 93-97, 2004.

Ginther OJ: Equine pregnancy: physical interactions between the uterus and conceptus, *Proc Am Assoc Equine Pract* 44:73-104, 1998.

Hackett ES, Orsini JA, Divers TJ: Equine emergency drugs (approximate dosages and adverse reactions. In Orsini JA, Divers TJ, editors: *Equine emergency treatment and procedures,* St Louis, 2008, Elsevier, 739-752.

Roberts SJ: *Veterinary obstetrics and genital diseases, theriogenology,* ed 3, Woodstock, VT, 1986, SJ Roberts.

Rooney JR: Internal hemorrhage related to gestation in the mare, *Cornell Vet* 54:11-17, 1964.

Rossdale PD, Ricketts SW: *Equine stud farm medicine,* ed 2, Philadelphia, 1980, Lea & Febiger.

Vandeplasssche M: The pathogenesis of dystocia and fetal malformation in the horse, *J Reprod Fertil* 35(Suppl):547-552, 1987.

Vandeplassche M, Spincemaille J, Bouters R: Aetiology, pathogenesis and treatment of retained placenta in the mare, *Equine Vet J* 3: 144-147, 1971.

Vandeplassche M, Spincemaille J, Bouters R et al: Some aspects of equine obstetrics, *Equine Vet J* 4:105-109, 1972.

Routine Management of the Neonatal Foal

CHAPTER 11

OBJECTIVES

While studying the information covered in this chapter, the reader should attempt to:
- Acquire a working understanding of procedures for evaluation of the newborn foal.
- Acquire a working understanding of the need for colostrum acquisition by the newborn foal, techniques for administration of colostrum to foals, and techniques for testing for failure of passive antibody transfer to foals.
- Acquire a working understanding of techniques for caring for the umbilical cord of the foal at the time of parturition and for preventing meconial impaction.

STUDY QUESTIONS

1. Describe the procedure for performing a physical examination of a newborn foal and include expected normal findings.
2. Describe the procedures for testing foals for passive antibody transfer failure and methods for administration of colostrum to foals to avoid this condition.
3. Describe the procedures used for treatment of passive antibody transfer failure in foals.
4. Describe the techniques involved in caring for the umbilical cord of the newborn foal.
5. Describe the clinical signs of meconium impaction in foals, methods used to differentiate meconium impaction from other causes of colic or straining in newborn foals, and methods for administration of enemas to prevent this condition.

The neonatal period is a vulnerable segment of foal development. The transition from a protected, intrauterine existence to a state of relative independence is subject to a myriad of interferences. The vast array of potential inherent defects and environmental assaults can be devastating to the viability of the newborn foal and in turn can lead to significant losses for the horse industry. Equine practitioners should be well versed in all aspects of neonatal care to properly assist broodmare owners in managing newborn foals.

The managerial recommendations described herein are arranged in a chronologic sequence that can be applied to care of foals on a large broodmare farm. The order of events often is altered, especially on smaller farms where a veterinarian is not present during parturition to evaluate foals in the first few hours of life.

The chronologic span of the neonatal period is not defined uniformly; descriptions vary by as much as several weeks. The most critical part of neonatal development occurs within the first 4 days of life, when the newborn foal attempts to establish somatovisceral homeostasis. This chapter discusses general management guidelines for the immediate postnatal period. Application of basic management principles during the immediate neonatal period can prevent many problems that may result from birthing or environmental insults.

EVALUATION OF RESPIRATORY AND CARDIAC FUNCTION

Airway clearance and the establishment of a normal respiratory-cardiac rhythm are crucial. When the amnion envelops the mouth and the nostrils at birth, it should be removed to prevent asphyxiation (see Figures 9-13 and 9-14). Excessive fluid in the nasal cavity can be partially removed by stripping the nostrils with the fingers and thumb. If necessary, gentle suction also can be applied.

Fetal passage through the birth canal promotes thoracic compression and resultant expulsion of fluid from the upper airway. If a cesarean section is performed, the newborn is apt to need additional assistance to remove these contents effectively. The foal can be placed in a lateral recumbent position in a well-bedded location with the forequarters in a lower plane than the hindquarters to facilitate dependent drainage of fluid. Some practitioners hold the foal up by the hind legs for a short period of time to promote better fluid evacuation; this procedure should be brief because abdominal viscera compress the diaphragm, limiting the ability of the foal to expand its lungs. The foal is dried with a towel or blanket and rubbed briskly to stimulate respiratory activity (Figure 11-1). The rate and intensity of the heart beat and peripheral pulse should be evaluated (refer to "Physical Examination" in this chapter).

VIABILITY ASSESSMENT AND RESUSCITATION PROCEDURE

The practitioner should look for signs indicative of a strong, vigorous animal. Weak or immature foals are more vulnerable to stressful influences of the extrauterine environment and thus need more intensive care to maximize their chances for survival. Fetal stress should be suspected when meconial staining of the amniotic fluid, fetal membranes, or foal is observed, which increases the risk of aspirated meconium, predisposing the animal to hypoxia and pneumonia.

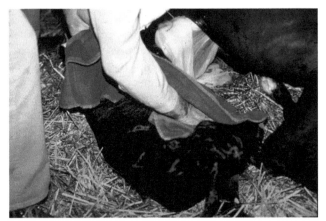

Figure 11-1   Respiratory activity can be stimulated by briskly rubbing the newborn foal with a towel.

The degree of neonatal stress and birth asphyxia can be evaluated in the newborn foal with a modification of the Apgar scoring system used in human neonatology (Table 11-1). The observations listed for the modified Apgar scoring system should be made 1 and 5 minutes after delivery. In infants, the 1-minute score correlates directly with umbilical cord blood pH and is an index of intrauterine asphyxia. The 5-minute Apgar score correlates more with the infant's eventual neurologic outcome.

Although the Apgar score has had limited use in equine neonatology, the criteria presented here provide a rational set of guidelines for evaluation of the degree of neonatal asphyxia and for determination of whether resuscitative measures are indicated. Early signs of asphyxia include increased rate and depth of respiration followed by a period of gasping and primary apnea. With severe asphyxia, the respiratory center becomes progressively depressed and is no longer responsive to sensory and chemical stimuli. The gasping episodes become weaker, and bradycardia develops, followed by a stage of secondary apnea.

Although much normal variation in foal adaptive responses occurs in the immediate postnatal period, comparison of foal responses with published values can provide some confidence that the foal is viable. The newborn foal should establish normal respiratory and cardiac rhythm within 1 minute of birth, and righting and suckle reflexes should be apparent within 5 minutes of birth. The suck reflex can be tested by placing a clean finger in the mouth of the foal. Most healthy foals begin attempting to stand within 30 minutes of birth and are able to stand without assistance by 1 to 2 hours of age. The newborn foal should be able to locate the mare's udder and nurse without assistance within 1 to 3 hours of birth.

Foals with signs of mild to moderate asphyxia (Apgar score 4 to 6) should be given moderate stimulation that includes brisk rubbing of the foal's back and sides with a dry towel, postural drainage in conjunction with gentle thoracic coupage, limb manipulation, and stimulation of the inside of the nares to elicit a sneeze or a cough. The induced cough helps to move secretions out of the lower airways. The neck should be gently hyperextended and the oropharynx cleared of mucus or amniotic fluid to ensure a patent airway. Suctioning of the oropharynx and the trachea can be performed with a 10F suction catheter (Regu-Vac, Becton Dickinson, Franklin Lakes, NJ). The foal must be preoxygenated (12 L/min through a catheter) before suction is applied to avoid causing respiratory distress, cardiac arrhythmias, or cardiac arrest. Prolonged periods of suction should also be avoided because they result in decreased arterial oxygenation. Suction (vacuum set at 80 to 120 mm Hg) should be applied only during withdrawal of the catheter from the airway.

Placement of the foal in a sternal recumbent position (Figure 11-2) helps decrease dependent lung atelectasis, thus minimizing the ventilation-perfusion inequalities

TABLE 11-1

Modified Apgar Scoring System for Evaluation of Foals 1 to 5 Minutes after Birth

Observation	Assigned Values*		
	0	**1**	**2**
Heart and pulse rate	Undetectable	<60 beats/min	>60 beats/min
Respiration (rate and pattern)	Undetectable	Slow, irregular	60 breaths/min, regular
Muscle tone	Lateral recumbency, limp	Lateral recumbency, evidence of some muscle tone	Able to maintain sternal recumbency
Nasal stimulation (with straw)	Unresponsive	Grimace with mild rejection	Cough or sneeze

*A value of 0, 1, or 2 is assigned for each of the four observations. Total score: 7 to 8, normal; 4 to 6, mild to moderate asphyxia; 0 to 3, severe asphyxia.
From Martens RJ: Pediatrics. In Mansmann RA, McAllister ES, Pratt PW, editors: *Equine medicine and surgery,* ed 3, vol 1, Santa Barbara, CA, 1982, American Veterinary Publications.

created by prolonged lateral recumbency. Supplemental oxygen (humidified) can be delivered via a nasal cannula or a face mask at a flow rate of 5 to 10 L/min. A nasal cannula should be passed in the ventral meatus to the approximate level of the medial canthus of the eye. A tight-fitting face mask requires a reservoir bag and adequate oxygen flow rates to prevent rebreathing of exhaled gases. Loose-fitting face masks result in lower inspired oxygen concentrations but still require a minimal oxygen flow rate of 10 L/min to prevent build-up of CO_2 in the mask. Sternal recumbent position, tactile and sensory stimulation, a judicious suction technique, and oxygen supplementation are sometimes sufficient therapy for foals with asphyxia or hypoxia.

Foals with severe asphyxia (Apgar score 0 to 3) need rapid, aggressive intervention to stimulate and support ventilation. Manual mouth-to-nose resuscitation can be accomplished with the clinician using both hands to occlude one of the foal's nostrils and the mouth and then breathing rhythmically into the foal's patent nostril to expand its lungs. Assisted ventilation is probably best performed with an endotracheal tube directly attached to a ventilator, an oxygen demand valve (Hudson oxygen demand valve II, Hudson Oxygen Therapy Sales, Wadsworth, OH), or a 1-L nonrebreathing resuscitation bag (Lifesaver II manual resuscitator, A. J. Buck and Son, Owings Mills, MD or E-Z Breather Foal Resuscitator, Animal Reproduction Systems, Chino, CA.) (Figure 11-3).

Oral intubation of the trachea can be done in emergency situations if short-term ventilation is all that is necessary. Nasotracheal intubation is better tolerated

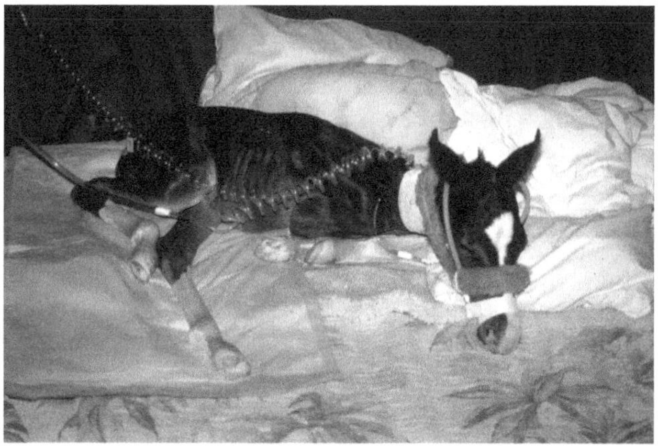

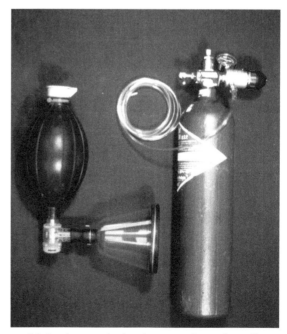

Figure 11-2 This premature (born at 315 days of gestation) foal was unable to maintain sternal recumbency and was propped up on its sternum to decrease dependent lung atelectasis. Supplemental oxygen was delivered via a nasal cannula.

Figure 11-3 A resuscitation bag, mask, and small oxygen tank with attached nasogastric tubing is shown. This equipment should be readily available at the time of parturition to help correct hypoxia in newborn foals.

for prolonged periods. Inert plastic or silicone rubber endotracheal tubes with high-volume, low-pressure cuffs (Aire-Cuf, Biovona Medical Technologies, Gary, IN) are preferred to minimize tracheal mucosal damage. A breathing rate of 20 to 30 breaths/min should be maintained. Excessive ventilatory pressure can result in overinflation with alveolar rupture and pneumothorax. Visual assessment of the foal's thorax is used to evaluate needed tidal volume.

Because the acidosis associated with terminal apnea usually is metabolic and respiratory in nature, administration of intravenous isotonic (1.3%) sodium bicarbonate solution at an initial dose of 2 mg/kg may help to correct the metabolic component. Administration of alkaline solutions without first ensuring that adequate ventilation is present can worsen the acidosis because sodium bicarbonate is converted to carbon dioxide and retained when poor ventilation-perfusion exists. Large volumes of hypertonic sodium bicarbonate solutions should be avoided; their use has been associated with hypernatremic and hyperosmotic states and with increased incidence of cerebrovascular accidents, especially in infants.

The ultimate outcome of severe, untreated asphyxia is myocardial and cerebral hypoxia, which result in death. Irreversible brain damage usually occurs after approximately 5 minutes of complete asphyxia. Therefore, the recognition and accurate, rapid treatment of asphyxia are vitally important.

INTERPRETATION OF CLINICAL LABORATORY DATA

Analysis of whole blood and serum from all newborn foals is customary on many well-managed broodmare farms. Blood samples for complete blood count (CBC), total protein, and fibrinogen as a component of the routine newborn foal examination provide a baseline for comparison if the foal has problems develop that become apparent later. In addition, despite the appearance of an apparently healthy foal, abnormal hematologic findings alert the veterinarian to the need for closer monitoring, or in some cases, the need to institute treatment (e.g., to control infection). Thus, proper interpretation of the laboratory results is reviewed here.

Normal hematologic, blood gas, and serum chemistry values for the newborn foal are cited in veterinary literature. Hematologic parameters of the newborn foal change during the first 2 weeks of life. Because of the shortened life span of erythrocytes in fetal and neonatal foals, the number of red blood cells peaks at term and then decreases during the next 10 days.

A relatively abrupt decrease in packed cell volume, hemoglobin concentration, and number of erythrocytes occurs within the first 12 to 24 hours post partum. The high hemoglobin concentration and packed cell volume at birth are attributed to the presence of peripheral

vasoconstriction in animals immediately after birth, which offers physiologic protection against shock, cold, and excessive blood loss from the umbilicus. After parturition, a gradual release from this vasoconstriction occurs, and circulatory volume increases with a concomitant drop in packed cell volume, number of erythrocytes, and hemoglobin concentration.

An increased leukocyte count during the first 24 hours after birth primarily results from an increase in the number of mature neutrophils, which can continue during the next 3 days. However, the finding of more than 5% to 10% band cells suggests underlying disease (infection). The lymphopenia present at birth might result from immature lymphatic organs or from the response to endogenous steroid release during parturition. Lymphocyte numbers should continue to rise in early postnatal life. Eosinophils, basophils, and monocytes are low in number or absent in the newborn foal. Premature foals tend to have lower numbers of leukocytes and neutrophils. Neutrophil counts of less than 4000/mm³ or more than 12,000/mm³, band neutrophil counts of more than 50/mm³, toxic changes in neutrophils, and fibrinogen concentrations of more than 500 to 600 mg/dL are predictive of sepsis or infection (Brewer and Koterba, 1990).

Concentrations of serum electrolytes remain relatively constant during the postnatal period. Liver enzyme concentrations generally are higher in neonates than in adults. The increased serum liver enzyme activity in foals is attributed to a relative increase in hepatic mass (as a percentage of total body weight) in the newborn and to a higher rate of enzyme production and release. The level of alkaline phosphatase is higher in foals up to 3 to 5 months of age because of osteoblastic activity of bone.

The dark yellow serum of newborn foals reflects increased postpartum bilirubin levels. An increase in the indirect bilirubin concentration accounts for the hyperbilirubinemia. Lower concentrations of glucuronyl transferase in the neonatal liver result in a slower conjugation of bilirubin during the first 5 days after birth. Bilirubin concentrations should approach adult values by 2 weeks of age. The bilirubin concentration is generally increased in foals with neonatal isoerythrolysis and may be of value in diagnosis of this condition when anemia, pallor, and tachypnea are present in newborns.

Serum creatinine concentrations during the neonatal period often are greater than adult values. This difference in creatinine levels probably reflects the initial immaturity of the renal transport and filtration systems. A markedly elevated serum creatinine concentration has been associated with both prematurity and neonatal maladjustment syndrome (NMS). Monitoring of creatinine levels is also necessary when drugs with a potential for renal toxicity, such as aminoglycosides, are administered to foals.

The blood glucose level of presuckle foals usually is lower than that in adults but increases after suckling.

Sepsis or insufficient energy intake should be suspected in foals with low blood glucose concentrations, and the clinician should be aware of the need for closer monitoring of nursing activity, the possible presence of agalactia, and the need for additional testing or examination for septicemia. Hypoglycemia can be treated by administering 5% to 10% dextrose solutions intravenously.

Interpretation of clinical laboratory data must be done with an understanding of the normal physiologic and biochemical adaptations that occur in the neonate. A precise history of peripartum events and a careful physical examination always should precede the interpretation of laboratory data.

PHYSICAL EXAMINATION

A thorough, systematic physical examination should be performed on every foal during the first day of life. Before actual physical examination, the clinician should begin by observing the foal from a distance to assess its alertness and behavior, ability to rise, coordination and strength, desire and willingness to nurse, and overall attitude. Rectal temperature should always be determined and is normally 99.5°F to 100.5°F (37.5°C to 38.5°C). When rectal temperature is less than 98.5°F, hypothermia should be suspected. When rectal temperature exceeds 101.5°F, infection should be suspected.

The actual physical examination should be systematic, beginning at the head and progressing to the hindquarters. It should yield prompt recognition of various maladies, including cleft palate, eye abnormalities (e.g., entropion, micropthalmia, cataract), fractured ribs, umbilical problems (e.g., swollen, wet, bleeding, hernia), inguinal hernias, and limb abnormalities (e.g., valgus, varus, contractures, laxities). The foal should possess a normal respiratory rate, heart rate, and rectal temperature. Its mucous membranes should be pink and moist. The veterinarian should also look for evidence that the foal has passed meconium and is suckling regularly (mare's udder is not full and turgid).

The foal's degree of maturity should be assessed. Signs that suggest prematurity include low birth weight, general weakness, inability to stand, decreased ability to suck and maintain body temperature, silky haircoat, floppy ears, soft lips, and increased passive range of limb motion with a decreased pastern slope. A premature foal also can have immature organ systems (e.g., pulmonary, endocrine, gastrointestinal, renal, immune, and hematopoietic system) and therefore need close observation and monitoring with appropriate supportive care.

Examination for Broken Ribs

With the foal standing and gently restrained, the thoracic cage is palpated in its entirety, usually with the practitioner standing over the foal and using both hands simultaneously, with the right hand on the right hemithorax and the left hand on the left hemithorax.

Each rib is followed dorsally to ventrally. Any irregularity (displacement) or movement (usually felt as a "popping" or "clicking" sensation) is noted and examined more closely. Fractures can occur anywhere in the ribs but are more common ventrally or near the costochondral junction. Suspected fracture sites should be examined with transcutaneous ultrasound for confirmation of fracture and degree of displacement (Figure 11-4) and for evidence of pleural disruption or hemorrhage. Most commonly, one or perhaps two ribs are involved, but sometimes several are fractured, which places the foal at great risk for puncture or laceration of the pleura, lungs, or heart. In many cases, confining the foal and the mare to a large well-bedded stall for 2 or more weeks is a satisfactory method of management of broken ribs. Certainly, risk of further injury exists for the confined foal and could result in death. However, the goal is to do everything possible to avoid trauma to the foal's thorax until the rib fracture is stabilized, thereby reducing risk of adverse consequences. Once firm callus formation around the fracture site has developed (confirmed with ultrasound examination and palpation of a stable thorax), the foal can be turned out with its dam in a small paddock for exercise. Separation from other mares and foals is necessary until satisfactory healing occurs, which is often evident within 4 to 6 weeks. Surgical techniques have been developed for fixation of fractured ribs and may be undertaken if chosen; however, even after surgery, accidents leading to pleural, lung, or cardiac puncture have occurred.

Neurologic Examination

A brief neurologic examination should be performed and should include a systematic evaluation of general behavior, mentation, cranial nerve function, posture, gait, coordination, and spinal reflexes. A healthy newborn foal is

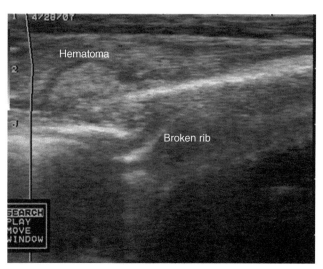

Figure 11-4 Transthoracic ultrasound view of fractured rib in a newborn foal. A hematoma has formed on the outer surface of the fracture site. (Courtesy Dr. Tom Seahorn, Lexington, KY.)

aware of and responsive to its environment soon after birth and shows close bonding behavior with the dam. Certain physiologic differences between the neonate and the adult should be acknowledged. Equine neonates normally have limb hyperreflexia, resting extensor hypertonia, crossed extensor reflexes, hypermetric gait, basewide stance, intention movements, and an absence of menace response. Neurologic abnormalities should be recognized, identified as to cause (e.g., developmental, infectious, or from vascular accidents within the central nervous system), and treated accordingly.

Peripartum asphyxia or hypoxia can result in a syndrome (hypoxic ischemic encephalomyelopathy [HIE]), often referred to as **maladjusment**, with variable clinical signs including abnormal behaviors, mentation (Figure 11-5), or seizures and secondary consequences, such as atelectasis and acidosis; thus, many cases should be managed in a neonatal intensive care hospital ward. The pathogenesis, diagnosis, and treatment of the disorder are discussed thoroughly in equine neonatology texts (e.g., Knottenbelt et al., 2004).

Cardiovascular System Examination

Evaluation of the cardiovascular system begins with examination of the visible mucous membranes, which should be pink and moist with a capillary refill time of 1 to 2 seconds. The jugular veins should not be distended but should fill readily when occluded at the thoracic inlet. Jugular pulsations reflect normal pressure changes within the right atrium and the thorax and should not extend beyond the level of the point of the shoulder. The apex beat, easily palpated over the left fifth intercostal space in the ventral third of the thorax, should be evaluated for intensity and for the presence of murmur-associated thrills.

Arterial pulses should be strong and readily palpable in the extremities, indicating adequate peripheral

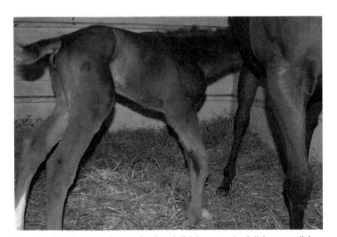

Figure 11-5 Newborn foal exhibiting typical "dummy" behavior caused by peripartum hypoxia. This foal had difficulty when searching for the mare's udder and attempted to nurse from the mare's hocks and tail. (Courtesy Dr. Tom Seahorn, Lexington, KY.)

perfusion. Percussion of the left hemithorax outlines a normal area of cardiac dullness that extends from the fourth intercostal space just below the point of the shoulder to the sternum at the sixth intercostal space. A smaller area of cardiac dullness is found over the right third and fourth intercostal spaces.

Auscultation of the heart base requires a general knowledge of the anatomic location of the four heart valves. Foals generally have loud heart sounds on auscultation because of their thin body wall and small size. The most commonly reported murmur in newborn foals is associated with blood flow through a persistent patent ductus arteriosus and is characterized by a continuous machine-like murmur that is loudest over the left heart base. The diastolic component of the murmur often is localized over the left third or fourth intercostal space, whereas the systolic component may be heard easily over the entire heart base. Continuous murmurs associated with a patent ductus arteriosus disappear in some normal foals by 24 hours of age and are considered abnormal if present beyond 4 days of age. Pulmonary hypertension can reduce the intensity of the diastolic component.

The heart rate of the foal is 40 to 80 regular beats/min initially but increases to 150 beats/min when the foal struggles to rise. It then falls to a rate of 70 to 95 beats/min. Sinus tachycardia can be associated with stress, excitement, fever, hypovolemia, or sepsis. Bradycardia can occur with hyperkalemia, hypertension, or increased intracranial pressure.

Respiratory System Examination

The respiratory rate, effort, and pattern should be examined carefully in the resting foal before handling (because any handling results in excitement of the foal). The rate decreases from a mean of 75 breaths/min at birth, to 50 breaths/min at 1 hour, and to 34 breaths/min at 12 hours of age. Lung sounds in the young foal typically are louder, harsher, and easier to hear than in the adult. The auscultation of moist rales in the neonate can stem from fluid accumulation in the lungs that has not yet dissipated completely. Decreased or absent lung sounds can be associated with lung atelectasis or consolidation related to lung immaturity or pneumonia.

Because auscultation alone is not the most accurate means of detecting pulmonary pathologic problems in the foal; other respiratory parameters should be monitored closely. Increased rate and effort of breathing in an unstressed foal are early indications of possible lung disease. Nonrespiratory factors such as fever, high environmental temperatures, metabolic acidosis, pain, excitement, hypotension, and neurologic disease also can result in tachypnea. Mucous membrane color should be evaluated but is not a reliable indicator of oxygenation because cyanosis usually is not observed until the partial pressure of arterial oxygen reaches very low levels. Thoracic ultrasound examination

(Figures 11-6 and 11-7), chest radiographs, and measurement of arterial blood gases are critical diagnostic aids in the workup of a foal with possible abnormal respiratory function.

Upper airway obstruction or abnormality can be another cause of moderate to severe tachypnea in the newborn. There should be equal airflow from each nostril. Congenital anomalies associated with respiratory distress in newborn foals include bilateral choanal atresia, subepiglottic cyst formation, abnormal function and conformation of the larynx and the arytenoid cartilages,

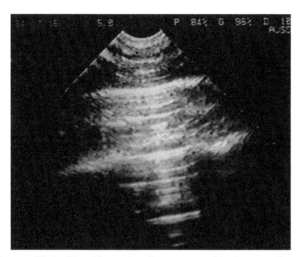

Figure 11-6 Transthoracic ultrasonographic image of normal air-filled lung in a foal. Air-filled lung parenchyma does not transmit ultrasound waves, so reverberation artifacts are evident. Reflections arise from the lung surface and fascial planes of the intercostal muscles. (Courtesy Dr. Tom Seahorn, Lexington, Ky.)

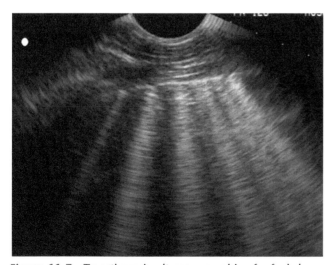

Figure 11-7 Transthoracic ultrasonographic of a foal showing the presence of many "comet tails," which are reverberation artifacts in the visceral pleura, indicating the existence of pleural irregularities. The presence of a few comet tails, particularly at the lower lung margins, is considered normal. The presence of many comet tails (as in this image), or the presence of larger comet tails, is suggestive of lung disease. (Courtesy Dr. Tom Seahorn, Lexington, Ky.)

and tracheal malformations. Severe upper airway obstruction necessitates emergency tracheotomy.

Gastrointestinal System Examination

The gastrointestinal system can be evaluated grossly with auscultation of the abdomen for normal borborygmi and observation to document the passage of dark, pasty meconium followed by softer, tan-colored feces associated with a milk diet. Absence of fecal passage might indicate meconium retention or impaction, or congenital anomalies such as atresia ani and atresia coli (Figure 11-8). Abdominal distention accompanied by colic can herald a variety of gastrointestinal disorders, including peritonitis, abnormal gut motility associated with enterocolitis, intestinal volvulus or intussusception, and gastrointestinal ulceration with or without perforation. The size and consistency of the umbilicus should be evaluated. Careful abdominal palpation is used to identify the presence of other congenital anomalies, including umbilical, inguinal, or scrotal hernias. Small hernias usually close spontaneously. Daily manual reduction of the hernia or bandaging of the area can hasten resolution of the defect. All hernias require regular monitoring because intestinal strangulation can occur; this usually necessitates prompt surgical intervention.

A foal that is straining to pass the meconium stands with its back arched and tail lifted. The foal becomes progressively more restless as it makes multiple attempts to defecate. With meconial impaction, colic signs, and eventually abdominal distention, occur. Gentle insertion of a lubricated finger (with care taken not to irritate the rectal mucosa) into the rectum may reveal the presence of a meconial ball, often just beyond the fingertip. Ultrasound examination of the caudal abdomen (just in front of the pelvis) may reveal the presence of retained meconial balls. The abdomen should also be evaluated (with palpation and ultrasonography) to determine whether abnormal amounts of gas or fluid are present.

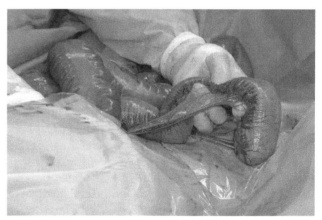

Figure 11-8 Rectal atresia apparent during abdominal surgery in a newborn foal.

Genitourinary System Examination

The genital tract should be examined to identify the foal's gender and to look for the presence of possible congenital defects. In males, the scrotum and the inguinal region should be palpated for the presence of the testicles. The testes often are within the scrotum at birth but might not descend for several weeks. Observation of normal micturition decreases the likelihood of uroperitoneum in the newborn. Urine specific gravity in normal nursing foals usually is low because urine is quite dilute.

Musculoskeletal System Examination

During examination of the musculoskeletal system, palpation for signs of trauma or distended joints should be performed. Any flexor or angular limb deformities should be assessed. Poor muscular tone ("floppy") can occur with sepsis. Excessive joint mobility (increased passive range of motion) is common with prematurity. Cuboidal bones of the carpus and tarsus may be radiolucent and soft (incompletely ossified) in premature foals, requiring stall confinement to prevent inadvertent crushing with permanent repercussions. Swollen joints, particularly if warm and painful, suggest infection, which may have been acquired in utero. Radiographs and aspiration of synovial fluid for culture and cytology may be indicated to guide treatment of septic joints or physes.

Ophthalmic Examination

An ophthalmic examination is best performed in a dark stall. The eyes of the newborn foal at birth are open with clear corneas. The pupils are circular and large, with a sluggish pupillary light reflex. Closer scrutiny of the chambers, the lens, and the fundus requires knowledge of normal adult and neonatal equine fundic anatomy.

The practitioner must not confuse pathologic processes with normal findings such as the Y-sutures of the lens or the hyaloid artery, both of which invariably are present in the newborn foal. The Y-suture of the anterior lens is inverted. The remnants of the fetal hyaloid artery, viewed as a fine dark line, are visible, attached to the posterior lens capsule, and floating freely in the vitreous body. Occasionally, this artery traverses the vitreous body to its posterior attachment at the optic nerve. The remnant usually degenerates as the foal ages. Persistent strands of pupillary membrane occasionally are observed in the midiris region.

Congenital cataracts are the most common congenital ocular defect in the foal. Cataracts associated with persistent hyaloid vasculature and Y-suture lines are of minor importance. Complete cortical and nuclear congenital cataracts are more serious and can cause partial or complete loss of vision.

Scleral, subconjunctival, or conjunctival hemorrhage usually is associated with rupture of the conjunctival or episcleral vessels from compressive or blunt trauma during birth. This type of hemorrhage should resolve without treatment in 1 or 2 weeks. If hyphema is present, a topical mydriatic agent should be used to prevent synechia formation. Occasionally, petechial and ecchymotic hemorrhages in this area can herald a generalized bleeding disorder resulting from disseminated intravascular coagulation or endothelial damage associated with septicemia.

The normal cornea is clear, with a smooth, intact epithelial surface. Entropion (Figure 11-9) can result in corneal irritation, keratitis, and ulceration, producing blepharospasm and lacrimation in the affected eye. Mild forms of entropion often are self-limiting. Temporary, nonabsorbable, vertical mattress sutures placed ventral to the lower lid margin usually correct the entropion (Figure 11-10); secondary corneal disease should be treated concurrently with topical antibiotics and a mydriatic agent as indicated. Hypotonia, corneal edema, miosis, hypopyon, and aqueous flare resulting in a

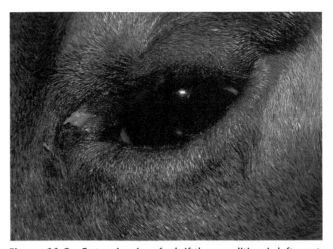

Figure 11-9 Entropion in a foal. If the condition is left unattended, corneal damage may occur. (Courtesy Dr. Joanne Hardy, Texas A&M University.)

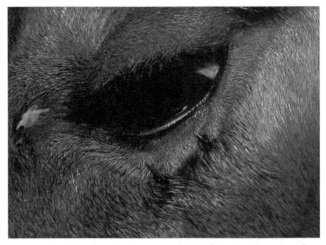

Figure 11-10 Surgical correction of entropion involves placement of one or two mattress sutures in the skin of the lower eyelid, rolling the inverted eyelid outward. Sutures can be removed in 7 to 14 days, depending on response. (Courtesy Dr. Joanne Hardy, Texas A&M University.)

green-yellow glow in the anterior chamber are characteristic signs of uveitis. Uveal inflammation usually is secondary to foci of infection elsewhere in the body and might result from bacteremia or septicemia.

Examination of Mare's Udder

Before the foal is allowed to nurse, the udder should be washed and checked for the presence of colostrum and for evidence of agalactia, mastitis, nonfunctional teats, or other malformations. The udder should be inspected routinely for signs of abnormal distention, which can be the first sign of decreased sucking and possible illness in the foal. The foal's blood glucose level can be checked to ensure that adequate suckling is taking place. A low blood glucose level should alert the clinician to the possibility of insufficient dietary energy ingestion.

CARE OF THE UMBILICAL CORD

The umbilical cord of the foal is intact as the foal emerges from the birth canal. To ensure maximum blood flow from the placenta into the newborn's circulation, the cord should remain attached for several minutes. It has been postulated that the foal may be deprived of up to 1.5 L of blood by premature separation of the umbilical cord. One study, however, suggests that this is not the case. In most circumstances, letting the cord break naturally is acceptable. This usually occurs when the mare or the foal attempts to rise. A predetermined break site is easily identifiable on the umbilical cord approximately 1 to 2 inches from the body wall (Figure 11-11).

If manual separation is necessary, the clinician should grasp the cord on each side of the intended break point and then twist and pull (from the placental side of the umbilicus) with the thumb and the forefingers to effect separation. Precautions must be taken to prevent undue tension on the ventral abdominal wall during this procedure. The cord should not be severed with a sharp instrument because this is more likely to result in excessive hemorrhage from the umbilical stump and possibly in a patent urachus (Figure 11-12). The umbilical stump should be observed after rupture for location of the break and for evidence of hemorrhage, urine, or abnormal swelling. The elastic, muscular walls of the two umbilical arteries allow prompt, prolonged constriction of the umbilical stump when it is separated through stretching. Failure of umbilical vessels to close when the cord breaks can lead to excessive blood loss, hemoperitoneum, or hypovolemic shock.

If hemorrhage is a problem, digital pressure should be applied to the stump for 30 to 60 seconds. If bleeding persists, an umbilical clamp or sterile, nonabsorbable ligature can be applied to the distal end of the stump, with removal in 6 to 12 hours. Prevention or treatment of shock may necessitate whole blood transfusion. Cardiovascular stabilization must preclude any surgical procedure that necessitates general anesthesia.

In all cases, the umbilical stump (navel) should be submerged without delay in a suitable disinfectant to minimize the opportunity for infectious organisms to ascend through the umbilical cord. A California study showed that 0.5% chlorhexidine solution (Nolvasan solution, Fort Dodge Animal Health, Fort Dodge, IA, is 2% chlorhexidine) is superior to 1% or 2% povidone-iodine solution or to 7% tincture of iodine for killing bacteria and preventing adverse umbilical tissue destruction in newborn foals. Disinfectant should be applied twice daily for 3 to 4 days. Contact of disinfectant (especially strong iodine) with the abdominal wall or the thighs must be avoided because it can have an irritating effect on these areas.

The umbilical stump should be evaluated daily for signs of omphalitis (including moistness, reddening, and swelling) (Figure 11-13), abscesses, or a patent urachus. If the umbilical region becomes abscessed or necrotic, it

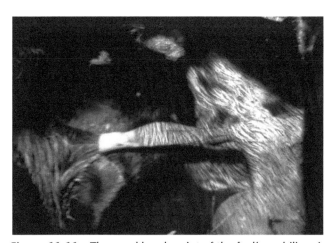

Figure 11-11 The usual break point of the foal's umbilicus is indicated by the pale, strictured area. If manual separation is necessary, the cord is grasped on each side of the intended break point. The cord is twisted and pulled until separated, with care taken to avoid undue tension on the ventral abdominal wall.

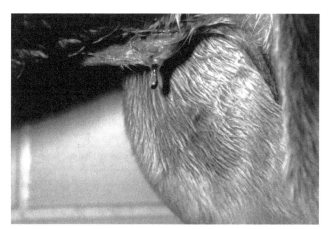

Figure 11-12 A moist umbilical stump with urine discharge is present in this foal with a patent urachus.

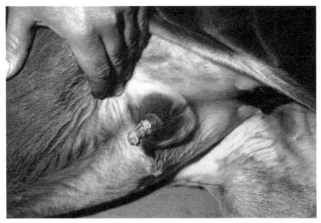

Figure 11-13 Omphalitis in a foal, as depicted by swelling at the base of the umbilical cord and reddening and necrosis of the tip of the umbilical stump.

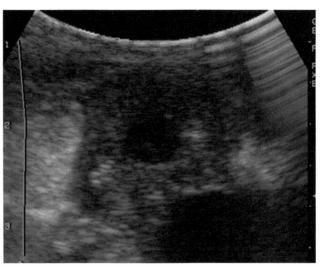

Figure 11-14 Transabdominal ultrasonographic image of infected umbilicus, with dilated urachus visible as the hypoechoic area in the center. (Courtesy Dr. Tom Seahorn, Lexington, Ky.)

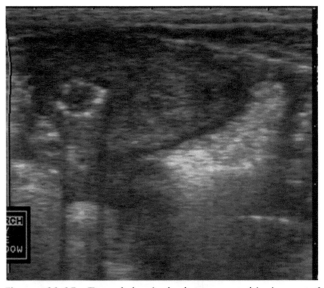

Figure 11-15 Transabdominal ultrasonographic image of infected umbilicus with the presence of gas evident as hyperechoic spots in center that casts shadows deeper within the image. The presence of gas may indicate anaerobic infection. (Courtesy Dr. Tom Seahorn, Lexington, Ky.)

should be surgically removed. In normal circumstances, the umbilicus appears as a dried stump 24 hours after birth. The dried umbilical stump usually falls off when the foal is between 1 and 2 weeks of age and the urachus remains sealed. In compromised neonates, the urachus may become patent (patent urachus) and drain urine when the stump falls off. In such cases, the umbilicus remains moist because of continuous urine dribbling. Patent urachus can also be congenital. Broad-spectrum antibiotics should be administered until urachal closure occurs because of the threat of ascending infection. If concurrent umbilical infection is not present, patent urachus often resolves spontaneously or with conservative therapy (e.g., mild cauterization applied 1 to 3 cm up into the urachal lumen two to three times per day for several days). If the urachus does not close, resection of the umbilical remnants and correction of urachal patency should be accomplished surgically.

Many umbilical infections can be detected with close examination of the umbilical stump and body wall. Palpation is sometimes helpful, but the absence of palpable abnormalities does not rule out infection of the umbilical vessels. Ultrasonography of the abdominal wall and umbilicus (Figures 11-14 and 11-15) should be performed when fever of unknown origin, chronic unthriftiness, or changes in the complete blood count (e.g., neutrophilia or hyperfibrinogenemia) suggest infection.

DAM-FOAL INTERACTION

Unnecessary disturbances to the dam and the foal during the immediate postnatal period should be avoided. Dam-foal interaction (sniffing, licking, and touching) is essential to the establishment of the bond between them (Figure 11-16). Interference during this period increases the likelihood of foal rejection by its dam, especially in nervous primiparous mares.

GIVING ENEMAS

Foals often have meconial impaction in the immediate postnatal period. Meconium consists of glandular secretions, swallowed amniotic fluid, and cell debris; it is dark brown to black in color and is present either in pasty consistency or as firm pellets. Meconium occupies the lumen of the rectum and the colon in the full-term fetus and, in normal circumstances, is not expelled until after birth (in utero stress can lead to meconial staining of amniotic fluid, fetal membranes, and the fetus). As the newborn foal passes meconium, fecal

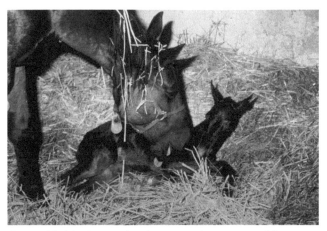

Figure 11-16 Interaction between the mare and her newborn foal is important to the establishment of a bond between them. Efforts should be made to avoid disturbing the mare or foal during this bonding period.

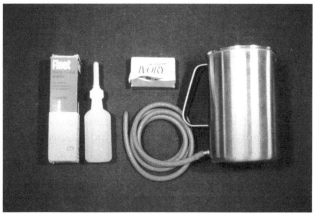

Figure 11-17 A commercially available phosphate enema and equipment commonly used for administration of a warm, soapy water enema, including an enema bucket and soft rubber tubing.

consistency changes to less tenacious, lighter brown material. Masses of meconium often are quite firm and large, resulting in various degrees of constipation and dyschezia in the first few days of postnatal life. Routine administration of enemas (C.B. Fleet Co, Richmond, Va.) to newborn foals tends to reduce the rate of occurrence of meconial impaction. The most commonly used types of enemas are 1 to 2 pints of warm, mild, soapy water, given via gravity flow through soft rubber tubing, and commercially available phosphate enemas (Figure 11-17). Extreme care should be taken during enema administration to prevent undue rectal trauma and perforation. Most instances of clinically apparent meconial impaction respond favorably to one or two enemas, often in conjunction with oral fluids containing mineral oil. Few impactions necessitate surgical intervention. Administration of more than one or two sodium phosphate enemas to a foal in the first 24 hours of life is not recommended because hyperphosphatemia may result.

A widely accepted method for treatment of meconial impaction resistant to one or two sodium phosphate or soapy water enemas is the administration of an acetylcysteine enema through a soft rubber tube (E-Z Pass Foal Enema Kit, Animal Reproduction Systems Chino, Calif.). Acetylcysteine apparently cleaves disulfide bonds in meconial mucoproteins, decreasing the consistency of the meconium and making it slippery. McCue (2006) recommends first sedating the foal and laying it on its side. A soft Foley catheter is then inserted 1 to 2 inches into the rectum, and the balloon is gently distended with air (maximum of 30 mL). Approximately 4 ounces of 4% acetylcysteine solution is slowly infused through the catheter, and the catheter is clamped to retain the solution, which is left within the rectum for 15 to 45 minutes (maximal acetylcysteine activity occurs by 45 minutes). The clamp is opened, the cuff deflated,

and the catheter removed after this time period. Meconial passage should occur within the next few hours. Sometimes, repeat administration is necessary. If this treatment is unsuccessful, or if colic does not resolve, surgical intervention may be required.

ANTIBIOTIC INJECTIONS

The use of a single, prophylactic injection of antibiotics to guard against infection is a topic of controversy. Proponents contend that it serves in a protective capacity when the foal is at a vulnerable stage and is exposed to a variety of organisms in the immediate environment and cite data that the leading cause of illness in neonatal units is bacterial infection (septicemia due most commonly to gram-negative bacteria). Adversaries assert that indiscriminate use of antibiotics can potentiate problems by prompting the development of antibiotic-resistant microorganisms. Madigan (1997) contends that short-term (48 to 72 hours) administration of broad-spectrum antibiotics (e.g., 20,000 U of procaine penicillin per kilogram of body weight intramuscularly every 24 hours and 6.6 mg of gentamicin per kilogram of body weight intramuscularly every 24 hours) is a prudent and effective, yet safe, means to treat exposure from bacteria across the gut wall in the newborn foal at risk for developing septicemia.

We do not recommend the prophylactic use of antibiotics in newborn foals except in extenuating circumstances. For example, foals with delayed ingestion of adequate colostrum during the first few hours of life, when there is evidence of placentitis, or for foals with complete or partial failure of passive antibody transfer. The clinician should make clients aware that proper hygiene, colostrum intake, and management cannot be replaced with prophylactic antibiotic administration.

Because no single physical examination or laboratory test finding confirms the presence of septicemia, a sepsis score was developed by Brewer and Koterba (1990) to aid in diagnosis of this condition. The scoring system ranks (from 0 to 4) neutrophil count, band neutrophil count, toxic changes of neutrophils, fibrinogen level, glucose level, immunoglobulin content, scleral petechiation or injection, rectal temperature, gestation length at birth, and other physical and historical data into an overall score. High and low scores were more than 90% and more than 85% accurate in predicting the presence or absence of sepsis, respectively. If infection is suspected, administration of broad-spectrum antibiotics should be initiated immediately. The spectrum of activity of the antimicrobials chosen should include effectiveness against gram-negative organisms most commonly associated with septicemia and against gram-positive organisms sometimes involved in neonatal infections. A combination of ampicillin (20 to 25 mg/kg of body weight intravenously every 6 hours) and amikacin (15 mg/kg of body weight intravenously every 24 hours) is used by some practitioners. Aseptically obtained blood cultures for identification of organisms associated with neonatal septicemia, and their antimicrobial sensitivity patterns, are useful for selection of appropriate antibiotics. If blood samples are collected for culture, sampling should occur before administration of the antibiotics.

NEONATAL VACCINATION

Protection of the newborn against specific infectious diseases should be provided by dam immunization in late gestation (booster immunizations with inactivated antigens 4 to 6 weeks before parturition). If the foal is not protected against indigenous pathogens through passively acquired immunity, neonatal vaccination can be provided when indicated and available. If low circulating levels of colostrum-derived tetanus antitoxins are suspected in the foal, tetanus antitoxin should be given to ensure protective levels during the first few weeks of life. However, the passive protection provided by antitoxin administration is short lived. The practitioner must recognize that vaccine response of foals varies by infectious agent and product used; however, the practitioner should also abide by the directions and precautions that accompany the vaccines.

In foals receiving adequate colostral protection from appropriately vaccinated broodmares, Wilson (1999) recommended that vaccination against equine herpesvirus 1 and 4 could begin at 4 months of age; vaccination against tetanus, Western equine encephalitis, and Eastern equine encephalitis could begin at 6 months of age; and vaccination against influenza could begin at 9 months of age. He recommended that vaccination against other potential pathogens (e.g., strangles, rabies, equine viral arteritis) be included in the foal immunization program when conditions of significant risk exist.

Current recommendations for active immunization of foals may change as more information on interference of colostrum-derived maternal antibodies with response to many vaccine antigens becomes available. Foals from vaccinated mares usually respond poorly to active immunization against common vaccine antigens begun at 3 months of age, even when repeated boosters are given. Most investigators agree that a more consistent response occurs if vaccines are not administered before 6 months of age and if three (rather than two) doses of the vaccine are given. Of additional concern with early vaccination is the finding that vaccination of foals against influenza before 6 months of age may induce tolerance that results in a poor response to vaccine administration later in life. In high-risk situations, particularly when colostral immunoglobulin transfer was poor, beginning vaccine administration at 3 months of age may be justified.

COLOSTRUM ACQUISITION

Although the equine fetus appears to be immunocompetent at mid gestation, at birth it is virtually devoid of circulating antibodies, except for small amounts of immunoglobulin M (IgM). The newborn foal adapts to the environment by producing its own antibodies, but these autogenous immunoglobulins are not evident for 1 to 2 weeks post partum and do not attain protective levels for as long as several weeks. Assurance that the neonate receives and absorbs an adequate supply of immunoglobulins therefore is of paramount importance. The passive immunity obtained via colostrum protects the newborn for several weeks while its own immune system is developing.

A foal must receive colostrum early in the first few hours of life. Absorption of intact antibodies through the intestinal epithelium of the newborn is a transient event that lasts approximately 24 hours. The efficiency of this process begins to decline approximately 6 to 8 hours after birth. Colostrum deprivation beyond this period increases the likelihood of a partial failure of passive immunoglobulin transfer to the foal. It is beneficial for all newborn foals to receive good quality colostrum within 2 hours after birth to maximize intestinal absorption of antibodies.

Colostrum can be delivered via bottle to newborn foals that are weak and unable to rise. When the suck reflex is absent, giving colostrum via nasogastric intubation is indicated. A foal that is unable to nurse the dam (because of dam agalactia, maternal death at parturition, foal rejection by the dam, or foal abnormalities such as neonatal maladjustment syndrome) should receive colostrum before placement on a receptive foster mare or hand feeding of mare milk or milk replacer.

A minimum of 1.5 to 2 L of high-quality colostrum currently is believed to be necessary to achieve a high postingestion serum level of passively obtained immunoglobulins. The newborn foal fed via bottle or nasogastric tube should receive colostrum at hourly intervals, with a maximum volume of 1 pint per feeding (Figure 11-18). Mares should be immunized properly during pregnancy and should be moved to the foaling premises 4 to 6 weeks before parturition to ensure high colostral levels of antibodies against the diseases of greatest concern to the equine population of the geographic location.

The immunoglobulin content of colostrum can be determined accurately but requires a tedious processing technique. Such verification is not routinely necessary but can be useful for evaluating colostrum to be stored or colostrum of questionable quality. Experimentation suggests that the specific gravity of colostrum is closely correlated with immunoglobulin content (>3000 mg/dL; specific gravity, >1.06); specific gravity of colostrum therefore might be a quick, reliable field test (>1.06 is desirable; determined with a colostrometer available from Jorgensen Laboratories, Loveland, CO.) (Figure 11-19) or a modified refractometer (Eclipse Model 45-03, Bellingham + Stanely, Lawrenceville, GA. or ECR-101, Animal Reproduction Systems). Sticky consistency typically indicates colostrum with a high immunoglobulin G (IgG) concentration, but determination of the approximate immunoglobulin content of colostrum based on the color of the sample is difficult. However, thick, yellow-orange colostrum tends to have a higher IgG content than white, milky-appearing colostrum.

If a source of fresh colostrum is not available, an alternative should be readily obtainable. The most feasible alternative is frozen equine colostrum from the same farm or a nearby farm or veterinary hospital. For such cases, colostrum from a mare is hygienically collected and stored at –20°C (–4°F) for future use. Colostrum preserved in this way maintains its antibody activity for

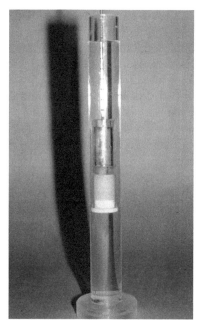

Figure 11-19 This colostrometer is used to measure the specific gravity of colostrum. The specific gravity of colostrum is highly correlated with immunoglobulin concentration.

at least 1 year. When needed, the frozen colostrum is thawed and warmed to body temperature by placing the receptacle in a warm (35°C to 37°C) water bath. Thawing of colostrum in a microwave should not be attempted; this results in destruction of the immunoglobulin proteins.

Only colostrum from the first postpartum milking should be used as an antibody source because it has the highest concentration of immunoglobulins; immunoglobulin content rapidly diminishes with subsequent milking. A maximum of 1 pint of colostrum should be removed from a single mammary gland of the donor mare at parturition. Attendants then should be certain that the foal nurses from the other mammary gland to ensure adequate ingestion of colostrum. Alternatively, some managers prefer not to milk out one teat until the foal has suckled.

Lyophilized equine IgG is an alternative to fresh or frozen equine colostrum. Foals need a dose of 40 to 60 g to elevate serum IgG concentrations to 400 to 1000 mg/dL. Serum or plasma can also be administered orally, but 6 to 9 L may be needed to obtain a satisfactory serum IgG concentration in the foal.

Colostrum and colostrum substitutes should be free of antierythrocyte antibodies (especially against the Aa and Qa blood group antigens) to prevent neonatal isoerythrolysis (see Chapter 10). The mare's serum can be tested (ideally during the last month of gestation) for the presence of antierythrocyte antibodies; if present, the colostrum should be discarded. An alternative source of antibodies has to be supplied to the foal—either colostrum tested against the foal's red blood cells (RBCs) with the jaundiced foal agglutination (JFA) test,

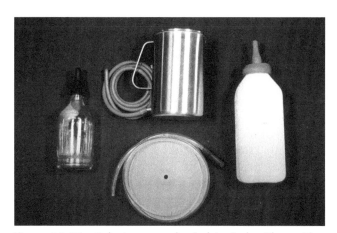

Figure 11-18 Colostrum can be fed to foals either with a bottle and nipple or through nasogastric tubing with an attached funnel. Enema buckets with attached tubing also work well for this purpose if properly cleaned before use.

or, preferably, serum or plasma known to not contain antierythrocyte antibodies (see "Failure of Passive Antibody Transfer" section).

The practitioner also should document that all foals have received an adequate amount of passively obtained antibodies by determining serum immunoglobulin levels at 16 to 24 hours of age.

FAILURE OF PASSIVE ANTIBODY TRANSFER

Passive antibody transfer failure is a primary underlying cause of infection in newborn foals. One study showed that approximately one quarter of all foals receive inadequate levels of passively obtained antibodies. The condition of such foals is precarious because they are not fully capable of warding off infectious assaults in the early weeks of life. Because the equine placenta does not permit transplacental transfer of maternal antibodies, the presuckle foal is virtually agammaglobulinemic.

At birth, the foal is capable of autogenous antibody synthesis against environmental antigens; however, a time lapse of several days is required for these actively obtained antibodies to be detected in the circulation. Protective levels of the antibodies might not be reached for weeks. The foal therefore relies entirely on passive immunity obtained through the colostrum as a defense against pathogens for the first weeks of life.

Colostrum acquisition by the foal is a time-dependent process. The antibody concentration of colostrum is depleted quickly after the first nursing and drops to negligible levels by 24 hours post partum. Furthermore, the intestinal wall of the foal is permeable to these antibodies for only approximately 24 hours. With adequate passive antibody transfer, the serum antibody levels of the foal should be approximately equal to those of its dam by 24 hours of age. From this time, passive protection is gradually eliminated (through immunoglobulin catabolism) concurrent with a steady rise in active immunity. Because the half-life of IgG reportedly is 3 weeks, passive protection reaches low levels by 6 to 8 weeks of age. Active immunization cannot be maximally stimulated until the titer of passive immunity is relatively low. Thus, foals reach a vulnerable stage in total immune status at approximately 1 to 2 months of age, during the transition to complete autogenous antibody protection. Because intestinal absorption of immunoglobulins is most expedient during the first few hours after birth and drops steadily thereafter, many potential opportunities exist for partial or complete failure of passive antibody transfer.

Causes

Causes of passive transfer failure can include the following: (1) weak, sick, or rejected foals that ingest an insufficient quantity of colostrum during the crucial 24 hours before the antibody absorptive function of the small intestine has ceased; (2) dysmature or premature foals that are too weak to nurse; (3) premature parturition, resulting in insufficient concentration of antibodies in the colostrum; (4) idiopathic low colostral IgG content in mares with no evidence of premature lactation, premature parturition, or subnormal serum IgG levels; and (5) depressed absorptive capacity of the foal's intestinal mucosa in the early hours of the postnatal period. Stress to the mare or the foal during the perinatal period is postulated as one mechanism behind intestinal malabsorption of antibodies. Increased endogenous steroid production, induced by stress, is believed to arrest intestinal absorption of immunoglobulins prematurely in other species. Ingestion of dirt or debris prior to colostrum ingestion, such as occurs with a nonhygienic udder, will also reduce antibody absorption.

Categories

Several gradations of passive transfer failure can occur. For practical purposes, two basic categories have evolved: partial failure of passive transfer (200 to 400 mg of IgG/dL of serum) and complete failure of passive transfer (<200 mg of IgG/dL of serum). Studies have shown that rate of occurrence and severity of illness are proportional to the amount of passive immunoglobulin deprivation. Approximately 25% of foals in the partial failure category become ill, whereas 75% of foals in the complete failure category contract infectious diseases. Few foals become ill when the serum level exceeds 400 to 800 mg/dL.

Detection

Early detection of passive transfer failure is an essential element in management of the disorder because prompt treatment helps alleviate encroaching infectious complications. If practical, diagnostic tests to determine IgG concentrations in foal blood at 8 to 12 hours of age can facilitate early detection of failure of passive transfer; this permits oral administration of high-quality colostrum to attempt to correct the immunodeficiency. Antibody absorption effectively nears completion at 18 to 24 hours of age; if the IgG concentration is low at this time, intravenous supplementation with plasma is necessary. A variety of kits are available for determination of the serum immunoglobulin concentration. Commonly used diagnostic kits are the single radial immunodiffusion test, the zinc sulfate turbidity test, semiquantitative immunoassays, and the glutaraldehyde coagulation test. Newer model densimeters (Models 590a and 591B, Animal Reproduction Systems Chino, Calif.), typically used for determination of sperm concentrations in semen, have software and kits available to measure IgG concentrations in foal serum.

Radial Immunodiffusion Test

The single radial immunodiffusion test uses equine IgG antisera and therefore is specific for measuring the IgG class of immunoglobulin. The test kit can be prepared by the practitioner or purchased commercially (Kit for the Quantitative Determination of Horse Immunoglobulin G, Miles Laboratories, Elkhart, IN; Equine IgG RID Kit, VMRD Inc, Pullman, WA; Equine IgG Test Kit, Kent Laboratories, Bellingham, WA). Accuracy is the primary advantage of this diagnostic technique. The test requires approximately 24 hours to perform. The commercially available test kit consists of agar gel plates, each of which can accommodate several samples for testing. The plates should be used only once; therefore, the cost per test sample increases as fewer samples are incorporated into the test plate.

Zinc Sulfate Turbidity Test

The zinc sulfate turbidity test is based on precipitation of salts created by the chemical combination of heavier globulins and trace metal ions. It can be interpreted with visual assessment or with spectrophotometry. Visual assessment offers the advantage of quick results (within 30 to 60 minutes) for a rough estimate of immunoglobulin protection. A precipitate gives the mixture a turbid appearance when the serum IgG concentration is at least 400 to 500 mg/dL, thus implying adequate IgG transfer. The degree of turbidity is directly proportional to the concentration of serum IgG. A more quantitative study is permitted when the absorbance of the mixture is determined with a spectrophotometer. The optical density of the sample is compared with a standard curve obtained with use of serial IgG dilutions of standardized serum. The zinc sulfate turbidity test is not specific for IgG but rather measures total immunoglobulin levels. Test results can be altered by sample hemolysis, carbon dioxide in the zinc sulfate solution, and time of interpretation; therefore, steps should be taken to prevent misinterpretation. Test kits can be fabricated at a veterinary hospital or obtained commercially (Equi-Z, Veterinary Medical Research and Development Inc, Pullman, WA). The procedure and necessary materials for the test are described in the literature.

Semiquantitative Immunoassays

A number of commercial kits are available to the practitioner for semiquantitative determination of foal IgG level (CITE Foal IgG Test, AgriTech Systems Inc, Portland, ME; Midland Plasma Foal IgG Quick Test Kits, Midland BioProducts Corp, Boone, IA; and Snap Foal IgG, Idexx Laboratories, Westbrook, ME). Test results can be obtained within 10 to 20 minutes up to 1 hour after venipuncture. Results of this test compare favorably with those of the single radial immunodiffusion test and the zinc sulfate turbidity test.

Glutaraldehyde Coagulation Test

The glutaraldehyde coagulation test is based on cross linkages formed by glutaraldehyde with basic proteins, which result in formation of insoluble complexes. A stock solution of 25% glutaraldehyde is diluted to 10% with deionized water, and 50 μL of this solution is added to 0.5 mL of test serum in a tube. The tube contents are examined at 5-minute to 10-minute intervals for evidence of coagulation. A positive reaction is evident as a solid gel that does not move when the tube is tilted. A positive reaction in less than 10 minutes is equivalent to more than 800 mg of IgG/dL, and a positive reaction between 10 and 60 minutes is equivalent to more than 400 mg of IgG/dL. The major advantage of the test is its low cost ($0.25/test), and the major disadvantage is the time needed to obtain results (i.e., the blood sample must be allowed to clot to obtain serum, and 60 minutes is required to get final results). A glutaraldehyde coagulation test is commercially available from Veterinary Dynamics Inc, Templeton, CA or Plassvacc USA Inc, Templeton, CA (Gamma-Chek-E).

In a recent study comparing performance of several commercially available assays for the diagnosis of failure of passive transfer (FPT) or partial FPT in foals, Florida workers (Davis and Giguère, 2005) found that most of the commercial test kits were generally adequate for detection of IgG levels less than 400 mg/dL, but some were less reliable in detection of IgG levels in the 400 to 800 mg/dL range, thus requiring further testing to determine the need for treatment. Practitioners should read this report to aid in a test kit that best fits their needs.

Treatment

Treatment measures for failure of passive antibody transfer vary depending on the stage of detection and the degree of immunoglobulin deprivation. If transfer failure is suspected less than 12 hours after birth, oral administration of colostrum is indicated. The foal should receive 500 mL of fresh or frozen/thawed colostrum at hourly intervals until a total intake of 1.5 to 2 L is achieved. To minimize the likelihood of neonatal isoerythrolysis or transfusion reactions, all colostrum must be checked for antierythrocyte alloantibodies before administration. Ideally, the IgG content of frozen colostrum is predetermined to ensure its quality.

If passive antibody transfer failure is detected more than 12 hours after birth, the foal should receive a plasma transfusion. The donor's plasma should be screened for compatibility with the foal's plasma. The ideal donor is Aa and Qa negative, with no alloantibodies to these blood group antigens. Depending on the IgG level of the foal and donor plasma, a plasma dose guideline is 20 to 50 mL of plasma per kilogram of body weight. This dose reportedly increases the foal's IgG content to 30% of that of the donor. Measurements for serum IgG should be repeated after transfusion because some foals may need a total of 2 to 4 L of plasma to attain satisfactory immunoglobulin levels. Specific guidelines for plasma collection are reported in the literature.

Because frozen (–20°C) plasma is thought to remain viable for several months to years, it may be advantageous to collect several liters of plasma from a universally compatible donor, determine the plasma IgG content, and then freeze it until needed. Properly immunized horses on the same premises that have antibody production against antigens indigenous to the area should be used.

Plasma for transfusions also is available through commercial laboratories (Foalimmune, Lake Immunogenetics, Ontario, NY; Equine Plasma, Veterinary Dynamics Inc, Templeton, CA). These products are generally screened for anti–red blood cell antibodies and certain immunoglobulins against a variety of equine diseases. Licensing of these commercial products implies substantiation of immunoglobulin content. These companies also provide custom formulating services to produce hyperimmune products that target specific diseases (e.g., *Rhodococcus equi*).

A healthy foal older than 3 weeks with 200 to 400 mg of IgG per deciliter of serum probably should not be given a plasma transfusion because this passively obtained antibody protection would hinder active immune development. Such foals should be monitored carefully, however, and placed in a clean, environmentally suitable area to minimize exposure to pathogens.

Prevention

Prevention of passive transfer failures consists of good management. All foalings should be attended, and the foal should receive colostrum by 6 hours of age. Routine serum evaluation of foals before 16 to 24 hours of age is necessary to check for adequate immunoglobulin transfer. If an inadequate circulating level of IgG is confirmed, appropriate therapeutic steps should be taken. Additional supportive measures for foals with passive transfer failure include isolation in a clean, protected, well-ventilated environment and antibiotic therapy when necessary.

ADMINISTRATION OF *RHODOCOCCUS EQUI* HYPERIMMUNE PLASMA

Texas workers have shown that transfusion of hyperimmune *R. equi* plasma, produced by harvesting plasma from adult horses repeatedly exposed to *R. equi* of newborn foals subsequently challenged with the aerosolized live organism, protects against the disease or attenuates response in a manner that better enables foals to overcome infection. Other studies have subsequently documented the value of transfusion of newborn foals with hyperimmune *R. equi* plasma in reducing disease incidence and death attributable to naturally occurring

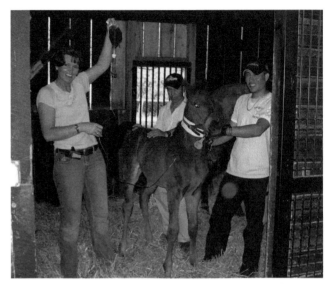

Figure 11-20 Transfusion of hyperimmune *R. equi* plasma to a 28-day-old foal as a component of a *Rhodococcus* control program.

infection. Certainly, the procedure is not completely (100%) effective. The optimal amount of plasma that needs to be transfused and the optimal age of foal at which transfusion needs to occur have yet to be determined. However, on farms endemically affected with *R. equi* pneumonia, intravenous administration of *R. equi* hyperimmune plasma (1 L) to newborn foals has become commonplace as a method to control clinical effects of this disease. One of the authors has transfused 1 L at 12 to 24 hours of age, plus another liter at 26 to 28 days of age, to all foals born on an endemically affected farm (Figure 11-20) with some perceived clinical success (i.e., reduced incidence of disease, reduced severity of disease, no deaths). When combined with a screening procedure (e.g., biweekly thoracic ultrasound evaluations for typical lesions; biweekly CBC analyses) used to detect early signs of infection, transfusion of *R. equi* hyperimmune plasma may provide an important component in the control of this disease on endemically infected farms. Those foals with early signs of disease detected by these methods are candidates for antimicrobial (e.g., azithromycin and rifampin) treatment. Early detection and treatment of *R. equi* infection can prevent permanent damage from developing.

BIBLIOGRAPHY

Brewer BD, Koterba AM: Development of a scoring system for the early diagnosis of equine neonatal sepsis, *Equine Vet J* 20:18-22, 1990.

Davis R, Giguère S. Evaluation of five assays for the diagnosis of failure of passive transfer of immunity in foals, *Proc 51st Ann Mtg Am Assoc Equine Pract* 43-44, 2005.

Knottenbelt D, Holdstock N, Madigan JE: *Equine neonatology: medicine and surgery,* Philadelphia, 2004, Saunders, 155-363.

Koterba AM: Physical examination. In Koterba AM, Drummon WH, Kosch PC, editors: *Equine clinical neonatology,* Philadelphia, 1990, Lea & Febiger.

LeBlanc MM: Immunologic considerations. In Koterba AM, Drummon WH, Kosch PC, editors: *Equine clinical neonatology,* Philadelphia, 1990, Lea & Febiger.

Madigan JE: Method for preventing neonatal septicemia, the leading cause of death in the neonatal foal, *Proc Am Assoc Equine Pract* 43:17-19, 1997.

Madigan JE: Physical exam of the neonate. In Madigan JE, editor: *Manual of equine neonatal medicine,* Woodland, CA, 1987, Live Oak Publishing.

Martens RJ: Pediatrics. In Mannsmann RA, McAllister ES, Pratt PW, editors: *Equine medicine and surgery,* ed 3, vol 1, Santa Barbara, CA, 1982, American Veterinary Publications.

Martens RJ, Martens JG, Fiske RA: *Rhodococcus equi* foal pneumonia: protective effects of immune plasma in experimentally infected foals, *Equine Vet J* 21:249-255, 1989.

McClure JJ: The immune system. In McKinnon AO, Voss JL, editors: *Equine reproduction,* Philadelphia, 1993, Lea & Febiger.

McCue PM: Meconium impaction in newborn foals, *J Equine Vet Sci* 26:152-155, 2006.

Rossdale PD, Ricketts SW: *Equine stud farm medicine,* ed 2, Philadelphia, 1980, Lea & Febiger, 277-305.

Traub-Dargatz JL: Postnatal care of the foal. In McKinnon AO, Voss JL, editors: *Equine reproduction,* Philadelphia, 1993, Lea & Febiger.

White SC: The use of plasma in foals with failure of passive transfer, *Proc Am Assoc Equine Pract* 35:215-218, 1989.

Wilson WD: Vaccination programs for foals and weanlings, *Proc Am Assoc Equine Pract* 45:254-263, 1999.

Semen Collection and Artificial Insemination with Fresh Semen

12

CHAPTER

OBJECTIVES

While studying the information covered in this chapter, the reader should attempt to:
- Acquire a working knowledge of procedures used for collection of semen from stallions.
- Acquire a working knowledge of proper breeding management of stallions and semen processing and handling techniques used in artificial insemination programs.

STUDY QUESTIONS

1. Discuss advantages and disadvantages of artificial insemination programs compared with natural breeding programs for horses.
2. Describe important components of a breeding shed to be used in an equine artificial insemination program.
3. Give advantages and disadvantages of the commonly used equine artificial vaginas.
4. Describe the technique for preparation of an artificial vagina for semen collection in the stallion.
5. List the advantages of use of a breeding phantom for semen collection.
6. Describe the role of semen extenders and temperature in maintenance of equine sperm viability in vitro.
7. Discuss the proper insemination dose (number of sperm and insemination volume), insemination timing, and insemination technique for artificial insemination in the mare.
8. Discuss indications for and advantages of low-dose insemination of horses.
9. Describe the technique for deep horn insemination with small inseminate volumes.
10. Describe the technique for hysteroscopic insemination directly onto the oviductal papilla.

Proper application of artificial insemination (AI) in an equine breeding program can dramatically improve operating efficiency and increase the availability of sires to the general public. This chapter addresses advantages and disadvantages of AI programs and provides a detailed description of the techniques involved.

Few breed registries in the United States do not currently permit the use of AI (e.g., the Jockey Club [Thoroughbreds]). The allowances and limitations regarding storage and transport of semen vary considerably among the breed registries that permit the use of

AI. One should contact specific breed registries before instituting an AI program to determine restrictions that might limit registration of foals produced.

ADVANTAGES AND DISADVANTAGES

AI offers numerous advantages over natural mating. For instance, division of an ejaculate into several insemination doses permits more efficient use of stallion semen, provided that the stallion has normal fertility. Accordingly, the number of mares that a stallion can impregnate during a breeding season or calendar year may be increased several-fold. The availability of stallion semen to mare owners is likewise increased within those breed organizations whose bylaws permit preservation and transport of stallion semen. Addition of antibiotics to semen extenders for AI minimizes venereal transmission of bacterial diseases to the mare where the stallion serves as a carrier. Transmission of potential pathogens from mare to stallion can also be reduced. Semen extenders contain supportive and protective factors for sperm that may improve the pregnancy rates of certain stallions. Use of a breeding phantom for collection of semen reduces the risk of breeding injuries. Collection of semen with an artificial vagina also allows scrutiny of semen quality before insemination and allows early detection of problems that may adversely affect the fertility of stallions. The development of low-dose insemination techniques further enhances the number of mares that can be bred with an ejaculate and can improve pregnancy rates for some subfertile stallions.

Certain disadvantages are inherent to AI programs. The success of such programs requires heightened knowledge and skill on the part of the stallion manager because ejaculated sperm are very susceptible to environmental injury. Improper semen collection, handling, processing, and insemination technique can lower pregnancy rates. Expenses related to the purchase of necessary equipment and supplies for AI can increase overhead costs of the breeding program. However, expenses incurred on a per mare basis are usually decreased because of the multiple inseminations possible with a single ejaculate. Another disadvantage is the somewhat increased risk of human injury during the process of semen collection with an artificial vagina (AV). Therefore, proper training of persons involved in the semen collection process is essential. Further training is needed to reach a level of competence to achieve satisfactory pregnancy rates with low-dose insemination techniques because semen processing and handling requirements are heightened. Finally, equipment costs for hysteroscopic insemination are relatively expensive compared with those required for manual insemination practices.

SEMEN COLLECTION

The semen collection procedure is an essential part of the AI program. Facilities and equipment that permit safe and efficient collection and handling of the semen are discussed.

Artificial Vagina Selection

A properly constructed and prepared AV increases the efficiency of semen collection in AI programs and optimizes the quality of ejaculated semen. Several well-designed AVs are available. Each type has distinct attributes and peculiarities, so AV selection is based on specific requirements and personal preference. AVs have also been homemade by users to meet their specific needs. When contemplating the purchase of an equine AV, one should consider initial and maintenance costs, durability, weight, temperature maintenance, and sperm losses incurred during semen collection.

Missouri Model Artificial Vagina

The Missouri model AV (NASCO, Ft. Atkinson, WI) (Figure 12-1) probably is the most widely used AV in the United States. It is composed of a double-walled rubber liner that contains a permanently sealed water chamber and a leather carrying case. This AV is relatively inexpensive, lightweight, and easy to assemble and clean. It has fairly good heat retention, and because the glans penis should be beyond the water jacket at the time of ejaculation, internal temperature of the AV may exceed the 45°C to 48°C sperm tolerance threshold without causing heat-related injury to ejaculated sperm. This property can be advantageous for stallions that prefer higher temperatures. This AV is equipped with an air valve so that it can be pressurized with water alone or with air and water to reduce its weight. Because the liner is made of heavy rubber and the water chamber is permanently sealed, there is little chance of water leakage contaminating the semen sample during collection. Latex liners are available for this AV in two lengths (16 inches and 22 inches). The occasional stallion with a large penis may prefer the longer liner.

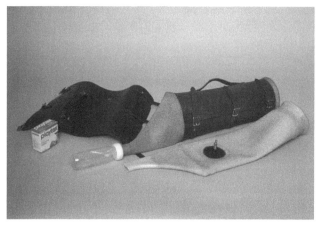

Figure 12-1 Missouri model artificial vagina: leather carrying case, double-layered latex rubber water jacket with attached latex rubber cone, bottle adapter, and collection bottle with semen filter inside. Disposable bottle liners *(shown)* can be used inside most collection bottles. (From Varner DD, Schumacher J, Blanchard TL, et al: *Diseases and management of breeding stallions,* Goleta, CA, 1991, American Veterinary Publications, 118.)

Japanese (Nishikawa) Model Artificial Vagina

The Japanese (Nishikawa) model AV (Figure 12-2) is composed of a small, rigid aluminum case and a single rubber liner, so it is lightweight and easy to maneuver. The Japanese model is no longer available commercially in the United States, but the Har-Vet model (Har-Vet, Spring Valley, WI) closely resembles the Japanese model, except that it has a plastic rather than an aluminum casing. The AV is easy to assemble and clean. Another attribute of this AV is the direct attachment of a semen receptacle to the casing. This design permits the ejaculate to be discharged directly into the receptacle, allowing only minimal contact of semen with the rubber liner. The liner must be secured tightly to the case with rubber bands before water is added to the chamber between the liner and the case. Water can leak out if this seal is not tight, reducing AV pressure and increasing the risk of water contamination in the ejaculate. The liner should be checked for defects before use because pinpoint holes in the rubber liner can develop, resulting in water leakage into the AV lumen.

Colorado Model Artificial Vagina

The original Colorado model AV is composed of two independent rubber liners and a heavy plastic case covered by a leather collar. It is more cumbersome to use than the previous two AVs but offers good heat retention. Because it has two rubber liners between the water chamber and the AV lumen, the likelihood of water contamination of the semen sample is greatly reduced. The water jacket of this AV is longer than the penis; therefore, the temperature must be carefully regulated to prevent undue heat damage to ejaculated sperm.

CSU Model Artificial Vagina

The CSU model AV (Animal Reproduction Systems, Chino, CA) (Figure 12-3) and Lane model AV (Lane Manufacturing, Denver) are modified versions of the original Colorado model. Both models are lighter than the original and have a rigid handle to facilitate AV manipulation. These versions have the advantages described previously for the Colorado model and come with an assortment of accessories, including several AV liners, semen filters and collection bottles, a thermometer to monitor internal temperature of the AV, and an insulated protector cone to cover the semen receptacle during the semen collection process.

Polish Model Artificial Vagina

The Polish model AV was designed as an open-ended AV for collection of only the sperm-rich fraction of the ejaculate from breeding stallions. This method of semen collection increases sperm concentration and, likewise, reduces the contribution (volume) of seminal plasma in ejaculates. The first three jets of an ejaculate contain 60% to 80% of the sperm present in total ejaculates, yet seminal volume is reduced more than 50%. The result of this semen-fractionation step is a significant increase in sperm concentration, sometimes exceeding 0.6 to 1×10^9 sperm/mL. The technique is considered useful for semen preservation programs because the sperm concentration can be increased without centrifugation and toxic influences of seminal plasma on sperm viability may be diminished. Collection of semen with this method often reduces contamination of ejaculates, whether by bacteria from the exterior of the penis, by urine from stallions affected by urospermia, or by blood from stallions with a penile injury. Removal of the coned

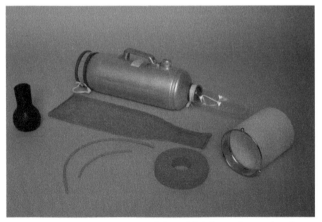

Figure 12-2 Japanese model artificial vagina: aluminum case with rigid handle, latex rubber liner, rubber bands for attaching the rubber liner to the aluminum case, collection bag and attached rubber band, insulating receptacle for the end of the artificial vagina, and rubber cushion (doughnut) for placement at the inside front of artificial vagina. The black rubber attachment can be used around the collection bag if desired. (From Varner DD, Schumacher J, Blanchard TL, et al: *Diseases and management of breeding stallions*, Goleta, CA, 1991, American Veterinary Publications, 119.)

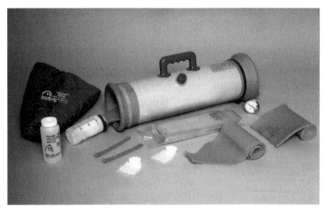

Figure 12-3 CSU model artificial vagina: rigid plastic case and handle with padded ends, outer latex rubber liner that forms the water jacket, inner latex rubber liner and cone, collection bottle and filter, and insulating bag for placement over the end of assembled unit. (From Varner DD, Schumacher J, Blanchard TL, et al: *Diseases and management of breeding stallions*, Goleta, CA, 1991, American Veterinary Publications, 120.)

end of the Missouri model AV (Figure 12-4) or shortening of the CSU model AV works well for this purpose. The glans penis is allowed to protrude from the AV, and as the semen is ejaculated, it is collected through a funnel system attached to semen receptacles or in urethral prosthetic devices attached to a bag (Figure 12-5), or by catching semen in individual receptacles.

Two other AVs are commercially available. The French (INRA) model (IMV International Corp, L'Aigle, France) is similar to but smaller than the Colorado AV and has two handles. The Roanoke artificial vagina (Roanoke AI Labs, Roanoke, VA) has a short, variable-diameter rigid casing designed to facilitate manual stimulation of the upper shaft of the penis.

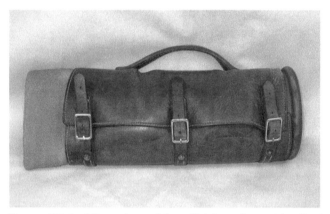

Figure 12-4 Missouri model artificial vagina with distal collecting cone removed (modified Polish or Krakow model). Removal of the collecting cone allows visualization and fractionation of the semen during the course of ejaculation.

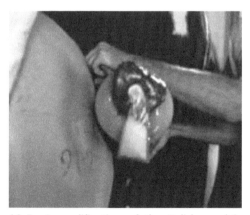

Figure 12-5 A modification of the Polish model artificial vagina (open-ended AV) is used to collect semen from a stallion. The AV is open at either end, permitting penile protrusion and collection of fractions of the ejaculate. The fractions ("spurts" or "jets") of the ejaculate can either be caught in hand-held containers or be collected in a prosthetic device attached to a sterile collection bag on the distal urethral process. (From Varner DD, Schumacher J, Blanchard TL, et al: *Diseases and management of breeding stallions*, Goleta, CA, 1991, American Veterinary Publications, 122.)

Artificial Vagina Maintenance

All AV components that come in contact with ejaculated semen must be nonspermicidal. Reusable items must be cleansed properly to render them chemically clean, then dried, and, if possible, sterilized between uses. Soaps or disinfectants should not be used to clean AV liners because the residue can be toxic to sperm during subsequent semen collections. The rubber AV liners should be cleaned with hot running water soon after use. If smegma within an AV is allowed to dry before cleaning, the chore becomes more difficult. Cleaned rubber liners can be submerged in ethyl or isopropyl alcohol for 0.5 to 24 hours for disinfection followed by air-drying in a dust-free cabinet. Any of the latex rubber liners can be gas sterilized with ethylene oxide as long as an adequate "air-out" period is allowed (i.e., 48 to 72 hours). Sterile, nontoxic disposable equipment should be used when possible to avoid chemical contamination of ejaculates or horizontal transmission of disease. Plastic disposable AV liners, with or without attached semen receptacles, are commercially available for most AVs. This equipment helps ensure a clean, nontoxic method of semen collection. Unfortunately, some stallions do not readily accept AVs fitted with a disposable plastic liner and seem to prefer the feel of the rubber liner.

Preparation of Artificial Vaginas for Semen Collection

Immediately before semen collection is attempted, the water jacket of the AV is usually filled with 45°C to 50°C water to provide an internal AV temperature of 44°C to 48°C (Figure 12-6). Providing an AV temperature above that of the body seems to aid in penile stimulation and facilitates ejaculation. Occasionally, some stallions may respond more favorably to semen collection with an AV if its luminal temperature is 50°C to 55°C. Sperm can be permanently damaged, however,

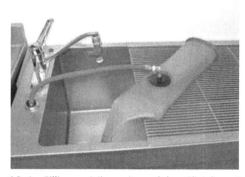

Figure 12-6 Filling a Missouri model artificial vagina with hot (45°C) water. An air nozzle attachment has been placed on the water hose and connects to the air/water valve inserted into the AV. This system avoids water spillage during the filling procedure. A dial thermometer can be placed within the lubricated AV to monitor temperature.

by contact with surfaces above 45°C. As mentioned previously, the luminal temperature of a Missouri model AV can exceed 45°C without damaging sperm, provided that the glans penis protrudes beyond the water jacket when ejaculation occurs.

Pressure of the AV should be adjusted to provide uniformly good contact around the penis, without interfering with penile penetration. Proper AV pressure accommodates expansion of the penis to full erection. Full insertion of the penis into the AV during the first penile thrust and then maintenance of the penis in this fully inserted position is important; otherwise, the glans penis dilates and may be too large to permit full penile penetration into the AV. The result is extended contact of ejaculated semen with the AV liner and elevated temperature en route to the semen receptacle or ejaculatory failure from inadequate penile stimulation. Both temperature and water pressure in the AV should be maintained relatively constant during semen collection to promote consistent stallion performance and maximal sperm harvest.

The inner surface of the AV should be lubricated with a sterile, nonspermicidal lubricant before penile insertion. The collection receptacle (Figure 12-7) should be maintained at body temperature during semen collection and transport to the laboratory to prevent cold shock to the sperm before they are placed in a protective extender. Semen should also be protected from light.

To maximize the number of sperm available from each semen collection, an appropriate filter should be incorporated into the collection receptacle. The filter allows most of the gel-free fractions to pass into the seminal receptacle but traps the gel (which is presented in the final fractions of an ejaculate). Although some sperm inevitably are trapped in the gel and filter, more would be lost if the semen were filtered after collection of the combined gel and gel-free portions or if the gel were aspirated from the gel-free portion with a syringe. Nylon micromesh filters (see Figure 12-7) are superior to polyester matte filters for separating gel from gel-free fractions because they are nonabsorptive and do not trap as many sperm. The filter with its contained gel should be removed immediately on collection of the semen to prevent seepage of gel into the gel-free portion of the ejaculate.

Use of Condoms for Semen Collection

A condom (Figure 12-8) is a poor alternative to an AV for semen collection but may be the only viable option if the stallion will not breed an AV or if an AV is unavailable. Stallions most reluctant to breed an AV are those accustomed to breeding mares by natural service and occasionally, those that have never bred before. The quality of semen collected in a condom is inferior to that obtained with an AV because of the marked contamination of the sample with bacteria and debris from the exterior of the penis.

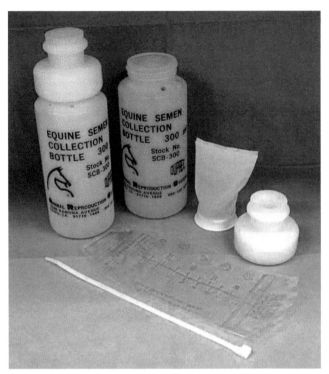

Figure 12-7 An efficient semen collection receptacle modified for use with the Missouri model artificial vagina. Vent holes have been punctured around the neck of the equine semen collection bottle (Animal Reproduction Systems) to allow semen to freely enter the disposable baby bottle liner (Playtex Products Inc, Westport, Conn.) placed inside the bottle. The plastic bottle adapter (NASCO) has been modified to permit attachment of the large semen collection bottle and is screwed onto the bottle top after the nylon mesh gel filter (Animal Reproduction Systems) has been inserted into the top of the bottle with the baby bottle liner inserted. This bottle adapter then fits into the latex coned end of the Missouri model AV. If the attachment is loose, a plastic snap tie can be used to prevent the assembled receptacle from detaching during the semen collection process. Finally, a collection bottle cover (Animal Reproduction Systems) is attached over the bottle with a drawstring when the AV is fully assembled. The insulated cover protects the semen against cold shock and light damage.

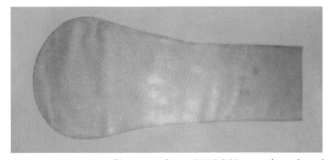

Figure 12-8 A stallion condom (NASCO) can be placed onto the stallion's penis before the stallion is permitted to breed a mare in estrus. After ejaculation and dismounting, the condom is removed, and semen is poured through a filter to remove gel and extraneous debris before the semen is processed.

Preparation of Stallion Mount

Semen collection with an AV ordinarily is performed by allowing the stallion to mount a mare or breeding phantom. In certain situations, however, stallions have been trained to ejaculate with an AV or manual stimulation while standing on the ground (Figure 12-9). To train a stallion for ground collection, the stallion is teased to erection, and the penis is washed and dried. The stallion is approached by the collector from the left shoulder, and the AV is placed on the stallion's penis. The AV is pushed toward the base of the penis to encourage thrusting. Stallions usually ejaculate after 5 to 10 pelvic thrusts. If the stallion does not ejaculate after the first attempt, the procedure is repeated until successful. As an alternative to ground collection, some practitioners prefer to use thin plastic mitts or rectal sleeves instead of an AV. The mitt is loosely placed on the penile shaft with 6 to 8 inches hanging beyond the end of the glans. Excess air is expelled from the mitt, and gentle pressure is applied to the glans penis to stimulate thrusting until ejaculation occurs. Application of hot compresses (6-inch squares of folded towels dipped in 50°C to 55°C water, squeezed to remove excess water from the compress), with one hand on the glans penis and one hand on the base of the penis, is often helpful in stimulating pelvic thrusting and ejaculation. A consistent, uniform method to which the individual stallion responds should be adopted. A modification of this technique can be used for chemical ejaculation (Figure 12-10). Chemical ejaculation is the method we use most often for stallions with ejaculatory problems associated with neurologic or musculoskeletal disorders that preclude mounting.

For standard semen collection protocols with the stallion mounted on a mare, either gonad-intact or ovariectomized mares can be used. Intact mares should not be used unless they are exhibiting strong signs of behavioral estrus and readily tolerate mounting and

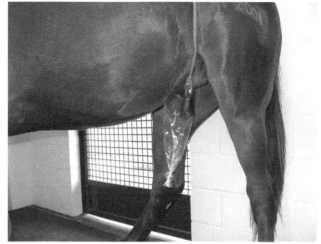

Figure 12-10 Use of a thin plastic mitt (or rectal sleeve) for collection of semen from a stallion standing on the ground. Hot compresses can be used to apply pressure to the glans penis and base of the penis to stimulate thrusting and ejaculation. In this particular stallion, the mitt has been hung over the penis for semen collection with chemical ejaculation. After sedation with detomodine, the stallion is left undisturbed until ejaculation occurs. Semen collected in this manner is highly concentrated and of low volume.

some nipping by the stallion. Ovariectomized mares generally are considered more appropriate than intact mares for daily semen collection activities because they are more predictable and can be used anytime. Mares should be selected as candidates for ovariectomy based on their degree of receptivity to a stallion while in estrus as intact mares. Ovariectomized mares rarely need exogenous hormonal therapy to display behavioral signs of estrus. When needed, a judicious use of 1 to 2 mg of estradiol cypionate can be given intramuscularly to intensify signs of behavioral estrus in ovariectomized mares. This regimen does not induce estrus in intact mares with a functional corpus luteum, and excessive use in ovariectomized mares can result in aggressive rather than receptive behavior.

Mares should be physically restrained before the stallion is allowed to mount. Leg hobbles and a twitch on the muzzle can be applied to mares (Figure 12-11). Rarely is tranquilization needed. If a mare's reactions to an approaching stallion are unknown or unpredictable, it is wise to allow a "teaser stallion" (with a breeding shield to prevent inadvertent breeding; Pinkston's Turf Goods, Lexington, Ky.) to mount the mare to test her response before permitting a more valuable stallion to mount for semen collection. If the mare reacts unfavorably, an alternative mount source should be used. It is equally important that the stallion not be allowed to savage the mare during breeding. This behavior usually can be controlled with a chain shank passed through the stallion's mouth (Figure 12-12). A muzzle can be fastened to the stallion's halter if

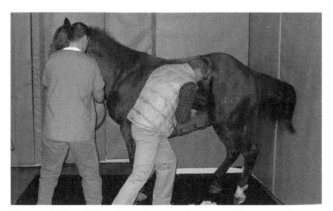

Figure 12-9 Collection of semen from a stallion standing on the ground (i.e., unmounted on a mare or phantom). Many stallions can be trained to ejaculate in such a manner, eliminating the need for a mount source.

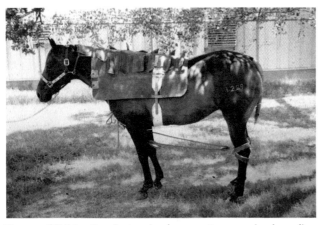

Figure 12-11 Ovariectomized mount mare in breeding hobbles; the tail is wrapped and a protective cape is fitted to protect the withers and neck of mare while the stallion is mounted.

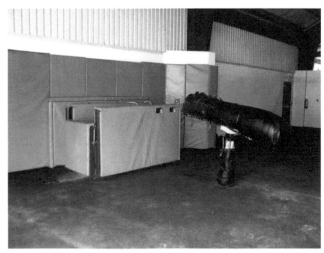

Figure 12-13 A commercial model of a breeding phantom (or dummy) commonly used for collection of semen from stallions.

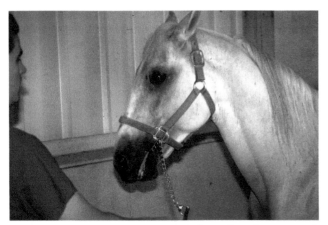

Figure 12-12 Chain shank placed through stallion's mouth to facilitate restraint during breeding.

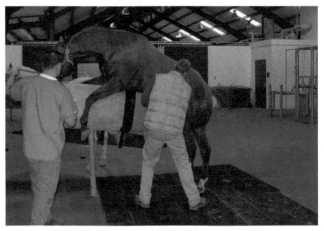

Figure 12-14 Collection of semen from a stallion mounted on a breeding phantom. The stimulus mare is placed in front of the breeding phantom in this breeding shed.

excessive biting cannot be controlled by other methods. If necessary, a leather breeding shroud can be secured around the neck of the mount mare so that the stallion bites this apparatus rather than the mare during breeding.

For most stallions, semen collection can be enhanced with use of a breeding phantom, or dummy (Figures 12-13 and 12-14). Although additional training is required to teach a stallion to mount one of these devices, the devices offer several advantages over an estrous or ovariectomized mount mare for semen collection. Breeding phantoms eliminate variability in the mount source, thereby allowing a more consistent semen collection protocol. They also greatly reduce the likelihood of stallion injury during semen collection and mare injury resulting from the vicious biting of some stallions. Stallions with rear limb or back maladies can mount a stationary breeding phantom more easily than a live mare. The height of the phantom can be adjusted to accommodate the stallion. In addition, the phantom can be thoroughly cleaned between

mounts, thereby minimizing horizontal transmission of disease.

The size, shape, and composition of breeding phantoms are quite diverse, ranging from padded hot-water tanks to sophisticated structures with mounted AVs and hydraulic controls for adjusting the height. Desirable elements of a dummy include the following:

- Adjustable height, with mid-height slightly shorter than the average height of the breed involved.
- Width sufficient to permit the stallion to grasp the dummy firmly with the forelegs (total width, including padding, usually should be 22 to 24 inches).
- Adequate padding with an overlying cover that is durable, nonabrasive, and easy to clean.
- A stand with a centrally placed upright support to prevent injury to the stallion's hind limbs or feet during collection.
- Installation in an area free of obstructions, with space for a live mare to stand adjacent to the dummy.

Most stallions readily accept the phantom as a mounting device. The novice stallion is trained by placing a mare alongside the phantom. The stallion is allowed to tease the mare over the end of the phantom. This stimulates mounting behavior in the stallion, but the stallion is diverted so that he mounts the phantom rather than the live mare. Very little training is required in most instances. Sometimes a mare in estrus must be close to the phantom to stimulate the stallion to mount it. On other occasions, the novice stallion remains reluctant to mount the phantom. For such a stallion, position him directly behind the phantom. Encourage him to rest his chin on the top with his chest touching the back of the phantom. Once the stallion is in this position, place the artificial vagina onto his penis. This usually results in the stallion thrusting forward and upward as he rears, landing him onto the phantom. After the first one or two collections are obtained in this manner, the procedure may no longer be necessary to encourage mounting. Once trained, some stallions do not need the presence of an estrous mare to mount the phantom. When properly constructed, breeding phantoms greatly improve the efficiency and safety of semen collection from the stallion.

General Semen Handling Techniques

Immediately after its collection, semen should be quickly transported to the laboratory with minimization of physical trauma, exposure to light, cold shock, or excessive heat. All materials that come in contact with the semen (including the semen extender) should be prewarmed to body temperature (37°C to 38°C). If an in-line filter was not fitted in the AV when semen was collected, the semen should be poured through a nontoxic filter to remove any gel or extraneous debris. The gel fraction of unfiltered ejaculate can also be removed via careful aspiration with a syringe. Loss of sperm is greater with the latter two methods than with use of an in-line, nylon micromesh filter (Animal Reproduction Systems), which is contained within the AV's collection bottle. Sperm concentration, volume and color of the gel-free semen, and the percentage of progressively motile sperm should be determined and recorded (Figures 12-15 to 12-18).

Whether the semen is to be used immediately or preserved, it should always be mixed with an appropriate extender within a few minutes after collection to maximize sperm longevity. An initial semen/extender dilution ratio of 1:1 to 1:2 is generally adequate if semen will not be stored for more than 1 to 2 hours before insemination. A warmed extender can also be placed in the semen receptacle before collection so that the sperm come in contact with this supportive medium immediately after ejaculation. This procedure can be beneficial for stallions whose seminal plasma seems to depress longevity of sperm motility or otherwise interfere with fertility. For accurate measurements

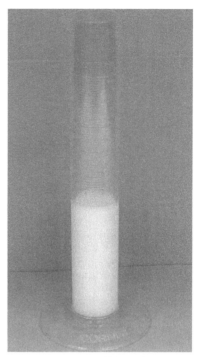

Figure 12-15 Measurement of filtered raw semen volume in a graduated cylinder.

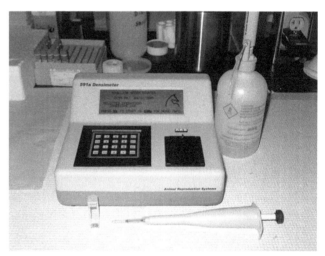

Figure 12-16 Determining the sperm concentration of raw semen with a Densimeter (Animal Reproduction Systems). After the Densimeter is standardized for 100% transmittance through a diluent-loaded cuvette, 180 μL of mixed gel-free raw semen is pipetted into the cuvette. The top of the cuvette is covered, and the cuvette is gently rotated to mix the semen evenly in the diluent. The cuvette is placed into the Densimeter, the door is closed, and the sperm concentration in the raw semen is read on the screen of the instrument.

of sperm concentration in extended semen with a spectrophotometer or similar photometric system, the extenders must be optically clear. If the extender used is not optically clear, a hemocytometer, flow cytometer, or NucleoCounter SP-100 (ChemoMetec,

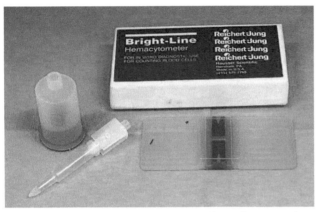

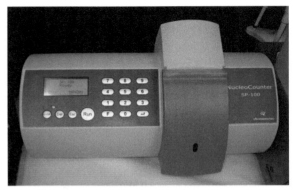

Figure 12-19 NucleoCounter SP-100 (ChemoMetec) used for determining sperm concentration. The instrument only identifies sperm based on cell size and staining of DNA with propidium iodide. Although it is more expensive than conventional photometric systems, the improved accuracy and the capability of use with extended semen offer distinct advantages.

Figure 12-17 The sperm concentration of semen (raw or extended) can be determined with a hemocytometer counting chamber (catalog no. 02-671-5; Fisher Scientific, Pittsburgh, Pa.) and the white blood cell/platelet Unopette system with 20-μL pipettes (catalog no. 13-680). The raw semen is gently mixed, and the pipette is loaded with the semen. The semen in the loaded pipette is aspirated into the diluent within the Unopette and mixed. The pipette is reversed, and the diluted semen is expressed into the cover-slipped hemocytometer chamber, allowing 5 minutes for sperm to settle. A phase-contrast microscope is used to enumerate the number of sperm in one of the nine large squares on the hemocytometer grid. This procedure is repeated on the other side of the hemocytometer, and the two counts are averaged. The averaged count represents the number of sperm (in millions) per milliliter of raw semen.

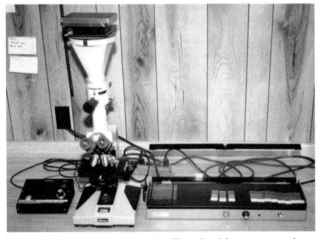

Figure 12-18 Raw semen is diluted with prewarmed extender for sperm motility assessment with a phase-contrast microscope with a warming stage. The percentage of sperm moving in a rapid, linear manner represents the percentage of progressively motile sperm in the ejaculate.

Allerød, Denmark; Figure 12-19) must be used to quantify sperm in the extended ejaculate.

Properly formulated semen extenders improve sperm survival during the interval between collection and insemination. Most commonly used equine semen extenders are milk based (Table 12-1). Some milk-based extenders are available commercially (Table 12-2). Addition of appropriate antibiotics to semen extenders aids elimination of bacteria, which invariably contaminate the semen sample during its collection. Polymyxin B sulfate (200 to 1000 U/mL), crystalline penicillin (1000 to 1500 U/mL), gentamicin sulfate (100 to 1000 μg/mL), amikacin sulfate (100 to 1000 μg/mL), ticarcillin (100 to 1000 μg/mL), and timentin (100 to 1000 μg/mL) are commonly used antibiotics. When gentamicin or amikacin is used in extenders, they must be 'reagent grade', not injectable formulations, which contain spermicidal preservatives, and sodium bicarbonate should be added to adjust the pH of the extender. An extender pH range from 6.6 to 7.2 may optimize sperm motility while avoiding premature capacitation of sperm, particularly during cool storage. Texas workers suggest that either a combination of potassium penicillin G (1000 U/mL) and amikacin sulfate (1 mg/mL) or timentin (1 mg/mL) in a milk-based semen extender may optimize longevity of sperm motility while providing good broad-spectrum antibacterial activity.

Various milk components in semen extenders are known to benefit sperm viability. Native phosphocaseinate is one such component and can be used in place of nonfat dried milk solids in equine semen extenders. Italian and Colorado workers recently found that native phosphocaseinate or casein formulated extenders were superior to an unfractionated nonfat dried milk solids extender (E-Z Mixin CST, Animal Reproduction Systems, Chino, CA) in maintaining sperm motility after cooled storage of semen for 24 and 48 hours. An additional useful characteristic of the extender is the lack of debris, in comparison with that typically present in nonfat dried skim milk solids extenders, which improves clarity for visualizing sperm motility microscopically. INRA96 extender (IMV Technologies, Maple Grove, Minn.), based on Hank's salts and native phosphocaseinate (used in

TABLE 12-1

Commonly Used Equine Semen Extenders

Name	Formula*
Kenney extender	1. Mix nonfat dry milk solids (2.4 g) and glucose (4.9 g) with 92 mL of denionized water. 2. Add crystalline penicillin G (150,000 U) and crystalline streptomycin sulfate (150,000 μg) or gentamicin sulfate (100 mg) mixed with 2 mL of 7.5% sodium bicarbonate.
Modified Kenney extender (TAMU† formula)	1. Mix nonfat dry milk solids (24 g), glucose (26.5 g), and sucrose (40 g) with 907 mL of deionized water. 2. Add potassium penicillin G (1,000,000 U) and amikacin sulfate (1 g). 3. Buffer to pH 6.8 to 6.9
Skim milk extender	1. Heat 100 mL of nonfortified skim milk to 92°C to 95°C for 10 minutes in a double boiler. Cool. 2. Add polymyxin B sulfate (100,000 U).
Cream-gel extender	1. Dissolve 1.3 g of unflavored gelatin in 10 mL of sterile deionized water. Sterilize. 2. Heat half and half cream to 92°C to 95°C for 2 to 4 minutes in a double boiler. Remove scum from surface. 3. Mix gelatin solution with 90 mL of heated half-and-half cream (100 mL total volume). Cool. 4. Add crystalline penicillin G (100,000 U), streptomycin sulfate (100,000 μg), and polymyxin B sulfate (20,000 U).
Modified cream-gel extender	1. Heat half and half cream (1 pint) to 85°C to 92°C in a glass flask in a double boiler for 10 minutes. Remove scum from surface. 2. Dissolve 6 g of unflavored gelatin in 40 mL of 5% dextrose and heat to 65°C in a water bath. 3. Add hot gelatin solution to cream and allow to cool covered to 35°C to 40°C. 4. Add potassium penicillin G (1,000,000 U) or amikacin sulfate (0.5 g).

*Many different antibiotics and antibiotic dosages have been used with these basic extenders, including potassium penicillin G (1000 to 2000 U/mL), streptomycin sulfate (1000 to 1500 μg/mL), polymyxin B sulfate (200 to 1000 U/mL), gentamicin sulfate (100 to 1000 μg/mL), amikacin sulfate (100 to 1000 μg/mL), ticarcillin (100 to 1000 μg/mL, or timentin (100-1000 μg mL). Use of reagent grade gentamicin sulfate or reagent grade amikacin sulfate may necessitate the addition of sodium bicarbonate to adjust the pH of the extender to 6.8 to 7.0. Gentamicin and amikacin must be 'reagent grade', and not the injectable formulations that contain spermicidal preservatives. The extenders can be stored in small packages at –20°C and thawed immediately before use.
†TAMU, Texas A&M University.

place of nonfat dried milk solids), was developed by French workers and is available commercially worldwide. It has become one of the most popular equine semen extenders used in the horse industry. However, the antibiotic levels in this extender do not appear adequate to fully suppress microbial growth, and our laboratory typically supplements this extender with timentin (1 mg/mL) when ejaculates are to be cooled and stored.

Processing Fresh Semen for Low-Dose Insemination

We commonly use one of two techniques for concentration of sperm in an ejaculate for preparing semen for low-dose insemination. The first method uses specially designed, 40-mL capacity, glass nipple-bottom centrifugation tubes (Pesce Lab Sales, Kennett Square, PA) (Figure 12-20). The tubes are reusable but should be washed, siliconized, and sterilized with dry heat (120°C for 2 hours) between uses. The nipple portion of the tubes is filled with 1.5 mL extended semen; then

30 μL of cushion medium (e.g., Eqcellsire Component B, IMV, Maple Grove, MN; Cusion fluid, Minitüb, Tiefenbach, Germany; or OptiPrep, Greiner Bio-One, Axis-shield, Oslo, Norway) is layered beneath the semen with a pipette. A further 35 mL of extended semen, usually containing approximately 1 billion sperm, is carefully added to the nipple tube so as not to disturb the cushion. Additional tubes can be prepared, or another tube filled with an equal amount of water, to balance the centrifuge. The nipple tubes are placed in specially designed centrifuge adapters (Thermo Scientific, Waltham, MA) and then balanced by weight and centrifuged (IEC Centra CL3, Thermo Scientific) with a swinging rotor at 400g for 20 minutes at ambient temperature. After centrifugation, the supernatatant is aspirated to the top of the nipple portion of the tube, and the sperm pellet is mixed with the 30 μL of cushion fluid. Alternately, disposable polypropylene 50-mL capacity conical-bottom centrifuge tubes (Corning Life Sciences, Lowell, MA) can be used for

Some Commercially Available Equine Semen Extenders*

Trade Name	Manufacturer	Comments
INRA 96 extender	IMV Technologies 11725 95th Ave North Maple Grove, MN 55369	Available only with gentamicin in low concentration. Should broader-spectrum antimicrobial activity be desired, timentin (100 to 1000 μg/mL) may be added immediately before mixing with semen.
E-Z Mixin	Animal Reproduction Systems 14395 Ramona Ave Chino, CA 91710	Available with or without different antibiotics.
Skim Milk Extender	Lane Manufacturing Co 2045 S Valentia St, Unit 1 Denver, CO 80231	Available with or without antibiotics.
Kenney Skim Milk Extender	Har-Vet Inc 219 S McKay Ave Box 39 Spring Valley, WI 54767	Available with or without antibiotics.
Kenney Extender	Hamilton Research Inc PO Box 2099 South Hamilton, MA 01982	Available without antibiotics.
Dr. Kenney Ready Mix Extender	Equine Breeders Services 1102 "S" Street Penrose, CO 81240	Available with or without antibiotics.
Next Generation Universal Stallion Semen Extender	Exodus Breeders Supply 5470 Mt Pisgah Rd York, PA 17406	Available with or without antibiotics.

*No endorsement of products is intended.

centrifugation. With use of these tubes, 35 mL of extended semen containing approximately 1 billion sperm is loaded into each tube, and 3.5 mL of cushion media is layered beneath the extended semen with a blunt-tipped 3.5-inch spinal needle (18-gauge), attached to a 5-mL syringe (Figure 12-21). After centrifugation at $1000g$ for 20 minutes at ambient temperature, the supernatant is removed to a preset volume mark of 5 to 7.5 mL, and then the major portion of the cushion medium is removed via aspiration with the blunt spinal needle and attached syringe, leaving the sperm pellet.

The resulting sperm pellet is mixed with a small amount of fresh semen extender, and sperm concentration is assessed. Further dilution, depending on the insemination dose (1 to 20 million sperm) and volume (0.2 to 1.0 mL) desired, is performed. Individual insemination doses can then be pipetted into small conical vials (maintained at ambient temperature in a dark environment) for later retrieval when insemination catheters are loaded immediately before insemination.

Density-gradient centrifugation is used to improve quality of semen for low-dose insemination and is commonly used in assisted reproduction for humans. Texas workers have adapted the technique for use in low-dose insemination procedures for stallions, particularly in an effort to improve fertility of some subfertile stallions. Sperm separation is based on isopycnic points (buoyancy). Some morphologically abnormal sperm are more buoyant, which causes them to be retained at the top of the centrifugation gradient; morphologically normal sperm pass to the bottom of the gradient during centrifugation. To accomplish density-gradient separation, a 15-mL polypropylene conical centrifuge tube (Corning Life Sciences) is loaded with 2 mL of EquiPure Bottom Layer (a silanated particle solution manufactured by Nidacon International AB, Mólndal, Sweden), followed by 2 mL of EquiPure top layer, and is finally overlaid with 1 mL of extended semen containing 250 to 500 million total sperm. The tube is centrifuged at room temperature at $200g$ for 30 minutes (Figure 12-22). A pipette is used to aspirate the sperm

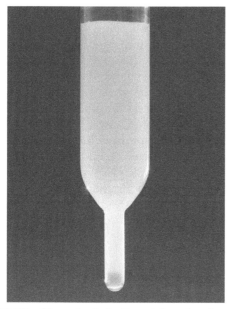

Figure 12-20 Glass nipple-bottom tube, showing a sperm pellet at bottom of tube after centrifugation in an opaque (milk-based) extender. Clear iodixanol solution (30 μL) (OptiPrep, Greiner Bio-One, Axis-shield) is directly underneath the sperm pellet.

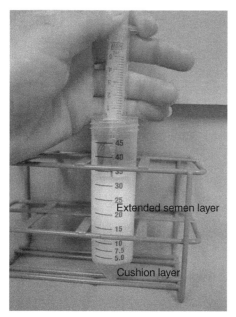

Extended semen layer

Cushion layer

Figure 12-21 Cushion medium (3.5 mL) is pipetted into a disposable conical centrifugation tube beneath 35 mL of extended semen, in preparation for centrifugation to concentrate sperm.

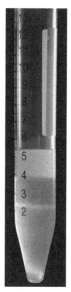

Figure 12-22 Plastic 15-mL conical polypropylene centrifuge tube after density gradient separation of equine sperm. The centrifuge tube was loaded with 2 mL of EquiPure bottom layer, followed by 2 mL of EquiPure top layer, and finally 1 mL of extended semen containing approximately 500 million sperm. The sperm at the bottom of the tube (sperm pellet) contains the population most free of morphologic defects, whereas the thin white line at the interface of the bottom and top layers of EquiPure contains sperm more likely to possess morphologic defects. The thick white line overlying the clear EquiPure layers contains extender and somatic cells, premature germ cells, and sperm with pronounced morphologic defects that resulted in markedly increased buoyancy.

ARTIFICIAL INSEMINATION

Insemination Timing and Breeding Frequency

In many AI programs, mares are inseminated every other day, beginning on the second or third day of estrus, until ovulation is detected or until the mare no longer exhibits signs of behavioral estrus. When semen from fertile stallions is used, acceptable pregnancy rates can sometimes be obtained when mares are inseminated within 72 hours before ovulation. Rarely do daily or twice-daily inseminations result in improved pregnancy rates, except for occasional stallions with reduced sperm longevity in ejaculated semen. Limiting the number of inseminations per estrous period improves the overall efficiency of the breeding program and reduces the risk of iatrogenic contamination of the mare's reproductive tract. Reduction of uterine contamination is especially important when mares with an increased susceptibility to uterine infections are bred. Ideally, regular genital tract examinations should be performed to more accurately predict time of expected ovulation so that the number of inseminations necessary is minimized. The goal should be to inseminate each mare once within 48 hours before ovulation. If a mare ovulates within

pellet. The sperm pellet is washed once by mixing it with 3 mL of fresh extender and centrifuging again at 400g for 15 minutes, after which the supernate is removed. The final sperm pellet is resuspended to the concentration and volume desired for low-dose insemination.

48 hours of breeding, further inseminations are not needed (Figure 12-23). However, if a mare has not ovulated after being bred 48 hours previously, the mare should be inseminated again.

Although good fertility has been reported when mares were bred after ovulation, a breeding strategy of postovulation breeding with fresh semen is not generally recommended. Wisconsin workers reported that mares bred 0 to 6 hours after ovulation had normal pregnancy rates (similar to mares bred 1 to 3 days before ovulation) and did not experience increased embryonic death rates. However, although mares bred 6 to 12 hours after ovulation had normal pregnancy rates, they experienced an increase in embryonic losses. Mares bred 12 to 24 hours after ovulation had both lower pregnancy rates and higher embryonic losses than those in mares bred before ovulation or within 6 hours after ovulation. Presumably, aging gametes can adversely affect developmental competence of the embryo.

Numerous studies have since been performed to compare pregnancy rates achieved with multiple versus single inseminations and preovulation versus postovulation inseminations, with both cooled and frozen semen. It is now widely accepted that single inseminations within a few hours (≤4 to 6 hours) after ovulation can result in acceptable pregnancy rates, so a single postovulation breeding strategy can be used successfully when semen must be conserved. If semen conservation is not needed, the extra effort and expense for frequent examinations necessary to ensure breeding occurs shortly after ovulation are not justified.

Insemination Dose (Number of Sperm)

Typically, mares in an AI program are inseminated with 250 to 500 million progressively motile sperm. Insemination of mares with 500 million progressively motile sperm helps ensure that acceptable pregnancy rates are achieved by allowing some margin for error in semen evaluation and handling when conditions are less than optimal. If semen is carefully handled and from a highly fertile stallion, the insemination dose can sometimes be reduced to 100 million progressively motile sperm without reducing fertility. Reducing insemination doses to less than 100 million progressively motile sperm is not recommended. For example, Texas workers recently achieved reduced pregnancy rates per cycle (30%) when using only 20 to 60 million progressively motile sperm in an insemination volume of 4 mL. Another study revealed that mares inseminated with 50 million motile sperm had a lower overall pregnancy rate (38%) than that achieved in mares inseminated with 500 million motile sperm (75%).

An exception to the use of 100 million or more progressively motile sperm in insemination doses is the recent finding that very low doses can be used when the sperm are placed near or on the oviductal papillae. This practice is referred to as low-dose insemination and is discussed subsequently.

Insemination Volume

The number of sperm in an insemination dose appears to be more critical than the volume of the inseminate that is infused into the uterine body. Although smaller or larger volumes can be used successfully, typical insemination volumes for fresh extended equine semen range from 10 to 30 mL. When timed closely with ovulation, insemination of frozen/thawed semen in volumes as low as 0.5 mL has resulted in pregnancies. Large insemination volumes are not advantageous because much of this volume may be lost through the mare's dilated cervix after insemination.

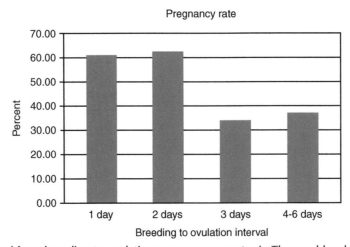

Figure 12-23 Effect of interval from breeding to ovulation on pregnancy rates in Thoroughbred mares bred via natural service on 902 estrus cycles. Pregnancy rates/cycle were 61.9% (206/333), 63.8% (326/511), 34.0% (16/47), and 36.4% (4/11) when breeding to ovulation interval was 1, 2, 3, and 4 or more days, respectively. Most mares were bred only once per estrus. Improved pregnancy rates that occurred with more than one breeding per estrus period resulted from shortening the interval from last breeding to ovulation.

Often, only a small number of mares are to be inseminated with an ejaculate, so it is commonly diluted with extender, with the total volume being equally divided among the mares to be bred. When a large number of mares are to be inseminated with a single ejaculate, insemination volume (IV) can be calculated by dividing the desired number of progressively motile sperm per insemination (PMS dose; e.g., 100 to 500 million) by the product of the sperm concentration in the extended semen (SC) and the percentage of progressively motile sperm in the ejaculate (%PM, expressed as a decimal):

$$IV \text{ (mL)} = PMS \text{ dose}/(SC \times \%PM)$$

Insemination Procedure

Sterile, nontoxic disposable equipment is recommended for AI procedures (Figure 12-24). Syringes with nonspermicidal, plastic plungers (Air-Tite, Vineland, N.J.) are preferable for AI because some rubber plungers may possess spermicidal properties. Individual stallion variation seems to exist regarding sperm sensitivity to the toxic effects of syringes with rubber plunger tips. Toxic effects are apparent in semen from some stallions with as little as 1 minute of contact with some syringe plungers. Washing and sterilization of syringes does not appear to affect sperm motility; therefore, properly prepared syringes may be reused as a cost-saving and ecologically sound approach to horse breeding.

Insemination of the mare should be performed in accordance with the minimum contamination techniques described by Kenney and coworkers (1975). The mare should be adequately restrained with her tail wrapped and diverted either to the side or over her rump. The perineal area is thoroughly scrubbed and rinsed, with particular attention paid to the vulva.

Any dirt or fecal material within the caudal vestibule should be removed during the washing process to prevent contamination of the proximal reproductive tract during insemination. Two to three scrubs with soap or a surgical scrub are recommended, followed by thorough rinsing to eliminate residual soap that may be spermicidal or irritating to mucous membranes.

For insemination of a mare, a sterile shoulder-length plastic sleeve is first placed over the arm used for insemination. The tip of a 20- to 22-inch insemination pipette is then positioned in the cupped hand, and a small amount of sterile, nonspermicidal lubricant is applied to the back of the hand. The covered hand and insemination pipette are passed into the cranial vaginal vault where the index finger identifies and penetrates the cervix. The insemination pipette is then advanced through the cervix to the midbody of the uterus. A syringe containing extended semen is attached to the insemination pipette, and the semen is slowly deposited into the uterine lumen (Figure 12-25). An alternative, but equally satisfactory, method of insemination is to pass the insemination pipette through the cervix with a lighted speculum preplaced in the vagina (Figures 12-26 and 12-27).

Low Dose Insemination

The perceived advantages of low-dose insemination are primarily to allow popular stallions to inseminate more mares with an ejaculate and to improve reproductive performance of some stallions that achieve suboptimal fertility with standard artificial insemination procedures. Although not critically tested to date, these two attributes of low-dose insemination are worthy of consideration. Recent studies have revealed that, with low-dose insemination, mares can be bred with a sperm number more than 100 times less than that of a traditional insemination dose (i.e., 1 to 5 million sperm as opposed to 500 million sperm), with good pregnancy

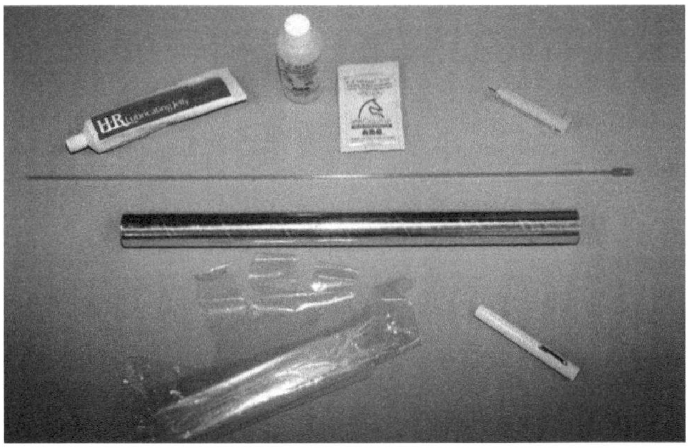

Figure 12-24 Equipment commonly used for artificial insemination of horses with fresh semen. *Clockwise from upper left:* sterile, nonspermicidal lubricant; semen extender; sterile nontoxic syringe; insemination pipette; disposable vaginal speculum; pen light for illuminating cervix through speculum; and plastic sleeve.

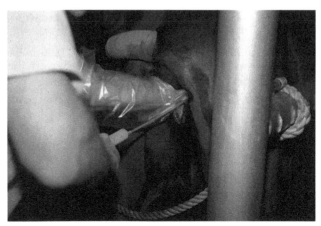

Figure 12-25 For performing artificial insemination, a pipette is carried in a lubricated, gloved hand into the cranial vagina and guided through the cervix into the uterine body where the extended semen is slowly deposited.

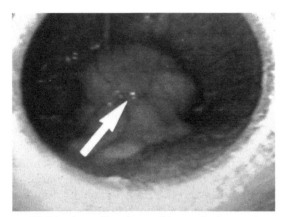

Figure 12-26 A sterile, disposable vaginal speculum and light can be used for artificial insemination of horses. The external os of the cervix is positioned at the end of the speculum as shown in this photograph.

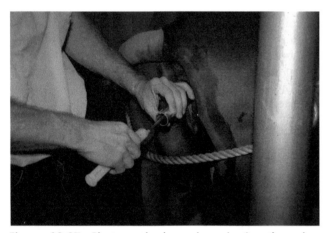

Figure 12-27 Photograph shows insemination through a vaginal speculum. The pipette has been passed through the cervix (shown in Figure 12-24) and the syringe is attached for insemination.

rates resulting. Improving the fertility of some stallions may also be possible by first concentrating the semen, or by removing a high percentage of the morphologically abnormal sperm, before low-dose insemination. The procedure does result in added expense for equipment and personnel, and those involved with providing this service require extra training on the procedural details.

With low-dose insemination techniques, the sperm number is typically reduced to 1 to 20 million sperm, with a corresponding reduction in inseminate volume, and semen is placed in the tip of the uterine horn, on or near the oviductal papilla which represents the opening from the uterus into the oviduct (or fallopian tube; fertilization occurs within the oviduct). Two techniques have been used to deliver the semen to this location. The hysteroscopic technique uses a videoendoscope that permits visualization of semen placement (Figure 12-28). The endoscope is passed transcervically into the uterine horn ipsilateral to the preovulatory follicle, which is then

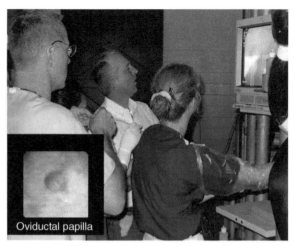

Oviductal papilla

Figure 12-28 Hysteroscopic insemination of a low dose of semen (typically 1 to 20 million sperm in 0.2 mL of extender). The *insert* shows the oviductal papilla, onto which the semen is deposited.

insufflated with air to distend the lumen. The tip of the endoscope is moved to the end of the uterine horn where the oviductal papilla is visualized. A catheter containing 0.1 to 0.2 mL of semen is passed through the biopsy channel of the endoscope, and the semen is expressed so that it pools onto and around the oviductal papilla. As the endoscope is withdrawn, air is carefully aspirated from the uterus. Another technique uses transrectally guided direction of a flexible insemination catheter to the tip of the uterine horn.

To perform deep horn insemination with a flexible, two-channel insemination pipette (Figure 12-29), the flexible end of the inner channel is attached to a 3-mL syringe (containing 2 mL of air), and the tip of the catheter is loaded with 0.2 to 1.0 mL of semen. The semen-loaded inner channel is inserted into the outer catheter until the tip locks in place (ensuring against leakage).

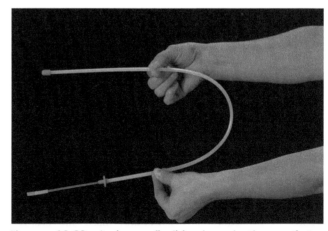

Figure 12-29 A long, flexible insemination catheter, with an interlocking inner tubing channel (available from Minitube of America, Verona, WI) that is used for transrectally guided, deep-horn insemination of small volumes (0.2 to 1.0 mL) of semen.

The instrument is passed transcervically into the base of the desired uterine horn (ipsilateral to the dominant follicle), and a hand is placed in the rectum to manipulate the tip of the catheter to the end of the uterine horn where the oviductal papilla is located. The hand in the rectum is then used to encircle and gently lift the middle portion of the uterine horn. The semen is slowly expelled, and the syringe is detached and refilled with air. The air-filled syringe is reattached to flush the catheter with air. The catheter is removed from the genital tract and checked to ensure semen was expelled. The midportion of the horn is held elevated for 1 to 2 minutes to help ensure that the semen remains at the tip of the uterine horn.

General Considerations

Semen from the stallion is normally delivered directly to the protective confines of the mare's reproductive tract at the time of breeding; therefore, if one plans to collect semen for in vitro storage and transport, it is necessary to first become fully aware of the vulnerability of sperm to the external environment. Sperm are very sensitive to many environmental factors, including temperature, light, physical trauma, and a variety of chemicals.

SUMMARY

Artificial insemination is an effective technique for improving the use of stallions in breeding programs. When proper semen handling and insemination procedures are used, optimal pregnancy rates are attainable. When AI techniques are used for mares and stallions with marginal fertility, pregnancy rates are sometimes improved over those achieved with natural mating.

BIBLIOGRAPHY

Batellier F, Vadament M, Fauquent J, et al: Advances in cooled semen technology, *Animal Reprod Sci* 68:181-190, 2001.

Brinsko SP: Insemination doses: how low can we go? *Theriogenology* 66:543-550, 2006.

Brinsko SP, Rigby SL, Lindsey AC, et al: Pregnancy rates in mares following hysteroscopic or transrectally-guided insemination with low sperm numbers at the utero-tubal papilla, *Theriogenology* 59:1001-1009, 2003.

Brinsko SP, Varner DD: Artificial insemination and preservation of semen, *Vet Clin North Am Equine Pract* 8:205-218, 1992.

Forney BD: How to collect semen from stallions while they are standing on the ground, *Proc Am Assoc Equine Pract* 45:142-144, 1999.

Kenney RM, Bergman RV, Cooper WL, et al: Minimum contamination techniques for breeding mares: techniques and preliminary findings, *Proc Am Assoc Equine Pract* 21:327-336, 1975.

Macpherson Macpherson ML, Blanchard TL, et al: Use of a silane-coated silica particle solution to enhance semen quality of stallions, *Proc 49th Ann Mtg Am Assoc Equine Pract* 347-349, 2003.

McDonnell SM, Love CC: Manual stimulation collection of semen from stallions: training time, sexual behavior and semen, *Theriogenology* 33:1201-1210, 1990.

Varner DD, Schumacher J, Blanchard TL et al: *Diseases and management of breeding stallions,* Goleta, CA, 1991, American Veterinary Publications.

Varner DD, Blanchard TL, Brinsko SP, et al: Low-dose insemination: table topic: reproduction: low dose inseminations: rationale and success, *AAEP Guardian* March:2-3, 2002.

Varner DD, Love CC, Brinsko SP, et al: Semen processing for the subfertile stallion, *J Equine Vet Sci* 28:1-9, 2008.

Woods J, Bergfelt DR, Ginther OJ: Effects of time of insemination relative to ovulation on pregnancy rate and embryonic-loss rate in mares, *Equine Vet J* 22:410-415, 1990.

Examination of the Stallion for Breeding Soundness

CHAPTER

OBJECTIVES

While studying the information covered in this chapter, the reader should attempt to:
- Acquire a working understanding of the anatomy and physiology of the reproductive organs of the stallion.
- Acquire a working understanding of how abnormalities of the reproductive organs, conditions associated with suboptimal general physical soundness, or disordered sexual behavior can adversely affect stallion fertility.
- Acquire a working understanding of procedures used for evaluation of a stallion for breeding soundness.

STUDY QUESTIONS

1. Describe the objective of a breeding soundness examination of a stallion.
2. List procedures that should be performed during a breeding soundness examination of a stallion.
3. Describe the anatomy of the normal reproductive tract of a stallion, including the prepuce, penis, scrotum and its contents, vas deferens, and accessory sex glands.
4. List potential venereal pathogens that may be transmitted by stallions.

5. Describe procedures used for evaluation of semen quality of stallions, including but not limited to:
   a. Gross evaluation of semen
   b. Sperm concentration
   c. Semen volume
   d. Number of sperm in ejaculate
   e. Semen pH
   f. Sperm motility
   g. Sperm morphology
6. Summarize minimal criteria for classification of a stallion as a satisfactory breeding prospect.

OBJECTIVE

The objective of a breeding soundness examination is to determine whether a stallion has the mental and physical faculties necessary to deliver semen that contains viable sperm but no infectious disease to the mare's reproductive tract at the proper time, ensuring the establishment of pregnancy in a reasonable number of mares bred per season. The examiner not only evaluates the quality and quantity of ejaculated sperm but also tests the libido and mating ability of a stallion, attempts to recognize congenital defects that may be transmissible to offspring or decrease a stallion's fertility, identifies infectious diseases that may be transmitted venereally, and searches for any other lesions that may reduce a stallion's longevity as a sire.

A record that summarizes results of the breeding soundness examination should be provided to the owner of the stallion after completion of the examination. An example of a form used for this purpose is shown in Figure 13-1.

Stallion Information:
Name: _____ Case #: _____
Age: _____ Breed: _____ Color: _____
Lip Tattoo #: _____ Registration #: _____
Markings / Brands: _____
_____
_____

Present Breeding Status:
□ Sexually rested   □ Actively breeding
□ At daily sperm output (DSO)
Intended Use: _____
_____
_____
_____

Owner / Agent: _____
Address: _____
_____
_____
_____
Telephone: _____
Fax: _____
Referring Veterinarian: _____
Address: _____
_____
_____
_____
Telephone: _____
Fax: _____

History: _____
_____
_____
_____

Physical Breeding Condition: _____
_____
_____
_____

External Genital Examination: Method(s) Used: □ Palpation   □ Ultrasound   □ Calipers   □ Other _____

● Testis: <u>Left</u>   <u>Right</u>
   $L \times W \times H$ (cm): _____ _____
   Volume (cm^3): _____ _____
   Consistency: _____ _____
● Epididymis: _____ _____
● Spermatic Cord: _____ _____
● Other Findings: _____ _____
_____

● Prepuce/Penis: _____
● Scrotum: _____
● Total Testicular Volume (cc): _____
● Actual sperm # ejaculated at DSO ($\times 10^9$): _____
● Estimated sperm # ejaculated at DSO ($\times 10^9$) (method): _____
● Predicted DSO based on testicular volume ($\times 10^9$): _____
● Spermatogenic efficiency (%): _____
● Sperm output/gram testis/day at DSO ($\times 10^6$): _____

Internal Genital Examination: □ Performed   □ Not performed
Methods(s) Used: □ Palpation   □ Ultrasound   □ Other _____

	<u>Left</u>	<u>Right</u>		<u>Left</u>	<u>Right</u>
● Inguinal Ring (size):	_____	_____	● Ampulla :	_____	_____
● Vesicular Gland:	_____	_____	● Prostatic Lobe:	_____	_____

Behavior and Breeding Ability:

<u>Temperament</u>	<u>Libido</u>	<u>Erection</u>	<u>Mounting</u>	<u>Intromission</u>	<u>Ejaculation</u>

Culture and Sensitivity:
□ Pre-Wash Penile Shaft: _____
□ Pre-Wash Fossa Glandis: _____
□ Post-Wash Urethra: _____
□ Post-Ejaculate Urethra: _____
□ Semen: _____
□ Other (_____): _____

Other Examination Findings: _____
_____

Additional Diagnostic Tests:

<u>Test</u>	<u>Date Performed</u>	<u>Result</u>
_____	_____	_____
_____	_____	_____
_____	_____	_____

Figure 13-1 Example of a stallion breeding soundness evaluation form.

Continued

Semen Evaluation	Ejaculate 1	Ejaculate 2	Ejaculate 3
Collection Time / Collection Method:			
Number of Mounts / Time to First Mount (minutes):			
Volume (mL) — gel-free / gel:			
Gross Appearance:			
Seminal pH (method) / Seminal Osmolarity(method):			
Initial Motility (% total / % progressive[velocity]) ☐ Raw (Vel. = 0-4 or µm/sec) Method used: _____ ☐ Extended			
Concentration ($\times 10^6$/mL) - Method used: _____			
Total Number of Sperm ($\times 10^9$):			
Total Number of Sperm $\times$ % Progressively Motile ($\times 10^9$):			
Sperm Morphology: ☐ Buffered Formol Saline ☐ Phase Contrast Microscopy ☐ Brightfield Microscopy ☐ Differential Interference Microscopy ☐ Stain: _____ ☐ Other: _____			
% Normal			
% Abnormal Heads			
% Abnormal Acrosomes			
% Tailless Heads			
% Proximal Droplets			
% Distal Droplets			
% Abnormally Shaped Midpieces			
% Bent Midpieces			
% Bent Tails			
% Coiled Tails			
% Premature (Round) (Germ Cells)			
% Other Abnormalities: _____			
Total Number Sperm $\times$ % Morphologically Normal ($\times 10^9$)			
Longevity (Viability) Test: Reported as Storage Time (Hours) / Motility (Total/Progressive[Velocity])			
Raw at ___ °C:			
_____ Extender at ___ °C: (dilution = _____)			
_____ Extender at ___ °C: (dilution = _____)			

Comments:_____

_____

Classification as Breeding Prospect: ☐ **Satisfactory**   ☐ **Questionable**   ☐ **Unsatisfactory**

☐ See attached letter   Signature: _____

Figure 13-1, cont'd.

HISTORY AND IDENTIFICATION

Collection of historical information about a stallion is an indispensable part of a breeding soundness examination. This information should be gathered in a methodical unassuming manner to ensure completeness and avoid inaccuracies. Possible environmental and heritable causes for the presenting problem should be addressed, and previous modes of therapy for an existing problem should be investigated when applicable. A historical review of stallions to be examined for breeding soundness should include their present usage, previous breeding performance, results of prior fertility evaluations, illnesses, injuries, and medications and vaccinations, with explicit information about previous and current reproductive management and medical programs.

Positive identification of the stallion, often considered a mundane procedure, is an integral part of the examination process, especially when sale of the horse is involved. Identification of a stallion must be accurate to avoid any ambiguity in identity at a subsequent date. Name, age, breed, and registration number of the stallion are recorded, in addition to identifying marks, such as lip tattoos, hide brands, color markings, and hair whorls. When possible, photographs of the stallion should be taken for permanent identification.

GENERAL PHYSICAL EXAMINATION

Although a breeding soundness examination focuses on the genital health of stallions, general physical condition cannot be ignored. An assessment of general body condition is done first. Particular attention should be given to abnormalities that affect mating ability (e.g., lameness, back pain, ataxia) or that are potentially heritable (e.g., cryptorchidism, parrot mouth, wobbler syndrome). All abnormalities are recorded. Examination of the various body systems (respiratory, cardiovascular, digestive, nervous, urinary, ophthalmic, and musculoskeletal) can be cursory, although abnormalities should be noted and pursued further diagnostically if the potential exists for interference with breeding ability or fertility. Common laboratory tests (Coggins test, hematologic analysis, serum chemistry, urinalysis, and fecal egg counts) can support physical examination findings in determination of the general health of a stallion.

PHYSICAL EXAMINATION OF REPRODUCTIVE TRACT

Knowledge of normal genital anatomy is essential to a competent physical examination of the stallion's reproductive tract. A thorough physical examination of both external and internal genital organs always should be incorporated into procedures for prediction of stallion fertility.

External Genitalia

The preferred method to allow close inspection of the penis (Figures 13-2 and 13-3) is to stimulate penile tumescence through exposure of the stallion to a mare in estrus. This procedure also permits assessment of sexual behavior, including erection capability. Manual extraction of the penis from the prepuce for examination is difficult and usually met with resistance from the stallion. In shy stallions, the penis can often be visualized from a distance while the horse urinates. Urination can sometimes be stimulated by placing the horse in a freshly bedded stall; shaking the bedding may increase the horse's urge to urinate. Tranquilization (acepromazine or xylazine) elicits penile prolapse, making the penis accessible; however, tranquilizers, especially those that are phenothiazine-derived (e.g., acepromazine), can cause penile paralysis or priapism and therefore should not be used indiscriminately. In addition, tranquilizers will probably render the horse ataxic which may interfere with mounting when collection of semen is attempted.

The penis may need cleansing before its inspection (Figure 13-4) because epithelial debris mixed with

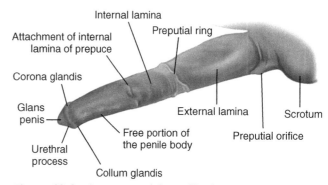

Figure 13-2 Structures of the stallion's penis and prepuce.

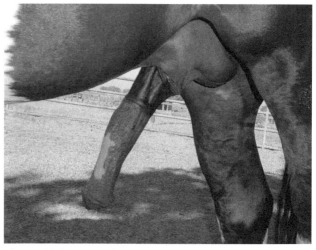

Figure 13-3 Normal external genitalia of a mature stallion.

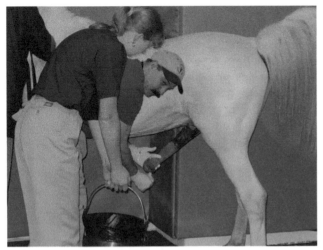

Figure 13-4 Cleansing the shaft of the penis of a stallion. Generally, only warm tap water and clean paper towels are needed to wash a stallion's penis. Soaps or disinfectants are not usually used, to avoid displacement of normal flora.

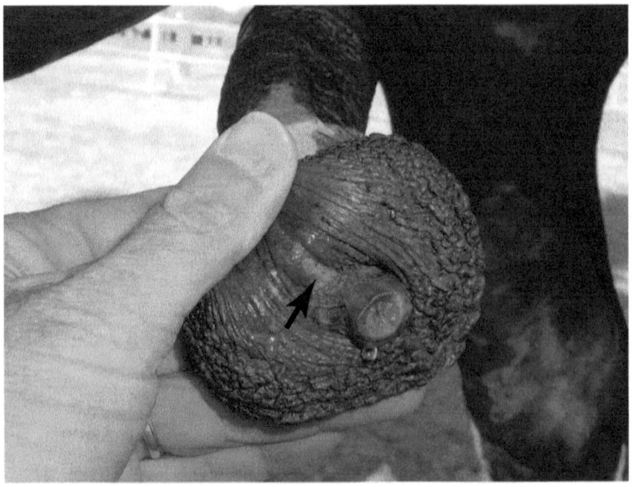

secretions from the preputial glands accumulates in the preputial cavity and on the exterior of the penis when it is unattended. The root and proximal body of the penis are buried in tissue, thereby limiting the examination to the exposed body and glans. The penis should be examined thoroughly, and any palpable or visual lesions should be recorded. Particular attention should be given to the fossa glandis and urethral process because they are partially concealed and smegma accumulates in these areas (Figures 13-5 to 13-7). Common penile lesions include those of traumatic origin and vesicles or pustules of equine coital exanthema, *Habronema* granulomas, squamous cell carcinomas, and papillomas (see Chapter 16).

During penile tumescence, the prepuce also is readily available for examination. If the stallion is excitable, it is often helpful to stand beside the horse with one hand on its withers while beginning to palpate the external genitalia with the other hand (Figure 13-8). The skin of the prepuce should be thin and pliable, with no evidence of inflammatory or proliferative lesions. Developmental abnormalities of the penis and prepuce are rare.

The scrotal skin should be thin and elastic, and the scrotum should have a distinct neck. The scrotum and its contents are normally pendulous (except during cold weather because of contractions of the tunica dartos) but may be drawn toward the body during palpation because of voluntary contractions of the cremaster muscles. Both testes and attached epididymides should be relatively symmetrical and freely movable within their respective scrotal pouches. Size, texture, and position of each testis always should be determined as part of a breeding soundness examination. Testicular size

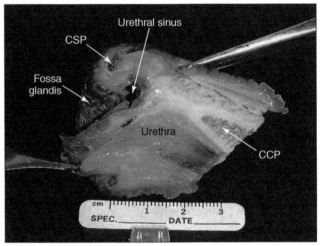

Figure 13-6 Dorsal aspect of the glans penis is reflected to show the urethral process, which is surrounded by the fossa glandis. The opening into the urethral sinuses (which may contain smegma in the form of "beans") is indicated *(arrow)*.

Figure 13-7 Longitudinal cross section of distal penis (glans) shows anatomic configuration of urethra, corpus cavernosum penis *(CCP)*, corpus spongiousum penis *(CSP)*, fossa glandis, and urethral sinus. (Courtesy Dr. Donald Schlafer.)

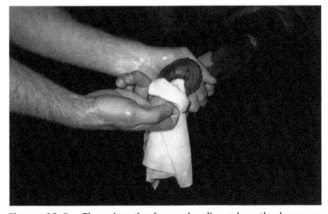

Figure 13-5 Cleansing the fossa glandis and urethral process of a stallion's penis.

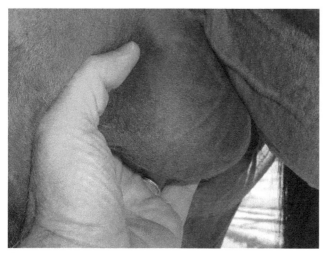

Figure 13-8 Palpation of the external genitalia of a stallion for identification of abnormalities.

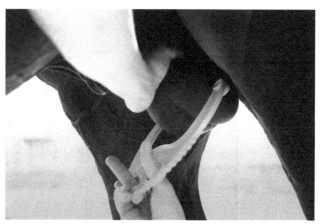

Figure 13-9 Measurement of scrotal width with use of calipers. The testes are gently held in the bottom of the scrotum while the widest measurement across both testes is taken.

correlates highly with daily sperm production and output, so this measurement helps predict a stallion's breeding potential. Testes of mature (≥4 years of age), fertile stallions generally are approximately 4.5 to 6 cm in width, 5 to 6.5 cm in height, and 8.5 to 11 cm in length; the total scrotal width (largest measurement taken across both testes and the scrotal skin) (Figure 13-9) generally approximates 9.5 to 11.5 cm (Table 13-1). Transcrotal ultrasonographic examination, including accurate measurement of size, can provide useful information about the normality of the scrotal contents (Figures 13-10 and 13-11). When length, width, and height of each testis are measured in centimeters (Figures 13-12 to 13-14), testicular volume (in cc) can be estimated with the formula for an ellipsoid (volume = 0.5233 × width × height × length). Volume should be computed for each testis, and the two volumes are added together to provide total testicular volume. Testicular volumes can be compared with averages established for horses of a similar age to give

the examiner an impression of whether the testes are small or not (Figure 13-15). The total testicular volume (TV) in cc can also be used to predict the range of expected daily sperm output (DSO) with the following formula:

$$\text{DSO (billions of sperm/day)} = (0.024 \times \text{TV}) - (0.76 \text{ to } 1.26)$$

When predicted DSO is significantly less than actual DSO, low spermatogenic efficiency from testicular dysfunction should be suspected. Low spermatogenic efficiency is associated with increased degeneration of testicular germ cells, which can contribute to ejaculation of low numbers of normal sperm.

In addition to its use in obtaining accurate testicular measurements, ultrasonography can be used to detect intratesticular masses and intrascrotal fluid accumulations and to examine the cavernous spaces of the penis (see Chapter 16). Ultrasonography is also a useful adjunct to examination per rectum (e.g., for evaluation

TABLE 13-1

Total Scrotal and Individual Testicular Widths (±Standard Deviation), Measured With Calipers, for 43 Horses Aged 2 to 16 Years

Age	TSW	LTW	RTW
2 to 3 yr	9.6 ± 0.8 cm	5.5 ± 0.5 cm	5.3 ± 0.5 cm
4 to 6 yr	10.0 ± 0.7 cm	5.7 ± 0.4 cm	5.5 ± 0.5 cm
≥7 yr	10.9 ± 0.7 cm	6.1 ± 0.4 cm	6.0 ± 0.5 cm

TSW, Total scrotal width; *LTW,* left testis width; *RTW,* right testis width.
From Thompson DL Jr, Pickett BW, Squires EL, et al: Testicular measurements and reproductive characteristics in stallions, *J Reprod Fert* 27(Suppl):13-17, 1979.

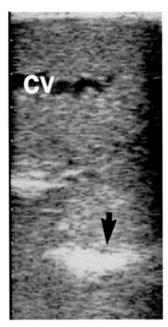

Figure 13-10 Transcrotal ultrasonographic image of stallion testes. The anechoic area in the near testis is the central vein *(CV)*. The *arrow* points to a hyperechoic area of the far testis. At castration, the testes were degenerated and the hyperechoic area was found to be fibrous tissue with some calcification.

of the accessory genital glands or abdominal/inguinal exploration for an undescended testis in a stallion suspected of being cryptorchid).

Both testes should be oval, with a smooth regular outline and a slightly turgid, resilient texture. The orientation of each testis within the scrotum can be determined accurately via palpation of the attached epididymis. The epididymis normally is palpable in its entirety as it courses over the dorsolateral surface of the testis; however, identification of its borders is sometimes difficult (Figure 13-16). The caudal ligament of the epididymis, a remnant of the gubernaculum, remains palpable during adult life as a small (~1 cm) fibrous nodule adjacent to the epididymal tail, which, itself, is attached to the caudal pole of the testis. This remnant serves as a landmark for determination of testicular orientation within the scrotum.

Exploration of the spermatic cord is possible via palpation through the neck of the scrotum, although its specific contents often are not definable. Transcrotal ultrasound examination can also be used to visualize these structures. Spermatic cords should be of equal size and uniform diameter (2 to 3 cm). Acute pain in this area usually is associated with inguinal herniation or torsion of the spermatic cord (see Figures 16-21 and 16-23). Inguinal herniation can usually be confirmed with ultrasonography, which reveals some degree of hydrocele (anechoic fluid accumulation between parietal and vaginal tunics) with hyperechoic gut wall patterns, in which fluid within the bowel lumen is some-

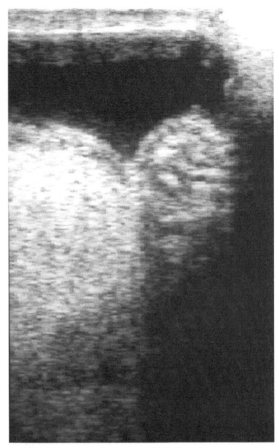

Figure 13-11 Lateral to medial longitudinal ultrasonographic image of the caudal half of the testis. The tail (cauda) of the epididymis is located at the right of the testis. The epididymis and testis are surrounded by fluid (hydrocele).

times visible (see Figure 16-20). Transrectal palpation or ultrasonography of internal inguinal rings confirms the herniation. Torsion of the spermatic cord can result in congestion of the affected testis (palpably turgid and slightly hyperechoic) with thickening and engorgement of the spermatic cord from vascular obstruction (see Chapter 16).

Internal Genitalia

The internal genital organs (Figure 13-17) can be examined via palpation per rectum. Although adequate restraint is of paramount importance to this procedure, minimal but effective restraint is the key to a safe examination and varies from stallion to stallion. The disposition of the stallion should be determined at the onset, and the examination should be canceled if the risk factor is high. Such precautions protect both the stallion and the operator from severe injury. Before the examination, the stallion should be placed in a stock, if available. Ideally, the stock should be equipped with a solid rear door to help prevent leg extension if the stallion decides to kick. The height of the door

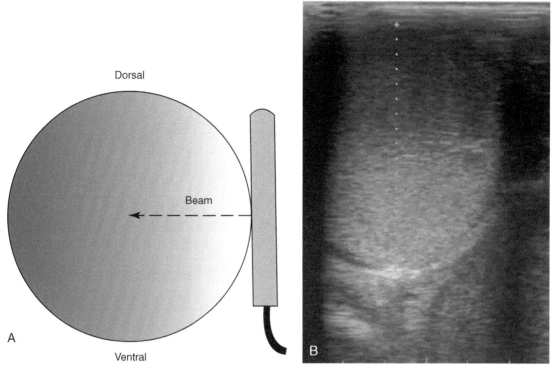

Figure 13-12 Ultrasonographic measurement of testicular width. The center of the testis was located with the probe, and the lateral-to-medial distance across the testicular parenchyma was measured (5.33 cm).

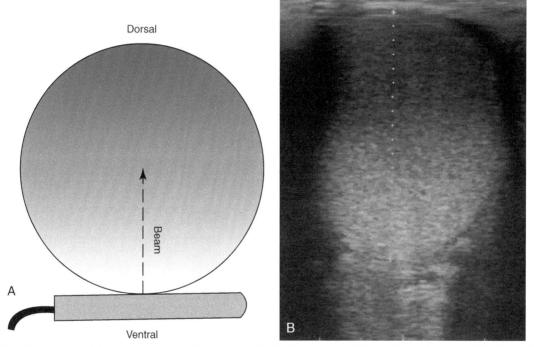

Figure 13-13 Ultrasonographic measurement of testicular height. The center of the testis was located with the probe, and the ventral-to-dorsal distance across the testicular parenchyma was measured (5.67 cm). A portion of the body of the epididymis is often visible on the bottom of the ultrasound screen (corresponding to the top of the testis) with this measurement.

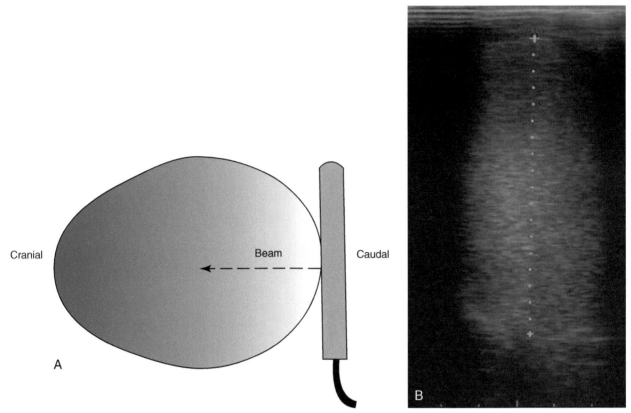

Figure 13-14 Ultrasonographic measurement of testicular length. The probe was placed in the back of the testis, just beside the tail of the epididymis, and the caudal-to-cranial distance across the testicular parenchyma was measured (8.8 cm).

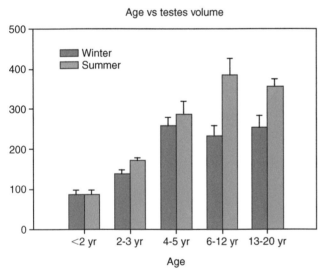

Figure 13-15 Mean testicular volume (in cc) for horses of differing age groups obtained at an abattoir during winter or summer. Weights of individual testes were doubled (to represent two testes) and converted to volume. (Modified from Johnson L, Thompson DL Jr: *Biol Reprod* 29:777-789, 1983.)

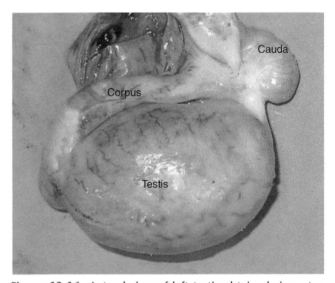

Figure 13-16 Lateral view of left testis obtained via castration. The corpus (body) and cauda (tail) of the epididymis should be readily palpable through the scrotum, confirming normal orientation within the tunics. A portion of the remnant of the gubernaculum is often palpable between the caudal pole of the testis and the tail of the epididymis.

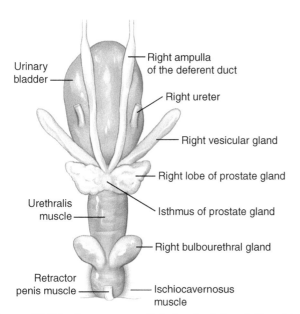

Figure 13-17 Accessory genital glands of the stallion (dorsal view). (Modified from Varner DD, Schumacher J, Blanchard TL, et al: *Diseases and management of breeding stallions,* St Louis, 1991, Mosby.)

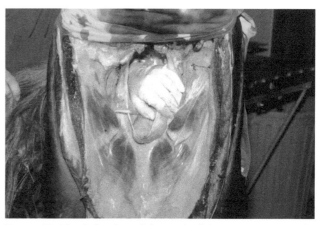

Figure 13-18 Palpation of the vaginal rings per rectum. The rectum has been removed to facilitate visualization.

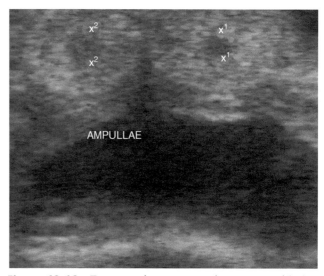

Figure 13-19 Transrectal transverse ultrasonographic image of the ampullae of a stallion. In some stallions, the lumen is visible as an anechoic central area within the ampulla.

should be level with the mid-gaskin region of the stallion's hindquarters.

Higher doors can damage the operator's arm if a stallion squats abruptly while the operator's arm is in the rectum. Lower doors permit the stallion to kick over this barrier. Poorly designed doors do not protect the examiner and increase the likelihood of injury to the stallion. If necessary, a twitch also can be placed on the stallion's muzzle for additional restraint. Sedation or tranquilization may be necessary to adequately restrain an anxious stallion. Remember, overrestraint can be as dangerous to the stallion and the operator as underrestraint.

The hand should be well lubricated, and all manure in the rectum and distal colon should be removed before evaluation of pelvic and abdominal structures is attempted. The two vaginal rings (abdominal orifices of the inguinal canals) are palpable as slit-like openings approximately a hand's breadth ventrolateral to the pelvic brim (Figure 13-18). The deferent duct and pulse of the testicular artery usually can be detected at the opening. The site is evaluated for size and for evidence of adhesions or herniation of viscera. The diameter of the opening is normally 2 to 3 cm. A larger opening may predispose the stallion to inguinal herniation or scrotal hydrocele. Some of the accessory genital organs (i.e., the ampullae and bilobed prostate gland) are also readily detected via palpation per rectum and transrectal ultrasonography (Figures 13-19 to 13-21). Lesions of the accessory genital glands, however, are uncommon in stallions.

OBSERVATION OF LIBIDO AND MATING ABILITY

Excellent semen quality in a breeding prospect is inconsequential unless that stallion also has the desire and ability to deliver the semen to the mare's reproductive tract or an artificial vagina. Sexual behavior can be evaluated by bringing the stallion in contact with a mare displaying behavioral estrus. Typically, a stallion with good libido shows immediate and intense desire for the mare, manifested by restlessness, pawing, vocalization, and intimate precopulatory activity, such as sniffing, licking, and nipping the mare; exhibition of the flehmen reaction (curling of the upper lip, primarily a response to sniffing of the mare's genitalia or

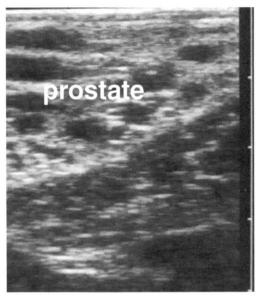

Figure 13-20 Transrectal longitudinal ultrasonographic image of the right prostatic lobe of a stallion. Acini are visible within the prostate.

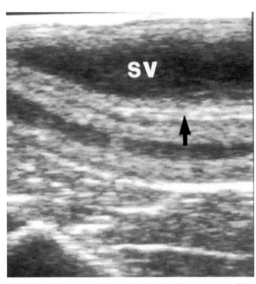

Figure 13-21 Transrectal longitudinal ultrasonographic image of the right seminal vesicle *(SV)* of a stallion. The stallion was teased to a mare in estrus before examination to ensure that the seminal vesicle would contain gel. Unless the stallion has been teased, the seminal vesicles are often difficult to palpate or visualize with ultrasonography. The ventral border of the seminal vesicle is denoted by the *black arrow*.

urine); and development of an erection (Figure 13-22). The onset, intensity, and duration of this courtship phase are affected by the stallion's genetic makeup, learned behavior (through both positive and negative experiences), seasonal variation, and disease. A common cause for reduced or arrested libido in stallions is mismanagement, especially overuse or repetitive abusive punishment for expression of sexual interest. Length of the courtship phase and number of mounts

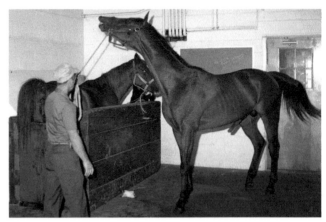

Figure 13-22 Exposure of a stallion to a mare in estrus, resulting in penile erection, vocalization, and display of the Flehmen reaction. (From Varner DD, Schumacher J, Blanchard TL, et al: *Diseases and management of breeding stallions,* St Louis, 1991, Mosby.)

necessary for ejaculation tend to increase in winter compared with summer. The physiologic mechanisms of stallion sexual behavior are not well understood but involve an intricate relationship between endocrine and neural systems.

The ability of a stallion to copulate normally (develop an erection, mount without hesitation, insert the penis, provide intravaginal thrusts, and ejaculate) should be assessed before the stallion is considered to be a satisfactory prospect for breeding. The most common physical abnormality associated with inability to mount is hind limb lameness (e.g., degenerative arthritis of the hock or stifle or even chronic laminitis). The specific cause of erection or ejaculatory failure, unrelated to psychologic malfunction, can be difficult to determine. Penile injuries, spinal cord lesions, and idiopathic organic dysfunctions can lead to impotence. For a thorough discussion of sexual behavior or ejaculatory dysfunction, the reader is referred to McDonnell (1992a, 1992b).

EXAMINATION FOR VENEREAL DISEASE

Several pathogenic microorganisms are transmitted by sexual contact, including bacteria, viruses, and protozoa. The role of fungi and *Chlamydia, Mycoplasma,* and *Ureaplasma* spp. in equine venereal disease is unknown but is not considered to be significant. Depending on the etiologic agent involved, venereal disease may manifest itself through overt clinical signs in the stallion, but more commonly, infected stallions are asymptomatic carriers.

Bacterial Genital Infections

Superficial bacterial colonization of the equine prepuce, penis, and distal urethra results in unavoidable contamination of the mare's reproductive tract during coitus. A variety of environmental bacteria can be isolated from these sites, many of which contribute to the normal nonpathogenic bacterial flora of healthy stallions. These commensal bacteria tend to prevent overpopulation of the external genitalia with potentially harmful organisms *(Klebsiella pneumoniae* or *Pseudomonas aeruginosa)*. Mismanagement of breeding stallions (through repeated penile washings with soaps or disinfectants or poor selection and upkeep of bedding) may convert the bacterial population on the surface of the penis from a mixed group of harmless bacteria to a population teeming with potential pathogens. The external genitalia of some stallions harbor large numbers of opportunistic bacteria. However, most bacteria are not considered pathogens unless they are recovered serially in heavy growth or unless postbreeding endometritis with the organism results in mares that have been bred to the stallion. The organism that causes contagious equine metritis, *Taylorella equigenitalis,* represents the only known bacterium capable of consistently producing venereal disease in horses. The stallion serves as a lesionless carrier of this disease, harboring the bacteria on its external genitalia, with subsequent horizontal transmission to the mare's reproductive tract at breeding.

Documentation of a bacterial infection depends on serial isolation of a pathogen, preferably in large numbers and in relatively pure culture. The exception is culture of *T. equigenitalis,* for which a single isolation is considered diagnostic (tests for *T. equigenitalis* must be conducted by an accredited veterinarian under the direction of a state or federal veterinarian). To identify organisms on the exterior of the penis or prepuce, swabbings of these areas should be taken for bacteriologic culture before the penis is cleansed to obtain urethral swabbings. Ideally, specimens should be retrieved from the fossa glandis, urethral sinus, free portion of the penile body, and folds of the external prepuce to provide an overall perspective of the microbial population. The stallion should be placed near a mare in estrus to achieve an erection and facilitate procurement of these samples for culture.

Internal Genital Infections

Internal genital infections in the stallion are rare but when they occur, are most often associated with seminal vesiculitis. Such infections are sometimes associated with hemospermia. Accumulation of leukocytes and the inciting bacteria in ejaculates is typical for stallions with internal genital infections.

If one is to gain insight into the cause of a possible infection of the internal genital tract, the penis and prepuce of the stallion should be washed meticulously with a surgical scrub before collection of appropriate samples for culture. Particular attention is given to removal of debris and organisms from the glans penis and fossa glandis. A thorough rinse should follow the scrub, and the procedure should be repeated twice. After the final rinse, the penis is dried thoroughly to

ensure that the urethral orifice is not contaminated. Briskly rubbing the glans penis during the washing process usually stimulates secretion of clear fluid (the presperm fraction of ejaculate), originating from the urethral or bulbourethral glands, into the urethral lumen. This procedure helps remove any bacterial contaminants that may have gained access via the external urethral orifice from the urethral lumen. Some of this fluid may be collected for culture and cytologic examination if an infection of the urethra or bulbourethral glands is suspected. A cotton swab is inserted 3 to 5 cm into the distal urethra to procure a sample for bacterial culture before semen collection (preejaculate swab) (Figure 13-23).

After collection of semen, the distal urethra is swabbed again immediately on removal of the penis from the artificial vagina; the urethral opening should not be contaminated before or during the swabbing process. Semen also can be sampled for bacteriologic culture, realizing that the semen has passed through the artificial vagina contaminated by the surface of the stallion's penis during thrusting. Collection of semen with an open-ended artificial vagina (Figure 13-24) minimizes contamination of the semen with organisms still residing on the exterior of the penis. Swabbings of semen collected into sterile containers with the open-ended artificial vagina are less likely to be contaminated and thus are more likely to yield meaningful cultures.

Vesicular gland fluid can be collected selectively for culture by first teasing the stallion vigorously to distend the lumen of these bladder-like glands with secretions. After aseptic preparation of the penis and distal urethra, a 1-cm × 100-cm sterile catheter with an inflatable cuff

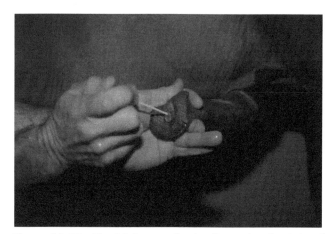

Figure 13-23 To obtain a urethral culture, the distal tip of the glans penis is first deflected dorsally with a thumb to allow better exposure of the urethral orifice for swab insertion. This procedure is performed immediately before (preejaculatory swabbing) and immediately after (postejaculatory swabbing) ejaculation to screen for potential internal genital infections. (From Varner DD, Schumacher J, Blanchard TL, et al: *Diseases and management of breeding stallions,* St Louis, 1991, Mosby.)

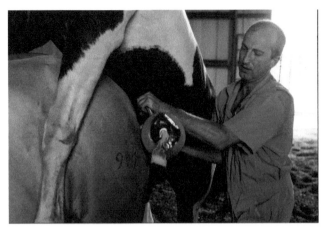

Figure 13-24 Collection of semen with an open-ended artificial vagina effectively reduces contamination of semen with microorganisms on the surface of the penis. Semen can be collected in sterile containers with a funnel or urethral prosthetic device.

is passed into the urethra to the level of the seminal colliculus (origin of the excretory ducts of the vesicular glands). The cuff is inflated, and the fluid in each vesicular gland is expressed manually per rectum for collection and study (Figure 13-25). Secretions from the prostate gland, ampullae, and ductus deferens may be cultured by swabbing semen collected in the first "spurt" or "jet" of an ejaculate with an open-ended artificial vagina, because this fraction of the ejaculate contains secretions originating primarily from these sites. Alter-

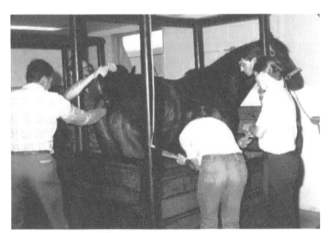

Figure 13-25 A sterile 100-cm flexible catheter has been passed into the pelvic urethra of this stallion. One examiner determines, via palpation per rectum, where to place the catheter tip and then expresses the fluid from each seminal vesicle in turn by using downward pressure with the digits, first from the blunt end and progressing toward the apical end, where the duct opening is located in the seminal colliculus. Fluid is collected through the catheter from each seminal vesicle in turn, which can also be examined further for evidence of infection (Courtesy Dr. Wendell Cooper.)

natively, the prostate and bulbourethral glands can be identified via transrectal ultrasonographic examination. After each gland is identified, the probe is retracted 2 to 3 inches while the digits are used to apply pressure to the gland of interest. Fluid expressed from the gland can be retrieved through a preplaced catheter or endoscope (Figure 13-26), and the gland can be immediately rescanned to confirm that fluid was expressed.

Infections that originate from the epididymides or testes usually induce changes that are palpable through the scrotum, except in severe cases in which scrotal edema is pronounced (Figure 13-27). The incriminating organism usually can be recovered from the semen, along with inflammatory cells recognized on cytologic

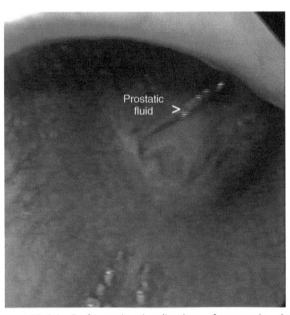

Figure 13-26 Endoscopic visualization of prostatic gland fluid being expressed per rectum. Fluid can be collected through a catheter passed through the biopsy channel of the endoscope or through a urinary catheter passed just into the pelvic urethra as described in the text.

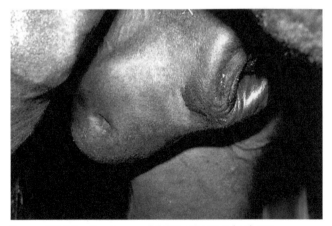

Figure 13-27 Pronounced (pitting) scrotal edema.

examination of stained semen smears. Chronic epididymitis or orchitis may result in azoospermia, as fibrous tissue proliferation can obstruct the epididymal duct. Adhesion formation between parietal and visceral tunics prevents free movement of the gonad within the scrotal tunics.

Viral Genital Infections

The two known venereal diseases attributed to viruses are equine coital exanthema, which is caused by equine herpesvirus 3, and equine viral arteritis (EVA), which is caused by a togavirus.

Equine coital exanthema, typically diagnosed via physical examination, produces characteristic blisters on the penile body and prepuce (Figure 13-28) that subsequently form pustules that ulcerate and eventually resolve in 2 to 4 weeks. The clinical disease is self-limiting, and fertility is not affected unless lesions are painful enough to interfere with breeding. Venereal transmission to mares is common during the active stage of the infection and results in similar lesions on the external genitalia of the mare (Figure 13-29). To avoid transmission of the virus, breeding can be delayed until lesions have healed. As with other herpesviruses, infection results in a lifelong carrier state with periodic outbreaks. However, for most stallions, recrudescence does not usually occur within the same breeding season.

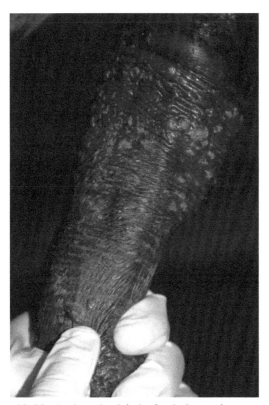

Figure 13-28 Lesions (vesicles) of coital exanthema, caused by equine herpesvirus 3, on the penile body in a breeding stallion.

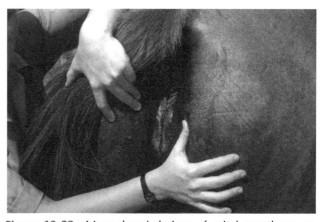

Figure 13-29 More chronic lesions of coital exanthema on the vulva and perineal area of a mare. This mare had been pasture bred during an equine herpesvirus 3 outbreak and was confirmed to be pregnant (35 days of gestation) at the time this photograph was taken.

Equine Viral Arteritis

Many strains of the equine arteritis virus are nonpathogenic. Infection with the pathogenic form of the virus only affects equids and most commonly results in subclinical infection but can cause a generalized illness 1 to 10 days after infection. Signs and symptoms include fever, lymphopenia, edema of the limbs, stiffness of gait, periorbital swelling with conjunctivitis and lacrimation, nasal discharge, maculopapular skin rash, edema of the scrotum and prepuce of the stallion and occasionally the mammary gland of the mare, abortion in the mare, and rarely a fulminating interstitial pneumonia in neonatal foals. EVA is spread via the respiratory route in most instances. The disease is of special interest to stallion managers because infected stallions can transmit the virus to susceptible mares during breeding (even via artificial insemination with cooled or frozen semen). Infected mares are then capable of transmitting the virus via the respiratory route to other susceptible horses they contact. Stallions infected with the equine arteritis virus can remain long-term asymptomatic carriers, with viral sequestration in the genital tract (particularly in the ampulla and vas deferens) and shedding in the semen (the sperm-rich portion of ejaculate is laden with virus). The venereal route appears to be the sole means of virus transmission from chronically infected stallions. Diagnosis of the disease in a stallion presumed to be a carrier is based on isolation of the causative virus from ejaculated semen or, alternatively, development of serum neutralization antibodies in seronegative mares that are bred to the suspect stallion.

Abortion (at 3 to 10 months of gestation) may occur during or shortly after the febrile period (1 to 4 weeks after infection) in affected mares, but it may also occur in exposed susceptible mares that display only mild or no premonitory clinical signs. The aborted fetus, membranes, and placental fluids are infective to susceptible horses and may help propagate an abortion storm in a herd of pregnant mares. During an outbreak, nasopharyngeal swabs, conjunctival swabs, or unclotted blood (ethylenediamine tetraacetic acid [EDTA] or citrate; not heparin) collected from acutely infected horses should be submitted for virus isolation. Infection of aborted fetuses can be confirmed with virus isolation, polymerase chain reaction (PCR) testing, or immunohistochemistry. The venereal mode of transmission is considered a major pathway for dissemination of the virus, but no evidence shows that mares exposed to semen from a carrier stallion will abort later in gestation.

Health regulation officials should be contacted for discussion and supervision of diagnosis and management of equine arteritis virus carrier or shedder stallions, which necessitates immunization of seronegative mares with a modified live-virus tissue culture adapted product (ARVAC; equine arteritis vaccine, Fort Dodge Laboratories Inc, Fort Dodge, IA) before breeding. Mares confirmed to be seronegative for equine arteritis virus are vaccinated. Vaccinated mares should be isolated from all other horses for 3 weeks to prevent infection of in-contact horses with the vaccine virus, which could cause seroconversion. After isolation requirements are met, vaccine-induced seroconversion is confirmed by repeating the blood test, and the mare can then be safely mated to the shedder stallion.

The vaccine is protective against the disease, but clients must have written, official certification of their horse's seronegative status from an approved laboratory before initial vaccination is used. In addition, documentation of vaccination in medical records is important in case it is required at some time in the future for health certificates, import, or export. The vaccine is thought to be safe for all ages of horses. Although it is not recommended for pregnant mares, especially in the last trimester, many pregnant mares were vaccinated without adverse effects during the recent 2006 outbreak in Quarter Horses. The American Association of Equine Practitioners strongly recommends that all male horses intended for breeding be vaccinated against EVA by 6 to 9 months of age, after colostral-derived antibodies have declined.

Protozoal Genital Infections

Trypanosoma equiperdum, the organism that causes dourine, is the only protozoan known to produce venereal disease in horses. The disease, which is not seen at present in the United States, is characterized initially by edematous swelling of the external genitalia, attendant mucopurulent discharge from the urethra, formation of 2- to 10-cm diameter urticarial cutaneous plaques, and progressive emaciation, sometimes in conjunction with penile paralysis. Diagnosis is based on a positive result on complement fixation testing and isolation of trypanosomes from the urethral exudate, blood, or urticarial plaques. Treatment is possible but generally impractical, and euthanasia is recommended.

COLLECTION OF SEMEN

Accurate assessment of semen quality depends heavily on proper semen collection techniques. Ejaculated semen is very susceptible to environmental influences, so mishandling of semen samples before evaluation negates their value for representing a stallion's innate fertility. The reader is referred to Chapter 12 for discussion of semen collection techniques and procedures.

EVALUATION OF SEMEN

To enhance the reliability of a semen evaluation, it should be performed in a thorough, methodic manner by an experienced person in an adequately equipped laboratory. Both routine and in-depth diagnostic tests are available and are selected based on time, availability of specialized equipment, and economic constraints of the stallion owner. Routine tests include gross evaluation of the sample, determination of semen volume and sperm concentration (to calculate total sperm number), and assessment of sperm motility, longevity, and morphology. More involved tests performed on selected stallions include chemical analysis of seminal plasma (including assay of alkaline phosphatase), electron microscopic study of sperm ultrastructure, a sperm chromatin structure assay, and various sperm function tests (e.g., membrane integrity, mitochondrial membrane potential, and the ability of sperm to undergo the acrosome reaction).

Gross Evaluation of Semen Quality

The gel is separated from the remainder of the ejaculate in the laboratory via aspiration into a syringe or pouring through a filter if an in-line filter was not placed in the artificial vagina to perform this function during semen collection. Filtration also helps to remove extraneous debris (e.g., smegma, hair, dirt) from the gel-free semen. The volume of gel-free semen is measured, and the color and consistency of the sample are noted. Although volume, by itself, is seldom an important determinant of fertility, it is used in calculation of total sperm number in an ejaculate. Consequently, accurate measurement of volume is essential. The filtered gel-free semen can be poured into 100-mL graduated cylinders to accurately measure volume (see Figure 12-15). Semen volume can be increased with excessive precopulatory teasing, but the total sperm number in the ejaculate usually remains unchanged. Ejaculate volume is affected by season (e.g., smaller volumes are produced in winter compared with summer) and sexual preparation time (i.e., prolonged teasing increases accessory sex gland secretions, which increase volume and decrease sperm concentration in the ejaculate). The gel-free portion of an ejaculate contains the majority of sperm, so the gel fraction usually is discarded without measurement of its sperm content after its volume is recorded. Gross evaluation of the semen sample provides a rough estimate of its sperm concentration and permits detection of color changes that may be associated with blood, urine, or purulent material in the ejaculate (Figures 13-30 and 13-31).

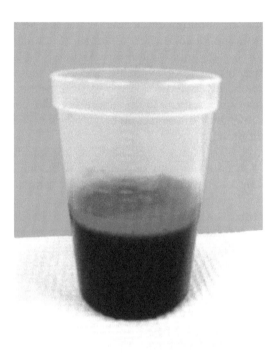

Figure 13-30 Cup containing bloody semen ejaculated by a stallion with hemospermia resulting from a pelvic urethral tear.

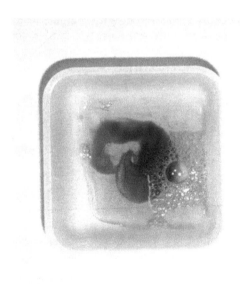

jet 2-3

Figure 13-31 Portion of fractionated ejaculate obtained with an open-ended artificial vagina from a stallion with ampullitis and seminal vesiculitis caused by *P. aeruginosa* infection.

SPERM CONCENTRATION

An accurate measurement of sperm concentration is critical because total sperm number in an ejaculate is derived by multiplying sperm concentration by semen volume. An imprecise estimate of sperm concentration produces a corresponding inaccurate calculated sperm number in an ejaculate. Such errors can produce misleading judgments and should be avoided. Sperm concentration of the gel-free semen can be determined with a hemacytometer (Bright-Line Hemacytometer, Hausser Scientific, Horsham, PA) (see Figure 12-17). Advantages of hemacytometer counting to determine sperm concentration include the following: it is a direct method for counting sperm visually identified under a microscope; discoloration of the sample does not affect accuracy of the count; and equipment expense is minor. Disadvantages of hemacytometer counting include that the counting takes a long time and variability from dilution and loading errors is common. For routine hemacytometer counting of sperm, the platelet/white blood cell Unopette system (Becton-Dickinson, Franklin Lakes, NJ) with 20-µL capillary pipettes can be used (see Figure 12-17). The capillary pipette is filled with semen, which is transferred to the Unopette (providing a 1:100 dilution). After thorough mixing, both sides of the cover-slipped hemacytometer chamber are loaded, and a few minutes are allowed for sperm to settle on the hemacytometer grid. The number of sperm within one of the nine large squares is counted (Figure 13-32), and this number is multiplied by 1 million to provide the number

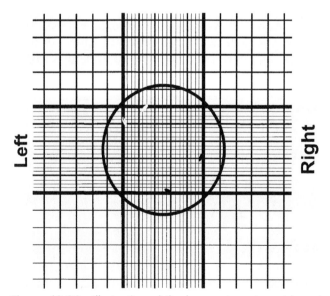

Figure 13-32 Illustration of the hemacytometer grid used for counting sperm. Nine large squares are present, with additional cross-hatched dividing lines within the center and central squares. All sperm present within the large center square are counted. For sperm heads lying on the lines, only those sperm heads lying on the upper and left lines are included in the count and not those lying on the lower or right lines.

of sperm per milliliter in the semen sampled. Both sides of separately loaded hemacytometer chambers should be counted and averaged. If the counts vary considerably (>10%), the dilution and loading procedures should be repeated, and the sample should be counted again.

Hemacytometer counting of sperm can be replaced by determination of sperm concentration with a spectrophotometer or photometric systems such as the densimeter (Animal Reproduction Systems, Chino, CA) (Figure 13-33). Besides the densimeter, other automated systems that use optical density to estimate sperm concentrations are commercially available (e.g., SpermaCue from Minitube of America Inc, Verona, Wis.; the model 10 sperm counter from Hamilton Research, Beverly, MA and Micro-Reader I from IMV, Maple Grove, MN). These instruments allow rapid measurement of sperm concentration in raw semen, and their accuracy is good if sperm concentration is not exceedingly high (>300 million/mL) or low (<100 million/mL) and the ejaculate is free of debris, blood, purulent material, or premature germ cells. Because these instruments measure optical density, the presence of contaminants or mixing semen with an extender that is not optically clear before measuring sperm concentration produces erroneous measurements. Dilution factors are automatically taken into account when commercially available optic density measuring systems are used (the exception is the SpermaCue, which requires no dilution of the raw semen).

A new instrument, the NucleoCounter SP-100 (ChemoMetec A/S, Allerød, Denmark) (see Figure 12-19), has been developed for assessment of sperm concentration in bulls and has recently been validated for use in the horse. The instrument uses the fluorescent probe propidium iodide, which binds to the DNA of the sperm. Although more expensive than instruments that use light impedance, it has proved to provide more accurate and repeatable measurements, particularly at both very high and very low sperm concentrations. Its use has an additional advantage in that debris (e.g., smegma, inflammatory cells, blood) does not interfere with sperm count. Another major advantage is that it can be used in semen samples already mixed with non-optically clear extenders (e.g., milk-based extenders or freezing extenders). This allows rapid and accurate determination of sperm concentration when adjusting dilutions for cooling or freezing semen or preparing small numbers of sperm for low-dose insemination. If a stallion has to be evaluated on a farm where laboratory equipment is not available, the extended semen can later be evaluated for sperm concentration when the practitioner returns to the laboratory. The count is then adjusted for dilution ratio to provide a raw semen concentration.

Total sperm number, calculated as the product of sperm concentration and semen volume, is one of the more important measurements used in estimating a stallion's fertility. Total sperm number per ejaculate is subject to seasonal variation but also is affected by numerous other factors that include rate of occurrence of ejaculation, age, testicular size, spermatogenic efficiency (i.e., number of sperm produced per cc of testis), size of extragonadal sperm reserves, and various forms of reproductive disease. Total sperm number in ejaculates obtained from mature stallions typically ranges from 4 to 12 billion but may exceed 15 to 20 billion in sexually rested stallions. For stallions ejaculating low numbers of sperm, an accurate estimation of actual DSO is advised. This usually requires determination of number of sperm present in ejaculates collected once daily for 7 to 10 days. After extragonadal sperm reserves are stabilized (requiring approximately 4 days of once-daily semen collection for stallions with smaller testes and 5 to 6 days of once daily semen collection for stallions with larger testes), the numbers of sperm recovered in ejaculates obtained on each of 3 consecutive days are averaged to provide the estimate of DSO. The stallion can be expected to ejaculate approximately this number of sperm each day when he is breeding regularly. DSO varies with age, testis size, and testicular health and season (reaching the highest values in the summer and lowest values in the winter).

SEMINAL pH

The pH of gel-free semen should be determined with a properly calibrated pH meter, preferably within 1 hour after semen collection. Measurements obtained with pH paper are less precise than those derived with a meter, so the former method of pH determination should be used only as a last resort. The pH of normal semen is slightly basic, with a reported range of 7.2 to 7.9. Louisiana workers determined that sperm motility was best when raw semen pH was 7.7 and significantly declined once pH was 7.9 or more.

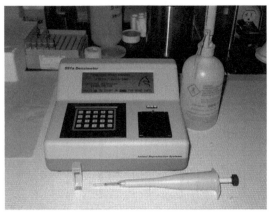

Figure 13-33 A densimeter (with accessories) is commercially available (Animal Reproduction Systems, Chino, CA) for estimation of sperm concentration in raw, gel-free stallion semen. The instrument can also be used to determine the volume of semen to use as an insemination dose after the percentage of progressively motile sperm has been entered.

Season of the year, rate of occurrence of ejaculation, and sperm concentration can affect the pH of normal stallion semen. An abnormally high semen pH value can be associated with contamination of the ejaculate by urine, soap, or excessive lubricant or with inflammatory lesions of the internal genital tract.

SPERM MOTILITY

Sperm motility generally reflects the viability of a sperm population. A positive relationship between sperm motility and fertilizing capacity has been shown in many species, although this correlation is not absolute. Several different instruments and methods have been developed for objective assessment of equine sperm motility, including time-lapse photomicrography, frame-by-frame playback videomicrography, spectophotometry, and computerized analysis (Figure 13-34). Computerized motility analysis provides a number of objective measures of sperm motion characteristics taken from tracks of large numbers of sperm, including percentage of motile sperm, percentage of progressively motile sperm (i.e., above a preset cutoff for speed and direction of movement), amplitude of lateral head displacement during forward movement, average path velocity in micrometers per second, and curvilinear velocity in micrometers per second. Subjective assessment of sperm motility via visual estimation, with a microscope equipped with phase-contrast optics and a warming stage (see Figure 12-18), is acceptable when personnel are experienced in analysis of sperm motility.

Visual assessment of sperm motility should include total sperm motility (percentage of sperm that exhibit motility of any form), progressive sperm motility (percentage of sperm that exhibit rapid, linear movement), and sperm velocity (on an arbitrary scale of 0 [immotile] to 4 [rapidly motile]). For example, a motility of 75/70 (4) indicates that 75% of sperm were motile and 70% of sperm were progressively motile, moving rapidly across the microscopic field. Rapid progressive

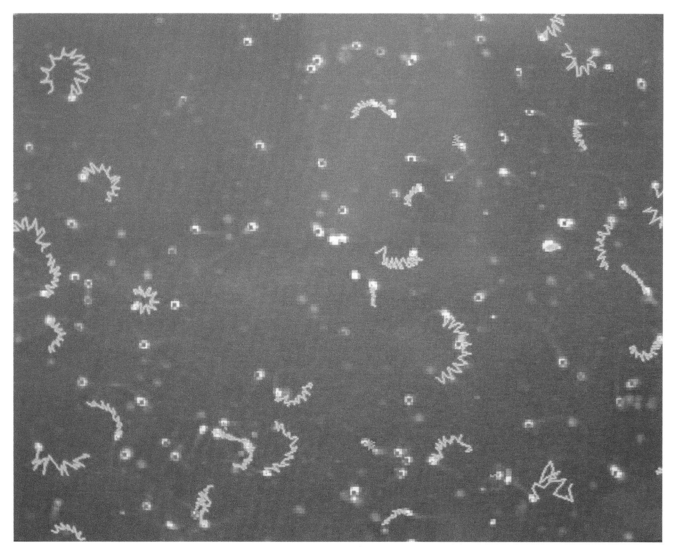

Figure 13-34 Image obtained from a Hamilton-Thorn computerized motility analyzer during assessment of sperm motility. The computer-identified tracks of moving sperm analyzed over a short time span are shown.

sperm motility generally is considered to be the most credible gauge of sperm motion for predicting the fertilizing capacity of a semen sample.

Both the initial sperm motility and the longevity of progressive sperm motility should be assessed and recorded. Initial sperm motility of raw (undiluted) semen samples can be estimated as a control for testing the possible detrimental effects of semen extenders on sperm motility. Accuracy and repeatability of the sperm motility evaluation are improved markedly by diluting the semen in an appropriate extender before analysis (see Tables 12-1 and 12-2). Warmed (37°C) nonfat dry skim milk-glucose extender, or native phosphocaseinate-based extender, serves this purpose well because it supports sperm motility and does not interfere with microscopic visualization of the sperm. To standardize the sperm motility testing protocol, all semen samples should be diluted with extender before analysis. We prefer to dilute semen to a standard concentration of 25 to 30 million sperm/mL for motility assessment. One advantage of use of a standard concentration of extended semen is that it conditions the viewer to see sperm at a consistent concentration among all stallion ejaculates evaluated. At higher concentrations, sperm motility tends to be overestimated. This concentration of sperm diluted in an appropriate extender has also been shown to maximize both immediate sperm motility and the longevity of sperm motility.

The longevity of sperm motility can be determined on raw semen samples stored at room temperature (20°C to 25°C) and on samples diluted in extender (preferably to a final sperm concentration of 25×10^6 sperm/mL) and stored at room temperature or refrigerated (4°C to 6°C). The longevity of sperm motility is enhanced by dilution of semen with extender and refrigerated storage. The Society for Theriogenology guidelines for evaluating the semen of prospective breeding stallions recommend that at least 10% progressive sperm motility be maintained in raw and extended semen samples maintained in a light-shielded environment at room temperature for 6 and 24 hours, respectively. If properly processed, semen from stallions that survives cooling well will have similar to slightly lower sperm motility after 24 hours of cooling compared to that semen when evaluated fresh. The relationship between longevity of sperm motility in samples maintained at room temperature is questioned by many investigators, whereas less dissension is found concerning the value of determining the longevity of the sperm motility in cooled samples when processed ejaculates are used for breeding with cooled, transported semen.

To accurately assess longevity of sperm motility in vitro, semen should be first be properly extended. This necessitates diluting semen so that less than 20% (volume:volume) seminal plasma (preferably 5% to 10%) remains in the extended samples, as excess seminal plasma depresses sperm membrane stability, DNA

quality, and motility over time. If raw semen concentration is too dilute to allow a 1:4 dilution (i.e., 1 part semen to 4 parts extender) without lowering final sperm concentration to less than 25 million sperm/mL, then excess seminal plasma must be removed after centrifugation. To maximize sperm recovery and minimize damage to sperm (Figures 13-35 to 13-38), semen is first

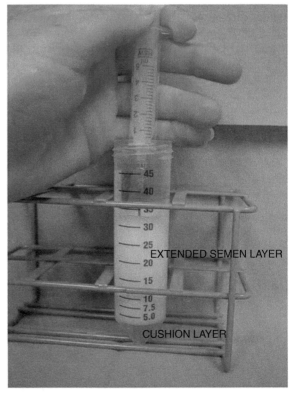

Figure 13-35 For preparation for centrifuging semen to remove excess seminal plasma, a 50-mL conical polypropylene centrifuge tube is filled with 35 mL of semen extended 1:1 or 2:1. An 18-gauge blunt spinal needle is used to place 3.5 mL of cushion fluid (Eqcellsire Component B, IMV) beneath the extended semen.

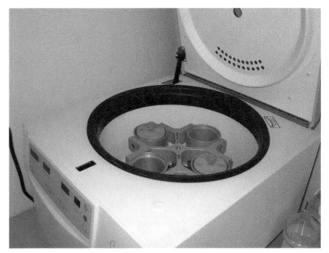

Figure 13-36 After balancing of the centrifuge, the loaded tubes are centrifuged at $1000 \times g$ for 20 minutes.

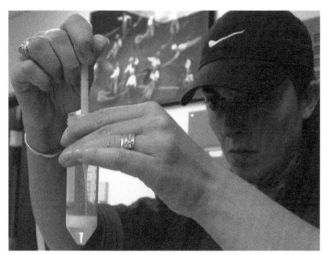

Figure 13-37 After centrifugation, the supernatant is aspirated down to the 7.5-mL mark on the conical tube.

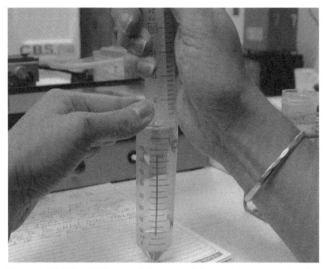

Figure 13-38 With the 18-gauge blunt spinal needle, the cushion fluid is carefully removed from the bottom of the centrifuge tube, leaving approximately 4 mL of concentrated extended semen. Sufficient fresh extender is added to the remaining sperm pellet to result in a final seminal plasma concentration of 5% to 10% (i.e., 36 to 76 mL of extender), and the finally diluted semen is gently mixed to ensure sperm are evenly distributed throughout.

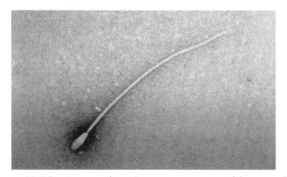

Figure 13-39 A normal equine sperm prepared for morphologic evaluation by mixing a drop of semen with a drop of eosin-nigrosin stain, smearing this mixture along a slide, allowing it to air dry, and examining the smear under oil immersion with a light microscope.

mixed with an equal volume of extender, and 35 mL of extended semen is placed in a 50-mL conical polypropylene centrifuge tube. Then, 3.5 mL of cushion fluid (e.g., Eqcellsire Component B, IMV Technologies, Maple Grove, Minn. or Cushion fluid, Minitúb, Tiefenbach, Germany) is placed beneath the semen in the bottom of the tube with a blunt 18-gauge spinal needle with attached syringe. The loaded tube is centrifuged at $1000 \times g$ for 20 minutes, and the supernatant is aspirated down to the 7.5 mL mark on the centrifuge tube. With the spinal needle, the cushion fluid is carefully removed, and the remaining sperm pellet is mixed with sufficient fresh extender to result in a final sperm concentration of 25 to 50 million sperm/mL yet still retain 5% to 10% seminal plasma (e.g., 4 mL of centrifuged semen was left after centrifugation, so addition of 36 mL extender results in a maximum of 10% seminal plasma being present). After the desired dilution is accomplished, the semen is used to fill nontoxic vials (or bags), ensuring all air is eliminated. The vials are placed in an insulated, dark environment for incubation at room temperature and also loaded into a container such as an Equitainer (Hamilton-Thorne Inc, Beverly, MA) for cooling and storage at 4°C to 6°C. Semen samples should be warmed to 37°C for 10 to 15 minutes before assessment of sperm motility after the appropriate incubation period.

SPERM MORPHOLOGY

The morphology (structural appearance) of sperm is typically examined with a light microscope at $1000 \times$ to $1250 \times$ magnification (under oil immersion). Standard bright-field microscope optics can be used to examine air-dried semen smears provided that appropriate stains are used in slide preparation. Specific stains for sperm include those developed by Williams and Casarett. General purpose cellular stains (e.g., Wright's, Giemsa, hematoxylin-eosin) also have been used to accent both germinal and somatic cells in semen smears. Background stains (e.g., eosin-nigrosin, India ink) probably are the most widely used stains because of their ease of use (Figures 13-39 and 13-40). Visualization of the structural details of sperm can be enhanced by fixing the cells in buffered formol-saline or buffered glutaraldehyde solution and then viewing the unstained cells as a wet mount with either phase-contrast (Figure 13-41) or differential interference-contrast microscopy (Figures 13-42 and 13-43). Sperm fixation also is simplified by this method, and the incidence of artifactual changes is reduced compared with that seen with stained smears. In one Texas study, droplet and midpiece abnormalities were underestimated in semen smears stained with eosin-nigrosin and examined under oil immersion with light microscopy compared with samples of the same ejaculates fixed in 2% buffered formol-saline

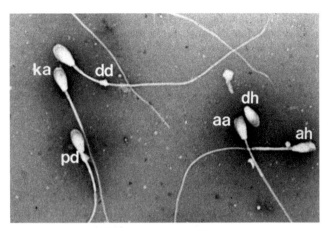

Figure 13-40 Morphologically abnormal equine sperm prepared for evaluation by staining with eosin-nigrosin. *ka,* Knobbed acrosome; *aa,* abnormal acrosome; *dh,* detached head; *pd,* proximal droplet; *dd,* distal droplet; *ah,* abnormal head.

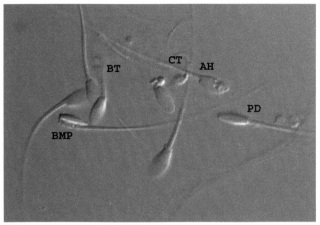

Figure 13-42 Equine sperm fixed in 2% buffered formol-saline solution and examined on a wet mount slide preparation under oil immersion with a differential interference contrast microscope. The morphologic defects of these sperm include proximal protoplasmic droplets *(PD),* reversed or bent tails *(BT),* coiled tails *(CT),* bent midpiece *(BMP),* and abnormal heads *(AH).*

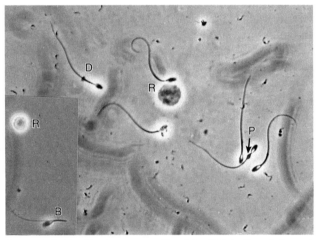

Figure 13-41 Equine sperm fixed in 2% buffered formol-saline solution and examined on a wet mount slide preparation under oil immersion with a phase-contrast microscope. Morphologic defects of these sperm include distal protoplasmic droplets *(D),* reversed or bent tails *(B),* proximal cytoplasmic droplets *(P),* and round spermatogenic cells *(R).* (From Blanchard TL, et al: Testicular degeneration in large animals: identification and treatment, *Vet Med* 86:537, 1991.)

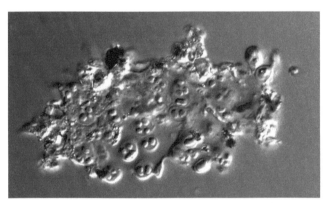

Figure 13-43 Numerous neutrophils are seen in this semen specimen fixed in 2% buffered formol-saline solution and examined on a wet mount slide preparation under oil immersion with a differential interference contrast microscope.

solution and examined under oil immersion with phase-contrast microscopy.

Over the years, a number of investigators have used the eosin-nigrosin stain to assess the percentage of live, acrosome-intact sperm in a semen sample. Those sperm stained with eosin (red) were considered to be dead or to have lost the acrosome. However, caution must be exercised in interpreting the significance of eosin-positive sperm because many artifactual changes can occur simply from cold or osmotic shock, or other handling errors, and can lead to an elevation in the percentage of sperm that stain with eosin. To decrease the incidence of artifactual eosin staining, the slides,

stain, and semen must be warm. A small drop of the stain should then be promptly mixed with a drop of semen and smoothly spread across the surface of the slide. If the preparation is too thick, the stained smear dries too slowly. In addition, recent experimental evidence has demonstrated that eosin staining for membrane integrity is less sensitive than once believed, and an overestimation of the number of sperm with intact membranes can occur. Therefore, we prefer to use fluorescent stains such as carboxyfluorescein diacetate (CFDA) or SYBR-14 in conjunction with propidium iodide (PI) to assess sperm membrane integrity.

At least 100 sperm should be evaluated for evidence of morphologic defects. The type and incidence of each defect (Figure 13-44) should be recorded. Abnormalities in sperm morphology traditionally have been classified

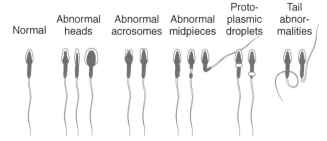

Figure 13-44 Drawing of morphologically normal and abnormal sperm. (From Blanchard TL, Varner DD: Evaluating breeding soundness in stallions: II: semen collection and evaluation, *Vet Med* February:144, 1996.)

as primary, secondary, or tertiary. Primary morphologic abnormalities were considered to be associated with a defect in spermatogenesis and, therefore, of testicular origin. Secondary morphologic abnormalities were considered to be created in the excurrent duct system. Tertiary morphologic abnormalities were considered to develop in vitro as a result of improper semen collection or handling procedures.

The current trend is to record the number of specific morphologic defects, such as detached heads, abnormal heads, knobbed acrosomes, proximal and distal protoplasmic droplets, bent or irregular midpieces, and bent or coiled tails. This method of classification is considered superior to the traditional system because it reveals more specific information about a population of sperm while avoiding erroneous assumptions about the origin of these defects, which is often unknown. Some morphologic abnormalities (e.g., detached heads) can be primary, secondary, or tertiary in nature, thereby introducing the possibility of error when this classification system is used exclusively. Another example is osmotic shock, which can cause bending of the tail so that an actual abnormality might be construed as a secondary defect rather than recognized as a tertiary morphologic abnormality.

The value of sperm morphologic studies in predicting the fertility of a stallion is met with a degree of skepticism because some stallions can have many sperm abnormalities yet still achieve good pregnancy rates when they are bred under good management conditions. Conversely, some stallions have decreased fertility even though the percentage of morphologically normal sperm in their ejaculates is high (based on light microscopic studies). Morphologically abnormal sperm are assumed to not have a negative influence on normal sperm in the ejaculate. Therefore, the total number of morphologically normal sperm in ejaculates may provide more information regarding the fertility of a stallion than the percentage of morphologically abnormal sperm.

CHEMICAL ANALYSIS OF SEMINAL PLASMA

Adverse effects of some stallion seminal plasma on sperm have been shown. Excess seminal plasma present in dilute ejaculates may damage sperm and has

been shown to adversely affect the longevity of sperm motility and sperm chromatin structure in cool-stored semen. Centrifugation and removal of excess seminal plasma, followed by extension of the sperm pellet in dried skim milk extender before cooling, have been shown to improve sperm motility and DNA stability (COMP α-t in sperm chromatin structure assays) of ejaculates of stallions with "poor cooling" semen. Also, the addition of seminal plasma from stallions with high post-thaw sperm motility to ejaculates from stallions with low post-thaw sperm motility enhanced both the post-thaw sperm motility and membrane integrity of these stallions.

Despite increasing work on the potential adverse effects of seminal plasma on stallion sperm, the factors present or absent in seminal plasma that cause problems are not well known. Chemical analyses of equine seminal plasma have been reported, but clear relationships among the various components of seminal plasma to sperm fertilizing capacity have not been established. One study revealed that electrolyte concentration, total protein concentration, or specific protein composition of seminal plasma does not provide good predictive information regarding post-thaw motility of cryopreserved sperm. However, Troedsson and coworkers (2002, 2005, 2006) have recently shown that seminal plasma modulates influx of neutrophils into the uterus, protects normal sperm within the uterus from being bound to neutrophils, and promotes binding and engulfment of dead or abnormal sperm by neutrophils to facilitate removal from the uterus. Their work showed that at least two separate seminal plasma proteins are components involved in these processes, and they have preliminary data that support differences in presence or absence of these proteins between some fertile and subfertile stallions. Further characterization of seminal plasma proteins that affect stallion fertility is ongoing.

The alkaline phosphatase activity of seminal plasma can be determined and is of proven practical use. The sources of alkaline phosphatase are primarily the testes and epididymides. Turner (1996) suggested that seminal plasma alkaline phosphatase activity of less than 100 U/L results from failure of testicular/epididymal secretions to reach the ejaculate and that values of more than 2500 U/L confirm complete ejaculation with normal contribution of the testes and epididymides to the ejaculate. This test is useful for evaluation of stallions producing azoospermic ejaculates (e.g., no sperm in the ejaculate with high alkaline phosphatase activity indicates a testicular problem with spermatogenesis, whereas no sperm in the ejaculate with low alkaline phosphatase activity either indicates failure to ejaculate or shows that testicular/epididymal products are not entering the ejaculate, which may occur with blockage of the excurrent duct system).

TRANSMISSION ELECTRON MICROSCOPIC EXAMINATION OF SPERM

Light microscopy affords limited magnification and, therefore, limited appraisal of sperm morphology. This obstacle can be overcome with use of scanning or transmission electron microscopic techniques. Although expensive, these two microscopic methods offer high-resolution detail and permit closer examination of sperm morphology. Subtle morphologic alterations, unapparent with light microscopy, often can be identified easily with electron microscopic analysis. Scanning electron microscopy offers three-dimensional visualization of entire spermatozoon (Figure 13-45). Transmission electron microscopy permits cross-sectional viewing of sperm and reveals the ultrastructure in detail (Figure 13-46). Both electron microscopic techniques may be economically justifiable diagnostic aids in selected circumstances.

EVALUATION OF THE ABILITY OF SPERM TO UNDERGO THE ACROSOME REACTION

Ejaculated sperm are not immediately capable of fertilizing an oocyte. Instead, they must undergo final maturational changes within the reproductive tract of the mare. Two of these events (thought to be accomplished

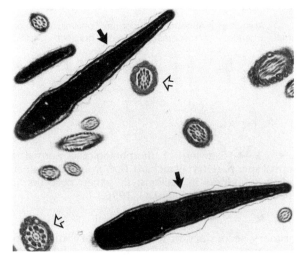

Figure 13-46 Transmission electron micrograph of stallion sperm, showing the head *(solid arrows)* and flagellar *(open arrows)* components. (Courtesy Dr. Larry Johnson. From Varner DD, Schumacher J, Blanchard TL et al: *Diseases and management of breeding stallions,* St Louis, 1991, Mosby.)

in the mare's oviduct) are completion of capacitation and the acrosome reaction. The acrosome reaction culminates in fusion and fenestration of the sperm's plasma membrane and outer acrosomal membrane, which allows acrosomal contents to be released and thus aids in penetration of the vestments of the oocyte and fusion with the oocyte's plasma membrane. These changes are necessary for fertilization to occur.

Some substances known to induce the acrosome reaction in vitro can be used in a variety of assays to quantitate the percentage of sperm that have reacted. Texas workers used a 3-hour incubation of ejaculated sperm with the ionophore A23187 (Calbiochem, San Diego, CA) and determined the percentage of sperm undergoing an acrosome reaction with transmission electron microscopy (Figures 13-47 and 13-48). With this assay, they noted that some highly subfertile stallions with otherwise normal semen quality apparently produce sperm incapable of undergoing the acrosome reaction.

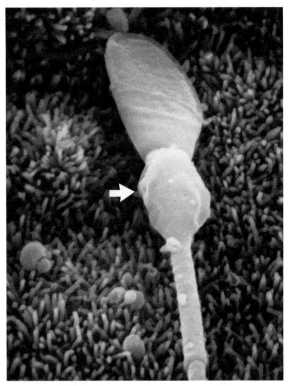

Figure 13-45 Scanning electron micrograph of an equine sperm from an efferent ductule. Note the proximal cytoplasmic droplet *(arrow)*. (Courtesy Dr. Larry Johnson. From Varner DD, Blanchard TL, et al: *Diseases and management of breeding stallions,* St Louis, 1991, Mosby.)

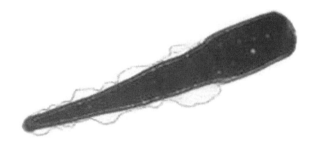

Figure 13-47 Transmission electron micrograph of a sagittal section through the head of a stallion sperm before incubation with calcium ionophore to induce acrosome reaction. No vesiculation of the outer acrosomal and plasma membranes is evident (i.e., the sperm has not undergone the acrosome reaction).

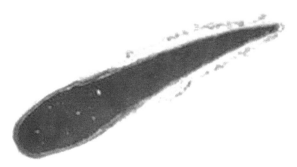

Figure 13-48 Transmission electron micrograph of a sagittal section through the head of a stallion sperm after 3 hours of incubation with calcium ionophore to induce acrosome reaction. Vesiculation of the outer acrosomal and plasma membranes is evident (i.e., the sperm has undergone the acrosome reaction).

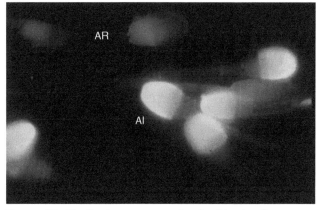

Figure 13-49 Equine sperm stained with the fluorescent dyes FITC-PSA and PI examined under a fluorescent microscope are shown. *AR,* Acrosome reacted; *AI,* acrosome intact.

California workers used progesterone to initiate the acrosome reaction in ejaculated sperm and determined that subfertile stallions had sperm with decreased ability to undergo the acrosome reaction compared with sperm of fertile stallions. At present, practitioners must work with research laboratories to have an acrosome reaction assay performed.

USE OF FLUORESCENT DYES IN EVALUATION OF SPERM COMPARTMENTS

Fluorescent dyes (available from Molecular Probes Inc, Eugene, Ore.) have been used in evaluation of membrane integrity, acrosomal status, and midpiece mitochohondria of fresh and preserved sperm. Proportions of sperm with different staining patterns can be assessed with epifluorescent microscopy, or with a flow cytometer (which allows evaluation of thousands of sperm instead of 100 to 200 that can routinely be evaluated microscopically).

The fluorescent dye fluorescein isothiocyanate (FITC) conjugated to pea *(Pisum sativum)* agglutinin (FITC-PSA) or peanut *(Arachis hypogea)* agglutinin (FITC-PNA), which bind to the acrosomal components of sperm, can be used to determine the acrosomal status of an equine sperm population (Figure 13-49). In some instances, ejaculates of subfertile stallions may contain high proportions of sperm that have prematurely acrosome-reacted. Stallions whose ejaculate contain a high proportion of prematurely acrosome-reacted sperm may be subfertile. These dyes can also be used in evaluation of semen processing or storage techniques, to guide selection of those practices that preserve acrosomal status of the processed sperm.

Both SYBR-14 and propidium iodide (PI) are commonly used in evaluation of membrane integrity, with penetration of the sperm membrane and binding to nucleic acids of the DNA. SYBR-14 penetrates intact membranes, binding with DNA and fluorescing green; PI penetrates damaged membranes and fluoresces red. The mitochondrial membrane probe JC-1 selectively penetrates mitochondrial membranes, fluorescing green in the presence of low membrane potential or red-orange in the presence of high membrane potential. Texas workers used SYBR-14/PI/JC-1 staining (Figure 13-50) to evaluate sperm populations in semen from fertile stallions and found good correlation between membrane integrity and total sperm motility (green heads with green or red midpieces versus total motility; $r = 0.98$). In that study, membrane-intact motile sperm had mitochondria expressing high and sometimes low membrane potential. A number of other fluorescent dyes are available for use in evaluation of different sperm compartments and have been applied to equine semen.

URETHRAL ENDOSCOPY

Urethral endoscopy generally is reserved for use in stallions with hemospermia or those with suspected specific urethral, bladder, or vesicular gland lesions. Use of a flexible endoscope is recommended because it easily negotiates the ischial arch when passed via the urethral orifice, avoiding the need for subischial urethrotomy. To permit easy passage through the urethral lumen, the endoscope should have a maximum outside diameter of 10 mm. A working length of 100 cm permits access to the bladder lumen if the penis is not fully erect. Proper preoperative disinfection of equipment and subsequent removal of potentially caustic disinfectants such as gludaraldehyde is critical. Endoscopic examination of the urethra and bladder may reveal mural and luminal abnormalities undetectable by other means. Urethral pathologic entities detectable with endoscopic examination include inflammation, ulcerations, lacerations (Figures 13-51 and 13-52), fistulae, strictures, growths, calculi, and foreign bodies. In stallions with seminal vesiculitis, lesions and purulent material may be visible (and sampled for culture/cytology) when viewed through the endoscope.

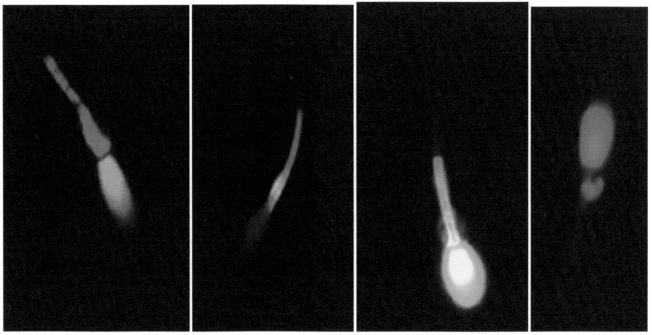

Figure 13-50 Equine sperm stained with the fluorescent dyes SYBR-14, PI, JC-1. DNA of sperm with damaged membranes are labeled with PI and fluoresce red, and sperm with intact plasma membranes are stained green by the SYBR-14. The dye JC-1 stains the mitochondria of the mid pieces orange if a high membrane potential is present or pale green if a low membrane potential is present. The midpieces of dead sperm or those with inactive mitochondria do not take up the JC-1 fluorescent label.

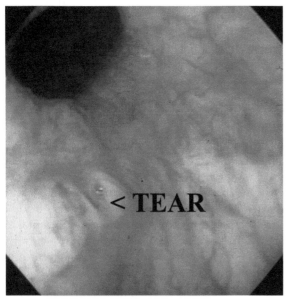

Figure 13-51 Urethral laceration evident during endoscopic examination of a stallion with profuse hemospermia.

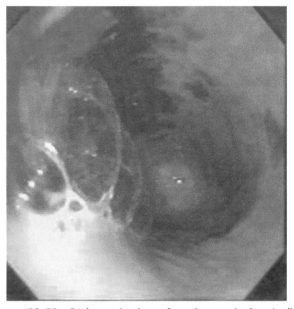

Figure 13-52 Endoscopic view of erosive seminal vesiculitis with accumulation of purulent material on the floor of the seminal vesicle in a stallion with purulent material present in ejaculates.

Repeated lavage (Figure 13-53), followed by infusion of the antibiotic of choice, of the infected seminal vesicle is often indicated because most antimicrobials do not have favorable fat solubility or pKa characteristics that permit penetration into accessory sex glands when administered systemically. Cystitis, bladder calculi, and bladder tumors also may be revealed with urethral endoscopy.

RADIOGRAPHY

Radiographic techniques have been used effectively in the stallion to evaluate patency of the urethra and ductus deferens. Contrast or double-contrast radiography also may be useful for evaluation of the corpus cavernosum penis. Urethrograms (contrast and

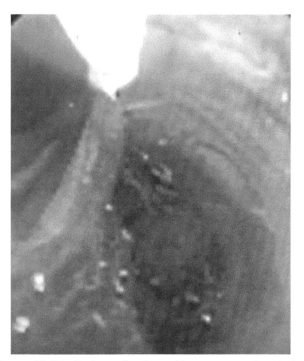

Figure 13-53 Endoscopic view of lavage procedure being performed in an infected seminal vesicle. After passage of the endoscope through the ejaculatory duct opening of the seminal colliculus and into the seminal vesicle, a catheter is passed through the biopsy port of the endoscope. Lactated Ringer's solution is used to lavage the vesicle until purulent material is removed, and the seminal vesicle is infused with the antibiotic of choice.

double-contrast radiography of the urethral lumen) have been used in diagnosis of urethral strictures and ulcerations, space-occupying lesions, and urethral fistulas. Contrast radiography has been used in detection of bilateral luminal obstructions of the ductus deferens, which cause azoospermia. A contrast radiographic study of the corpus cavernosum penis also may be useful to evaluate the patency of the corpus cavernosum penis after chronic penile paralysis or priapism.

CHROMOSOMAL ANALYSIS

Cytogenetics has become an increasingly popular area of clinical reproduction analysis in stallions. Oftentimes, the etiology of infertility and reduced fertility in the stallion is not disclosed with conventional diagnostic methods; therefore, investigators rely more heavily on chromosomal studies to isolate genetically derived causes for such problems. Karyotyping permits scrutiny for numeric or structural changes in chromosome composition that could affect reproductive performance. Pennsylvania workers karyotyped 62 fertile, subfertile, and infertile stallions and identified chromosomal defects (including mosaicism with sex or autosomal deletions or duplications) in 18 of these stallions (Kenney et al., 1991). To perform karyotyping, a cytogenetics laboratory needs

aseptically obtained blood samples shipped at room temperature overnight. In some instances, the cytogeneticist may request that an aseptically obtained skin biopsy specimen be placed within a tube that contains whole blood and transported at room temperature overnight, which facilitates culture of fibroblasts to improve the karyotyping capability.

SPERM CHROMATIN

A flow-cytometric procedure has been developed to evaluate the structural integrity of sperm chromatin. The potential of the sperm chromatin structure assay (SCSA) for prediction of fertility has been evaluated in stallions with encouraging results. This assay system measures the susceptibility of sperm nuclear DNA to acid denaturation in situ. The extent of denaturation is determined with flow cytometry, measuring the red and green fluorescence emitted from acid-treated sperm stained with the metachromatic dye acridine orange. Green fluorescence is emitted on laser excitation when the stain is intercalated into the native (stable), double-stranded DNA; red fluorescence is emitted when the stain is bound to denatured, single-stranded DNA. The extent of sperm chromatin acid denaturation is negatively correlated with fertility. The COMP α-t value (percentage of abnormal cells outside the main population) is calculated after large numbers (>5000) of sperm are counted (Figures 13-54 and 13-55). In one Pennsylvania study, the COMP α-t was found to be 16% in fertile stallions (seasonal pregnancy rate of 86%) and 41% in very subfertile stallions (seasonal pregnancy rate of 38%). Stallions with a COMP α-t value between 16% and 41% often demonstrate lesser reductions in fertility. The SCSA requires freezing of semen (usually raw) on dry ice or in liquid nitrogen, followed by frozen transport to an appropriate laboratory.

ANTISPERM ANTIBODIES

Equine antisperm antibody tests have been developed to assess the potential role of these antibodies in the infertility of stallions and mares. Antisperm antibodies are hypothesized to interfere with sperm transport and gamete interaction, resulting in fertilization failure and perhaps even early embryonic death. There is some suggestion that damage to the testis, particularly degeneration, may culminate in the formation of antibodies against sperm as a result of disruption of the blood-testis barrier. At present, no commercial laboratories offer these tests.

HORMONAL ANALYSES

The goal of reproductive endocrine assessment in stallions is detection of which components in the hypothalamic-pituitary-gonadal system may contribute to abnormal reproductive function. The hypothalamus

Stallion with high fertility:
90% SPR; 60% PR/cycle

Sperm Chromatin Structure Assay:
Mean α-t = 230
Standard deviation α-t = 60
COMP α-t = 10%

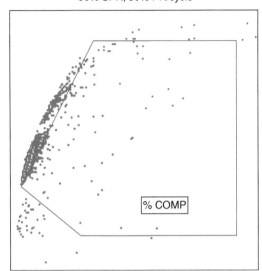

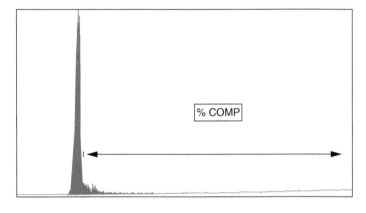

Figure 13-54   Sperm chromatin structure assay cytogram *(left)* of a fertile stallion's sperm stained with acridine orange and measured with flow cytometry. Green fluorescence is on the y-axis and red fluorescence in on the x-axis. A corresponding α-t frequency histogram with the number of cells on the y-axis is presented on the *right*. The cells in the region denoted by the *arrow* are denatured and fall outside the main (normal) population; they are termed the COMP α-t cells.

Stallion with low fertility:
55% SPR; 20% PR/cycle

Sperm Chromatin Structure Assay:
Mean α-t = 270
Standard deviation α-t = 80
COMP α-t = 45%

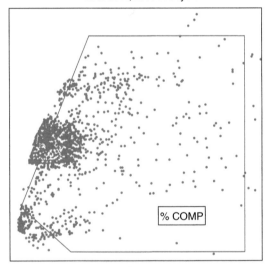

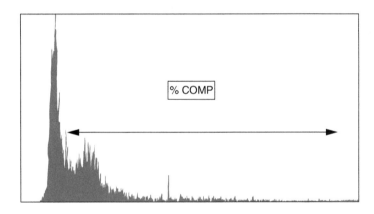

Figure 13-55   Sperm chromatin structure assay cytogram *(left)* of a subfertile stallion's sperm stained with acridine orange and measured with flow cytometry. Green fluorescence is on the y-axis, and red fluorescence is on the x-axis. A corresponding α-t frequency histogram with the number of cells on the y-axis is presented on the *right*. The cells in the region denoted by the *arrow* are denatured and fall outside the main (normal) population; they are termed the COMP α-t cells.

secretes gonadotropin hormone-releasing hormone (GnRH), which stimulates the pituitary gland to secrete follicle-stimulating hormone (FSH) and luteinizing hormone (LH), which in turn stimulate their respective target cells in the testis. The primary effect of LH is to indirectly promote spermatogenesis by stimulating Leydig cells in the testicular interstitium to produce testosterone. Stallion Leydig cells also produce large amounts of estrogens, most of which are conjugated. High concentrations of intratesticular testosterone are thought to be necessary for spermatogenesis to proceed normally. High circulatory testosterone feeds back to the brain and inhibits LH secretion. Sertoli cells within the seminiferous epithelium initiate and maintain spermatogenesis in response to FSH and testosterone. Sertoli cells also produce the protein hormone inhibin (which decreases pituitary gland secretion of FSH) and the protein hormone activin (which increases pituitary gland secretion of FSH). Although research is improving our understanding of more intricate endocrine control of spermatogenesis in horses and other species, clinicians can effectively use this endocrine control model (Figure 13-56) when attempting to diagnose an endocrine abnormality associated with subfertility or infertility in stallions.

The reader should note, however, that an endocrinologic basis for reproductive malfunction in stallions has not been firmly established. An exception is the administration of exogenous testosterone or anabolic steroids, both of which adversely affect spermatogenesis. One unrefuted application of a hormonal assay is to aid in diagnosing of cryptorchidism in horses without scrotal testes. In cryptorchids, baseline concentrations of testosterone and estrogens are often, but not always, elevated. However, a twofold or threefold increase in testosterone concentration in response to administration of 10,000 IU of human chorionic gonadotropin (hCG) (i.e., hCG stimulation test) indicates the presence of testes.

An abnormally high plasma concentration of FSH, sometimes accompanied by a high plasma concentration of LH, has been postulated to indicate testicular degeneration in older stallions. Conversely, a low

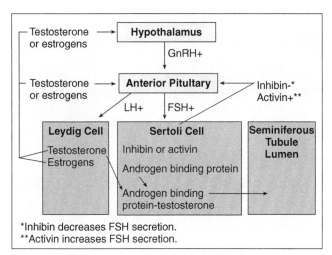

*Inhibin decreases FSH secretion.
**Activin increases FSH secretion.

Figure 13-56 A proposed model for reproductive hormone feedback control in a stallion. An elevated testosterone level in the bloodstream feeds back on the hypothalamus and anterior pituitary gland to suppress discharge of GnRH and thus LH, causing Leydig cells to produce less testosterone. As testosterone levels in the blood decline, the inhibiting effect of a high testosterone level on release of GnRH and LH is removed, permitting bursts of secretion to occur. In this model, estrogens are assumed to be produced primarily by the Leydig cells and to have a negative feedback effect similar to that of testosterone. Circulating FSH acts directly on Sertoli cells, which secrete the protein hormones inhibin and activin. When the FSH level is high, inhibin secretion rises, causing a subsequent decrease in the amount of FSH secreted by the anterior pituitary gland. As FSH secretion declines, activin secretion rises and causes a subsequent increase in FSH secretion by the anterior pituitary gland. Testosterone and FSH concentrations must be adequate to stimulate a Sertoli cell environment conducive to spermatogenic cell support and development. (From Blanchard TL, Varner DD: Evaluating breeding soundness in stallions: IV: hormonal assay and testicular biopsy, *Vet Med* April:358, 1996.)

plasma LH concentration has been associated with poor fertility in young stallions. Some investigators also contend that low libido or impotence in stallions may be related to low plasma concentrations of LH and estradiol-17β in the presence of normal testosterone values. Contradictory reports indicate that stallions with low plasma concentrations of LH and estradiol-17β can have excellent libido and semen quality. When collecting blood samples for hormone assays, one should remember that most hormones are released into the bloodstream in an episodic fashion; therefore, assays of single blood samples may not be truly representative of the endocrine status of the stallion. We recommend hourly collection of heparinized blood samples from 9 AM through 1 PM because this time is when gonadotropin and testosterone concentrations normally peak in the stallion. Plasma is harvested and kept chilled, and equal volumes of plasma from each sampling are mixed together to represent a pooled sample (from the 4-hour sampling), which is frozen and shipped overnight to the endocrine laboratory. The pooled samples should more closely represent a true average (i.e., "smooth out" the peaks and troughs) for each hormone assayed. Separate pooled samples are submitted for each hormone of interest because not all assays may be performed on a given day, and thus samples do not have to be thawed and refrozen. For this type of baseline screening, we request assays of LH, FSH, estradiol, testosterone, and inhibin in the pooled plasma samples. Poor semen quality is sometimes associated with low estradiol and inhibin concentrations and high FSH concentration in stallions with abnormal testicular function. On occasion, low testosterone and high or low LH concentrations also exist.

To pursue whether the endocrine anomaly is associated with hypothalamic, pituitary, or testicular abnormality, hormone stimulation tests can be performed. Intravenous administration of 5 to 25 μg of GnRH to normal stallions typically stimulates LH release (≥50% increase) in 15 to 30 minutes, followed by testosterone release (≥100% increase in 1 to 2 hours) (Figure 13-57). We recommend obtaining samples before administration of GnRH and at 15, 30, 60, and 120 minutes thereafter. Only LH and testosterone assays need to be performed on GnRH stimulation tests. If LH or testosterone response is inadequate, the stimulation can be repeated with larger doses (50 to 250 μg) of GnRH to determine whether the pituitary and testicular Leydig cells are capable of responding. Roser (1995) proposed that hCG stimulation testing should be done to determine whether an abnormality exists at the testicular level. Blood samples are collected before drug administration, then 10,000 U of hCG is administered intravenously and blood samples are collected 1, 2, and 48 hours later for testosterone assay. Testosterone concentrations should reach 3 to 6 ng/mL in 1- to 2-hour samples and may reach 9 to 12 ng/mL in 48-hour samples from

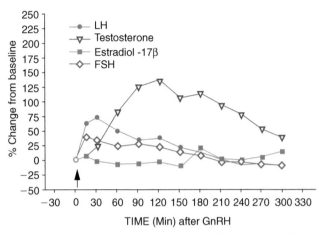

Figure 13-57 Results of intravenous administration of 15 µg of GnRH to a group of eight reproductively normal stallions. The *arrow* represents the time of GnRH administration.

stallions with a normal Leydig cell response. Failure of significant testosterone secretion to occur confirms that a primary testicular endocrine abnormality exists (most likely as a result of atrophied Leydig cells).

TESTICULAR BIOPSY

Although testicular biopsy has been recommended by some investigators as an innocuous diagnostic procedure for stallion infertility, we do not endorse it for routine use. Postoperative complications, such as sperm granuloma formation or intratesticular hemorrhage with an attendant increase in intratesticular pressure, could cause irreparable interference with spermatogenesis. However, biopsy provides the only method for direct assessment of testicular tissue parameters (e.g., hormone concentrations, stages of spermatogenesis, sperm production rates, and the presence of space-occupying lesions) and therefore provides useful information in some circumstances.

An aspiration biopsy is potentially less damaging than a punch biopsy but usually does not offer useful information about spermatogenesis. Aspiration biopsy may help in differentiation among causes of testicular enlargement, such as neoplasia, trauma, or septic orchitis. To provide a better sample of tissue for histologic interpretation, we prefer to use a spring-loaded biopsy instrument (e.g., Bard Biopty biopsy instrument, C.R. Bard Inc, Covington, GA) (Figures 13-58 and 13-59). Similar disposable biopsy instruments are also available (14- to 18- gauge). The technique can be performed using profound sedation with the horse standing; local anesthesia of the scrotum is unnecessary. The scrotum is disinfected, and the sterile biopsy instrument is pushed through the scrotal skin and fascia just through the outer tunica albuginea in the mid region of the cranial one third of the testis. The testis is held firmly, the instrument is triggered, and the needle is withdrawn (Figure 13-60). The tissue is transferred to a suitable fixative (Bouin's, Davidson's, paraformaldehyde, or glutaraldehyde); left

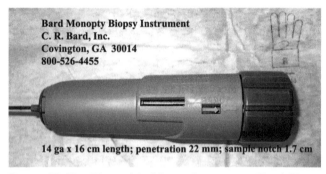

Figure 13-58 Disposable biopsy instrument (Bard Biopty biopsy instrument, C.R. Bard Inc) used to obtain testicular punch biopsy from the stallion. The needle punch end is not shown.

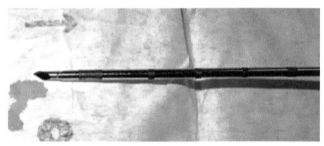

Figure 13-59 Needle-punch end of Bard Biopty biopsy instrument shown in Figure 13-58.

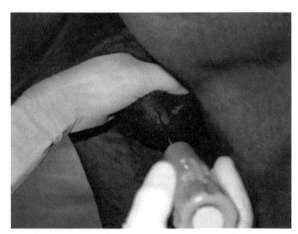

Figure 13-60 Procedure for procuring punch-biopsy specimen from the stallion testis. The stallion is sedated, and the scrotal skin scrubbed and disinfected. The testis is grasped firmly by one hand of the operator, and the needle of the "cocked" punch-biopsy instrument is inserted through the skin and tunics and into the outer parenchyma of the testis. The button trigger is pushed on the biopsy handle, which automatically forces the needle cutting surface inward and retracts the parenchymal sample back into the needle guide. The instrument is removed, and the biopsy sample is gently teased into fixative solution.

for 24 hours; transferred to alcohol; and processed for staining. Sufficient testicular tissue is present in biopsy specimens procured in this manner to evaluate whether qualitatively normal spermatogenesis is occurring (Figures 13-61 and 13-62). Pronounced testicular degeneration or the failure of spermatogenesis to proceed to sperm formation is also easily determined.

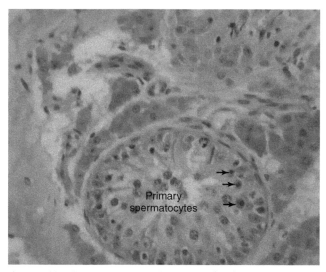

Figure 13-61 A representative testicular biopsy specimen procured with the Bard Biopty biopsy instrument from a stallion with azoospermia. The specimen was stained with periodic acid Schiff-hematoxylin. Spermatogenesis was not proceeding to completion, and several degenerating germ cells *(arrowheads)* were noted.

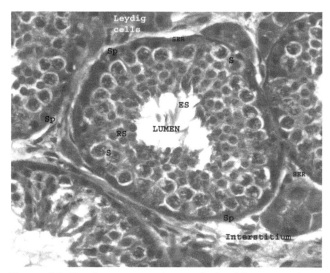

Figure 13-62 A representative testicular biopsy specimen (periodic acid Schiff-hematoxylin stain) procured with the Bard Biopty biopsy instrument. Normal seminiferous tubules are present, with Sertoli cells *(SER)*, spermatogonia *(Sp)*, spermatocytes *(S)*, round spermatids *(RS)*, elongating spermatidis *(ES)*, and Leydig cells in the interstitium.

INTERPRETATION OF FINDINGS: BREEDING SOUNDNESS EXAMINATION

An inherent drawback of a stallion fertility examination (or breeding soundness examination [BSE]) is imprecision stemming from the biologic nature of the specimens under consideration. Although the examination process has scientific merit, precision is impossible. In addition, factors other than innate stallion fertility, including mare fertility and management procedures, markedly influence pregnancy and foaling rates for a given stallion and often are difficult to control or assess.

The purpose of a fertility examination is to estimate a stallion's capability as a sire. Ideally, the testing process should produce sufficient information about a stallion to permit approximation of the number of mares to which that stallion can safely be booked during a breeding season. An indispensable ingredient in this formulation is the stallion's estimated daily sperm output (DSO). Numerous other factors also must be considered before a reasonable judgment can be made about a "stallion book."

Stallions typically are classified as satisfactory, questionable, or unsatisfactory breeding prospects. In general, to be classified as a satisfactory breeding prospect, stallions must be free of undesirable and potentially heritable defects, behavioral disorders, or transmissible diseases (venereal or otherwise); possess no physical traits that would interfere with mating ability, semen quality, or sperm output; and ejaculate 1×10^9 or more progressively motile, morphologically normal sperm in the second of two ejaculates collected 1 hour apart after 1 week of sexual rest. The categorizations are usually predicated on a stallion's ability to produce a seemingly low season pregnancy rate of 60%, but this percentage coincides with conditions for payment of fertility insurance the first year in which insured stallions stand at stud. This pregnancy rate assumes that the stallion breeds a standard number of mares (e.g., 40 to 45 mares by natural service or 120 to 140 mares by artificial breeding during a typical breeding season of 135 to 150 days). An additional stipulation is that the stallion be bred to mares of normal fertility under good management conditions. It is now known that most normal stallions can produce satisfactory pregnancy rates with much larger books of mares. Specific criteria that must be met before a prospective breeding stallion can be appropriately classified are discussed in depth in the Society for Theriogenology's *Manual for Clinical Fertility Evaluation of the Stallion.* The reader should refer to this official manual for a thorough discussion of the subject.

Although the breeding soundness examination serves as a guideline for prepurchase examination of a stallion intended for breeding purposes, we most commonly use information gained from the breeding soundness examination to develop management strategies that maximize pregnancy rates achieved by the stallion examined. It is rare, in our experience, for a stallion to be completely and irreversibly sterile (infertile), except for the old stallion with pronounced degeneration and shrinking of the testicles. Therefore, development of specific breeding management protocols for an individual stallion, based in large part on information gained from the BSE, can maximize the breeding usefulness of the stallion.

BIBLIOGRAPHY

Blanchard TL, Kenney RM, Timoney PJ: Venereal disease. In Blanchard TL, Varner DD, editors: Stallion management, *Vet Clin North Am Equine Pract* 8:191-203, 1992.

Blanchard TL, Varner DD, Miller C, et al: Recommendations for clinical GnRH challenge testing of stallions, *J Equine Vet Sci* 20:678-682,686,731-737, 2000.

Dahms BJ, Troedsson MHT: The effect of seminal plasma components on opsonisation and PMN-phagocytosis of equine spermatozoa, *Theriogenology* 58:457-460, 2002.

Hurtgen JP: Evaluation of the stallion for breeding soundness. In Blanchard TL, Varner DD, editors, Stallion management, *Vet Clin North Am Equine Pract* 8:149-166, 1992.

Kenney RM, Evenson DP, Garcia MC, et al: Relationships between sperm chromatin structure, motility, and morphology of ejaculated sperm, and seasonal pregnancy rate, *Biol Reprod Monogr* 1:647-653, 1995.

Kenney RM, Hurtgen JP, Pierson H, et al: *Manual for clinical fertility evaluation of the stallion*, Hastings, NE, 1983, Society for Theriogenology, 1-100.

Kenney RM, Kent MG, Garcia MC, et al: The use of DNA index and karyotype analyses as adjuncts to the estimation of fertility in stallions, *J Reprod Fertil* 44(Suppl):69-75, 1991.

Love CC, Garcia MC, Riera FR, et al: Evaluation of measures taken by ultrasonography and caliper to estimate testicular volume and predict daily sperm output in the stallion, *J Reprod Fertil* 44(Suppl):99-105, 1991.

Love CC, Garcia MC, Riera FR, et al: Use of testicular volume to predict daily sperm output in the stallion, *Proc 36th Ann Mtg Am Assoc Equine Pract* 15-21, 1990.

McCue P: *Equine viral arteritis [client information bulletin]*, Fort Collins, 2006, Colorado State University; available at www.cvmbs. colostate.edu/bms/ERL/evaupdate_f)6.pdf.

McDonnell SM: Normal and abnormal sexual behavior. In Blanchard TL, Varner DD, editors: Stallion management, *Vet Clin North Am Equine Pract* 8:71-90, 1992.

McDonnell SM: Ejaculation: physiology and dysfunction. In Blanchard TL, Varner DD, editors: Stallion management, *Vet Clin North Am Equine Pract* 8:57-70, 1992.

Meyers SA: Diagnosis of subfertility in stallions: evaluation of sperm function, *Proc Soc Theriogenol* 271-277, 1996.

Pickett BW, et al: *Procedures for collection, evaluation and utilization of stallion semen for artificial insemination*, Colorado State University experiment station animal reproduction laboratory general series bulletin, Fort Collins, 1987, Colorado State University.

Pickett BW, et al: *Management of the stallion for maximum reproductive efficiency: II*, Colorado State University experiment station animal reproduction laboratory general series bulletin, Fort Collins, 1989, Colorado State University.

Ramirez J: Equine viral arteritis, *Compendium Equine* 3:456-465, 2008.

Roser J: Endocrine profiles in fertile, subfertile, and infertile stallions: testicular response to human chorionic gonadotropin in infertile stallions, *Biol Reprod Monogr* 1:661-669, 1995.

Timoney PJ: Equine viral arteritis: is the disease a cause for industry concern? *Impulsion* 4-7,9-10, 2005.

Timoney PJ, McCollum WH: Equine viral arteritis, *Vet Clin North Am Equine Pract* 9:295-309, 1993.

Troedsson MHT, Desvousges AL, Hansen PJ, et al: Equine seimal plasma proteins protect live spermatozoa from PMN-binding and phogocytosis, while providing a mechanism for selective sperm elimination of apoptotic and dead spermatozoa, *Proc 9th Int Symp Equine Reprod Animal Reprod Sci* 94:60-61, 2006.

Troedsson MHT, Desvousges A, Alghamdi AS, et al: Components in seminal plasma regulating sperm transport and elimination, *Animal Reprod Sci* 89:171-186, 2005.

Turner RM: Alkaline phosphatase activity in stallion semen: characterization and clinical implications, *Proc Am Assoc Equine Pract* 42:284-293, 1996.

Varner DD, Schumacher J, Blanchard TL, et al: *Diseases and management of breeding stallions*, St Louis, 1991, Mosby, 61-96.

Varner DD, Brinsko SP, Blanchard TL, et al: Subfertility in stallions associated with spermatozoal acrosomal dysfunction, *Proc Am Assoc Equine Pract* 47:221-228, 2001.

Semen Preservation

14

CHAPTER

OBJECTIVES

While studying the information covered in this chapter, the reader should attempt to:
- Acquire a working understanding of the advantages and disadvantages of breeding with transported, cooled, or frozen equine semen.
- Acquire a working understanding of techniques and procedures used to process equine semen for cooling or freezing and to manage or breed mares with cooled or frozen equine semen.

STUDY QUESTIONS

1. List the ingredients in semen extenders that protect equine sperm against cold shock.
2. Discuss desirable cooling rates for minimizing damage to sperm in extended equine semen.
3. List the steps (in order) to be followed to prepare equine semen for cooling and shipment.
4. List the steps (in order) to be followed to freeze equine semen.
5. Discuss the reasons for, methods of, and expected fertility related to cryopreservation of epididymal sperm.
6. Discuss the methods for inseminating mares with cooled or cryopreserved semen.

EQUINE SEMEN PRESERVATION: COOLED AND FROZEN SEMEN

Most equine breed registries within the United States condone pregnancies achieved via artificial insemination. Many of the registries also permit artificial insemination with cooled or frozen semen. Before embarking on an artificial insemination program, particularly with cooled or frozen semen, one must obtain the current regulations for the breed registry of interest, because regulatory allowances may change without widespread notification.

Transported, cooled semen is used increasingly for breeding purposes in the United States, and most U.S. breed registries currently permit the use of cooled or frozen semen for off-site use. Preserved semen may be more commonly used outside the United States. It has been used on a large scale for artificial insemination in China, where hundreds of thousands of mares have been inseminated with transported frozen or cooled semen in recent years. In European countries, preserved semen is used predominantly for Warmblood, draft, and Standardbred breeds.

Sperm are sensitive to many environmental factors, including temperature, light, physical damage, and a variety of chemicals. Accordingly, the semen preservation process begins with the semen collection process; one should use precautions to thwart any environmentally induced injury to sperm (see Chapter 12). Damage to sperm from cold shock is attributed primarily to temperature-induced membrane perturbations and oxidative stress.

Cooling of extended semen for transport is generally successful if the initial quality of the semen is good, a proper storage technique is used, and insemination is not delayed beyond 24 hours. For some stallions, good pregnancy rates can be obtained with semen stored for 48 to 72 hours before insemination.

Currently, frozen preservation of stallion sperm generally yields poorer fertility than cooled storage and is also far less successful than frozen preservation of sperm from dairy bulls. Direct extrapolation of techniques used to freeze bull semen has yielded discouraging results with stallion semen, an outcome probably related to compositional differences between the sperm of the two species. Research has revealed that sperm of dairy bulls are unusually resistant to the effects of cryopreservation. This phenomenon is probably attributed to years of careful selection of bulls with sperm capable of surviving the freezing and thawing processes, a practice not followed in horse-breeding circles.

The economic incentives for improving techniques of semen preservation in stallions are becoming increasingly evident, as major breed registries now permit its use. Previously, limited financial support for research in this field had slowed progress in development of superior methods for preserving stallion semen, in both cooled and frozen forms. Advancements now being made in this area may lead to more prolonged storage intervals for cooled semen and successful cryopreservation of semen from a larger percentage of stallions.

GENERAL CONSIDERATIONS

Preservation of semen begins with the actual collection process. To ensure that sperm quality is optimized, semen should be collected as described in Chapter 12. Regardless of the technique of semen preservation to be used, semen must be placed in a suitable extender within a few minutes after collection from the stallion. To maximize success with preserved semen, one should screen for ejaculates of poor quality. If the quality of fresh stallion semen is poor (see Chapter 13) or if fertility achieved by breeding with fresh semen is poor, successful results are highly unlikely to be obtained by breeding with preserved semen.

Figure 14-1 provides an example of a processing form to be sent with the transported, cooled semen as a method of quality control. Copies of this form can be kept in a log book for the stallion owner to help maintain accurate records of mares being bred.

COOLED SEMEN

Extended semen from fertile stallions can oftentimes be stored in a cooled state for hours to days before insemination, without a significant reduction in pregnancy rate. Guidelines for maximizing the longevity of sperm viability after cooled storage follow.

Dilute Semen with a High-Quality Extender

Semen extenders contain protective ingredients that permit survival of sperm outside the reproductive tract. Lipoproteins, such as those contained in milk or egg yolk, protect sperm against cold shock by stabilizing cellular membranes. Metabolizable substrates, such as glucose, provide a plentiful source of energy for sperm. Antibiotics are added to extenders to retard or eliminate growth of bacterial organisms. The osmotic pressure and pH of extenders can be adjusted to maximize sperm survival. The osmolarity of milk-based extenders should be between 300 and 400 mOsm/L, with 350 mOsm/L considered to be optimal. The pH of semen extenders can probably range from approximately 6.5 to 7.2 without affecting the longevity of sperm viability during storage, but a pH of 6.7 to 6.9 may optimize sperm track linearity (i.e., a computerized motility assessment measure of the straightness of sperm movement). Extenders may be homemade formulations (see Table 12-1) or commercially available preparations (see Table 12-2). Nonfat dried milk solids–glucose (NFDMS-G) extender maintains better sperm motility in cooled semen than does heated skim milk extender, although fertilizing capacity may not differ between the two extenders. The NFDMS-G extender also maintains cooled sperm motility better than a sucrose-bovine serum albumin extender. No conclusive studies have been done to determine whether cream-gel– or egg yolk–based extenders are more or less desirable than milk-based extenders for enhancing either sperm viability or fertility in cooled equine semen. Milk-sugar extenders are the most popular formulations in the United States, and milk-based extenders are more commonly used worldwide than are egg yolk–based extenders. A commercial extender that has become quite popular in recent years in the United States is the French-developed INRA 96 extender (available though IMV Technologies, Maple Grove, Minn.). This extender contains native phosphocaeseinate derived from milk as the sole source of protein-based sperm membrane protection against cold shock. Other milk components were excluded from the composition of this extender because some were considered to be detrimental to sperm function.

The proper selection of antibiotics to include in the semen extender enhances the viability of stored semen.

Stallion Information: Name: Breed: Lip tattoo #: Registration number: Markings/Brands:	Owner/Agent: Name: Address: Telephone: Fax:
Processor Information: Name: Address: Telephone: Fax:	Referring Veterinarian: Name: Address: Telephone: Fax:

Semen information:

- Date and time of semen collection:
- Volume of raw gel-free semen (cc):
- Concentration of raw gel-free semen ($\times 10^6$/mL):
- Semen extender used:
- Antibiotic used:
- Dilution ratio:
- Sperm concentration of extended semen ($\times 10^6$/mL):
- Initial sperm motility (total/progressive):
- Initial sperm velocity (0-4):

- Date and time of semen shipment:
- Volume of extended semen shipped (cc):
- Total sperm number shipped ($\times 10^9$):
- Total number of progressively motile sperm shipped ($\times 10^9$):

- Recommended volume/insemination (cc):
- Number of insemination doses shipped:

Signature _____   Date _____

Figure 14-1 An example of an equine cooled semen transport form to accompany transported semen.

A combination of amikacin sulfate (1 mg/mL) and potassium penicillin G (1000 U/mL) was shown in one Texas study to be effective for control of bacterial growth and optimization of sperm motility of cool-stored semen. This antibiotic combination has also yielded excellent fertility in breeding trials. Timentin (ticarcillin disodium–clavulanate potassium; Glaxo-SmithKline, New York; 1 mg/mL) and Naxel (ceftiofur sodium; Pfizer Animal Health, Research Triangle Park, NC; 1 mg/mL) have also shown good control of aerobic bacterial growth and maintenance of sperm motility in laboratory conditions. One may wish to evaluate other antibiotics for inclusion in semen extender, because variations among individual stallions may

exist. It is important to use only antibiotics and antibiotic dosages that are not detrimental to sperm function. The objective of use of an antibiotic is elimination of all bacterial growth without hampering sperm viability. Antifungal drugs may be needed to control fungal growth, especially if the storage temperature exceeds 10°C to 12°C.

Ideally, semen should be mixed with a prewarmed (37°C) extender within 2 to 5 minutes after ejaculation. A minimum ratio of 1:1 (extender to semen) is recommended for immediate inseminations. If semen is to be stored for a period of 2 to 4 hours or longer before insemination, greater dilution (i.e., a higher extender-to-semen ratio) is usually necessary. A final concentration of 25 to 50 million sperm/mL in extended semen generally maximizes sperm survivability in vitro. To maximize sperm survival, a minimum of a 1:4 (i.e., 1 part semen to 4 parts extender) dilution should be obtained to ensure that the final seminal plasma concentration in extended semen is less than 20%. For dilute ejaculates (<100 million sperm/mL), centrifugation of the semen may be necessary to remove excess seminal plasma; resuspension of the sperm in extender may be necessary to ensure that no more than 20% seminal plasma remains in the extended semen and the final sperm concentration is at least 25 million sperm/mL.

The seminal plasma of some stallions can have a detrimental effect on sperm viability, even when the seminal plasma concentration is adjusted to 5% to 10% (volume/volume [v/v]) in the extended semen. In these circumstances, centrifugation of the semen after its initial dilution with extender can become necessary, followed by removal of virtually all of the seminal plasma. The pellet of sperm can then be resuspended in extender preloaded with sperm-free seminal plasma (5% to 10% [v/v]) from a fertile stallion that is known to possess good quality seminal plasma. In this circumstance, it is important to ensure that the seminal plasma of the donor is free of organisms that cause transmissible disease, such as equine viral arteritis, equine infectious anemia, or contagious equine metritis. Although sperm are best preserved when customary milk-based extenders contain 5% to 10% seminal plasma, a centrifuged sperm pellet devoid of seminal plasma can be placed in an extender type developed at Cornell University (Kenney extender with modified Tyrode's medium [KMT]). The composition of this extender (Table 14-1) is such that it eliminates the need for seminal plasma in the extender. Fertility trials with semen centrifuged to remove seminal plasma, followed by dilution of sperm in KMT extender and cooled storage, have yielded excellent results.

COOL SEMEN TO REFRIGERATED TEMPERATURE FOR STORAGE

Extended semen should be promptly removed from the incubator (37°C) because extensive sperm death occurs within a few hours if sperm are maintained at this temperature. Cooling extended semen to 4°C to 8°C for storage is superior to storage at room temperature (i.e., 20°C to 25°C) for breeding 1 to 2 days later. The longevity of sperm viability is probably improved by storage at near-refrigeration temperature compared with storage at higher temperatures because of a corresponding reduction in metabolic activity. Sperm fertilizing capacity is often maintained for 24 to 48 hours or longer when extended semen is stored at refrigerated temperature. Normal fertility has been reported after refrigerated storage of semen for periods of 72 to 96 hours for selected highly fertile stallions. If semen is stored at room temperature, fertility is often reduced after 12 to 24 hours. Some studies have suggested that a storage temperature of approximately 15°C may be superior for semen from some stallions, but more research is needed to determine whether this is the case.

When stallion semen is extended for transport and subsequent artificial insemination, a rapid change to temperatures of less than 18°C to 20°C causes sperm to undergo cold-shock damage. Currently, only passive cooling/transport systems are commercially available for use with stallion semen. Passive cooling systems generate variable rates of cooling (i.e., cooling rates become progressively slower as the target semen temperature is approached). Cooling rates may also vary according to environmental temperatures, initial temperature of semen, and volume of extended semen being cooled (Figure 14-2). Experimental studies have shown that an initial cooling rate of –0.3°C/min is most desirable for maximizing sperm viability. This cooling rate is achieved with the Equitainer I or Equitainer II (Hamilton Research Inc, South Hamilton, MA). Cooling rates from 20°C to 8°C are thought to be more critical for stallion sperm survival than are cooling rates from 37°C to 20°C, and a range of –0.05°C/min to –0.17°C/min is currently

TABLE 14-1

Formula for Kenney Extender Containing Modified Tyrode's Medium (KMT)*

NaCl	420 mg
KCl	187 mg
NaHCO$_3$	210 mg
NaH$_2$PO$_4$	5 mg
Na lactate (60% syrup)	0.31 mL
CaCl$_2$ • 2 H$_2$O	29 mg
MgCl$_2$ • 6 H$_2$O	8 mg
HEPES	238 mg
Na Pyruvate	11 mg
Amikacin sulfate	100 mg
Potassium penicillin G	1×10^5 units
Bovine serum albumin (fraction V)	600 mg
Deionized distilled water	qs 100 mL
Kenney extender containing modified Tyrode's medium	Mix MTM with a Kenney-type extender at a ratio of 35% MTM and 65% Kenney-type extender

MTM, Modified Tyrode's medium.
*Modified from Padilla AW, Foote RH: Extender and centrifugation effects on the motility patterns of slow-cooled stallion spermatozoa. *J Anim Sci* 1991;69:3308-3313.

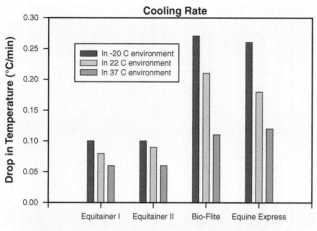

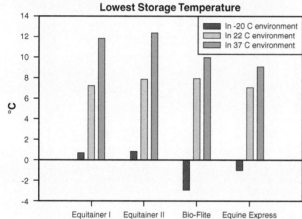

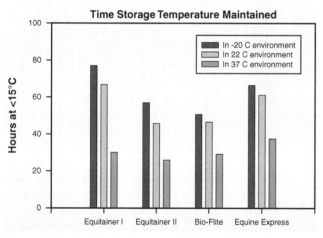

Figure 14-2 Effect of storage container on internal temperature when exposed to three different ambient storage conditions. Tests were performed on 40-mL volumes of extended semen. All extended semen was packaged according to manufacturer's recommendations. Containers were initially stored for 6 hours to mimic environmental conditions during shipment (i.e., in a freezer [–20°C] to mimic airline transport at high altitudes or ground transport in cold climates; at room temperature [22°C] to mimic ground transport in mild climates; and in an incubator [37°C] to mimic ground transport in hot climates). Containers in freezers for 6 hours were then moved to room temperature for the remainder of the storage period.

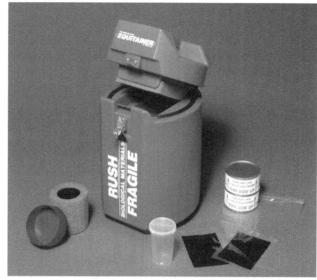

Figure 14-3 Components of the Equitainer I semen cooling/transport system: thermal container, coolant cans, cup and isothermalizer, plastic bag, and ballast bags.

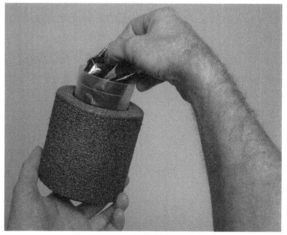

Figure 14-4 Placement of a prewarmed (37°C) ballast bag into the cup in the isothermalizer of the Equitainer. Each ballast bag contains 60 mL of diluent, and one or two ballast bags are used to bring the total volume of liquid placed into the isothermalizer to 120 to 170 mL, an amount necessary to ensure that the proper cooling rate is established for the extended semen.

recommended to maximize the maintenance of sperm motility. Final storage temperatures of 4°C to 8°C are currently thought to be superior to temperatures of 0°C to 2°C, but more studies are needed to determined whether this the case.

Commercial systems for semen storage, such as the Equitainer I, Equitainer II, and Equitainer Clipper (Hamilton Research Inc) (Figures 14-3 to 14-9); the Equine Express II (Exodus Breeders Corporation, York, PA) (Figure 14-10); and the Equine Semen Transporter (EST-SH, EST XL–SH, EST-S, and EST XL; Plastilite Corporation, Omaha, NE; Figure 14-11), greatly simplify transport of cool-stored stallion semen. Semen

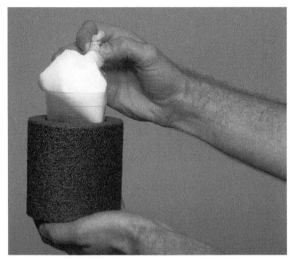

Figure 14-5 Placement of a double-bagged extended semen sample into the cup inside the isothermalizer of the Equitainer I. Residual air has been expressed, and bags have been sealed with tightly wrapped rubber bands.

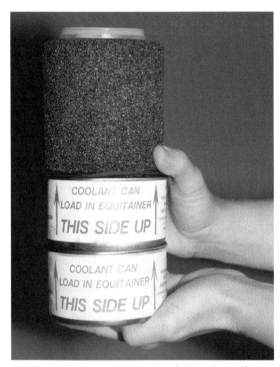

Figure 14-6 Placement of the loaded isothermalizer, which contains a capped semen cup with extended semen and ballast bag, on top of two cooling cans (frozen upside down in a freezer for 24+ hours before use).

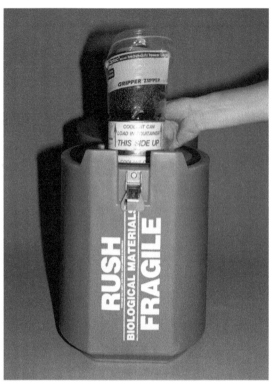

Figure 14-7 All components are loaded in the order shown in Figure 14-6 into a plastic bag to be inserted into the Equitainer, permitting easy removal of contents when the mare is to be bred.

is generally packaged in either plastic bags or all-plastic syringes before loading into semen shipment containers (Figure 14-12). The package type is dependent on the style of container used for semen transport. Heat sealing of packages provides a nice product, but should be done in such a manner that the heat-sealing process does not damage semen (Figures 14-13 and

14-14). Labels should be affixed to packaged semen so that pertinent information regarding the stallion identification, semen collection date, and mare to be inseminated is easily identified (Figure 14-15). Additional information should be made available on the accompanying semen transport form (see Figure 14-1).

Regulations for interstate shipment of semen are not well defined, so packaged semen is usually transported via air carrier throughout the United States without accompanying health certificates. Authorized shipment of semen outside the United States requires that specific regulations of the importing country be met. Health authorities responsible for importation of semen into other countries should be contacted to ensure that requirements are met before arrangement for semen transportation is made. Some countries require that extensive health screening (e.g., serologic testing, culturing of reproductive tract or semen, vaccination, inspection of premises and animals by regulatory officials) be performed before semen is collected for preservation.

Quarantine measures sometimes must be used for the stallion, farm, and mares maintained at the farm where the stallion stands to meet semen importation requirements. Cooled semen has been successfully imported into the United States from abroad for prompt insemination of mares, but considerable regulatory requirements must be met before shipments are authorized.

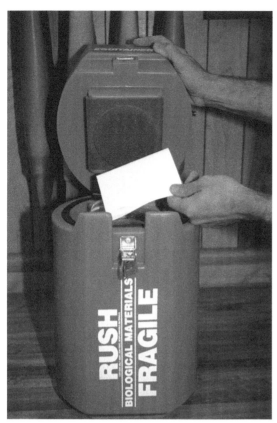

Figure 14-8 Placement of the record of semen shipment into the Equitainer I before closing and latching of the container. The latch should be secured before shipment. A record of semen shipment should be made regardless of the transport system used. Duplicate records should be maintained by the stallion owner/manager for reference if fertility or shipment problems arise. For an example of this form, refer to Figure 14-1.

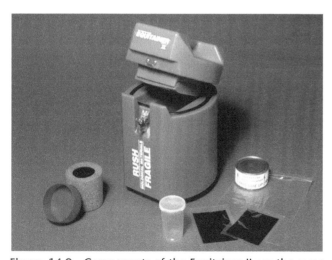

Figure 14-9 Components of the Equitainer II are the same as those for the Equitainer I, with the exception that only one coolant can is used. Both the Equitainer I and Equitainer II are also available with a lead shield in the cap that may aid to protect the semen against radiation damage during security screening.

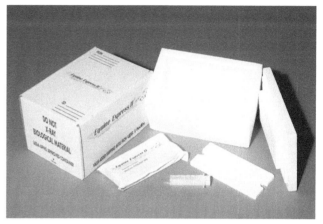

Figure 14-10 Components of the Equine Express II cooled semen transport system. *Clockwise from left:* cardboard shipping box, Styrofoam insulation box with lid, coolant pack, rubber caps for syringe tips, sterile syringes, and Styrofoam plank for separation of syringes from coolant pack. Two 30-mL or 50-mL all-plastic syringes are filled with warm (35°C to 37°C) extended semen, capped to prevent leakage, and placed into the Styrofoam box. The Styrofoam plank is placed over the semen-loaded syringes, and the frozen (24+ hours) coolant pack is placed on top of the Styrofoam plank. The Styrofoam lid is placed on top of the Styrofoam insulation box, and the entire assembly is boxed and prepared for shipment.

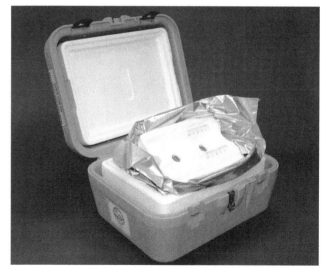

Figure 14-11 Components of the Equine Semen Transporter (EST XL–SH) reusable shipper for transported semen. This container accommodates either two polyethylene containers for bagged semen or two 50-mL all-plastic syringes. A lead-foil shield is also available for protection against airport security radiation. Extended semen is placed in plastic bags, the filled bags are placed in jars with cotton balls for impact protection, and the jars are placed in the tray. Syringes can be used instead of the jars for holding semen. The lid is placed on the tray, and rubber bands are placed around the tray. The coolant pack that has been frozen for at least 24 hours is placed in the bottom of the shipper, and the tray is placed (holes down) on top of the coolant pack. The lid is placed on the shipper and secured with logo labels to hold the lid tight on the base cooler. Documentation of the processed semen shipment is placed in a zipped bag and inserted into the interior lid recess. The corrugated box and luggage carrying case are then closed and secured for shipment.

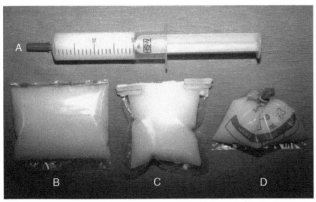

Figure 14-12 Packages for cooled-semen transport. *A,* All-plastic syringe. *B,* Baby-bottle liner sealed with heat-sealing instrument. *C,* Whirl-Pak bag. *D,* Baby-bottle liner sealed by twisting end and securing with rubber band. Storage of semen in capped all-plastic syringes or heat-sealed plastic bags *(A and B)* is probably preferable because these methods reduce the likelihood of semen leakage during transport.

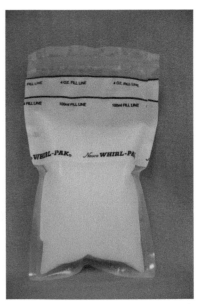

Figure 14-14 Heat-sealed plastic bag containing extended semen. Note that all air is removed from the plastic bag before sealing, and the heat seal is created away from the extended semen. This procedure protects the semen from heat-related injury without resulting in air-related injury to sperm during transport and also allows easy opening of the plastic bag without spillage of extended semen.

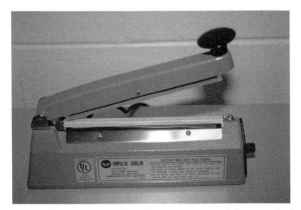

Figure 14-13 Heat-sealing instrument used for producing hermetic seals on plastic bags.

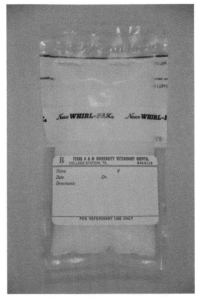

Figure 14-15 Heat-sealed bag containing extended semen. Note that the bag is equipped with an appropriate label so that information can be provided to the recipient of the semen regarding stallion identification, semen collection date, and mare to be inseminated. Additional information is available on the semen-transport form (see Figure 14-1).

Cool-transported semen that is transported "counter-to-counter" by commercial airlines may be subjected to radiographic security screening. One study revealed no adverse effects of x-radiation at doses up to 10 μSv (an exposure level similar to that of conventional airport security screening systems) on equine sperm motility (either initial motility or longevity of motility), sperm morphology, or fertility of irradiated semen. Mares bred with x-irradiated semen also delivered normal foals at term. However, recommendations for screening luggage on commercial flights in the United States may result in new radiographic screening requirements that could increase the amount of radiation exposure to 300 times or more than that currently used. Effects of exposure of horse semen to this amount of radiation remain unstudied. Hamilton Thorne Research Inc (Beverly, Mass.), provides a lead shield for their reusable transport systems that may protect semen from potential radiation damage; however, the shield overlies the top of the container and does not prevent radiation exposure to the

sample if the transport container is exposed to radiation from the side. The container is labeled to caution airport luggage screening personnel to only allow the container to be opened for less than 2 minutes during examination. The manufacturer has found that opening the container for less than 2 minutes does not interfere with the cooling rate or holding temperature of the stored extended semen. Plastilite Corp provides lead-foil shields for their reusable and disposable semen shipping systems.

The most accurate method for determining the inseminate dose (i.e., sperm number) necessary for transport for breeding is to conduct semen cooling trials for individual stallions. The semen is diluted in an appropriate extender as described previously and cooled for 24 hours in semen transport containers to be used by farm management personnel. The cooled semen sample is gently remixed after this cooling period, and an aliquot is warmed to 37°C. Sperm motility is evaluated 15 minutes after warming, and the percentage of progressively motile sperm obtained is used as a guideline to ensure that future shipments provide a minimum of 500 million progressively motile sperm after 24 hours of cooling. For example, if after 24 hours of cooling, the progressive sperm motility is 50%, 1 billion total sperm would need to be prepared for shipment to ensure that an insemination dose of 500 million progressively motile sperm was available for breeding a mare. The procedure can also be performed on semen cooled for 48 hours if demand for 48-hour cooled semen is suspected. If justified, more extensive studies of cooled semen can be conducted by reference laboratories, such as objective measurement of sperm motion, chromatin quality, membrane integrity, intact acrosomes, and morphology after cooled storage.

It has become common practice for some stallion owners/managers to prepare two insemination doses of extended semen for shipment: one to be used for an initial insemination on arrival, and one to be held for insemination again the next day. For many stallions, the longer the semen is held at a refrigerated temperature, the poorer sperm motility becomes. In addition, fertility of semen cooled for 48 hours tends to be reduced compared with that of semen cooled for only 24 hours. Except for special cases, we believe it is generally better to inseminate a mare with the transported semen as soon as practical after it arrives rather than to wait for breeding or to inseminate the mare twice, 24 hours apart, with the semen in that shipment. More research must be performed before convincing evidence shows that fertility is improved by holding a second insemination dose for breeding the day after the first insemination. Certainly, if two large doses of good-quality semen arrive, breeding the mare twice at 12- to 24-hour intervals might be advantageous. However, if sperm motility is poor when the semen arrives, it is unlikely that the second dose will survive an additional 12 to 24 hours of cooling. If the practitioner chooses to hold semen for breeding again the next day, precautions should be taken to maintain the cooled semen at 4°C to 6°C until the time of the second insemination. To ensure

that the temperature of the second dose of semen left in the shipping container does not increase above 10°C, causing premature sperm death, the remaining semen dose can be repackaged and the container placed in a refrigerator (4°C to 6°C) until it is opened for breeding the next day. Alternatively, the remaining packaged semen can be removed from the shipping container, wrapped in an insulting paper towel, and placed in a refrigerator that is set at approximately 4°C.

Breeding the Mare with Cooled Semen

When the cooled semen arrives for insemination of the mare, current recommendations are as follows:

1. Prepare the mare for breeding (see Chapter 12).
2. Open the shipping container, carefully remove the chilled semen, and gently mix it. Carefully aspirate the semen into a syringe (if the semen was not stored in a syringe during shipment), and attach an insemination pipette.
3. Inseminate the mare by infusing the semen into the mare's uterus. Uterine body breedings are adequate in most instances. Deep uterine horn inseminations may have an advantage when semen quality is poor or the mare is subfertile (see Chapter 12).
4. A small aliquot of the extended semen should be warmed to 37°C, and sperm motility should be assessed and recorded for quality control purposes. If sperm motility is poor, inquiries can be made to determine whether this was an unexpected problem. If sperm motility in additional shipments is consistently poor and the mare fails to conceive on repeated breedings, the stallion may possibly be incapable of producing sperm that survive the cooling/transportation process well. In such instances, use of a different semen extender or dilution ratio or experimentation with centrifugation and removal of excess seminal plasma might prove beneficial for improving livability of sperm harvested from that particular stallion.

Overseas workers often recommend warming the chilled semen to body temperature before insemination of the mare. In the United States, the chilled semen is usually placed directly into the uterus as soon as possible after the shipping container is opened. Because no detrimental effects on pregnancy rate have yet been determined by inseminating mares with as much as 170 mL of chilled semen, at present, we see no reason to prewarm the chilled semen before insemination.

CRYOPRESERVATION OF SEMEN

A variety of protocols are available for cryopreservation of stallion semen. Controlled studies that might disclose the most successful of these techniques have not been conducted. Marked variation exists among stallions with respect to "freezability" of semen and response to different cryopreservation extenders, so cryopreservation protocols probably need to be individualized to accommodate these idiosyncrasies. Pregnancy rates are reported to range from 0 to more than 70% per cycle when frozen-thawed stallion semen is used for insemination, with pregnancy rates per cycle in the 25% to 40% range for a high percentage of stallions. Some studies, however, have reported similar per-cycle pregnancy rates in mares inseminated with cooled versus frozen semen. Although the technique works well for select stallions, much improvement is needed in the technique so that semen can be successfully frozen from a larger percentage of stallions. Intensified reproductive management of mares (e.g., repeated palpations and ultrasound examinations to ensure insemination close to ovulation, deep uterine horn breeding, and postbreeding uterine therapy) may also be necessary to enhance pregnancy rates achieved by breeding with frozen-thawed semen.

Semen cryopreservation implies storage of sperm at subzero (i.e., frozen) temperatures. The cryogen normally used for this task is liquid nitrogen (–196°C). If sperm withstand the freezing and thawing process, sperm integrity may be maintained almost indefinitely in liquid nitrogen because metabolic activity of sperm is considered to be negligible at this temperature. If sperm from a given stallion respond favorably to the freeze-thaw cycle, they possibly may retain their function for centuries when maintained at –196°C. Cells at this temperature are in a form of suspended animation, and cellular reactions are generally limited to that associated with free radical formation and background ionizing radiation.

Semen cryopreservation has the potential of adding a new dimension to the horse breeding industry by allowing long-term preservation of sperm from superior stallions and permitting distribution of this semen to breeding establishments worldwide. Such a breeding policy would maximize usage of select stallions and greatly reduce mare shipping/boarding costs and transmission of contagious diseases. Geographic constraints would be abolished; thus, mare owners could select semen from a larger pool of stallions, including deceased stallions from which semen had been stored frozen.

Undesirable aspects related to the use of cryopreserved semen are also apparent. For instance, pregnancy rates are typically reduced for a high percentage of stallions, given the existing technology in this area. An increased number of progeny of popular stallions may arise if good pregnancy rates are achieved with their cryopreserved semen, as compared with that of other stallions. Reduction in the genetic pool is also possible if all mare owners have access to semen of select sires. Opportunities for errors and corruption would also increase but could be held in check by quality control during processing steps and incorporation of techniques for documenting parentage.

Several features of sperm are considered important for fertilization and must be retained after cryopreservation if normal fertilizing capacity is to be expected: progressive motility, normal metabolism, intact cellular membranes, the presence of acrosomal enzymes, intact surface-associated proteins responsible for sperm-egg interactions, and uninjured nucleoprotein. Cryopreserved sperm undergo tremendous stresses associated with freezing, thawing, and insemination that could render them nonviable. Fertility of stallions is often compromised when cryopreserved semen is used for insemination of mares. Although individual stallion variation exists, a fairly large percentage of a sperm population sustains fatal injury as a result of the freeze-thaw cycle. A subset of processed sperm incurs sublethal disturbances that render these cells incapable of fertilization or, possibly, may lead to postfertilization failure. Functional disturbances are ascribable primarily to perturbations in membrane properties (including lipid rearrangements, protein clustering, and alterations of membrane receptor sites), disruption of cytoskeletal elements, and disturbances of nuclear composition. The alterations in these subcellular constituents result from susceptibility of sperm to temperature changes, osmotic and oxidative stressors, and the intrinsic toxic properties imparted by cryoprotectants. Given the destructive forces associated with cryopreservation, that any sperm could survive the process seems amazing.

The technique for cryopreservation of stallion sperm involves several steps.

Increasing Sperm Concentration and Reducing Seminal-Plasma Concentration

This procedure is conducted to increase sperm concentration such that insemination doses can be loaded into small packages (Figure 14-16), while reducing the percentage of seminal plasma contained in the resuspension medium. The centrifugation process can be circumvented by collecting only the initial portion of the ejaculate (sperm-rich portion) in an artificial vagina to increase sperm concentration; however, the use of cushioned centrifugation techniques (see Chapter 12) greatly enhances sperm harvest and permits a more sensible method for adjusting seminal plasma concentration in resuspended semen to the desired level (generally 5% to 10%). If centrifugation is performed, the semen must first be mixed with an appropriate centrifugation medium (Tables 14-2 and 14-3; see also Tables 12-1 and 12-2) to minimize cellular injury. Centrifugation time and force should be adjusted to maximize sperm yield while maintaining sperm viability. A centrifugation force of $500 \times g$ for 10 minutes is generally a safe centrifugation technique

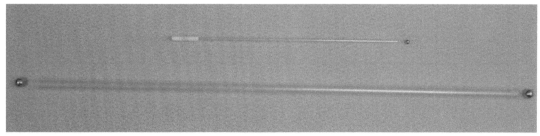

Figure 14-16 Five-mL German macrotubes and 0.5-mL French-style straws are the most commonly used packages for cryopreservation of stallion semen. Sealing balls for both types of straws are shown. The 5-mL macrotubes can also be cut in half before filling to create straws with a 2.5-mL capacity.

TABLE 14-2

German Centrifugation and Cryopreservation Media Used for Freezing Equine Sperm

Centrifugation Medium (Merck I Extender)

D-Glucose	60.00 g
Trisodium citrate dihydrate	3.75 g
Disodium ethylenediaminetetraacetic acid (EDTA)	3.70 g
Sodium bicarbonate	1.20 g
Potassium penicillin G	1,000,000 U
Amikacin sulfate	1.00 g
Deionized distilled water	qs 1000 mL

Adjust pH to 6.9 with sodium bicarbonate
Extender can be frozen at –20°C in smaller aliquots until used

Cryopreservation Medium

D-Lactose solution (11% w/v)	50.0 mL
Centrifugation medium (Merck I extender)	25.0 mL
Egg yolk	20.0 mL
Glycerol	5.0 mL
Equex STM (Nova Chemical Sales, Scituate, Mass.)	0.8 mL

w/v, weight/volume.

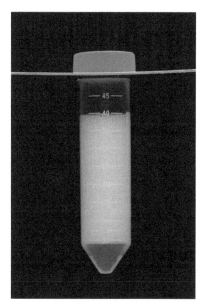

Figure 14-17 Fifty-mL conical centrifugation tube containing extended semen *(white)* and underlying cushion fluid *(clear)*. After centrifugation, the sperm relocate to the area directly overlying the cushion fluid. The sperm pellet is recovered by first aspirating the semen extender down to a line midway between the 7.5-mL and 5.0-mL marks on the tube and then aspirating the cushion fluid with a long small-bore open-ended catheter or blunt spinal needle.

for 40 to 45 mL of extended semen in 50-mL centrifuge vials. The centrifugation rotor should have swinging buckets to ensure that the pellet of sperm is in the bottom of the tube after centrifugation is performed. A centrifugation technique that is becoming more popular is referred to as cushioned centrifugation; this technique uses a cushion fluid during centrifugation (Figure 14-17). The addition of a relatively high-density cushion fluid permits increased centrifugation force and time, thereby improving sperm recovery rate without an attendant drop in sperm viability (see Chapter 12). After centrifugation, most of the seminal plasma is removed from above the sperm pellet. Although the technique is not studied intensively, workers generally recommend that some seminal plasma is retained in the resuspended semen sample, such that the final seminal plasma concentration is approximately 5% (v/v) in the semen extended in cryopreservation extender.

Adding Cryopreservation Medium

The extenders for cryopreservation (examples in Tables 14-2 to 14-5) of stallion semen generally consist of various mixtures of egg yolk, milk, sugars, buffers,

TABLE 14-3

Skim Milk–Based Centrifugation and Cryopreservation Media for Freezing Equine Sperm

Modified Kenney (TAMU) Centrifugation Medium

Nonfat dry milk solids (e.g., Sanalac)	24.0 g
Glucose	26.5 g
Sucrose	40.0 g
Potassium penicillin G	1,000,000 U
Amikacin sulfate	1.0 g
Sodium bicarbonate (1 mEq/mL)	6.0 mL
Deionized distilled water	qs 1000 mL

This extender may be frozen at –20°C until used

Cryopreservation Medium

Centrifugation medium (listed above)	93.0 mL
Egg yolk	4.0 mL
Glycerol	3.0 mL

Once egg yolk and glycerol are added, do not refreeze

TAMU, Texas A&M University.

electrolytes, antibiotics, and a cryoprotectant, such as glycerol. The cryopreservation medium is added back to the pellet of sperm after the initial centrifugation and supernatant aspiration, and the sperm are gently resuspended in sufficient cryopreservation medium to achieve the desired concentration of sperm. A variety of semen extenders are available commercially that can be used for cryopreservation of stallion semen. Oftentimes, these extenders are clarified so that the processing personnel can more readily visualize sperm microscopically after thaw. In addition, various cryoprotectants (e.g., glycerol, methylformamide, dimethylformamide, or dimethylsulfoxide) may be used, singularly or in combination, at variable concentrations.

The final sperm concentration in cryopreservation medium can range from 100 million sperm/mL to 1.6 billion sperm/mL, depending on straw size and number of straws desired for a complete insemination

TABLE 14-4

INRA 96–Based Cryopreservation Media for Freezing Equine Sperm

INRA 96 Extender	96.5 mL
Clarified egg yolk	2.0 mL
Glycerol	2.5 mL

TABLE 14-5

Some Commercial Sources of Extenders Used for Cryopreservation of Equine Semen in the United States

E-Z Freezin – "LE" Extender; E-Z Freezin – "MFR5" Extender	Animal Reproduction Systems 14395 Ramona Avenue Chino, CA sales@arssales.com
INRA Freeze	IMV USA 11725 95th Avenue North Maple Grove, MN contact@imvusa.com
EquiPro CryoGuard Complete	Minitube of America Gent Extender PO Box 930187 Verona, WI usa@minitibe.com
Botu-Crio	Biotech Botucatu João Passos 573 – Center São Paulo, Brazil bbiotechnotucatu@yahoo.com.br Product available in the United States

dose. A breeding dose of 400 to 800 million total sperm is common when traditional insemination techniques are used. Measurement of sperm concentration can be achieved with a hemacytometer (see Figures 12-17 and 13-32), but a newly developed commercial instrument, the NucleoCounter (Chemometec A/S, Allerod, Denmark) (see Figure 12-19), is well adapted for quick and reliable measurement of sperm concentration in opaque solutions, such as cryopreservation medium.

Packaging Semen

Stallion sperm most commonly are packaged in small-volume straws (0.5-mL or 5-mL capacity) (see Figure 14-16). The 5-mL straws generally contain 600 to 800 million total sperm, and one straw is used per breeding. The 0.5-mL straws usually contain considerably fewer sperm (50 to 100 million), so more than one straw may have to be used to provide an adequate insemination dose (often six to eight straws). Recent studies suggest that the insemination dose may be reduced when applying low-dose insemination techniques (see Chapter 12). Cryopreservation of semen in 0.5-mL straws provides a more uniform freeze rate than that offered in 4- to 5-mL straws, and some studies indicate that postthaw semen quality is enhanced when semen is frozen in the 0.5-mL straws. Other studies indicate that post-thaw semen quality is not affected by package diameter.

Straws should be labeled with pertinent data such as stallion identification, breed registration number, processing date, and laboratory identification. Bar codes can also

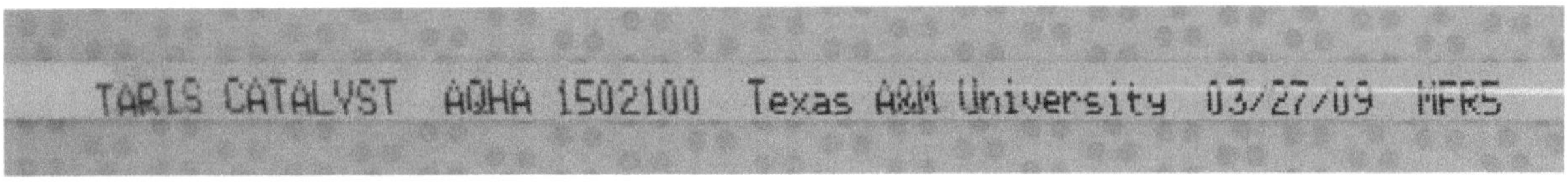

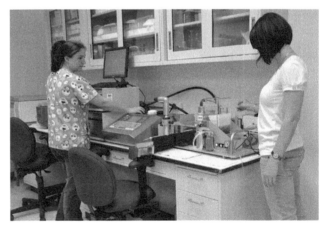

Figure 14-18 A 0.5-mL straw labeled with stallion identification, breed registry, registration number, semen-processing location, date of processing, and cryopreservation extender used.

be printed on the straws, in certain instances. Commercial equipment is available for this purpose (Figure 14-18), but companies that distribute straws often offer a service of prelabeling straws for specified purposes. Straw loading can also be done manually or with semiautomatic equipment (Figure 14-19) or fully automated equipment (Figure 14-20) that is available commercially. Straws must be hermetically sealed before initiation of the freezing process (Figure 14-21), and an air space should be present in the straws before sealing to permit expansion of the frozen contents. After sealing of the ends of the straws, the air space is shaken to the center before initiation of the freezing sequence to reduce likelihood of liquid nitrogen access into the straw lumen during storage (Figure 14-22).

Freezing Semen

The most common cryogen for semen cryopreservation is liquid nitrogen. Packaged semen can be placed horizontally in static nitrogen vapor at a recommended level (1 to 4 cm) above the liquid-gas interface, with use of a specially designed rack (Figure 14-23). Alternatively, packaged semen can be frozen in a programmable nitrogen freezer (Figures 14-24 and 14-25). Processing personnel are encouraged to use the prefreeze cooling technique and the freezing technique recommended by the manufacturer when commercial cryopreservation extenders are used. We have observed that, with glycerol-based cryopreservation extenders

used in our laboratory, post-thaw sperm viability is enhanced when semen is subjected to a 90-minute prefreeze cooling period before being subjected the freezing process. We have also observed that a programmable freezer can result in a more repeatable freezing curve and can result in improved post-thaw sperm viability, when compared with a static vapor freeze. In our laboratory, loaded straws are placed in the chamber of a programmable liquid nitrogen cell freezer (CBS Freezer 2100 Series; Custom Biogenics Systems, Shelby Township, MI). The chamber cooling/freezing ramps that we typically use in this system are $-2.0°C/min$ from approximately $25°C$ to $22°C$; $-0.3°C/min$ from $22°C$ to $10°C$; $-0.2°C/min$ from $10°C$ to $4°C$; and $-60°C/min$ from $4°C$ to $-140°C$. These cooling and freezing ramps are based on studies conducted by French workers.

Figure 14-20 Example of a fully automatic straw filler that can be used for rapid filling, sealing, and labeling of straws. This instrument is available from IMV USA.

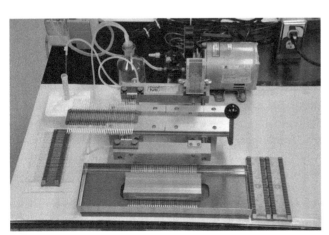

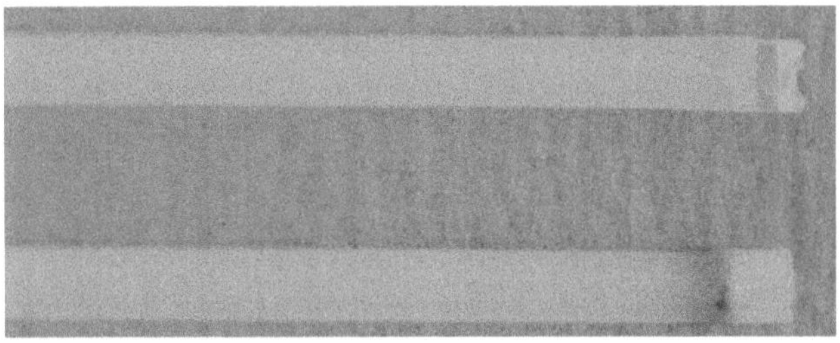

Figure 14-19 Example of a semiautomatic straw filler that can be used for moderately rapid filling and sealing of straws that have been prelabeled. This instrument is available from Minitube of America, Verona, Wis.

Figure 14-21 Image of 0.5-mL straws sealed with ultrasonic seal (with instrument in Figure 14-20) or stainless steel ball (with instrument in Figure 14-19).

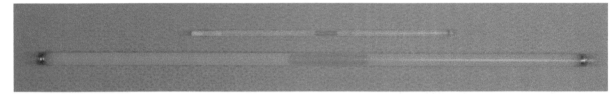

Figure 14-22 Straws (0.5-mL and 5-mL) that are loaded with extended semen, following by moving the air bubble to the center of the straw to help prevent movement of liquid nitrogen into the straw lumen. Access of liquid nitrogen into the straw lumen likely results in rapid expansion of the compressed gas during thawing and destruction of the straw and contained semen.

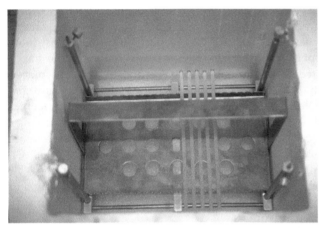

Figure 14-23 Semen-loaded 5–mL straws are placed on a rack before being suspended in liquid nitrogen vapor. Once the contents of the straws have been frozen (e.g., after 15 to 20 minutes in the nitrogen vapor), the straws are plunged directly into the liquid nitrogen for several minutes before the straws are transferred to a liquid nitrogen holding tank.

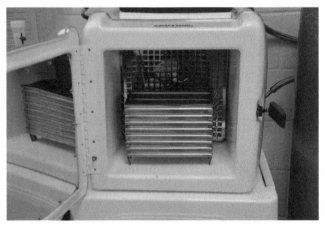

Figure 14-25 Straw racks can be designed for stacking so that hundreds of straws can be frozen simultaneously when placed in the chamber of a programmable freezer. Personnel in our laboratory prefer a programmable freezer with a side-loading chamber, as opposed to a top-loading chamber. Racks with straws containing semen are placed within the freezer chamber and the door is closed. Nitrogen vapor is emitted into the chamber to permit freezing of semen. The rate at which vapor is emitted into the chamber to control for specific cooling and freezing rates can be set via computer.

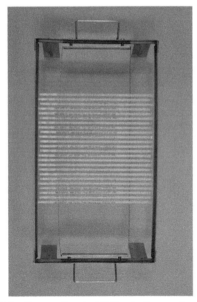

Figure 14-24 Semen-loaded 0.5-mL straws placed on a rack designed for cryopreservation.

Storing Semen

Semen is submerged in liquid nitrogen (–196°C) contained in specially designed storage tanks (dewars) to maintain sperm in a dormant state (Figure 14-26). Although 5-mL straws are generally placed directly into dewar canisters, 0.5-mL straws are most suitably placed into plastic goblets, which are then attached to canes before placement into canisters (Figure 14-27). Alternatively, straws can be loaded into small color-coded goblets contained within large outer goblets for direct placement into canisters of liquid nitrogen dewars (Figure 14-28).

A straw of the cryopreserved semen from each freezing should be thawed and warmed to 37°C for 10 to 15 minutes to determine post-thaw sperm motility. Some workers consider that post-thaw motility after longer periods of incubation may be a better measure of sperm function. Frozen semen can also be sent to a

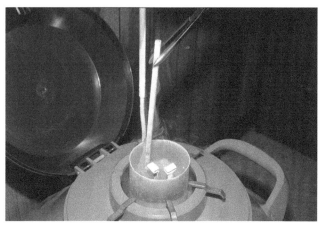

Figure 14-26 Liquid nitrogen storage tank (dewar) fitted with six canisters for holding straws of semen. Five-mL straws are generally placed directly into canister for storage, and 0.5-mL straws are generally placed in goblets attached to aluminum canes (shown within canister).

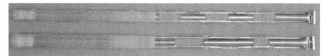

Figure 14-27 Small (0.5-mL) straws are generally placed into plastic goblets, which are then snapped onto aluminum canes before placement in the canisters of liquid nitrogen dewars. Goblets are available in different sizes. Shown are a goblet containing six straws (*upper*) and a goblet containing 10 straws (*lower*).

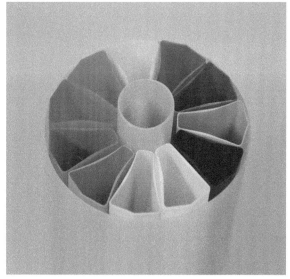

Figure 14-28 For maximized storage space within canisters of liquid nitrogen dewars, 0.5-mL straws can be stored in numerous small color-coded goblets within encompassing outer goblets. These goblets can then be stacked in dewar canisters to avoid the use of aluminum canes.

reference laboratory for more extensive testing of post-thaw sperm quality. A record of this post-thaw sperm viability should be kept, and a form containing semen-freezing information should accompany transport of semen sent to a storage facility (Figure 14-29).

Thawing Semen

Packaged semen is thawed in a water bath. Bath temperature and immersion time are generally designated by the company or individual responsible for freezing the semen. The thawing method is generally dictated by straw size, specifically the straw diameter. In most instances, 0.5-mL straws can be thawed in a 37°C water bath for 30 seconds. Sperm survivability is probably enhanced with a rapid thawing method, and some investigators have suggested that thawing 0.5-mL straws in a 75°C water bath for 7 seconds may yield higher post-thaw sperm motility. Others have recommended thawing 0.5-mL straws in a 46°C water bath for 20 seconds. Although this may be the case, the submersion time must be critically monitored to prevent overheating of straw contents with a water bath set at values above 37°C. For 5-mL "macrotube" straws, the thawing rate is generally 40 to 42 seconds in a water bath set at 50°C. Accurate measurement of submersion time is advisable with this technique, as is inversion of the straw during the thawing process, such that sperm in the periphery of the straw are not overheated.

Insemination

Immediately after thawing, packaged semen is inseminated, with the technique prescribed by the company or individual responsible for freezing the semen. For most stallions, the best pregnancy rates are probably achieved when mares are inseminated within 0 to 12 hours before ovulation or within 6 to 8 hours after ovulation. This can be achieved with frequent transrectal monitoring of the mare's ovarian state and use of ovulation-inducing drugs. Although this method has proven to be reliable and reduces wastage of cryopreserved semen, studies have also shown that timed insemination can yield similar fertility results. Daily transrectal examination with insemination at 24 and 40 hours after administration of an ovulation-inducing drug has become a popular method of insemination timing, and trials indicate that pregnancy rate is similar to that of postovulatory insemination. When this technique is used, mares are generally inseminated with a half dose of frozen-thawed semen at each of the two insemination times, such that the total sperm number in the inseminate is similar to that used with postovulation insemination. Others have reported acceptable fertility with timed insemination at 32 and 40 hours, or at 30 and 48 hours, after administration of an ovulation-inducing drug.

The standard insemination dose has customarily been set at 400 to 800 million total sperm. If post-thaw

Stallion Information: Name: Breed: Registration #: Age: Present breeding status: ☐ Sexually rested ☐Actively breeding ☐DSO Total testicular volume (cc): Estimated daily sperm output ($\times10^9$): Additional information:	Client:	Veterinarian:

Semen Collection:
Date of collection:
Volume (cc):
[Sperm] ($\times10^6$/mL):
Total sperm # ($\times10^9$):
Initial motility (total/progressive [velocity]):
Sperm morphology (%):

Normal:	Abn heads:
Abn. Acrosomes:	Det. Heads:
Abn M/P:	Bent Midpieces:
Prox. Drop.:	Dist. Drop.:
Bent tails:	Coiled tails:
P.G.C.:	Other:

Total number of morphologically normal, progressively motile sperm ($\times10^9$):

Centrifugation:
Centrifugation extender used:
  ☐ German ☐ TAMU ☐ Other:
Antibiotic used:
  ☐K$^+$ pen. G ☐ Amikacin sulfate ☐ Other:
Centrifugation tubes used:
  ☐50-mL plastic ☐ 50-mL glass
Centrifugation time: G-force:
Sperm number recovered in pellet ($\times10^9$):
Sperm recovery rate:

Straw Information:
  ☐ Stallion name:
  ☐ Stallion breed:
  ☐ Registration number:
  ☐ Processing date:
  ☐ Processing location:
  ☐ Extender used:
  Additional information:

Freezing Technique:
Freezing extender used:
  ☐ German Number of straws:
  ☐ TAMU Number of straws:
  ☐ Other Number of straws:
Antibiotic used:
Straw size: ☐ 0.5 mL ☐ 5 mL ☐ Other:
Method: ☐ Static vapor ☐ Programmable freezer
Sperm per straw ($\times10^6$):

Microbiological information:
Equine Viral Arteritis (EVA) test and vaccination: ☐ Test not performed ☐ Vaccination not performed
  Test: Date: Results:
  Vaccine used: Date:
Semen bacterial culture results (bacteria isolated): ☐ Test not performed
  Pre-freeze semen:
  Post-thaw semen:
Other tests performed: ☐ None
  Test: Date: Results:
  Test: Date: Results:

Post-thaw sperm evaluation:
Number of straws evaluated:
Water bath: Temperature: °C Time: Sec.

Extender		
% Motile sperm		
% Progressively motile sperm		
Sperm velocity (0-4)		
Number motile sperm/straw		
Number prog. motile sperm/straw		

General assessment:

Extender:
  ☐ Post-thaw sperm viability appears good
  ☐ Post-thaw sperm viability appears marginal
  ☐ Post-thaw sperm viability appears poor
Extender:
  ☐ Post-thaw sperm viability appears good
  ☐ Post-thaw sperm viability appears marginal
  ☐ Post-thaw sperm viability appears poor

Figure 14-29   Example of equine frozen semen processing form.

progressive sperm motility is 35%, then the insemination dose extrapolates to 140 to 280 million progressively motile sperm. Similar to that with fresh or cooled semen, considerable individual stallion variation probably exists regarding the threshold insemination dose that maximizes fertility with frozen-thawed semen. One report from the United Kingdom revealed a high pregnancy rate (64%) when mares were inseminated conventionally with only 14 million motile sperm from two pony stallions. A French study indicated that pregnancy rate was no different when mares were inseminated with 400 million versus 800 million sperm when breeding was performed once, within 24 hours before ovulation. Similarly, another European study indicated no difference in fertility for mares inseminated with 100 million or 800 million frozen-thawed sperm when post-thaw progressive motility was more than 35%.

Direct insemination near the tip of the uterine horn on the side ipsilateral to the ovulating follicle has become popular in recent years in an effort to improve pregnancy rate with frozen-thawed semen or to reduce the sperm dose necessary to achieve commercially acceptable fertility. This has been accomplished with advancement of a double-lumen catheter via transrectal guidance to the tip of the uterine horn for semen deposition or via video endoscope-directed (i.e., hysteroscopic) deposition of semen on or near the oviductal papilla at the tip of the uterine horn (i.e., at the uterotubal junction). With the latter technique, a specially designed insemination catheter is passed through the biopsy channel of the video endoscope. On the basis of findings in the literature, these two deep-horn insemination techniques currently tend to yield similar results, but extensive studies have not been conducted to determine definitively whether either of these techniques yields an advantage over conventional insemination in the uterine body when the inseminate contains more than approximately 15 to 25 million progressively motile sperm. One experimental trial did reveal that hysteroscopic insemination yielded higher fertility than conventional uterine body insemination when the insemination dose was lowered to 3 million frozen-thawed sperm. Please refer to Chapter 12 for more information on low-dose insemination techniques.

Cooling Semen for Transport Before Cryopreservation

Many facilities do not have experienced personnel or equipment for cryopreservation of semen, so a likely alternative is transport of the semen to a referral laboratory where the cryopreservation procedures can be performed. Earlier studies yielded lowered post-thaw sperm viability when stored for 24 hours before cryopreservation. More recently, however, cooled storage of extended semen for 18 to 24 hours before cryopreservation has yielded pregnancy rates similar to those of semen immediately subjected to cryopreservation without prior cooled storage.

The best method for processing of semen before cooled storage is not yet resolved. Fertility similar to that with control frozen-thawed semen (i.e., that not subjected to a prolonged period of cooled storage) has been achieved when semen was centrifuged before cooled storage, followed by addition of glycerol and cryopreservation. Likewise, good fertility results have been realized when semen was simply diluted and subjected to cooled storage, followed by centrifugation at room temperature and semen cryopreservation. Milk-based extenders, or milk egg yolk–based extenders, have been used successfully for cooling semen before cryopreservation. Skim-milk egg-yolk freezing extender and Botu-Crio (Biotech Botucatu, São Paulo, Brazil) freezing extender have yielded acceptable pregnancy rates for cool-stored semen, and these extenders may be superior to lactose ethylenediamine tetraacetic acid (EDTA) freezing extender, based on existing laboratory results. Research directed at comparing these extenders in fertility trials is needed.

Freezing Epididymal Sperm

The untimely loss of a breeding stallion, such as that associated with catastrophic injury, acute illness, or sudden death, may necessitate that epidymal sperm be cryobanked for future use. This procedure has also been applied to sexually naive stallions subjected to elective castration. In this circumstance, the owner of the stallion may be reluctant to have the stallion exposed to a sexual environment (such as with those stallions in athletic competition) but wish to castrate the stallion and preserve its germ plasma for future use. Our success (i.e., number of normal sperm and post-thaw sperm motility) when epididymides are flushed from chronically ill stallions has been poor.

Most experimental studies indicate that the fertility of cryopreserved epididymal semen is much lower than that of cryopreserved ejaculated semen, but the reason for this disparity is presently not known. One recent Brazilian report, however, revealed a high pregnancy rate (69%; 9 of 13) with cryopreserved epidymal semen preserved in Botu-Crio extender.

If the facility where the stallion is located does not have the personnel or equipment required for isolation and cryopreservation of epididymal sperm, the surgically removed testes and accompanying epididymides can be shipped to a referral center for processing. The castration method should be performed in a manner such that the epididymis is not damaged during the procedure and the ductus deferens is transected at a location approximately 8 to 10 cm distal to its junction with the cauda epididymis. The distal end of the ductus deferens should then be ligated to prevent loss of sperm from the ductus lumen (Figure 14-30). The testis

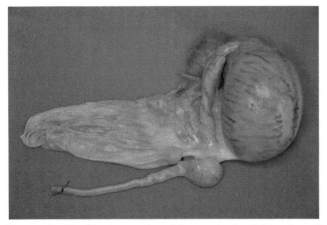

Figure 14-30 Equine testis, with attached epididymis and ductus deferens. The common (parietal) tunic has been open and reflected to allow easy visualization of these structures. The location at which the ductus deferens is ligated before shipment (black suture material) is also shown.

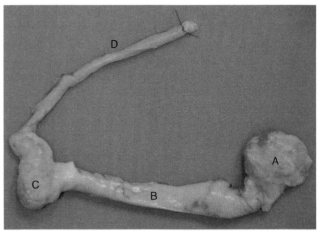

Figure 14-31 Equine epididymis and ductus deferens after dissecting free from testis and other connecting tissues. *A,* Epididymal head (caput); *B,* Epididymal body (corpus); *C,* Epididymal tail (cauda); *D,* Ductus deferens.

and attached epididymis/ductus deferens can then be rinsed with isotonic saline solution or other balanced salt solution, then placed in a sealed plastic bag for transport. For shipment to a referral center, the bagged contents should be shipped at refrigerated temperature (i.e., approximately 4°C to 6°C). This can be accomplished by placing the tissues in a passive-cooling container, such as an Equitainer, that has been fitted with frozen coolant cans. The tissues should be separated from the coolant cans with some paper towels to prevent direct contact of the tissues with these cans.

Alternatively, the plastic bag containing the tissues can be wrapped in paper towels, then placed in a Styrofoam container fitted with frozen gel packs used for transport of biologic materials. Research reports suggest that the tissues can be stored at refrigerated temperature for 24 hours, or possibly 48 hours, without significant damage to the epididymal sperm.

Controversy exists regarding the method to extract sperm from the epididymis and the need for mixing seminal plasma with the epididymal sperm before cryopreservation. Most of the sperm in the extragonadal ducts are generally stored within the tail (cauda) of the epididymis and the adjoining segment of the ductus deferens, and the sperm number in each epididymal tail and ductus deferens can be as high as 20 to 30 billion. These two sites are considered to be the storage depot for mature sperm, whereas sperm in the more proximal regions of the epididymis (body or corpus, and head or caput) are immature and probably not capable of fertilization without assisted reproductive techniques, such as intracytoplasmic sperm injection (ICSI). Therefore, only sperm within the epididymal tails and ductus deferentia should be collected for processing (Figure 14-31).

Techniques reported for harvesting sperm from the epididymis include the "flotation" (or "float-up") method and the "retrograde flushing" method. The flotation method entails separating the cauda epididymis and adjoining ductus deferens from the remaining portions of the epididymis and then slicing these tissues abundantly with a sharp scalpel while they are suspended in extender. The mixture is gently agitated for approximately 10 minutes in an effort to allow sperm to escape into the medium from the confines of the epididymal and deferent ducts. The retrograde flushing technique entails isolating the epididymis from the testis. The distal end of the ductus deferens opening can be threaded with a tomcat catheter (2.5F) or a blunt 16- to 18-gauge needle for retrograde flushing of medium (Figure 14-32). These devices should be secured in position to create an air-tight seal when the flushing procedure commences. An alternative is to thread the end of the ductus deferens with a 100- to 200-μL air-displacement pipette tip that is properly fitted to the Luer tip of a plastic syringe. In this instance, digital pressure can be applied to ensure an air-tight seal at the pipette tip–ductus deferens interface when flushing is attempted.

Before flushing, the epididymal duct can be dissected free of overlying fascia in the region of the epididymal cauda, then the epididymal cauda can be transected with a sharp scalpel blade (Figure 14-33). The contents of the epididymis only exit from one duct of the transected epididymis because it is a singular highly coiled duct. The contents of the ductus deferens and epididymal cauda are then removed by flushing with approximately 10 to 12 mL of medium, with care taken to prevent spillage of the contents outside the collection reservoir (Figures 14-34 and 14-35). Our laboratory uses the retrograde flushing method of

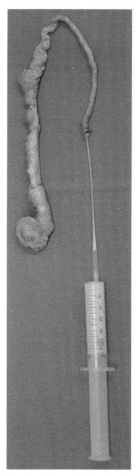

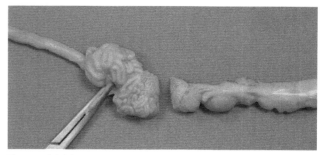

Figure 14-33 Transection of the epididymal cauda with a scalpel blade, showing the majority of the epididymal cauda and attached epididymis *(left)* separated from a portion of the epididymal cauda and epididymal corpus *(right)*. The cauda was transected within the cauda, as opposed to the junction of the cauda and corpus, to avoid including immature sperm in the flush contents. Approximately 12.4 billion sperm were recovered after retrograde flushing of this epididymal cauda and ductus deferens.

Figure 14-32 Catherization of the ductus deferens with a tomcat catheter. The catheter is inserted into the end of the ductus deferens immediately after transecting the site proximal to the ligation point (see Figure 14-30). The catheter is inserted approximately 1 cm into the ductus deferens and is firmly secured in position with two tight ligatures. An all-plastic syringe containing 12 mL of semen extender is attached to the catheter. Note the passage of epididymal semen into the catheter when the catheter is inserted into the lumen of the ductus deferens. This is the reason behind ligating the ductus deferens before shipment (i.e., to avoid unnecessary loss of sperm during transport).

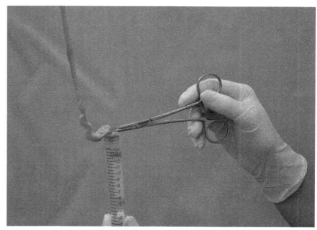

Figure 14-34 Positioning of epididymis and ductus deferens for retrograde flush. One attendant slowly pushes fluid into the ductus deferens while another attendant positions the cut end of the epididymal cauda into the opening of a 15-mL capacity tube. The epididymis is held in position with a pair of forceps, and care is taken not to grasp any portion of the epididymal duct, as this would occlude the lumen and prevent sperm from exiting.

sperm recovery because the resulting sample is less likely to be contaminated with blood.

The ideal medium to be used for flotation or retrograde-flush methods of sperm recovery is subject to debate. Arguments exist in the literature both for and against exposing epididymal sperm to seminal plasma, in an effort to simulate sperm exposure to conditions consistent with ejaculated semen. Media used for harvesting epididymal sperm have included fresh-semen extenders, cryopreservation extenders, seminal plasma, and balanced salt solutions. Although no consensus exists regarding the most appropriate medium to be used, the best fertility results reported to date for cryopreserved equine epididymal sperm were obtained with retrograde flushing of the epididymal ducts with a milk-based extender containing no seminal plasma.

Recovered epididymal sperm are subjected to cryopreservation, with the methods described previously. One Brazilian study revealed that post-thaw motility of epididymal sperm was better when Botu-Crio was used as the cryopreservation extender, as compared with other commonly used cryopreservation extenders (INRA 82 and lactose EDTA).

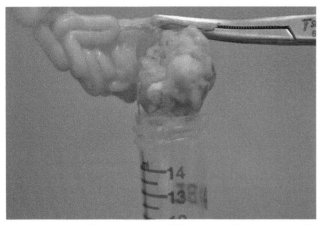

Figure 14-35 Close-up view of Figure 14-34, showing the distention of the ductus deferens and adjoining epididymal duct as semen extender is pushed through the lumen. Semen is seen exiting the epididymal duct and is captured in the plastic tube. Care is taken to direct the flow of epididymal semen directly into the tube with no splashing of semen outside the tube.

SUMMARY

Preservation of stallion semen in the cooled or frozen state may reduce the costs and potential health hazards incurred by transporting mares and provides easier access to genetic material that may otherwise be unavailable. Acceptable pregnancy rates are consistently obtained with cooled semen. Conversely, techniques for cryopreservation of stallion semen require more refinement before the procedure can be considered successful over a large population of otherwise fertile stallions. Cryopreservation of epididymal sperm can be attempted as a last course of action to preserve the germ plasma of a stallion lost for breeding purposes. The fertility of cryopreserved epididymal sperm, however, has generally been significantly lower than that of frozen ejaculated semen.

BIBLIOGRAPHY

Aurich C: Recent advances in cooled-semen technology, *Anim Reprod Sci* 107:268-275, 2008.

Backman T, Bruemmer JE, Graham JK, et al: Pregnancy rates of mares inseminated with semen cooled for 18 hours and then frozen, *J Anim Sci* 82:690-694, 2004.

Ball BA: Oxidative stress, osmotic stress and apoptosis: impacts on sperm function and preservation in the horse, *Anim Reprod Sci* 107:257-267, 2008.

Barbacini S, Loomis P, Squires EL: The effect of sperm number and frequency of insemination on pregnancy rates of mares inseminated with frozen-thawed sepermatozoa, *Anim Reprod Sci* 89:203-205, 2005.

Brinsko SP, Varner DD: Artificial insemination and preservation of semen. In Blanchard TL, Varner DD, editors: Stallion management, *Vet Clin North Am Equine Pract* 8:205-218, 1992.

Brinsko SP, Varner DD, Love CC, et al: Effect of feeding a DHA-enriched nutriceutical on the quality of fresh, cooled and fozen semen, *Theriogenology* 63:1519-1527, 2005.

Brinsko SP, Crockett EC, Squires EL: Effect of centrifugation and partial removal os seminal plasma on equine spermatozoal motility after cooling and storage, *Theriogenology* 54:129-136, 2000.

Brinsko SP, Rowan KR, Varner DD, et al: Effects of transport container and ambient storage temperature on motion characteristics of equine spermatozoa, *Theriogenology* 53:1641-1655, 2000.

Brum AM, Sabeur K, Ball BA: Apoptotic-like changes in equine spermatozoa separated by density-gradient centrifugation or after cryopresevation, *Theriogenology* 69:1041-1055, 2008.

Clulow JR, Mansfield LJ, Morris LH, et al: A comparison between freezing methods for the cryopreservation of stallion spermatozoa, *Anim Reprod Sci* 108:298-308, 2008.

Crowe CAM, Ravenhill PJ, Hepburn, et al: A retrospective study of artificial insemination of 251 mares using chilled and fixed time frozen-thawed semen, *Equine Vet J* 40:572-576, 2008.

Kayser JP, Amann RP, Shideler RK, et al: Effects of linear cooling rate on motion characteristics of stallion spermatozoa, *Theriogenology* 38:601-614, 1992.

Kloppe LH, Varner DD, Elmore RG, et al: Effect of insemination timing on the fertilizing capacity of frozen/thawed equine spermatozoa, *Theriogenology* 29:429-439, 1988.

Leipold SD, Graham JK, Squires EL, et al: Effect of spermatozoal concentration and number on fertility of frozen equine semen, *Theriogenology* 49:1537-1543, 1998.

Love CC, Brinsko SP, Rigby SL, et al: Relationship of seminal plasma level and extender type to sperm motility and DNA integrity, *Theriogenology* 63:1584-1591, 2005.

Loomis PR, Graham JK: Commercial semen freezing: individual male variation in cryosurvival and the response of stallion sperm to customized freezing protocols, *Anim Reprod Sci* 105:119-128, 2008.

Melo CM, Papa FO, Fioratti AISB, et al: Comparison of three different extenders for freezing epididymal stallion sperm [abstract], *Anim Reprod Sci* 107:30, 2008.

Melo CM, Zahn FS, Martin I, et al: Effects of cooling stallion semen for 24 h before freezing on fertility rates, *Anim Reprod Sci* 89:250-252, 2005.

Metcalf ES: The efficient use of equine cryopreserved semen, *Theriogenology* 68:423-428, 2007.

Miller CD: Optimizing the use of frozen-thawed equine semen, *Theriogenology* 70:463-468, 2008.

Moran DM, Jasko DJ, Squires EL, et al: Determination of temperature and cooling rate which induce cold shock in stallion spermatozoa, *Theriogenology* 38:999-1012, 1992.

Morris LHA, Tiplady C, Allen WR: Pregnancy rates in mares after a single fixed time hysteroscopic insemination of low numbers of frozen-thawed spermatozoa onto the uterotubal junction, *Equine Vet J* 35:197-201, 2003.

Palmer E: Factors affecting stallion semen survival and fertility [abstract], *Proc 10th Int Congress Anim Reprod* 377, 1984.

Papa FO, Melo CM, Fioratti EG, et al: Freezing of stallion epididymal sperm, *Anim Reprod Sci* 107:293-301, 2008.

Pillet E, Batiellier F, Duchamp G, et al: Freezing stallion semen in INRA96-based extender improves fertility rates in comparison with INRA82, *Dariy Sci Technol* 88:257-265, 2008.

Reger HP, Bruemmer JE, Squires EL, et al: Effects of timing and placement of cryopreserved semen on fertility of mares, *Equine Vet Educ* 15:101-106, 2003.

Rigby SL, Brinsko SP, Cochran M, et al: Advances in cooled semen technology: seminal plasma and semen extender, *Anim Reprod Sci* 68:171-180, 2001.

Saragusty J, Gacitua H, Pettit MT, et al: Directional freezing of equine semen in large volumes, *Reprod Domest Anim* 42:610-615, 2007.

Sieme H, Harrison RA, Petrunkina AM: Cryobiological determinants of frozen semen quality, with special reference to stallion, *Anim Reprod Sci* 107:276-292, 2008.

Sieme H, Schäfer T, Stout TAE, et al: The effects of different insemination regimes on fertility in mares, *Theriogenology* 60:1153-1164, 2003.

Squires E, Barbacini S, Matthews P, et al: Retrospective study of factors affecting fertility of fresh, cooled and frozen semen, *Equine Vet Educ* 18:96-99, 2006.

Varner DD, Blanchard TL: Current perspectives on handling and storage of equine semen, *Proc Am Assoc Equine Pract* 40:39-40, 1994.

Varner DD: Developments in stallion semen evaluation, *Theriogenology* 70:448-462, 2008.

Vidament M, Ecot P, Noue P, et al: Centrifugation and addition of glycerol at 22°C instead of 4°C improves post-thaw motility and fertility of stallion spermatozoa, *Theriogenology* 54:907-919, 2000.

Waite JA, Love CC, Brinsko SP, et al: Factors impacting equine sperm recovery rate and quality following cushioned centrifugation, *Theriogenology* 70:704-714, 2008.

Surgery of the Mare Reproductive Tract

15

CHAPTER

O BJECTIVES

While studying the information covered in this chapter, the reader should attempt to:
- Acquire a working knowledge of the conformational defects acquired through injury during parturition or that develop insidiously in aged, multiparous mares.
- Acquire a working understanding of the surgical procedures and techniques used to correct conformational abnormalities that contribute to infertility in the mare.

S TUDY Q UESTIONS

1. Discuss injuries that occur during parturition and result in abnormal conformation of the genital tract.
2. Discuss conformational defects of the urogenital tract that occur in aged, multiparous mares and contribute to infertility.
3. Describe procedures and techniques for a Caslick's vulvoplasty.
4. Describe the procedure for a breeding stitch in the vulva.
5. Describe the procedure for a perineoplasty (i.e., vestibuloplasty).

6. Describe the procedure used to create a urethral extension for treatment for urine pooling.
7. Describe the procedure used to treat a mare with a third-degree perineal laceration.
8. Describe the procedure used to treat a mare with a rectovaginal fistula.
9. Describe the procedure for treating a mare with a cervical laceration.
10. List preoperative and postoperative considerations for urogenital surgery in the mare.

Surgical procedures performed on the mare reproductive tract (with the exceptions of cesarean section, surgical correction of uterine torsion, and ovariectomy) are performed primarily to correct urogenital abnormalities that contribute to contamination of the reproductive tract. Contamination results from injuries that occur during parturition or from conformational changes that occur as mares age. This chapter discusses only the most common surgical procedures performed to reconstruct vulvar, vestibular, and cervical abnormalities. For more detailed descriptions of

these and other surgical procedures involving the reproductive tract, the reader should refer to veterinary medical-surgical texts.

SELECTION OF CANDIDATES FOR SURGERY

Mares with conformational changes of the urogenital tract that can be corrected with surgical reconstruction are candidates for surgery, provided that the results of a thorough breeding soundness examination indicate that the procedure has a good chance of restoring the mare's fertility. An exception to the need for a breeding soundness examination is a mare with a rectovestibular laceration or fistula, because these injuries nearly always arise in fertile, young mares during foaling as a result either of fetal malposture during delivery or inadequate dilation of the caudal birth canal sufficient to allow foal passage without tissue disruption. Indeed, such a mare has no reason to be infertile once contamination of the reproductive tract is prevented by surgical reconstruction. However, for other procedures used for surgical correction of reproductive abnormalities, a breeding soundness examination is indicated to assess the breeding potential of the mare. If severe and irreparable damage to the endometrium, cervix, vagina, or vestibule has occurred, the owner may elect not to invest time and money into surgery and aftercare.

Before any surgical procedure is performed, the practitioner should ensure that the mare has been adequately immunized against tetanus.

Defects commonly corrected with reconstructive surgery of the reproductive tract include the following:
- **Pneumovagina** caused by a cranially sunken anus and tipping of the vulva (see Figure 1-12).
- **Urovagina** caused by cranioventral deviation of the vagina, which pulls the urethral orifice cranially, resulting in urine splashing into the vestibule and vagina during urination (see Figure 4-19).

Perineal injuries occur during foaling and are characterized by tearing of the shelf between the rectum and vestibule (Figure 15-1). **Third-degree perineal lacerations** or **rectovestibular lacerations** (the most severe type of perineal injury) are those

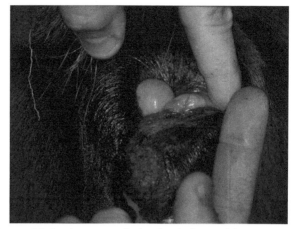

Figure 15-2 A rectovestibular fistula located just cranial to the anal sphincter. A finger has been passed through the fistula from the vestibule into the rectum to illustrate the location of the fistula. Fistulas can be small or large. They may be located in the vagina, but most are located in the vestibule.

that extend from the vestibule into the lumen of the rectum and through the perineal body. A laceration through the dorsal aspect of the vestibule that perforates the rectum but does not disrupt the perineal body is termed a **rectovestibular fistula**. The fistula often results in contamination of the vestibule and vagina with feces, but because the perineal body is intact, the laceration may not be readily apparent (Figure 15-2). Cervical lacerations arise from tearing of an insufficiently dilated cervix during normal delivery or during dystocia (see Figure 4-12).

PNEUMOVAGINA

Pneumovagina is a condition leading to constant fecal contamination of the vestibule and vagina because of conformational faults that cause a mare to aspirate air into the tubular portion of the reproductive tract. The condition is commonly called "wind sucking" and usually culminates in ascending infection of the vagina, cervix, and endometrium. Causes of pneumovagina include tearing or stretching of the vulvar seal or the vulvovaginal sphincter (see Chapter 1) and a sunken perineal body, characterized by cranial displacement of the anus and resulting in tipping of the vulva cranially over the brim of the pelvis (see Figure 1-12). The condition is quite common in underweight, aged, pluriparous mares.

The most common surgical procedure used to correct pneumovagina is the **Caslick's operation**, sometimes referred to as a **vulvoplasty**. For a Caslick's vulvoplasty, the mare is placed in a stock, and her tail is wrapped and directed away from the perineum. The perineum and vulva are scrubbed with a disinfectant soap, rinsed, and dried, and the dorsal aspect of the mucocutaneous margin of each labium is desensitized with a local anesthetic solution, such as lidocaine. The

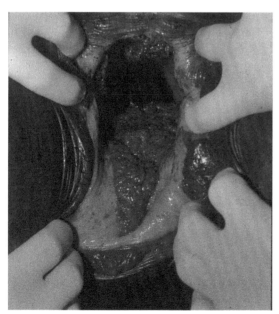

Figure 15-1 Third-degree perineal laceration in a mare. The perineal body and rectovestibular shelf were breached during foaling. Extensive fecal contamination is apparent.

mare can be sedated, or a twitch can be applied to its upper lip to prevent the mare from moving excessively during infiltration of the labia with local anesthetic solution. The local anesthetic solution is injected subcutaneously at the dorsal commissure of the vulva (Figure 15-3) and infiltrated along the margin of each labium to slightly below the floor of the ischium. The level to which the margins of the labia are sutured ventrally can be determined by placing firm pressure with the fingers on either side of the vulva and pressing down to locate the ischium. If the labia are not sutured to slightly below the floor of the ischium, the vulva may migrate far enough cranially, as the mare moves, to permit air to be aspirated into the vagina. Care should be taken to ensure that the ventral portion of the vulva remains spacious enough to allow urine to escape during urination, insertion of the stallion's penis during copulation, and insertion of a vaginal speculum, if the mare is to be bred via artificial insemination. If the ventral aspect of the vulva is sufficiently spacious, the surgeon should be able to easily insert four fingers into the vulvar opening after the operation is completed.

After the mucocutaneous margin of the right and left labia is infiltrated with local anesthetic solution, a thin strip of tissue, approximately 0.5 cm wide, is removed at the mucocutaneous junction of each labium with scissors (Figure 15-4). Removal of strips wider than this results in a large scar, which complicates subsequent Caslick's operations. The margins of the labia are apposed intimately with no. 0 or 00, nonabsorbable sutures (Figure 15-5). The type of suture pattern used is not important, if the labial margins are closely apposed, because little tension is exerted on the suture line. Patterns commonly used include simple continuous, continuous interlocking, and continuous horizontal mattress. Sutures should be removed at 10 to 14 days, at which time the wound should be healed.

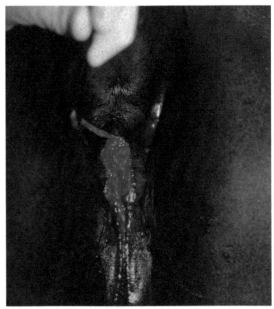

Figure 15-4 Caslick's operation. A thin strip of skin at the mucocutaneous junction of vulvar lips is excised to prepare for suturing.

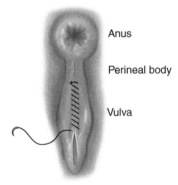

Figure 15-5 Caslick's operation. The debrided vulvar lips are apposed intimately with suturing. A simple continuous pattern is shown in this illustration, but a continuous interlocking suture pattern is more commonly used.

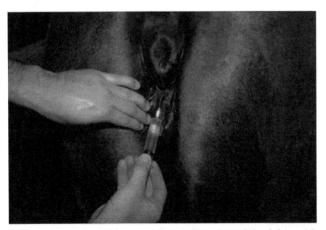

Figure 15-3 Caslick's operation. Infiltration of the labia with a local anesthetic solution. The area anesthetized should extend from the dorsal commissure of the vulva to just below the floor of the ischium.

If the labia must be opened for breeding, for vaginal examination, or for unobstructed foaling, they should be reapposed when a large vulvar opening is no longer necessary. A **breeding stitch** is a single, simple interrupted suture sometimes placed at the ventral aspect of the vulvar closure to preclude the need to open the sutured labia of a mare that must be bred (Figure 15-6). Umbilical tape or heavy, polymerized caprolactam suture (e.g., Vetafil, S. Jackson Co, Washington, D.C.) is commonly used for the breeding stitch. The suture bite should extend at least 1 cm abaxial to the margin of each labium, and the deep portion of the suture should be buried in the labial submucosa so that it does not abrade the stallion's penis during breeding. The suture is placed loosely enough to allow stretching of the ventral aspect of the sutured labia, but not so loosely that it allows the sutured tissue to tear.

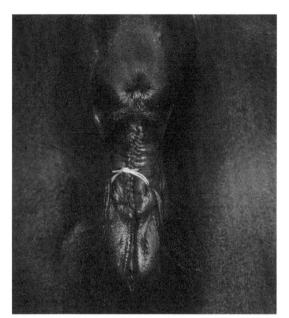

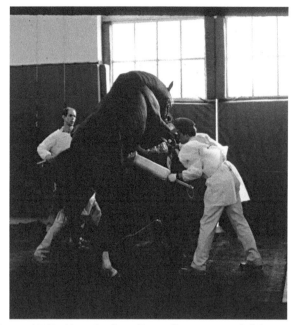

Figure 15-6 A breeding stitch is sometimes placed at the ventral aspect of the vulvoplasty to preclude the need to open the vulvoplasty if the mare must be bred with natural service. A single, simple interrupted suture is placed at the ventral edge of the vulvoplasty with a large, nonabsorbable suture, such as Vetafil. The suture bite should extend at least 1 cm abaxial to the vulvar labia, and the deep portion of the suture should be buried in tissue so that it does not abrade the stallion's penis during copulation. The suture is tied loosely so it provides tension only when the vulvar opening is stretched.

Figure 15-7 Use of a breeding roll to prevent full intromission of the stallion's penis into the vagina during natural service. The roll is inserted above the base of the penis, between the groin of the stallion and the rump of the mare, during breeding.

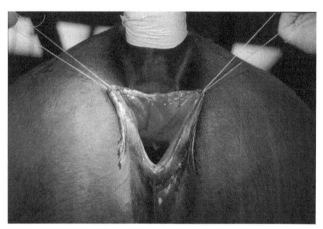

Figure 15-8 Modified perineoplasty as described by Dr. Steven Slusher. After the surgical area is desensitized, retraction sutures are placed to the right and left of the dorsal commissure of the vulva. The dorsal aspect of the labia are retracted caudally and dorsally to expose the dorsal mucosal surface of the vestibule.

Use of a breeding roll helps to limit the extent of penile intromission during natural service to avoid tearing of the sutured tissue or the breeding stitch (Figure 15-7).

The entire vulva of a mare with an extremely sunken anus and perineal body may be deviated so far cranially and ventrally that the vulvar cleft assumes a nearly horizontal position over the ischium. A Caslick's suture may not correct pneumovagina in such mares or may prevent the mare from adequately expelling urine. For prevention of both pneumovagina and urine pooling caused by this extreme conformational abnormality, the perineal body must be reconstructed (i.e., **perineoplasty** or **vestibuloplasty**). We often perform a modified vestibuloplasty, as described by Slusher (1986). This vestibuloplasty entails removal of an isosceles triangle of mucosa from the dorsal aspect of the vestibule.

In preparation for reconstruction of the perineal body, as described by Slusher (1986), the mare is sedated, and the perineum is desensitized with administration of 2% lidocaine or mepivacaine (1 to 1.25 mL/100 kg) through an 18- or 20-gauge, 1.5-inch (3.8-cm) needle inserted into the epidural space. The dorsal aspect of the vestibule is exposed by retracting each labium laterally, with a loose suture or Backhaus towel clamp placed through the labium at the juncture of its dorsal one third and ventral two thirds and with retraction of the dorsal

commissure of the vulva dorsally and caudally, also with a loose suture or towel clamp (Figure 15-8). A point on the dorsal aspect of the vestibule that lies directly beneath the anus is marked to serve as the apex of a triangle of mucosa to be removed. The distance between this mark and the dorsal commissure of the vulva is measured, and one half of this distance from the dorsal commissure of the vulva is marked on the mucocutaneous margin of each labium. A line between these two points on the labia serves as the base of the mucosal triangle to be removed (Figure 15-9).

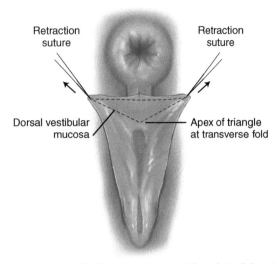

Figure 15-9 Modified perineoplasty. The *dotted line* indicates the area of dorsal vulvar mucosa to be excised.

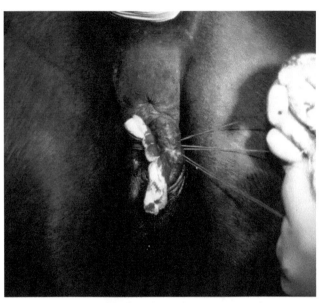

Figure 15-11 Modified perineoplasty. Two or three retention sutures are placed horizontally in a line from the apex to the base of the triangle shown in Figure 15-10. Small rolls of gauze or rubber tubing can be placed in the loops of the retention sutures to distribute pressure and avoid pressure necrosis.

The points of the triangle are connected with a scalpel, and the mucosa overlying this area is removed (Figure 15-10). Two or three, no. 1 or 2 nonabsorbable sutures are placed horizontally through the perineum in a line from the apex of the triangle to the base, as shown in Figure 15-11. Small rolls of gauze swabs work well as stents to prevent the sutures from pulling through the skin. Just enough tension is placed on the sutures to bring the triangular area into a vertical position. Sutures are removed in 5 to 10 days. Excessive tension placed on the sutures can cause tissue necrosis. If sutures begin to cause tissue necrosis, they can be removed, one daily or at alternate-day intervals, to relieve pressure. This surgical procedure effectively increases the area of the perineal body and returns the vulva to a more vertical position (Figure 15-12), but the sunken position of the anus remains unchanged. If the procedure is done properly, the vulvar opening is not diminished appreciably, and the mare can be bred with natural service.

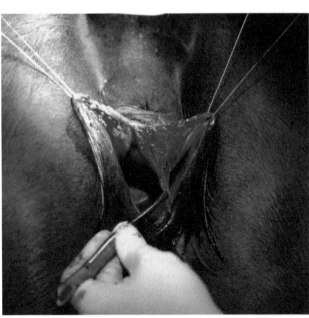

Figure 15-10 Modified perineoplasty. A triangular area of dorsal vulvar mucosa is excised with forceps and scissors.

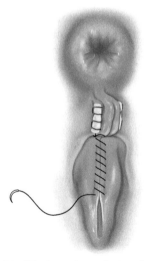

Figure 15-12 Modified perineoplasty. Completed placement of retention and Caslick's sutures. This procedure elevates the perineal body and returns the vulva to a more vertical position.

UROVAGINA

Old, pluriparous mares sometimes have reflux of urine into the vagina during urination, attributable to conformational changes that result from progressive descent of the vestibule and vagina into the abdomen from repeated stretching (during pregnancy) of the tissues that suspend the uterus and birth canal. These conformational changes cause the external urethral orifice to be positioned cranial and ventral to the brim of the pelvis and dorsal to the cranial portion of the vagina, leading to pooling of urine in the vaginal fornix. Pooling of urine *(urine pooling)* into the vagina is termed **urovagina** or **vesicovaginal reflux**. The constant presence of urine is irritating and contributes to inflammation and sometimes infection of the uterus and birth canal (i.e., vaginitis, cervicitis, and endometritis; see Figure 4-19). Severely affected mares dribble urine chronically from the vulva. The skin of the tail, ventral aspect of the vulva, and the inner aspect of the thighs may become chronically irritated, which causes exudate to accumulate in these areas (Figure 15-13). Before surgery is performed to alleviate urine pooling, the endometrium should be biopsied for histologic examination. If the mare has severe, widespread periglandular fibrosis of the endometrium, which permanently lowers the mare's ability to conceive and carry a viable foal to term, the owner of the mare may choose not to proceed with surgery. The mare is a more suitable candidate for corrective surgery if the endometrium is not severely and permanently damaged.

Different surgical techniques have been described for correction of urovagina in mares, including caudal retraction of the transverse fold, as described by Monin, and the McKinnon and Brown techniques of urethral extension. For correction of urovagina, we prefer the urethral extension technique described by Brown et al. (1978). This technique involves forming a tunnel that extends caudally along the floor of the vestibule from the external urethral orifice to the labia. The mare is prepared for surgery with systemic administration of a sedative and desensitization of the perineal region by instillation of 2% lidocaine or mepivacaine (1 to 1.25 mL/100 kg) through an 18- or 20-gauge, 1.5-inch (3.8-cm) needle inserted into the epidural space. The tail is wrapped and tied dorsally, and the perineal area is scrubbed with an antiseptic soap. Sterile tissue retractors, either hand-held or self-retaining, are used to expose the lumen of the vestibule and the urethral orifice. The transverse membranous fold (i.e., the hymen remnant) is sutured to the dorsal aspect of the vestibule, and the mucosa on the ventral surface of the transverse membranous fold is incised 1 to 1.5 cm dorsal to the urethral orifice so that it encircles the cranial half of the urethral orifice (Figure 15-14). Each side of the incision is continued caudolaterally and slightly dorsally so that the mucosal extension is wider caudally than cranially, preventing buildup of pressure

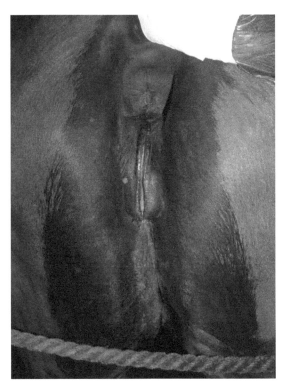

Figure 15-13 Urine scalding caused by constant dribbling of urine between the thighs of a mare with severe urovagina.

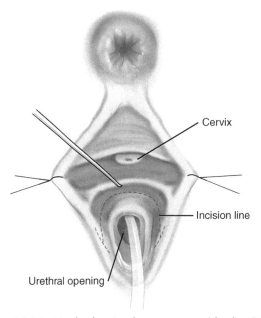

Figure 15-14 Urethral extension surgery with the Brown technique. The incision *(dotted line)* for the surgery is shown. The hymen fold can be tacked to the dorsal aspect of the vestibule to expose the urethral orifice and improve visualization.

during urination, which can lead to dehiscence. The incision is closed in three layers in the following order:

- The right and left ventral edges of the mucosal incision are apposed with no. 0 or 00 absorbable suture material with use of a continuous horizontal mattress suture pattern, which inverts the sutured mucosal edges into the lumen of the extended urethra (Figure 15-15).
- Submucosal tissue on the right and left sides of the vestibule exposed by the incision is apposed with no. 0 or 00 absorbable suture material with use of a simple continuous suture pattern (Figure 15-16).

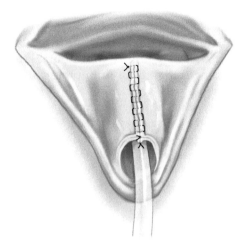

Figure 15-17 Urethral extension. The outer mucosal layer of the urethral extension is everted into the lumen of the vagina, with a continuous horizontal mattress suture pattern.

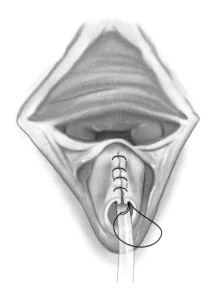

Figure 15-15 Urethral extension. The inner layer of vestibulovulvar mucosa is inverted into the lumen, with a continuous horizontal mattress suture pattern, to form the inner most layer of the extension of the urethra.

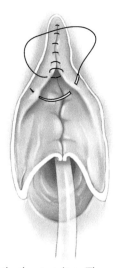

Figure 15-16 Urethral extension. The middle (submucosal) layer of the urethral extension is created by apposing the subcutaneous tissue in the right and left sides of the vestibular incision with a simple continuous suture pattern.

- The right and left dorsal edges of the mucosal incision are apposed with no. 0 or 00 absorbable suture material with use of a continuous horizontal mattress suture pattern, which everts the sutured mucosal edges into the lumen of the vestibule (Figure 15-17).

A Caslick's suture is placed in the vulva if the mare also has pneumovagina, a condition that commonly accompanies urovagina. Some mares may also need vestibuloplasty, as described previously. Aftercare consists of administration for 3 to 5 days of a broad-spectrum antimicrobial drug that is eliminated through the urine (e.g., trimethoprim-sulfamethoxazole). Administration of a nonsteroidal antiinflammatory drug (e.g., phenylbutazone or flunixin meglumine) for 12 to 24 hours after surgery may help to relieve postoperative pain.

PERINEAL LACERATIONS AND FISTULAS

Perineal lacerations are classified as first, second, or third degree. A **first-degree perineal laceration** involves the mucosa, submucosa, and skin of the dorsal aspect of the vestibule. A first-degree laceration may go unnoticed unless the mare is closely examined after foaling. A **second-degree perineal laceration** extends through the musculature of the constrictor vulvae muscle and the perineal body, compromising the ability of these muscles to constrict the vestibule. Disruption of the musculature causes the perineum to sink cranially and ventrally, predisposing the mare to pneumovagina and urine pooling.

Third-degree perineal lacerations, or **rectovestibular lacerations**, occur predominately in primiparous mares, probably because the annular fold of the hymen of primiparous mares is more prominent than that of pluriparous mares. The strong abdominal press that ensures delivery of the foal forces complete disruption of the roof of the vestibule, the floor of the rectum, and the perineal body. If a contributing malposture is corrected in time (e.g., returning a protruding foot to the birth canal) before delivery, the perineal body may be spared but a rectovestibular fistula will remain. A rectovestibular laceration creates a common rectal and vestibular vault, permitting direct fecal contamination that results in bacterial infection of the vagina, cervix, and uterus. Although the condition is commonly referred to as a rectovaginal laceration, the laceration is more commonly rectovestibular.

A mare with a first-degree perineal laceration can be treated with a Caslick's vulvoplasty, but mares with a second-degree perineal laceration need more extensive treatment because the perineal musculature is disrupted. If only a Caslick's vulvoplasty is used to repair a second-degree perineal laceration, the perineum sinks, predisposing the mare to pneumovagina and urine pooling. Repair of a second-degree perineal laceration is sometimes called a **vestibuloplasty**. The aim of vestibuloplasty is to reduce the diameter of the abnormally enlarged vestibule by 30% to 50%; the technique is similar to that used to treat mares with pneumovagina caused by faulty perineal conformation. If a second-degree perineal laceration cannot be sutured immediately after parturition, surgery should be delayed until bruising and swelling have subsided.

A mare with an acute, third-degree perineal injury should receive tetanus prophylaxis and should be treated with administration of a broad-spectrum antimicrobial drug, a nonsteroidal antiinflammatory drug, and a stool softener (e.g., raw linseed oil or mineral oil) for several days. Devitalized tissue can be excised to speed contraction and epithelialization of the wound. Attempts to repair the laceration immediately after injury are usually unsuccessful because the lacerated tissue rapidly becomes inflamed and edematous and because contraction of the muscles of the rectum and vestibule rapidly widen and lengthen the wound. Waiting at least 3 to 4 weeks before attempting repair is common to allow swelling to resolve and the wound to decrease in size by contraction. This permits epithelial regrowth to cover the damaged tissue. Postponing repair of a third-degree perineal laceration until the foal is weaned avoids potential nosocomial infection of the foal while the mare is hospitalized and problems that may be associated with reduced milk production resulting from the need to alter the mare's diet (see subsequent discussion).

Mares with a third-degree perineal injury need more preoperative preparation and more postoperative care than do mares with a first-degree or second-degree perineal laceration because the rectum is involved in the injury. Before the mare is prepared for surgery, the reproductive tract should be examined per vaginum and per rectum to detect cervical laceration, pregnancy

(if running at pasture with a stallion), uterine adhesions, filling of the uterus with manure, or pyometra. Surprisingly, although fecal contamination of the vagina and adjacent structures is constant, the uterus is unlikely to be permanently damaged, provided that surgical repair is performed in an effective and timely manner.

A major factor that affects the outcome of the surgery is softness and bulk of the mare's stool. The stool must remain soft and unformed to minimize stress on the healing tissues during defecation. Simply allowing the mare to graze lush, green pasture may be all that is necessary to keep the stool soft. If lush pasture is not available, the mare should receive a diet of alfalfa pellets (beginning several days before surgery) to decrease the bulk of the stool, plus administration of a stool softener before surgery and for at least 10 days after surgery. The diet of pellets should be fed in amounts sufficient to allow the mare to maintain body weight. Administration of 2 to 4 L of mineral oil via nasogastric intubation for 1 to 2 days before surgery generally ensures that the stool is soft and pliable at surgery. Administration of several ounces of raw linseed oil once or twice daily in the feed is another effective method of softening the stool. A broad-spectrum antimicrobial drug should be administered within several hours before surgery.

A third-degree perineal injury can be repaired with the mare sedated and standing, after the perineal region is desensitized with epidural anesthesia, or with the mare anesthetized and in dorsal recumbency. Most surgeons perform the surgery with the mare standing. The two stages of reconstruction—rectovestibular reconstruction and anoperineal reconstruction—can be performed during the same operation, or anoperineal reconstruction can be completed 3 to 4 weeks or more after rectovestibular reconstruction. Less stress is placed on the reconstructed rectovestibular tissue during defecation if anoperineal reconstruction is postponed until the reconstructed rectovestibular tissue has healed. However, performance of both stages of reconstruction during the same operation minimizes expense and time needed for recovery.

For preparation for repair of the rectovestibular laceration, the tail is wrapped and tied dorsally, and the rectum is emptied of feces as far as the operator can reach. A tampon, made from a 3-inch or 4-inch stockinette filled with cotton, can be placed in the rectum cranial to the defect to prevent feces from contaminating the surgical site during repair, but the presence of a rectal tampon may cause some mares to strain. The vagina, vestibule, and rectum are cleaned with cotton soaked in dilute povidone-iodine solution, and the perineal area is scrubbed with a disinfectant soap. The laceration is exposed by suturing or clamping (with Backhaus towel clamps) the dorsal aspect of each labium and the ventrolateral aspect of the right and left sides of the anus to the skin adjacent to the perineal body (Figure 15-18).

Long surgical instruments are helpful in rectovestibular reconstruction. To reconstruct the rectovestibular tissue, the submucosa between the ventral aspect of the rectum and the dorsal aspect of the vagina (at the cranial border of the laceration) is split cranially in a transverse plane with scissors for 5 to 10 cm (Figures 15-19 and 15-20). Dissection is continued with a scalpel caudolaterally along the right and left walls of the

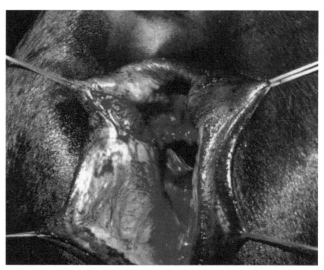

Figure 15-20   Repair of a third-degree perineal laceration. Dissection is carried cranially into the remaining rectovestibular shelf for 5 to 10 cm to separate the rectum from the vagina.

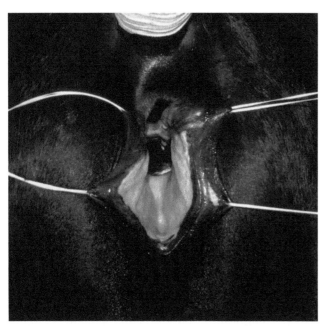

Figure 15-18   Repair of a third-degree perineal laceration. Retention sutures are placed in the dorsolateral aspect of the labia and ventrolateral aspect of the anal sphincter.

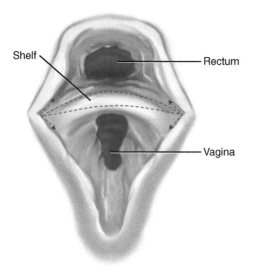

Figure 15-19   Repair of a third-degree perineal laceration. The path of dissection lies along scar tissue from the torn rectovestibular shelf located along the cranial and lateral borders of the defect.

common vault of the rectum and vestibule, to the point at which the labia normally should join at the dorsal commissure of the vulva. Then, with scissors, the incision along each wall of the vestibule is deepened dorsolaterally to form right and left flaps. The flaps are used to recreate both the ventral aspect of the rectum and the dorsal aspect of the vestibule. Dissection is continued until right and left flaps can be apposed without significant tension. At this point in the surgery, several techniques can be used to reconstruct the rectum and vestibule. We prefer the Goetz six-bite technique (described in detail by Walker and Vaughan, 1980). With this technique, interrupted, six-bite sutures of no. 1 or 2 absorbable monofilament suture material, placed 0.5 to 1 cm apart, are used to appose the rectal and vestibular shelves (Figure 15-21). This pattern causes the edges of the vestibular shelves to invert into the vestibular lumen and the edges of the rectal shelves to invert into the rectal lumen. The interrupted, six-bite sutures can be alternated with no. 0 or 00 monofilament absorbable suture, inserted just beneath the rectal mucosa in an interrupted or continuous Lembert pattern to provide additional insurance that the edges of rectal mucosa will have good apposition, thereby reducing the likelihood of leakage of rectal contents into the healing tissue.

The rectovestibular shelves are apposed with the six-bite and Lembert suture patterns until the region of the perineal body is reached. The perineal body is reconstructed with a technique similar to that described for vestibuloplasty. A right triangle of tissue is removed from each side of the common rectal and vestibular vault. One side of the triangle is the perineal skin between the dorsal aspect of the labium and the anus.

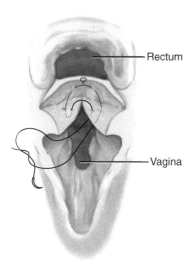

Figure 15-21 Repair of a third-degree perineal laceration. An inverting (i.e., into rectal lumen) suture pattern is placed just beneath the rectal mucosa, ensuring that no suture material is exposed to the rectal lumen. An interrupted, six-bite suture pattern is used to close the defect in the rectovestibular shelf.

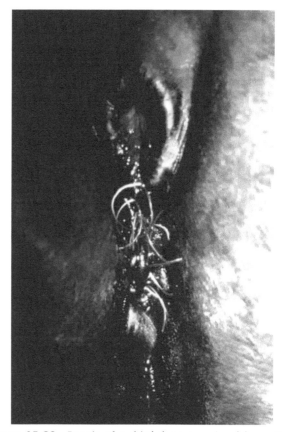

Figure 15-22 Repair of a third-degree perineal laceration. The perineal body and vulva have been sutured, illustrating how the procedure restores the normal configuration to the anal sphincter and vulva.

The dorsal aspect of the triangle is an incision between the end of the newly created rectovestibular shelf and ventral aspect of the torn anus. The hypotenuse of the triangle is the incision that extends from the rectovestibular shelf to the dorsal aspect of the labium. The pale, vestibular musculature should be exposed with removal of this triangle of tissue. The vestibular mucosa that forms the hypotenuse of one triangle is sutured to that of the opposite triangle with no. 1 absorbable monofilament suture with use of a continuous horizontal mattress pattern, so that the sutured edges are inverted into the vestibular lumen. The rectal mucosa of one side of the triangle is sutured to that of the opposite triangle with no. 00 absorbable monofilament suture with use of a continuous Lembert pattern, so that the sutured edges are inverted into the rectal lumen. The submucosa and musculature exposed in the center of one triangle are sutured to that of the other triangle with no. 2-0 or 0 absorbable monofilament suture with use of multiple simple interrupted sutures or multiple rows of simple continuous sutures. Nonabsorbable sutures are placed in the skin of the perineal body. Finally, to ensure a good labial seal, a Caslick's vulvoplasty is performed (Figure 15-22).

RECTOVAGINAL FISTULAS

A rectovaginal laceration or fistula occurs at parturition when the annular fold of the hymen at the vaginovestibular junction obstructs passage of the foal's forefoot or nose. The injury occurs when the birth canal does not dilate sufficiently to accommodate passage of the foal. A rectovaginal or rectovestibular fistula should not be converted into a third-degree perineal laceration for repair purposes unless it is exceptionally large (i.e., greater than 3 fingers in diameter). A fistula 3 fingers or less in diameter can be repaired with Forssell's technique, which spares complete disruption of the intact perineal body (Walker and Vaughan, 1980) (Figure 15-23). With this technique, the skin of the perineum is incised in a frontal plane, midway between the ventral aspect of the anus and the dorsal commissure of the vulva (Figure 15-24). The incision is extended cranially through the perineal body to 3 to 4 cm beyond the fistula, separating the rectovaginal defect into a dorsal hole (in the rectum) and a ventral hole (in the vagina/vestibule) (Figure 15-25). The rectal hole is closed in a transverse plane (because the musculature of the rectum is primarily circular and sutures placed perpendicular to the muscle fibers are subject to less stress than are sutures placed parallel to the direction of the muscle fibers) with no. 00 or 0 absorbable monofilament suture placed in an interrupted or Lembert or Halsted suture pattern (Figure 15-26). Preplacing all sutures and then tying the sutures from the center outward may allow for more uniform placement of sutures. Care must be taken to place all sutures into

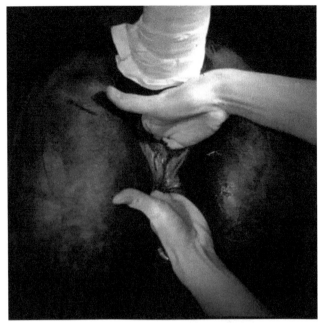

Figure 15-23 The rectovaginal fistula can be located by inserting fingers into the defect from both the rectal and vaginal sides.

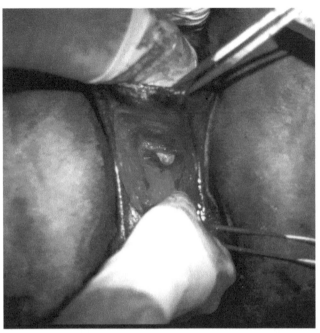

Figure 15-25 Repair of a rectovaginal fistula. Dissection between the rectum and vagina is carefully continued cranially beyond the fistula, permitting the dorsal rectal defect to be separated from the ventral vaginal defect. Fingers have been inserted into the rectal and vaginal openings.

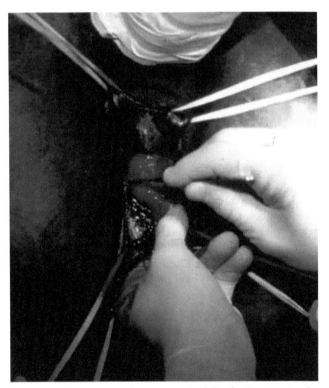

Figure 15-24 Repair of a rectovaginal fistula. To prepare the site for reconstruction, a scalpel and scissors are used to dissect horizontally through the perineal body midway between the anal sphincter and the dorsal commissure of the vulva.

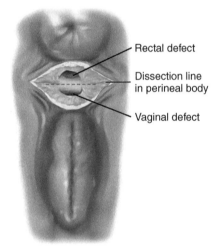

Rectal defect

Dissection line in perineal body

Vaginal defect

Figure 15-26 Drawing of a rectovaginal fistula showing the line of dissection in the perineal body between the rectal and vaginal defects.

submucosal tissue to avoid tearing when the sutures are tightened. The vaginal hole is closed in a sagittal plane (because its muscle fibers are primarily longitudinal) with no. 00 or 0 absorbable monofilament suture placed in an interrupted Lembert or Halsted suture pattern (Figure 15-27). Closing the openings of the rectum and vestibule/vagina at right angles to each other reduces the likelihood of rectal contents leaking into the repair site (Figure 15-28). The dead space

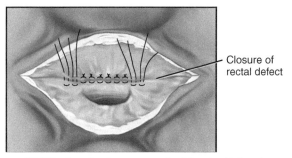

Figure 15-27 Repair of a rectovaginal fistula. Halsted sutures are placed in a longitudinal direction in the submucosa of the rectal defect. Sutures are preplaced and then tied from the middle outward, closing the defect transversely.

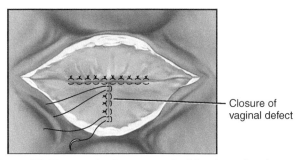

Figure 15-28 Repair of a rectovaginal fistula. Halsted sutures are placed in a transverse direction in the submucosa of the vaginal defect. Sutures are preplaced and then tied from the middle outward, closing the defect longitudinally.

remaining between the rectum and vestibule/vagina is then closed with simple interrupted sutures of no. 0 or 1 absorbable suture material. The incised skin of the perineal body is closed with interrupted nonabsorbable monofilament sutures, which are removed 10 to 14 days later. The frontal plane of dissection is difficult to close and may be left unsutured to heal by second intention.

Postoperative treatment of the mare after repair of a rectovaginal laceration or fistula usually includes administration of a broad-spectrum antimicrobial drug and a nonsteroidal, antiinflammatory drug for several days. The mare should receive tetanus prophylaxis, if she has not received it previously. Feces should be kept soft and scanty for at least 10 days by modification of diet and administration of a fecal softener (e.g., mineral oil or raw linseed oil). Repair can usually be safely evaluated on the 9th or 10th postoperative day. Defects in the repair are best detected with palpation of tissue between a hand inserted into the rectum and a hand inserted into the vestibule. Mares that strain excessively after surgery should receive epidural anesthesia and sedation, and the cause of straining should be eliminated. Causes of straining include fecal impaction of the rectum and bacterial cystitis.

Mares that are reproductively healthy before development of a rectovaginal laceration or fistula are usually able to eliminate bacteria from the tubular genital tract within one estrous cycle. In mares that still have a functional vestibulovaginal seal after a rectovestibular laceration or fistula, endometritis may not develop, provided that the tear is caudal to the seal. Those mares that have endometritis develop appear to be capable of rapidly resolving inflammation after perineal repair. Natural breeding should not be allowed for at least 3 months after repair of a third-degree perineal laceration. After 2 to 4 weeks of convalescence, sufficient healing should have occurred to permit safe examination of the reproductive tract per rectum and passage of an insemination pipette through the cervix.

CERVICAL LACERATIONS

A cervical laceration occurs during parturition and often goes undetected until it is discovered during routine postpartum examination or during examination for determination of the cause of infertility or repeated uterine infection. A cervical laceration may cause the cervix to appear short, persistently dilated, or adhered to the vagina. In this case, the prognosis for correction is poor. However, most cervical lacerations are longitudinal tears in the cervical muscle. These longitudinal tears are best identified with palpation of the cervical wall between the index finger inserted into the cervical lumen and the thumb placed on the vaginal aspect of the cervix. The defect is often pie-shaped and may or may not extend entirely through the wall of the cervix. Occasionally, more than one cervical defect can be detected.

Cervical repair may not be necessary if the laceration does not extend beyond more than half the length of the cervix and the internal cervical os remains competent. Cervical competency is best evaluated when the mare is in diestrus when a competent cervix typically must be dilated to allow a finger to be passed through it into the uterine lumen. Alternatively, 300 mg of progesterone in oil can be administered intramuscularly daily for 5 to 7 days to cause the cervix to close. If the cervix has not closed sufficiently after progesterone administration, the cervix must be repaired to restore fertility. Because the repaired cervix is incapable of dilating completely, scar tissue at the site of repair is usually disrupted during subsequent parturition. Therefore, the owner should be forewarned that another repair is likely needed after each subsequent parturition.

Preparation for repair of a cervical defect (Brown et al., 1984) is similar to that for repair of a third-degree perineal laceration (i.e., sedation, epidural anesthesia, tail wrap and tie, and so on). The tear is most easily repaired when the mare is in diestrus or anestrus or has been administered progesterone as described previously. A two-bladed speculum that opens later-ally (Figure 15-29) and long surgical instruments are required. Two retention sutures are placed in the exter-nal cervical os, one on each side of the cervical tear (Figure 15-30). The cervix is retracted caudally, and each retention suture is tied to one side of the base of the speculum. The mucosa is excised from the pie-shaped defect, with scissors, until the cervical muscu-lature is identified (see Figure 15-30). The cervical de-fect is closed in three layers.

- The inner mucosal layer (i.e., toward the cervical lumen) is sutured first with no. 0 or 00 absorbable suture placed in an inverting (i.e., into the cervical lumen) continuous horizontal mattress pattern (Figure 15-31). Suturing begins at the cranial end of the defect and continues caudally to the external os.

- The middle, muscular layer is sutured with no. 0 absorbable suture inserted in a simple continuous pattern (Figure 15-32). This is the critical layer of closure, so sufficient tissue must be procured to ensure that the layer remains intact after healing. Thickness can be checked periodically during

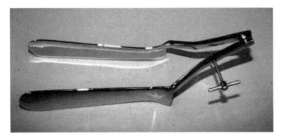

Figure 15-29 Two-bladed vaginal speculum used in the repair of cervical lacerations.

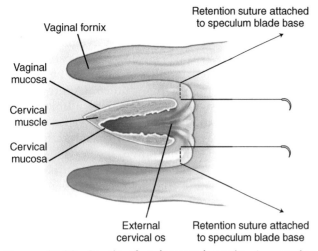

Figure 15-30 Repair of a lacerated cervix. A retention suture is placed in the external cervical os on each side of the cervical defect to be repaired. The retention sutures are retracted and tied to the base of each speculum blade to spread the defect and to retract the cervix to as near the vulvar opening as possible. The pie-shaped cervical defect is debrided to expose the muscular layer. (Modified from Brown JS, et al: Surgical repair of the lacerated cervix in the mare, *Theriogenology* 22:351, 1984.)

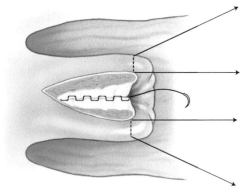

Figure 15-31 Repair of a lacerated cervix. The inner muco-sal edges of the laceration are apposed with a continuous horizontal mattress pattern so that the sutured edges are inverted into the cervical lumen. (Modified from Brown JS, et al: Surgical repair of the lacerated cervix in the mare, *Theriogenology* 22:351, 1984.)

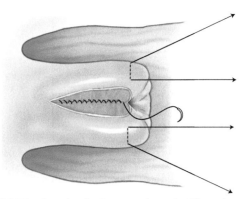

Figure 15-32 Repair of a lacerated cervix. The edges of the middle, muscular layer of the laceration are apposed with a simple continuous pattern. (Modified from Brown JS, et al: Surgical repair of the lacerated cervix in the mare, *Therio-genology* 22:351, 1984.)

insertion of this suture line by inserting a finger into the cervical lumen.

- The outer mucosal layer (i.e., toward the vaginal lumen) is sutured cranially to caudally in an everting manner (i.e., into the vaginal lumen) with no. 0 or 00 absorbable suture material inserted in a continuous horizontal mattress pattern (Figure 15-33).

The retention sutures are removed, and the vagina and the external cervical mucosa are covered with an oily, antimicrobial preparation. The mare should undergo a Caslick's vulvoplasty, if necessary. A suitable, broad-spectrum, antimicrobial drug can be admin-istered to the mare for 3 to 5 days if infection is a concern. The mare should receive sexual rest for 1 month, and the cervix should be examined for competency and patency before the mare is bred.

ENDOMETRIAL CYST REMOVAL

If endometrial cysts necessitate removal (see Chapter 5), they can be removed through an endoscope with use of a snare passed through the biopsy channel and looped

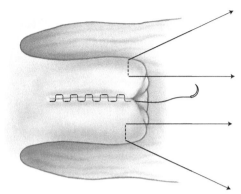

Figure 15-33 Repair of a lacerated cervix. The outer mucosal edges of the laceration are apposed with a continuous horizontal mattress pattern so that the sutured edges are everted into the vaginal lumen. (Modified from Brown JS, et al: Surgical repair of the lacerated cervix in the mare, *Theriogenology* 22:351, 1984.)

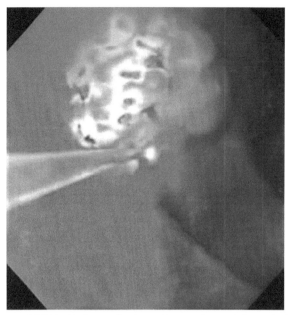

Figure 15-35 Endoscopic view of an endometrial cyst being removed with YAG laser surgery. Extensive cauterization of cyst epithelium is necessary to ensure sufficient sloughing of the cyst wall occurs to prevent refilling of the cyst with fluid.

around the base of a pedunculated cyst. In some cases in which a cyst is located just cranial to the cervix, blind transcervical removal of the cyst may be accomplished with either a snare or biopsy punch. For most endometrial cysts, however, laser-surgical (Nd YAG or Diode) removal via endoscopy is recommended. Ideally, the procedure is performed when the mare is in diestrus so that the closed cervix aids in maintaining sufficient distention of the uterine lumen with air or fluid for visualization. Once the cysts are visualized (Figure 15-34), sufficient tissue in the wall of the cysts are burned (with care taken not to damage the rest of the endometrium) to cause necrosis and sloughing of the cyst (Figure 15-35).

Postsurgical uterine lavage and infusion of broad-spectrum antimicrobials are recommended at intervals for up to a week, to minimize chances of intraluminal adhesions developing, to remove sloughed necrotic cyst tissue, and to prevent infection. Because underlying uterine problems may contribute to further cyst formation, treated mares should be bred as soon as possible after endometrial healing.

BIBLIOGRAPHY

Brown JS, Varner DD, Hinrichs K, Kenney RM. Surgical repair of the lacerated cervix in the mare, *Theriogenology* 22:351, 1984.

Brown MP, Colahan PT, Hawkins DL: Urethral extension for treatment of urine pooling in mares, *J Am Vet Med Assoc* 173:1005, 1978.

Slusher S: *Modified perineoplasty,* presented at the Western States Veterinary Conference, Las Vegas, February 17-18, 1986.

Walker DR, Vaughan JT: *Bovine and equine urogenital surgery,* Philadelphia, 1980, Lea & Febiger.

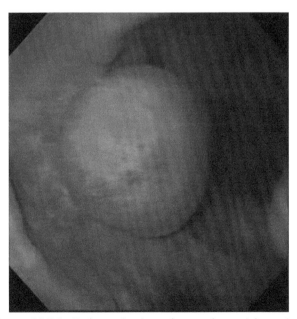

Figure 15-34 Endoscopic view of an endometrial cyst in a mare before removal with laser surgery.

Surgery of the Stallion Reproductive Tract

OBJECTIVES

While studying the information covered in this chapter, the reader should attempt to:
- Acquire a working knowledge of the types of reproductive disorders of stallions that can be corrected with surgery.
- Acquire a working understanding of the surgical procedures or treatments used to correct disorders of the stallion genital tract.

STUDY QUESTIONS

1. Discuss indications, techniques, and potential postoperative complications of castration of stallions.
2. Discuss methods used to diagnose and correct cryptorchidism in stallions.
3. Describe the surgical procedures or treatments that can be used for the following disorders:
   a. Inguinal herniation
   b. Torsion of the spermatic cord
   c. Hydrocele
   d. Hematocele
   e. Testicular neoplasia
   f. Penile and preputial injuries
   g. Paraphimosis/penile paralysis
   h. Phimosis
   i. Neoplasia of the penis and prepuce
   j. Cutaneous habronemiasis
   k. Priapism
   l. Hemospermia and hematuria

CASTRATION

Orchiectomy, castration, emasculation, gelding, and *cutting* are terms for surgical removal of the testes. Castration is one of the most commonly performed equine surgical procedures, and its complications are among the most common causes of malpractice claims against veterinarians.

General Considerations

Castration prevents or decreases objectionable sexual behavior and aggressive temperament and prevents stallions of inferior quality from reproducing. Castration removes the major source of circulating androgens and estrogens responsible for male sexual behavior. Castration may be indicated for removal of a testicular tumor or because one or both testes have been irreparably damaged. During repair of an inguinal (or scrotal) hernia, the ipsilateral testis is usually removed.

Horses can be castrated at any age, but the age at which a horse is castrated is usually determined by managerial convenience. Most horses are castrated when they are between 1 and 2 years old, when objectionable sexual behavior most commonly commences. The operation may be delayed until male characteristics develop or until the owner can determine whether the horse may have value as a sire. Castration before puberty may delay closure of the growth plates of the long bones, causing the horse to grow to a height greater than it would have had it not been castrated.

Before the horse is castrated, its scrotal region should be inspected closely to document the presence of two normal scrotal testes and the absence of an inguinal (or scrotal) hernia. The scrotal region should be palpated after the horse is sedated, if the region cannot otherwise be palpated safely. The absence of either testis or detection of intestine in the inguinal canal (or scrotum) may alter the method of anesthesia or the technique of castration.

Orchiectomy may be performed with the open, closed, or half-closed technique, regardless of whether the horse is castrated while standing or recumbent. With the open technique of castration, the parietal (or common vaginal) tunic is not excised, but with the closed and half-closed techniques of castration, the portion of the parietal tunic that surrounds the testis and distal portion of the spermatic cord is excised along with the testis.

Several different emasculators are available for equine castration. Some of the more commonly used emasculators are shown in Figure 16-1; individual preference governs which one is used. We prefer the Reimer emasculator.

Both tetanus antitoxin and tetanus toxoid should be administered to the horse before or after castration, if the horse has not been previously immunized with tetanus toxoid. A tetanus toxoid booster should be given to a previously vaccinated horse if more than a year has elapsed since the horse was vaccinated. Prophylactic antimicrobial therapy is usually not necessary, provided that the horse is castrated with aseptic technique and the horse's surroundings are clean, but a survey of practitioners to determine factors that influence the incidence of complications associated with castration indicated that infection may be less likely to develop at the site of surgery if horses receive perioperative antimicrobial treatment.

The castrated horse should be confined to a clean stall for the first 24 hours after surgery to diminish the likelihood of hemorrhage from the severed spermatic vessels. Thereafter, the horse should be exercised to the degree necessary to prevent excessive preputial and scrotal edema. A typical regimen of exercise is 15 minutes of vigorous activity twice daily for 10 days. Although the ejaculate is unlikely to contain enough viable sperm to permit impregnation 1 week after castration, the horse should be isolated from mares for at least 2 to 3 weeks to avoid copulation. Abdominal forces during copulation could allow viscera to traverse a vaginal ring.

Castration in Lateral Recumbent Position

A variety of safe, short-term anesthetic agents can be administered intravenously, alone or in combination, to induce a recumbent position for castration. Thiopental, an ultra–short-acting thiobarbiturate, used alone or after administration of an α-2 agonist (e.g., detomidine HCl, xylazine HCl, or romifidine) provides a short period of general anesthesia but no analgesia. When used with an alpha-2 agonist, muscular relaxation is satisfactory. Recovery usually is satisfactory if only a single dose of thiopental is administered. Guaifenesin (5% to 10%) in combination with thiopental or ketamine HCl (with xylazine administered as a preanesthetic agent) provides good analgesia with smooth induction and recovery. This combination can also be used as a constant-rate infusion, if the length of anesthesia must be extended. Other anesthetic drug combinations include the standard xylazine-ketamine regimen, with the addition of butorphanol or valium. The use of the neuromuscular blocking agent succinylcholine alone to provide restraint during castration is inhumane because the drug provides no analgesia or sedation.

After general anesthesia is induced, the horse is positioned in a lateral recumbent position with the upper hind limb drawn cranially toward the shoulder by a loop of rope, encircling the pastern and hock that extends from another loop of rope encircling the base of the neck. The rope maintains the hind limb in a flexed position (Figure 16-2). For the right-handed operator, the castration is most easily performed with the horse in left lateral recumbent position.

The scrotum and sheath are prepared for aseptic surgery. Removal of the bottom of the scrotum (Figure 16-3) to expose the testes provides better drainage, resulting in fewer complications, than if the testes are exposed through an incision over each scrotal sac. For removal of the bottom of the scrotum, traction is placed on the scrotal raphe, and the tented tissue is excised with careful dissection with a scalpel. To avoid transection of large vessels, dissection should be relatively superficial through the scrotal fascia as opposed to cutting straight across the tented tissue. Alternatively, the median raphe can be tensed by pulling the

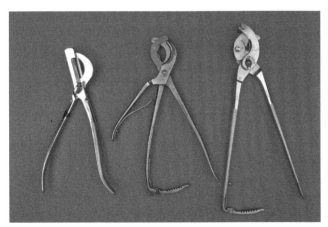

Figure 16-1 Emasculators commonly used for equine castrations. *Left to right:* Improved White, Reimer, Serra. (From Varner DD, Schumacher J, Blanchard TL, et al: *Diseases and management of breeding stallions,* St Louis, 1991, Mosby.)

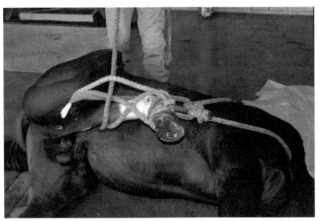

Figure 16-2 The horse is cast in left lateral recumbent position with the right hind limb tied forward to expose the scrotum for castration.

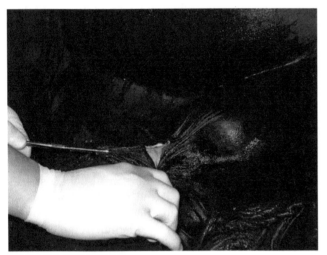

Figure 16-3 For removal of the bottom of the scrotum, a tissue forceps is attached to the midscrotal raphe, tension on the forceps "tents" the scrotum, and skin and scrotal fascia are excised with a scalpel. Care is taken to ensure that excessive tissue is not removed and the tissue removed is in the center of the scrotum. Dissection should remain superficial, to avoid transecting large vessels.

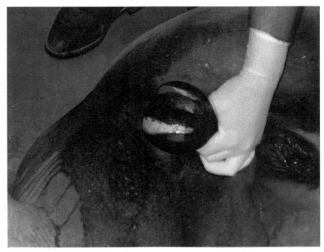

Figure 16-4 Two longitudinal incisions can be made in the scrotum after it is tensed by pulling the sheath craniad and upward.

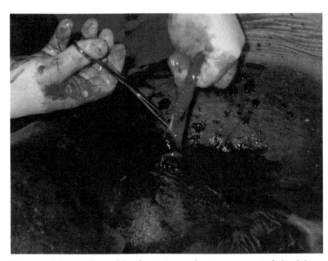

Figure 16-5 The skin between the two scrotal incisions should be removed for better drainage.

cranial end of the sheath forward and upward with one hand while making a longitudinal incision on each side of the median raphe with a scalpel in the other hand (Figure 16-4). The incision is extended through the skin, tunica dartos, and underlying scrotal fascia. If an open technique of castration is used, the common vaginal (parietal) tunic of each testis is also incised. The skin between the two incisions can be excised to provide better drainage (Figure 16-5).

When an **open technique of castration** is used, the common vaginal (parietal) tunic is not removed. Instead, the common vaginal tunic is incised, and the caudal ligament of the epididymis (a remnant of the gubernaculum), which affixes the common vaginal tunic to the epididymal tail and attached testis, is severed. The spermatic vessel and ductus deferens are transected close to the superficial inguinal ring with an emasculator.

When a **closed castration technique** is used, the common vaginal tunic is not opened, except at the point at which the spermatic cord is transected. The common vaginal tunic, its contents (i.e., the testis, epididymis, and spermatic cord) and attached cremaster muscle are freed from the surrounding scrotal fascia with blunt dissection and removed by transecting the cord and attached cremaster muscle close to the superficial inguinal ring with an emasculator. The closed technique of castration can be modified (i.e., the **modified-closed technique of castration**) with a longitudinal incision, 3 to 4 cm long, in the common vaginal tunic proximal to each testis (Figure 16-6). The left thumb (of a right-handed operator) is inserted through

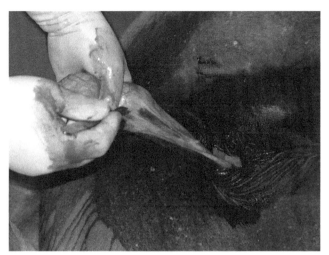

Figure 16-6 A small longitudinal incision is made through the parietal tunic proximal to the testis in preparation for a modified-closed castration.

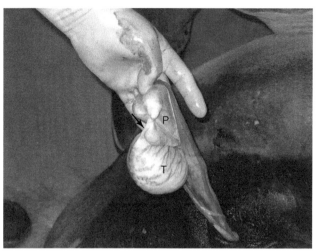

Figure 16-8 Exteriorizing the testis *(T)* inverts the parietal tunic *(P)* because the caudal ligament of the epididymis *(arrow)* is attached to its internal surface. Fingers are inserted into the sac created, allowing tension to be easily maintained on the parietal tunic.

the incision into the vaginal cavity and traction is applied to the tunic with the thumb while the fingers of the left hand force the epididymis and testis through the incision (Figure 16-7). Because the ligament of the tail of the epididymis affixes the fundus of the common vaginal tunic to the epididymis and attached testis, the fundus inverts and follows the testis through the incision (Figure 16-8). The left index and middle fingers are placed into the inverted fundus to maintain tension on the common vaginal tunic, and the left thumb is wrapped around the spermatic cord firmly to assist in traction. The spermatic cord and attached cremaster muscle are bluntly dissected free from scrotal fascia

and transected near the superficial inguinal ring with an emasculator. By opening the common vaginal tunic, this modified-closed, or half-closed, technique of castration allows observation of all enclosed structures (i.e., testes, epididymis, ductus deferens, and spermatic vessels).

Because the common vaginal tunic is removed with closed and modified-closed castrations, the likelihood of infection of the spermatic cord and of formation of a hydrocele is decreased. If the horse has a scrotal or inguinal hernia, use of the closed technique of castration and placement of a ligature around the spermatic cord proximal to the site of transection prevent evisceration. The closed or modified-closed technique is indicated when the condition for which the horse is being castrated involves the common vaginal tunic. Such a condition could include neoplasia, periorchitis, and torsion of the spermatic cord.

Proper application of an emasculator that is in good working order is crucial to successful castration. The jaws of the emasculator are placed around the distal end of the spermatic cord, if the castration is closed (Figure 16-9), or around the contents of the spermatic cord, if the castration is open. The jaws are closed tightly enough to prevent inclusion of skin in the emasculator's jaws but loosely enough to allow proximal movement of the emasculator to the site of transection near the superficial inguinal ring. The emasculator must be applied with the crushing portion of the instrument positioned proximal to the cutting portion. That is, the wing nut of the emasculator is directed toward the testis ("nut-to-nut" configuration). Tension on the spermatic cord is released before transection. To promote satisfactory hemostasis, the spermatic cord

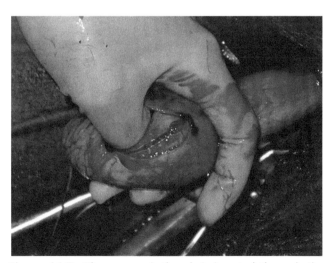

Figure 16-7 The surgeon's thumb is inserted through the incision of the parietal tunic and into the vaginal cavity. The incision is stretched with the thumb so that the contained testis can be exteriorized.

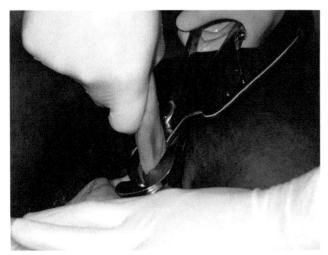

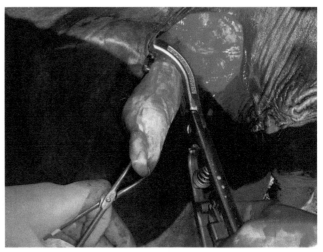

Figure 16-9 For a closed castration, the scrotal fascia is stripped from the common vaginal (parietal) tunic, and the emasculator is placed around the spermatic cord with the crushing portion of the instrument positioned proximally (i.e., in the "nut-to-nut" position) near the superficial inguinal ring.

Figure 16-10 Proper placement of the Henderson instrument. The instrument is clamped to encompass the entire spermatic cord just proximal to the testicle. (Courtesy Dr. Cleet Griffin.)

should be divided transversely rather than tangentially, and the emasculator should be left in place for 30 to 60 seconds, depending on the size of the cord. If the cord is large, the ductus deferens and spermatic vessels can be separated from the common vaginal tunic and cremaster muscle and the two components transected separately.

Fascia or tunic that could protrude from the scrotal incision when the horse stands should be removed with scissors. The scrotal wound is usually left unsutured to allow drainage, but the wound can be sutured to permit healing by first intention, provided that orchiectomy has been performed aseptically. Complete hemostasis is necessary when the scrotal incision is primarily closed, so a ligature should be placed around the cord proximal to the intended point of transection, before the spermatic cord is transected with emasculators. The skin incision is closed with synthetic absorbable suture material with a continuous intradermal pattern. No attempt is made to close dead space.

The use of the Henderson castrating instrument (Stone Manufacturing & Supply Co, Kansas City, Mo.) has been gaining popularity among equine practitioners. The instrument is used in combination with a standard 14.4-V, variable-speed cordless hand drill; it was originally introduced in 1994 for castration of bulls but was recently redesigned for castration of stallions. Patient preparation and surgical approach are essentially the same as for the closed castration technique with emasculators in the recumbent animal. Instead of emasculators, however, the Henderson instrument, attached to the drill, is clamped to encompass the entire spermatic cord just proximal to the testicle (Figure 16-10). Then, without any tension placed on the cord, the drill is judiciously powered to

provide a slow to moderate rotational speed in a clockwise direction. The cord initially shortens as it twists but then elongates just before severance, which usually occurs after 15 to 20 turns. The tight twisting and tearing action seal the spermatic cord and result in hemostasis (Figure 16-11). The second testicle is removed in a similar manner. The scrotal incision can be sutured to heal by primary intention or left open to allow drainage. This technique is reported to result in fewer complications than with the use of emasculators.

Castration Performed with the Horse Standing

Standing castration can be performed safely and efficiently if the surgeon is technically proficient, candidates for standing castration are selected prudently, and the spermatic cords and scrotum are desensitized adequately with local anesthetic solution. Sedation or

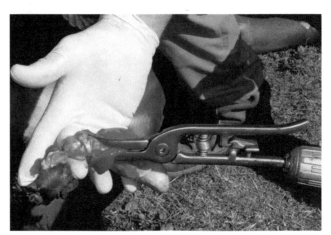

Figure 16-11 Testis removed with the Henderson instrument attached to a variable speed cordless drill. Tight twisting and tearing action sealed the spermatic cord and resulted in hemostasis. (Courtesy Dr. Cleet Griffin.)

tranquilization for standing castration is optional but strongly recommended. Suitable drugs include an α-2 agonist (e.g., detomidine HCl, xylazine HCl, or romifidine) and butorphanol tartrate. These drugs often are used in various combinations. Acetylpromazine is commonly administered to tranquilize stallions for standing castration or before induction of general anesthesia for castration, but its administration to stallions should be discouraged because it can result, on a rare occasion, in penile paralysis or priapism.

The surgical site is desensitized by infiltrating the subcutaneous scrotal tissue with 10 to 15 mL of local anesthetic solution (e.g., 2% lidocaine HCl or mepivacaine HCl) on each side of the scrotal raphe, followed by deposition of 10 to 15 mL of the anesthetic solution into each spermatic cord. Direct injection into the spermatic cord occasionally causes a hematoma at the site of injection, which may interfere with transection of the cord. Alternatively, 15 to 30 mL of local anesthetic solution can be injected into the parenchyma of each testis and allowed to diffuse proximally into the cord.

Before injection, the scrotal and inguinal areas should be scrubbed thoroughly, and the tail should be wrapped to prevent contamination of the surgical site. Even if the horse has been tranquilized or sedated, a twitch should be applied to its muzzle to prevent the horse from moving when the surgical site is infiltrated with local anesthetic solution. The right-handed surgeon generally works from the left side of the horse, leaning into the horse's side and avoiding the horse's kicking range. After the scrotum and spermatic cord are desensitized, a final scrub is applied to the operative site.

The standing horse can be castrated with an open, closed, or modified-closed technique, as described for the recumbent horse. With castration with the horse standing, the risks of general anesthesia are avoided, drug expense is usually less, and the procedure is shorter because no recovery time from general anesthesia is needed. Risks to the surgeon are greater, however, so candidates for the procedure should be selected carefully. Standing castration should be reserved for well-mannered stallions with well-developed scrotal testes and no history of recurrent scrotal swellings. If the testes cannot be palpated easily and safely and are not within the scrotum, the horse should be anesthetized and castrated while recumbent. Donkeys, mules, and small ponies are castrated more easily and safely with general anesthesia.

Laparoscopic Castration

Testes of entire stallions have been removed with a laparoscopic technique with the horse sedated and standing or, if intractable, anesthetized and in dorsal recumbent position. For laparoscopic removal of a scrotal testis, the vaginal ring is incised with scissors, and the testis is retracted into the abdomen with application of traction to the mesorchium. The ligament of the tail of the epididymis is severed, the testicular artery and vein are ligated and divided, and the testis is pulled from the abdomen. The vaginal ring is closed with staples or sutures.

A scrotal testis can also be left in situ and destroyed by disrupting its blood supply with electrocautery or ligation. The epididymis and the outer layer of the tunica albuginea remain viable, but the parenchyma of the testis undergoes avascular necrosis. Although the testis can still be palpated for up to 5 months, it is incapable of producing sperm and hormones. Failure to destroy the testicular parenchyma by disrupting the testicular blood supply, resulting in preservation of stallion-like behavior, has been reported. The advantages of laparoscopic castration include a rapid return of the horse to function and few complications.

Postoperative Complications of Castration

Hemorrhage

Excessive hemorrhage is the most common, immediate, postoperative complication of castration and is often caused by an improperly applied or malfunctioning emasculator. The spermatic vessels, especially the spermatic artery, may not be crushed sufficiently if scrotal skin is included accidentally in the jaws of the emasculator or if the spermatic cord is exceptionally large. The spermatic cords of mature and old stallions often must be transected with the technique known as "double emasculation." With this technique, the spermatic vessels and deferent duct are isolated from the common vaginal tunic and cremaster muscle and are transected separately with the emasculator.

The scrotal vessels can be lacerated when the practitioner incises the scrotum or excises scrotal fascia. This hemorrhage is usually not serious and stops spontaneously. An excited horse, however, often has increased blood pressure, which could result in excessive hemorrhage from the spermatic artery. For this reason, horses caught with difficulty or after a long pursuit should be allowed to cool down before they are castrated. Similarly, frightened horses should be calmed before the operation. Excessive estrogens produced by grazing some lush pastures also may interfere with hemostasis.

Severe hemorrhage occurs if the emasculator is applied upside down because the cord is severed proximal to the crushed portion. If the blade of the emasculator is too sharp, the spermatic vessels may be severed and retract before they are properly crushed. Severe hemorrhage should be assumed to originate from the spermatic artery.

If blood flow from the spermatic cord does not diminish after the horse stands quietly for 20 to 30 minutes, the severed end of the cord can be grasped with fingers and stretched and a crushing forceps, ligature, or emasculator applied to it. If the horse was castrated while recumbent, the cord is not anesthetized when the horse stands, and the horse is likely to resist attempts to grasp the sensitive, severed spermatic cord. In this case, administration of a sedative (e.g., xylazine HCl or detomidine HCl) and analgesic drug (e.g., butorphanol tartrate) is indicated before the inguinal canal is explored. Intractable horses may have to be anesthetized again. Laparoscopic intraabdominal ligation of the testicular vasculature has been used in standing or anesthetized and recumbent horses to stop excessive hemorrhage after castration.

If the end of the severed spermatic cord is inaccessible, sterile, rolled gauze can be packed tightly through the scrotal incision into the inguinal and scrotal cavities. The skin incision is then closed with closely placed sutures or towel clamps. The pack can usually be removed the next day. If hemorrhage continues despite packing, the hemorrhaging vessel must be located and ligated or crushed, usually with the horse anesthetized.

Intravenous administration of 10 to 15 mL of 10% formalin in 1 L of physiologic saline solution, through a catheter, may promote hemostasis by increasing the rigidity of the red blood cells (RBCs). In one experiment, this dose of formalin decreased coagulation time by 67%. In another evaluation of the effects of intravenously administered formalin on hemostasis, however, no benefit was detected. Although we have noted a dramatic reduction of hemorrhage immediately after administration of formalin in our clinical practice, the safety and efficacy of this treatment have not been established.

Swelling

Swelling of the prepuce and scrotum is expected after castration and, unless excessive, is no cause for alarm. Insufficient exercise after castration results in poor drainage from the open scrotum and promotes excessive scrotal and preputial swelling. Beginning on the day after surgery, the horse should be exercised vigorously every day to promote drainage and to discourage premature closure of the scrotal wound. Turning the horse into a large clean field may aid in controlling swelling but does not guarantee the horse will exercise at a level that is beneficial.

The prepuce can be massaged manually to reduce swelling, provided that the horse tolerates palpation in this area. If the scrotal wound seals prematurely, it should be opened with gentle massage of surrounding scrotal skin or dilated with a gloved finger to remove blood clots or serum from the scrotal cavity. Hydrotherapy may help prevent the scrotal incision from sealing prematurely, thereby decreasing scrotal and preputial edema, but a survey of practitioners conducted to investigate results of techniques of castration indicated that horses that receive hydrotherapy after castration may be prone to infection of the scrotum.

Infection

Postoperative swelling may be caused by bacterial infection of the surgical site. Tissues of the scrotal cavity can become infected because the open incisions expose injured tissue to contamination from the environment. Sepsis of the scrotal tissue usually resolves after systemically administered antimicrobial therapy and establishment of proper scrotal drainage. Forced exercise promotes drainage of septic fluid from the scrotal cavity.

Clostridial infection of castration wounds is particularly catastrophic because it causes toxemia and severe tissue necrosis. Clinical signs vary with the clostridial species involved. Affected horses are usually treated with systemic administration of large doses of penicillin and a nonsteroidal anti-inflammatory analgesic agent, supportive therapy, and radical debridement of necrotic tissue from the scrotal wound.

Infection of the spermatic cord, or septic **funiculitis**, can occur as an extension of a scrotal infection, from repeated crushing of the spermatic cord, or from bacterial contamination of the emasculator or ligature. Signs of septic funiculitis include scrotal swelling, pain, and fever. Antimicrobial treatment, drainage, and hydrotherapy may resolve the infection, but removal of the infected stump is usually necessary, especially if the cord has been ligated.

If an affected horse is not treated, the stump of the cord is likely to remain infected, even though the scrotal wound may heal. The stump may become very large because of excessive formation of fibrous tissue, which contains abscesses that may drain continuously or periodically to the exterior. A hard, chronically infected stump of the spermatic cord is sometimes called a scirrhous cord and can be caused by any pyogenic bacterium. Scirrhous cord caused by *Staphylococcus* spp. is sometimes termed botryomycosis. Fungi also have been recovered from infected spermatic cords. The scirrhous cord adheres to the scrotal skin, and draining tracts are usually present. The horse may display only mild or no signs of pain when the mass is palpated, and chronically affected horses are usually afebrile. A large scirrhous cord may cause hind limb lameness and, in extreme cases, may be palpable per rectum.

Removal of a scirrhous cord usually results in uncomplicated recovery. The infected cord is removed with the horse anesthetized and in dorsal recumbent position. An incision is made over the mass, and the affected portion of cord, along with a section of normal cord, is exposed. Isolation of the scirrhous cord may be difficult if the infection is long standing because of numerous large vessels that invade the mass. The spermatic cord is transected proximal to the mass with an écraseur or emasculator, and the wound is left open to heal by second intention. Postoperative management is the same as that for routine castration.

Septic Peritonitis

Although reported rarely, septic peritonitis can occur after castration because the cavity of the vaginal process (i.e., the vaginal cavity) communicates with the peritoneal cavity. Extension of infection from the vaginal cavity to the peritoneal cavity (or from the peritoneal cavity to the vaginal cavity) is rare because the funicular portion of the vaginal process is collapsed as it courses obliquely through the abdominal wall. Signs of septic peritonitis include fever, depression, weight loss, tachycardia, hemoconcentration, colic, and constipation or diarrhea. Development of any of these signs after castration may warrant gross and cytologic examination of peritoneal fluid. Results of analysis of peritoneal fluid must be interpreted carefully because nonseptic peritonitis occurs in many horses as a result of castration. Nonseptic peritonitis may be related to postoperative, intraabdominal hemorrhage, because free blood within the peritoneal cavity incites inflammation of the peritoneum. A nucleated cell count in the peritoneal fluid of more than 10,000/mL indicates peritoneal inflammation. Counts of more than 10,000/mL are common for 5 or more days after uncomplicated castration, and counts of more than 100,000/mL are occasionally noted. A diagnosis of septic peritonitis should not be based on a high peritoneal nucleated cell count alone. The presence of degenerate neutrophils or intracellular bacteria in the peritoneal fluid is more indicative of peritoneal sepsis, and when accompanied by clinical signs of septic peritonitis, antimicrobial therapy and lavage of the peritoneal cavity are indicated.

Hydrocele

A hydrocele, also called a vaginocele or water seed, may appear several months after castration as a circumscribed, fluid-filled, painless swelling of the scrotum. The scrotum may appear to contain a testis or may resemble a scrotal hernia. If neglected, the fluid-filled scrotum can become as large as a football. Sterile, clear, amber-colored fluid is obtained via needle aspiration of the scrotum. During ultrasound examination of the scrotum, anechoic to semiechoic fluid is seen within the vaginal tunic. Scrotal enlargement is the result of a slowly increasing collection of fluid within the vaginal cavity. The condition is uncommon, and the specific cause is unknown. Hydrocele can occur in stallions and in castrated horses, but the highest incidence rate of the condition may be in castrated mules. The open technique of castration predisposes the gelding to the condition because with this technique, the vaginal tunic is not removed. Removal of the vaginal tunic in castration of a mule may therefore be prudent. Removal of the vaginal tunic is the treatment indicated for castrated horses in which a hydrocele develops.

Evisceration

Evisceration after castration of a horse with normally descended testes is an uncommon but potentially fatal complication. It may occur up to 1 week after castration but usually happens within hours and may be precipitated by the horse's attempt to rise from general anesthesia. A horse that eviscerates after castration probably has a preexisting, inconspicuous, inguinal hernia that a preoperative examination failed to reveal. Standardbreds, draught horses, Tennessee walking horses, and American saddlebred horses may be more frequently affected by postoperative evisceration because they have a higher incidence of congenital inguinal herniation.

If intestine appears in the scrotal incision after castration, the horse should be anesthetized immediately. If not, the eviscerated intestine soon becomes contaminated and damaged during the violent struggle that ensues from the accompanying pain. A balanced electrolyte solution should be administered intravenously in amounts adequate to combat hypotensive shock. The horse should be positioned in dorsal recumbent position, and the intestine should be cleaned meticulously with copious amounts of physiologic saline solution or a balanced electrolyte solution. Damaged mesentery and intestine should be repaired or resected, and the eviscerated intestine should be reduced into the abdomen as soon as possible to prevent its vascular supply from being damaged. Intraabdominal traction on the intestine at the vaginal ring through a paramedian or ventral midline celiotomy may be necessary to reduce the eviscerated intestine. If the vaginal sac was not removed at the time of castration or was shredded during reduction of the eviscerated intestine, it is ligated with absorbable suture material and transfixed to the medial crus of the superficial inguinal ring. The superficial ring is then closed with doubled absorbable suture material (no. 2 or 3) with a continuous pattern. The superficial layers of the wound are left unsutured if the wound is grossly contaminated.

As a poor alternative to suturing the superficial inguinal ring, sterile rolled gauze can be packed into the inguinal canal. Care should be taken to avoid introducing the gauze into the abdomen. The gauze is held in position for 48 to 72 hours with suturing of the scrotal incision. The vaginal ring should be palpated per rectum before the gauze packing is removed to confirm that the ring has decreased to a size that is no longer capable of permitting the escape of intestine and to confirm that intestine has not adhered to the pack.

Antimicrobial treatment, administered parenterally, should be initiated, and if signs of septic peritonitis develop, the abdominal fluid should be evaluated. The peritoneal cavity should be lavaged once or twice daily for at least several days with a balanced electrolyte solution if the horse has septic peritonitis develop.

Escape of Omentum

Omentum occasionally escapes through the vaginal ring and scrotal incision after castration. If this occurs, the vaginal ring should be palpated per rectum to determine whether intestine has also exited the vaginal ring. Exposed omentum can be removed with emasculators, usually with the horse standing. Because the omentum plugs the vaginal ring, suturing of the superficial inguinal ring may not be necessary. The horse should not be exercised for 48 hours, to prevent further escape of omentum. If omentum continues to escape through the scrotal incision, the superificial inguinal ring should be sutured with the horse anesthetized.

Continued Stallion-like Behavior

Continued stallion-like behavior is a common complication of castration. Geldings that display stallion-like behavior are sometimes called *false rigs*. False rigs may display masculine behavior ranging from genital investigation and squealing to mounting and even copulation. False rigs are often said to have been *proud cut*, indicating that epididymal tissue, responsible for the stallion-like behavior, was left with the horse at the time of castration. It is improbable that the epididymis is partially excised during castration of scrotal testes because the epididymis is closely attached to the testis. In fact, few, if any, false rigs have epididymal tissue. Regardless, the epididymis is incapable of producing androgens, and geldings with epididymal tissue are endocrinologically and behaviorally indistinguishable from geldings without epididymal tissue. Spermatic cord remnants have been removed from false rigs to abolish sexual behavior, but because the cords contain no androgen-producing tissue, the efficacy of this procedure is doubtful.

The plasma concentration of luteinizing hormone is increased after castration in response to a decreasing plasma concentration of testosterone, and this increase in concentration of luteinizing hormone has been postulated to stimulate production of androgens by the adrenal cortex. False rigs, however, have no higher circulating concentrations of testosterone than those in normal quiet geldings, and administration of adrenocorticotropic hormone to false rigs does not increase the plasma concentration of testosterone. Adrenal production of androgens is therefore unlikely to contribute to the persistence of stallion-like behavior after castration.

Because some sexually experienced stallions castrated late in life continue to display masculine behavior, stallion-like behavior in geldings has been attributed to learned behavior. Many false rigs, however, have been castrated as juveniles. A retrospective survey found no difference in the prevalence of stallion-like behavior between horses castrated before puberty and those castrated after puberty. In that study, 20% to 30% of each group displayed stallion-like behavior at least 1 year after castration. Persistent sexual behavior in geldings may therefore be part of the normal social interaction between horses and may be completely independent of the presence of testes. Changes in management or stricter discipline may alleviate sexual behavior or reduce it to a tolerable level.

Immunologic Castration

Stallion-like behavior in an entire stallion (i.e., a stallion with two descended testes) or a cryptorchid stallion can be alleviated temporarily by immunizing the stallion against gonadotropin-releasing hormone (GnRH) or luteinizing hormone (LH) to decrease the serum concentration of testosterone. Stallions vary in response to immunization against GnRH or LH, but the usual effects, in addition to diminution of sexual behavior, are a decrease in the concentrations of testosterone and estrogen in the serum, a decrease in the size of the testes, and a decrease in semen quality. Repeated immunization is necessary to maintain sufficient binding titer for complete neutralization of GnRH and inhibition of the reproductive endocrine axis. Although no commercial vaccine against GnRH or LH is currently available in the United States, a vaccine against gonadotropin releasing factor (GnRF or GnRH) is available in Australia (EQUITY, Pfizer Animal Health, West Ride, NSW, Australia), and was recently investigated by Canadian workers for its ability to induce ovarian atrophy and anestrus in cyclic mares. Two injections, administered 4 weeks apart, resulted in almost all treated mares entering anestrus lasting the rest of the breeding season. This vaccine could be a valuable tool for temporarily decreasing undesirable sexual behavior of a stallion that competes in athletic endeavors. Vaccination could be discontinued when the stallion was determined to be suitable for breeding.

CRYPTORCHIDISM

Cryptorchidism is a condition in which one or both testes fail to descend into the scrotum. The undescended testis is termed **cryptorchid**, and by extension of the term, stallions with one or both testes in a location other than the scrotum are said to be cryptorchid. Other terms for horses with an undescended testis include *rig*, *ridgling*, and *original*. If the testis has passed through the vaginal ring but not the superficial inguinal ring, the horse is termed an **inguinal cryptorchid** or *high flanker*. A **retractile** testis is a testis that can be palpated in the inguinal area but can be manipulated into the scrotum. It should be distinguished from a truly inguinal cryptorchid testis. The retractile testis may reside in a position remote from the scrotum until the horse reaches puberty, when growth of the testis causes the testis to be maintained permanently within the scrotum. A subcutaneous testis that cannot be displaced manually into the scrotum is termed **ectopic**. The horse is termed a

complete abdominal cryptorchid if the testis and epididymis are both within the abdomen. The horse is termed a **partial abdominal cryptorchid**, if the testis is within the abdomen but a portion of the epididymis lies within the inguinal canal.

A horse with two testes, one descended and one cryptorchid, is sometimes described incorrectly as being monorchid. The term **monorchid** should be reserved to describe a horse that has only one testis, regardless of that testis' location. The most common cause of monorchidism is failure of the surgeon to remove both testes at the time of castration, but the condition can also occur from unilateral testicular agenesis or from degeneration of an abdominal testis caused by torsion of its spermatic cord.

Retained testes are aspermic because spermatogenesis is inhibited by elevated temperature. The temperature of the scrotal skin is typically maintained 3°C to 4°C lower than body temperature. Bilateral testicular retention, therefore, results in elevated testicular temperature culminating in germ cell degeneration, testicular atrophy, and sterility. However, because the androgen-producing Leydig cells of cryptorchid testes remain functional (secrete androgens), cryptorchid horses have secondary sexual characteristics and exhibit male sexual behavior.

Cryptorchidism is a sex-limited, complex developmental condition, the cause of which is not completely understood. It is the most common disorder of sexual differentiation in male horses and one of the most common congenital abnormalities in male mammals. In one retrospective study, one of every six 2- to 3-year-old colts referred to 16 North American veterinary university teaching hospitals for medical attention was cryptorchid. The condition was most prevalent in Percherons and least prevalent in Thoroughbreds. Quarter Horses ranked third, behind the Palomino, in relative risk. The mechanisms of testicular differentiation and descent in domestic animals and in men are similar. The details of this process in horses have been studied but remain poorly understood.

Causes of Cryptorchidism

Testicular descent is a complex process, and thus, the causes of abnormal descent are probably varied and difficult to document. Reported mechanical causes of abnormal testicular descent in stallions include failure of the testis to regress sufficiently in size to traverse the vaginal ring; overstretching of the gubernaculum; insufficient abdominal pressure to cause expansion of the vaginal process; inadequate growth of the gubernaculum and related structures, resulting in inadequate dilation of the vaginal ring and inguinal canal for the testis to pass through; and displacement of the testis into the pelvic cavity, where abdominal pressure prevents its passage through the inguinal canal.

Several reports suggest a genetic basis for cryptorchidism in horses. Some postulated methods of inheritance cryptorchidism in the horse include transmission by a simple autosomal recessive gene, transmission by an autosomal dominant gene, and transmission by at least two genetic factors, one of which is located on the sex chromosomes. All of the published studies dealing specifically with genetic aspects of cryptorchidism in horses suffer from the same weakness: the data presented are not adequate to support the models advocated for genetic transmission. Although cryptorchidism in many affected horses probably has a genetic basis, a definitive study dealing with a plausible genetic mechanism has yet to be performed; perhaps more than one pattern of inheritance exists. The effects of maternal environment and other factors, such as dystocia, on the development of cryptorchidism in horses have not been examined.

Retrospective studies of large numbers of cryptorchid horses indicate that retention of the right and left testis occurs nearly equally, but that unilateral retention occurs about nine times more often than does bilateral retention. Most (about 60%) retained right testes are located inguinally, whereas abdominal retention more commonly occurs with the left testis. Bilateral abdominal retention of testes is nearly 2.5 times more prevalent than bilateral inguinal retention. The occurrence of both abdominal and inguinal testes in the same horse is relatively uncommon.

Diagnosis of Cryptorchidism

Cryptorchidism is easily diagnosed if no attempt has been made to castrate the horse. External palpation of the scrotum reveals the absence of one or both testes. Gonadal agenesis is extremely rare, and so, if the history that the horse has not been castrated is reliable, the retained testis must be in an ectopic, inguinal, or abdominal position. Horses purchased as geldings but displaying stallion-like behavior pose more of a diagnostic challenge. One must determine whether the horse is cryptorchid and, if so, whether one or both testes are retained.

Palpation

Examination of a suspected cryptorchid begins with palpation of scrotal contents and the inguinal region. The scrotum should be inspected for scars, but a scrotal scar indicates only that an incision has been made, not that a testis has been removed. If both testes cannot be palpated, the horse should be administered a sedative and its genital area should be palpated again. Sedation may relax the cremaster muscles, thereby making a subcutaneous or inguinal testis more accessible. Because the average length of the inguinal canal is about 10 cm, testes high within the canal are difficult to palpate. An inguinal testis lies in the canal with its long axis in a vertical position. Because its epididymal tail precedes the testis during descent into the inguinal canal, the tail of the epididymis of a partial abdominal cryptorchid can be mistaken for a small, inguinal testis during palpation.

If external palpation fails to reveal both testes, the abdomen can be palpated per rectum to locate an abdominal testis. Male horses are at greater risk for rectal tear during palpation of the abdomen per rectum than are mares because male horses are seldom palpated per rectum and may resist more violently. Most cryptorchids are seen at a young age, and young horses are more prone to rectal tear because they have a smaller rectum and more nervous disposition and they strain more. Administration of caudal epidural anesthesia, the antispasmodic Buscopan (Boehringer Ingelheim, Ridgefield, Conn.), or sedation to the horse can facilitate palpation per rectum. The risks of injury to the rectum must be measured against the diagnostic value of the information to be gained from examination per rectum.

During palpation per rectum, the examiner attempts to trap the testis between the hand and abdominal wall just beyond the brim of the pelvis or to grasp the testis while sweeping the caudal area of the abdominal cavity. Actual palpation of an abdominal testis, however, is difficult because abdominal testes are small, flaccid, and often mobile. Locating the vaginal ring on the side of the suspected retained testis may be informative. The lateral aspect of the wrist should be positioned on the pubic brim near the pelvic symphysis. The fingertips are pressed against the abdominal wall, and the middle finger is flexed and extended in a cranioventral direction until it enters the slit-like vaginal ring (see Figure 13-18). If the area is palpated by flexing the fingers caudally, the medial border of the ring tends to close, causing the fingers to slide over the ring. Structures converging at the vaginal ring can sometimes be identified with palpation per rectum. The ductus deferens is the most readily palpable structure, and if the testis or epididymis has descended, it can usually be palpated as it exits the caudomedial aspect of the vaginal ring. The ipsilateral vaginal ring of a horse with complete abdominal retention of a testis is usually difficult to identify with palpation per rectum. If the vaginal ring can be identified, the testis, or at least the epididymis, has probably descended into the inguinal canal. A partial abdominal cryptorchid is difficult to differentiate from a horse whose epididymis and testis have both descended through the vaginal ring.

Ultrasonography

Ultrasonography is reported to be a more useful diagnostic method than palpation for locating a retained testis in either the inguinal canal or abdominal cavity. Transrectal scans are initiated at the pelvic brim and continued cranially with a to-and-fro scanning pattern between the midline and lateral aspect of the abdominal wall. Inguinal ultrasonography is ineffective in location of an abdominal testis, and abdominal ultrasonography, performed per rectum, is ineffective in location of an inguinal testis. The ultrasonographic image of a retained testis often appears less dense (i.e, less echogenic) than that of a normally descended testis, but retained testes are still identified easily and measured accurately (Figure 16-12). A 5-MHz transrectal transducer is used for ultrasonographic examination of a retained testis. It is sometimes possible, with a transabdominal ultrasound curvilinear scanning probe, to ultrasonically visualize an inguinally retained testis (Figure 16-13). The probe head is pushed inward in the groin area, pointing upward into the inguinal canal.

Hormonal Assays

Hormonal assays have considerable diagnostic value when the castration history is not known and examination of the external or internal genitalia is inconclusive. The concentrations of testosterone or estrogen can be measured in the serum or plasma to help differentiate geldings from cryptorchids. Although values may vary among laboratories, typically a serum concentration of testosterone of less than 40 pg/mL indicates absence of testicular tissue, a serum concentration of 40 to 100 pg/mL is nondiagnostic (i.e., equivocal), and a concentration of more than 100 pg/mL indicates the presence of testicular tissue.

The concentration of testosterone in the serum or plasma of young colts (<18 months of age) should be interpreted cautiously because young colts often have

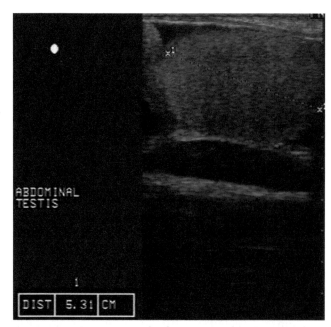

Figure 16-12 Transrectal ultrasonographic image of an abdominally retained testis in a cryptorchid horse. The testicular parenchyma has the typical homogeneous echogenic appearance seen in a scrotal testis.

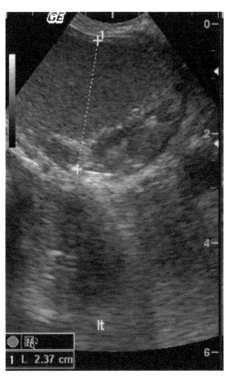

Figure 16-13 Ultrasonographic image of an inguinally retained testis obtained with a sector scanning probe. (Courtesy Dr. Barry David.)

a testosterone concentration of less than 100 pg/mL. The concentration of testosterone in the serum or plasma of normal adult stallions during the winter can be as low as 200 to 400 pg/mL. For more precise determination of whether a suspected cryptorchid stallion has testicular tissue, a human chorionic gonadotropin (hCG) stimulation test can be performed with administration of 10,000 U of hCG intravenously. Blood samples are obtained immediately before and then 2 or 24 hours after administration of hCG. If the horse has testicular tissue, hCG causes the serum or plasma concentration of testosterone to increase, usually twofold or threefold, above the baseline (i.e., prestimulation) concentration.

Because the testes of stallions that have reached sexual maturity produce an unusually high amount of estrogen, quantification of the concentration of total estrogen in the plasma or serum can be used to detect the presence of a retained testis in horses 3 years old and older. Horses with an estrone sulfate concentration less than 50 pg/mL in plasma or serum should be considered geldings, and concentrations more than 400 pg/mL (depending on the individual laboratory) indicate that the horse has testicular tissue. Evaluation of baseline estrone sulfate concentration has been reported to be more reliable than evaluation of baseline testosterone concentration for diagnosis of cryptorchidism in horses. To maximize the chances of endocrinologic confirmation of cryptorchidism, many practitioners

measure the serum concentration of estrone sulfate, the basal serum concentration of testosterone, and the concentration of testosterone, 2 hours after administration of hCG.

Removal of a Cryptorchid Testis

An abdominally retained testis can be removed through an inguinal (or scrotal), parainguinal, suprapubic paramedian, or flank approach. Only the inguinal (or scrotal) and parainguinal approaches allow removal of an inguinally retained testis. For all approaches, except those through the flank, the horse must be anesthetized. Although an immature or fractious stallion should be anesthetized for laparoscopic removal of an abdominally retained testis, an abdominally retained testis of many stallions can be removed through the flank, with a laparoscopic technique, with the horse standing. Regardless of the approach, the retained testis should always be excised before the descended testis is removed. Removal of the descended testis may complicate removal of the retained testis, performed at another time, because removal of the descended testis may cause the remaining retained testis to undergo some compensatory hypertrophy.

For the inguinal approach, the horse is placed in dorsal recumbent position and a cutaneous incision made directly over the superficial inguinal ring of the affected side. Alternatively, the bottom of the scrotum can be excised, and both the cryptorchid and scrotal testes (or two cryptorchid testes) removed from the single scrotal incision. The superficial inguinal ring is exposed with digital dissection. An inguinal testis is readily encountered during exposure of the superficial inguinal ring, but if the testis is located in the abdomen, the vaginal process should be located. The vaginal process of the partial abdominal cryptorchid lies everted within the inguinal canal and is readily encountered, whereas the vaginal process of the complete abdominal cryptorchid lies inverted within the abdominal cavity, along with the epididymis and testis, and must be everted into the inguinal canal. An everted process is white and glistening and usually about the size and shape of a small fingertip. A hypoplastic cremaster muscle can be observed on its lateral aspect.

An inverted vaginal process can be everted into the inguinal canal by exerting traction on the inguinal extension of the gubernaculum testis (IEGT), which attaches the vaginal process to the scrotum. The IEGT can be located on either the medial or lateral border of the superficial inguinal ring, at the junction of the middle and cranial third of the ring. Traction on the ligament everts the inverted vaginal process into the canal (Figure 16-14). An inverted vaginal process can also be everted into the canal by inserting a sponge forceps through the vaginal ring into the lumen of the vaginal process and grasping the fornix of the vaginal process

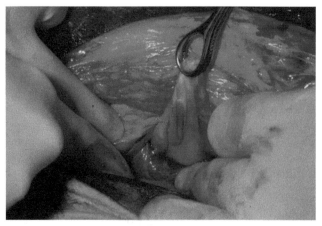

Figure 16-14 With use of the inguinal approach for cryptorchid castration, a forceps has been applied to the inguinal extension of the gubernaculum testis, and the vaginal process has been everted into the inguinal canal. (Courtesy Dr. Peter Rakestraw.)

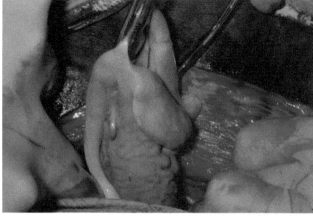

Figure 16-16 Traction is applied to the proper ligament of the testis, which attaches the tail of the epididymis to the caudal pole of the testis, to pull the testis through the vaginal ring. (Courtesy Dr. Peter Rakestraw.)

with the jaws of the forceps. Traction on the forceps everts the process into the inguinal canal.

The everted vaginal process is incised to expose the epididymis contained within (Figure 16-15). The proper ligament of the testis, which attaches the tail of the epididymis to the testis, is located, and with application of traction to this ligament, the testis is pulled through the vaginal ring (Figure 16-16). Often, the vaginal ring must be dilated with a finger to allow passage of the testis. The vaginal ring of immature stallions is usually more easily dilated than the vaginal ring of mature stallions. After the testis has been exteriorized, its spermatic vessels and ductus deferens are severed with an emasculator or an écraseur, or the cord is ligated and transected with scissors distal to the ligature.

Precautions to prevent evisceration after the testis has been removed are usually not necessary if the vaginal ring accommodates no more than the tips of two fingers. If the ring has been dilated beyond this diameter, the superficial inguinal ring should be sutured to

prevent evisceration. The cutaneous inguinal or scrotal incision can be sutured after the superficial inguinal ring is closed or left open to heal by second intention. Activity should be restricted to hand walking for several days before forced exercise is imposed.

For removal of an abdominal testis with the parainguinal approach, a 4- to 6-cm incision, centered over the cranial aspect of the superficial inguinal ring, is made in the skin 1 to 2 cm medial and parallel to the ring. The aponeurosis of the external abdominal oblique muscle is incised in the same direction, the internal abdominal oblique muscle underlying this aponeurosis is bluntly separated, and the peritoneum is penetrated with a sharp thrust of the index and middle fingers. The epididymis is located by sweeping the fingers around the vaginal ring, which is located caudolateral to the point of entry into the abdomen. The epididymis is grasped between the index and middle fingers and exteriorized. Traction on the proper ligament of the testis, which connects the tail of the epididymis to the testis, pulls the testis through the incision. After the testis is excised, the incision in the aponeurosis of the external abdominal oblique muscle is closed with heavy absorbable suture material. The subcutaneous tissue and skin are usually sutured.

The flank and the paramedian approaches are more invasive than are the inguinal or parainguinal approaches. The inguinal and parainguinal approaches allow the abdominal testis to be removed through small, finger-sized abdominal perforations, which makes surgery rapid and convalescence short. Abdominal testicular retention should be confirmed before either the paramedian or flank approach is used to remove a cryptorchid testis, because retraction of an inguinal testis into the abdomen is difficult.

Laparoscopy (Figures 16-17 and 16-18) may be useful to evaluate and castrate a horse that displays stallion-like

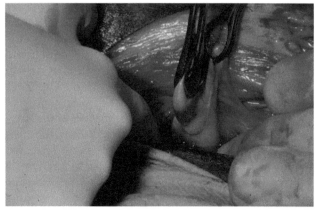

Figure 16-15 The everted vaginal process has been incised to expose the epididymis. (Courtesy Dr. Peter Rakestraw.)

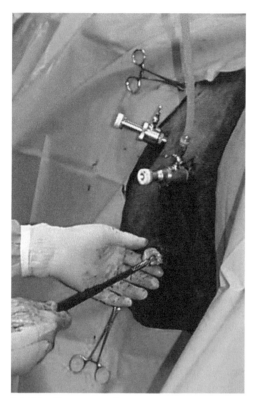

Figure 16-17 Three portals are necessary for laparoscopic cryptorchidectomy. One portal is used to insert the laparoscope, one portal is used to insert forceps to grasp the testicle, and one portal is used to insert an instrument to sever the spermatic cord. In this figure, the testis is being removed through the ventral portal. Laparoscopic cannulas are still in place in the two most dorsal portals, with the more caudal cannula attached to tubing used to insufflate the abdomen. (Courtesy Dr. Reese Hand.)

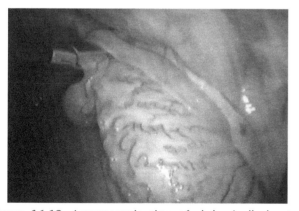

Figure 16-18 Laparoscopic view of abdominally located testis, with a LigaSure (Covidien, Boulder, Colo.) being applied to the spermatic cord. Application of the instrument seals the vessels in the cord. The LigaSure is then removed, and laparoscopic scissors are inserted to cut the tissue. This is repeated until the entire spermatic cord is cut. A new model of the LigaSure can cut tissue, and seal vessels, eliminating the need to insert a separate instrument to cut the tissue. (Courtesy Dr. Reese Hand.)

behavior but whose history of castration is unknown and whose scrotal appearance is that of a gelding. It may also be helpful when a scrotal testis of a cryptorchid horse was removed but the side of testicular retention was not recorded and is not known. Use of laparoscopy to remove an abdominal testis allows early return to exercise because the incisions into the abdomen are small. The disadvantages of laparoscopic cryptorchidectomy include the expense of the equipment and the need to determine the location of the testis (i.e., abdominal or inguinal) before surgery. A viscus can be penetrated if the instruments are not inserted carefully into the abdomen. If laparoscopic cryptorchidectomy is performed with the horse anesthetized, the hindquarters should be elevated to displace the viscera cranially, making positive-pressure ventilation necessary.

INGUINAL HERNIATION

A stallion experiences inguinal herniation when intestine, usually the ileum or distal portion of the jejunum, enters the vaginal sac or cavity (i.e., the inguinal canal) through the vaginal ring. This hernia is sometimes referred to as scrotal, rather than inguinal, when the intestine extends into the scrotum. Inguinal hernias of stallions are sometimes improperly called "indirect hernias," a term used to describe a somewhat similar condition in men.

Ruptured Inguinal (Scrotal) Herniation and Inguinal Rupture

Ruptured inguinal (scrotal) herniation occurs when the viscera within the hernia protrude through a rent in the vaginal sac into the subcutaneous tissue of the scrotum. **Inguinal rupture** is protrusion of viscera into the subcutaneous tissue of the inguinal canal or scrotum through a rent in the peritoneum and musculature adjacent to the vaginal ring. Inguinal ruptures of horses are sometimes inappropriately called "direct hernias," a term borrowed from a somewhat similar condition in men. Direct hernias in men, however, are caused by weakening of the inguinal musculature and are lined by peritoneum, whereas inguinal ruptures of horses are not lined by peritoneum. Direct herniation predominates in men, whereas *herniation into the vaginal cavity* occurs much more commonly in stallions than does inguinal rupture.

Causes of Inguinal Herniation and Rupture

Inguinal hernias of foals are usually congenital and are considered to be hereditary. They occur when the vaginal ring is so large that it permits viscera to enter the vaginal sac. Congenital inguinal hernias of foals may occur unilaterally (usually on the left side) or bilaterally and may occur more often in Standardbreds, Tennessee Walking Horses, and American Saddlebreds. Ruptured inguinal hernias occur most commonly in newborn foals and may be caused by the high abdominal pressure generated during parturition. Inguinal hernias of adult stallions are generally considered to be acquired, but the underlying cause may be a congenitally enlarged vaginal ring. Herniation has been reported to occur during breeding or exercise, but it has also been identified in stallions being transported or confined to a stall. The incidence rate of acquired inguinal herniation is reported to be higher in Standardbreds than in other breeds; the higher incidence rate in this breed may be caused by herniation of viscera through a congenitally enlarged vaginal ring. Inguinal ruptures of horses occur rarely and usually after a traumatic incident. Geldings rarely have inguinal herniation develop because their vaginal rings decrease in size soon after castration.

Diagnosis

Inguinal hernias (Figure 16-19), ruptured inguinal hernias, and inguinal ruptures cause a noticeable increase in the size of the scrotum. Palpation of the scrotum of an affected horse may elicit a sensation of crepitus, and peristalsis of entrapped intestine may cause movement of scrotal skin. Viscera outside the abdomen can be identified during transscrotal ultrasonographic examination (Figure 16-20). Congenital inguinal hernias in foals, because of the relatively large size of the affected vaginal ring, are rarely strangulated and reduce easily. Rupture of a congenital inguinal hernia should be suspected if the viscera cannot be reduced, if the scrotum is cold and edematous, or if signs of colic accompany the hernia.

Acquired inguinal herniation is usually first recognized when the stallion begins to show signs of severe colic caused by strangulation of the herniated intestine.

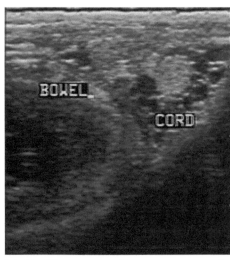

Figure 16-20 Ultrasonographic appearance of intestine present in the scrotum of a stallion with an inguinal hernia. Anechoic fluid is present within the vaginal cavity. The hyperechoic intestinal wall surrounds anechoic fluid within the intestinal lumen.

Scrotal and testicular edema usually accompany an acquired inguinal hernia because the vasculature of the spermatic cord becomes compressed. Intestine entering a vaginal cavity through a vaginal ring can be palpated per rectum. Omentum may also enter the vaginal cavity independently or with intestine.

Foals with a congenital inguinal hernia should be monitored regularly for signs of strangulation of the hernia contents. The hernia often resolves spontaneously by the time the foal is 6 months old, but the mechanism by which this occurs is not well understood. Application of a truss may hasten resolution. The truss is applied with the foal in dorsal recumbent position after the hernia has been manually reduced (Figures 16-21 and 16-22). Care should be taken to avoid interfering with urination by compressing the

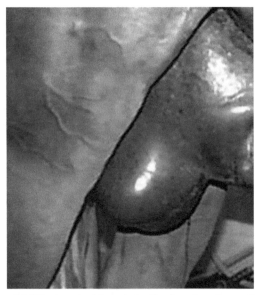

Figure 16-19 Inguinal hernia in the hemiscrotum of a stallion. Unilateral enlargement of the hemiscrotum is apparent.

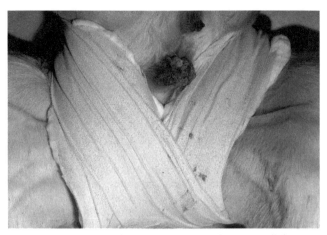

Figure 16-21 Ventral view of a foal with a truss ("diaper") to correct bilateral inguinal hernias. (From Varner DD, Schumacher J, Blanchard TL, et al: *Diseases and management of breeding stallions,* St Louis, 1991, Mosby.)

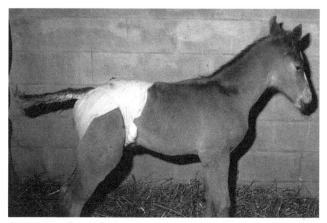

Figure 16-22 Standing view of a foal with a truss ("diaper") to correct bilateral inguinal hernias. (From Varner DD, Schumacher J, Blanchard TL, et al: *Diseases and management of breeding stallions,* St Louis, 1991, Mosby.)

penis. The truss is usually changed at 3- to 5-day intervals, and the hernia is often corrected within 1 to 2 weeks after application of the truss. Surgical correction of congenital herniation is necessary only if intestinal strangulation is detected or if the hernia fails to resolve.

Surgical Reduction

If an inguinal hernia ruptures into the subcutaneous tissue of the inguinal canal or scrotum, the entrapped viscera strangulate rapidly, necessitating immediate surgical correction. Stallions with an acquired inguinal hernia, inguinal rupture, or ruptured inguinal hernia need immediate attention because intestine that has escaped from the abdomen is nearly always strangulated. Reduction via external manual manipulation or by means of rectal traction on inguinally incarcerated intestine has been described but is difficult and not commonly successful unless undertaken soon after incarceration occurs. An acquired inguinal hernia should be reduced surgically if the viability of the testis or incarcerated intestine is uncertain.

For surgical reduction of inguinally incarcerated intestine, the stallion should be anesthetized, placed in dorsal recumbent position, and prepared for inguinal exploration and for celiotomy at the ventral midline. The scrotal skin and subcutaneous tissue are incised, and the parietal (common vaginal) tunic and its contents are exposed with blunt dissection. The parietal tunic is incised to expose the testis and its spermatic cord and the incarcerated intestine.

The incarcerated intestine should be reduced through the vaginal ring into the abdomen. Reduction is most easily accomplished by placing traction on the incarcerated intestine through a small ventral midline or suprapubic paramedian celiotomy. Often, the vaginal ring is so constricting that replacement of the intestine is impossible without first enlarging the ring. The ring is most easily

enlarged by cutting it with a curved bistoury. Devitalized intestine can be resected and anastomosed at the inguinal incision, but resection and anastomosis are usually more easily accomplished after the intestine is exteriorized through the celiotomy.

An attempt to save the testis is impractical unless it and its vasculature appear undamaged. For removal of the testis, the parietal tunic and its contents are isolated, and the scrotal ligament, which attaches the tail of the epididymis to the caudal aspect of the scrotum, is severed. The spermatic cord is transected with an emasculator or is ligated with heavy absorbable suture and severed distal to the ligature. The parietal tunic and overlying cremaster muscle can be excised with scissors or the emasculator, with care taken not to damage intestine that has not yet been reduced into the abdomen.

The superficial inguinal ring is closed with heavy, absorbable suture material with use of a continuous or interrupted pattern. Inguinal fascia and skin can be sutured or left unsutured to heal by second intention. The remaining testis often hypertrophies within a few months after the affected testis has been excised, and fertility is usually maintained.

For preservation of a viable testis with prevention of escape of intestine from the inguinal canal, the cranial half of the superficial inguinal ring can be sutured toward the caudally located spermatic cord. Another method of salvaging the testis, while preventing intestine from escaping through the vaginal ring, is to laparoscopically implant a mesh over the deep inguinal ring, with the horse anesthetized and in dorsal recumbent position. Another laparoscopic technique used to salvage the testis is to insert a coiled mesh through the vaginal ring, with the horse standing, and staple the mesh to the ring. Fibrous reaction to the mesh obliterates the vaginal ring. These laparoscopic procedures are performed after the horse has recovered from previous surgery to reduce the hernia.

TORSION OF THE SPERMATIC CORD

Torsion of the spermatic cord occurs when the spermatic cord rotates around the vertical axis of the testis. Torsion of 180 degrees or less seems to cause no discomfort to stallions and is often considered to be an incidental finding. Torsion of 180 degrees, however, may have a detrimental effect on testicular function, even in the absence of clinical signs of substantial vascular compromise. Torsion of 360 degrees or more causes acute occlusion of the testicular blood supply, and if the rotation is not corrected quickly, the testis and spermatic cord distal to the torsion become gangrenous. Torsion of the spermatic cord in the stallion apparently occurs intravaginally. Torsion may result from an abnormally long caudal ligament of the epididymis (ligament of the tail of the epididymis) or an abnormally long proper ligament of the testis. The same gubernacular attachments of the contralateral testis may also be abnormally long, making that testis prone to torsion. The spermatic cord of an abdominal testis is prone to torsion.

Signs of torsion of the spermatic cord in stallions include scrotal swelling and signs of colic. Other diseases that involve the testis and associated structures, such as inguinal herniation, orchitis, and epididymitis, produce similar signs, but these diseases can usually be excluded with palpation of the contents of the scrotum, with palpation of the vaginal rings per rectum, and with ultrasonographic examination of the scrotum and its contents. Horses with gangrenous necrosis of an abdominal testis caused by torsion of the spermatic cord may display no clinical signs of torsion.

Normally, the head of the epididymis lies on the cranial pole of the testis, the tail lies at the caudal pole, and the body attaches to the dorsolateral border of the testis. With torsion of 180 degrees, the tail of the epididymis lies cranially in the scrotum, but with torsion of 360 degrees, the testis and epididymis may appear to be correctly positioned except that the cranial pole of the testis is pulled more dorsally than usual because twisting shortens the cord. The affected testis and cord are enlarged and firm, and the testis may be surrounded by fluid. During ultrasound examination of the scrotal contents, increased fluid can be seen throughout the affected side of the scrotum, and compared with its normal counterpart, the affected testis appears enlarged and hyperechogenic (Figures 16-23 to 16-26).

A 360-degree torsion of the spermatic cord usually necessitates removal of the affected testis because of vascular compromise (Figure 16-27). If the testis is salvageable (i.e., infarction has not occurred), orchiopexy, with nonabsorbable suture material, can be performed

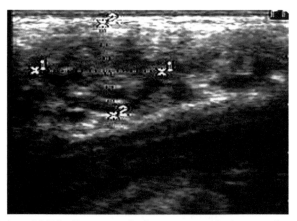

Figure 16-24 Transscrotal ultrasonographic image of normal spermatic cord of nonaffected contralateral testis in a horse with unilateral spermatic cord torsion. The spermatic cord cross section measured 2.4 × 1.9 cm. Vascular distention is not apparent.

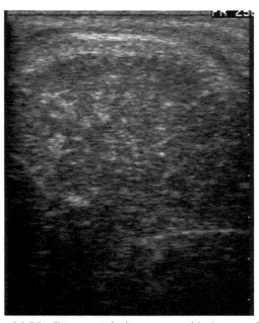

Figure 16-25 Transscrotal ultrasonographic image of congested right testis (note hyperechoic spots within parenchyma) of a stallion with unilateral spermatic cord torsion.

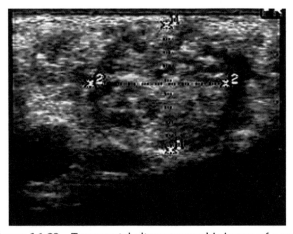

Figure 16-23 Transscrotal ultrasonographic image of a congested spermatic cord of a stallion with unilateral spermatic cord torsion. The cord measured 2.7 × 3.0 cm. Compare diameter, increased echogenicity from congestion, and vascular distention with image of nonaffected spermatic cord in Figure 16-24.

to permanently fix the testis in its proper position once the torsion has been corrected and the testis is oriented correctly within the vaginal tunics. One suture can be placed at the cranial aspect of the testis, and one at its caudal aspect. The suture is passed through the adjacent dartos tissue, vaginal tunic, and tunica albuginea. A salvaged testis should be observed periodically for atrophy caused by vascular damage at the time of torsion. In men, if the torsion is not recognized quickly and surgically corrected within 4 to 6 hours, extravasation of sperm occurs, which leads to formation of antisperm antibodies from disruption of the blood-testis barrier. The antisperm antibodies are thought to contribute to immunologic damage to the unaffected contralateral

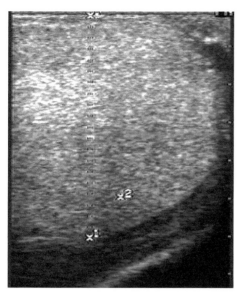

Figure 16-26 Transscrotal ultrasonographic image of normal nonaffected contralateral testis in a horse with unilateral spermatic cord torsion. Echogenicity of testicular parenchyma is uniform throughout the image.

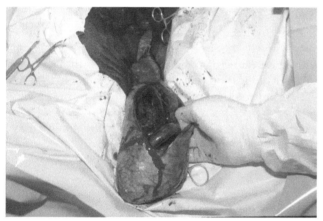

Figure 16-27 Infarcted testis resulting from spermatic cord torsion.

testis. The effect of transient torsion of the spermatic cord on the production of antisperm antibodies or the release of other factors that may affect fertility of stallions is not known.

HYDROCELE

A hydrocele is a pathologic accumulation of serous fluid between the visceral and parietal layers of the vaginal tunic. Because of the insulating effect of the fluid, temperature-induced dysfunction of spermatogenesis of one or both testes may occur, the outcome of which can be poor semen quality causing subfertility. The vaginal tunic secretes fluid, and this fluid is resorbed through the lymphatic vessels and veins of the spermatic cord. Hydrocele may result when production of fluid is increased or its resorption decreased.

A hydrocele can accompany testicular neoplasia or scrotal trauma, or it may be idiopathic. Idiopathic hydrocele may occur during hot weather and resolve when the ambient temperature drops. Because the vaginal cavity communicates with the peritoneal cavity, hydroceles also form as a result of passage of abdominal fluid through the inguinal canal. Migration of parasites into the vaginal cavity and associated structures has been implicated as a cause of hydrocele.

A hydrocele appears as a painless, fluid-filled scrotal enlargement that is often misinterpreted by owners as testicular enlargement (Figure 16-28). It may occur bilaterally or unilaterally and may develop acutely or insidiously. If development is chronic, the testis within the affected tunic is usually smaller than normal as a result of atrophy (Figure 16-29). A hydrocele can usually be differentiated from other diseases that cause scrotal enlargement with palpation of the contents of the scrotum, with transscrotal ultrasonography, and with palpation of the vaginal rings per rectum. During ultrasound examination of a hydrocele, anechoic to semiechoic fluid is seen surrounding the testis (Figure 16-30). Diagnosis can be verified with aseptic aspiration of a serous, amber-colored transudate from the vaginal cavity (Figure 16-31).

Initial treatment should consist of application of ice packs or gentle cold water hydrotherapy (10 to 15 minutes twice daily), plus administration of flunixin meglumine. Exercise often causes a hydrocele to decrease in size, at least temporarily, and occasionally hydroceles resolve spontaneously. Administration of 10 to 20 mg dexamethasone, once, may also be of benefit. Aspiration of fluid from a hydrocele usually provides only transient relief because the fluid soon reaccumulates.

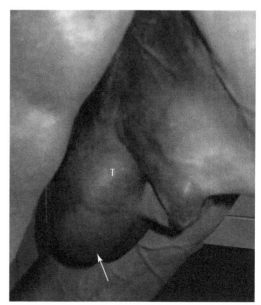

Figure 16-28 Stallion with scrotal enlargement from pronounced hydrocele. The testis *(T)* is dorsal to the pendulous fluid accumulation in the ventral scrotum *(arrow)*.

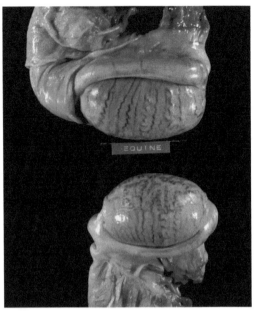

Figure 16-29 Normal and atrophied testes removed from a stallion with unilateral hydrocele. Fluid was chronically present surrounding the atrophied testis.

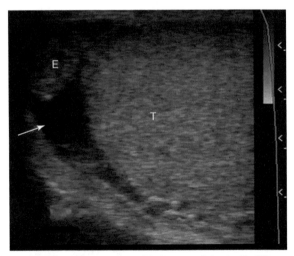

Figure 16-30 Ultrasonographic image of the testis *(T)*, cauda epididymis *(E)*, and vaginal cavity *(arrow)* of a stallion with mild hydrocele.

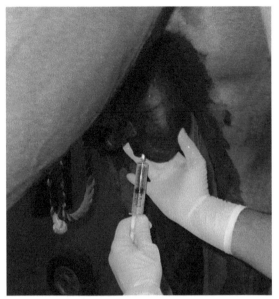

Figure 16-31 Aseptic aspiration of a serous, amber-colored fluid from the vaginal cavity of a stallion with hydrocele.

However, culture and cytologic assessment of the character of hydrocele fluid may be important in some more severe cases. If an infectious component is suspected, systemic administration of an antimicrobial that penetrates well into reproductive tissues (e.g., enrofloxacin, 7.5 to 10 mg/kg once daily, intravenously) can be instituted while awaiting culture and sensitivity results. Although treatment of an affected horse should be focused on removal of the cause of the hydrocele, the cause is rarely identified. Therefore, horses with a persistent, unilateral hydrocele are often treated by excising the affected testis and vaginal tunic to spare the contralateral testis from the adverse effects on

spermatogenesis resulting from the insulating effect of the excessive fluid. Prognosis for fertility is poor if a bilateral hydrocele persists, but reestablishment of fertility is likely if both hydroceles resolve. Sclerotherapy with tetracycline or polidocanol injected into the vaginal cavity, plication (parallel folding of affected vaginal tunic), and removal of redundant portions of the vaginal tunic have been used to treat men affected with hydrocele. To our knowledge, these treatments have not been evaluated in stallions with hydroceles.

HEMATOCELE

A hematocele resembles a hydrocele but is a collection of hemorrhagic fluid within the vaginal cavity (Figure 16-32). Scrotal swelling associated with hematocele can be quite pronounced. A hematocele is usually caused by trauma to the scrotum or its contents, but because the peritoneal and vaginal cavities of the horse communicate, a hematocele can also occur as an extension of hemoperitoneum.

A hematocele caused by acute trauma to the scrotal contents is usually associated with signs of pain. Ultrasonography may help differentiate hematocele from hydrocele and other causes of scrotal enlargement (Figure 16-33). Some causes of hematocele, such as rupture of the tunica albuginea of the testis, can sometimes be detected with ultrasonographic examination. Diagnosis is confirmed with aseptic aspiration of blood or sanguineous fluid from the vaginal cavity (Figure 16-34).

A small hematocele may cause no problem with fertility and may dissipate without treatment, but a large hematocele may insulate the testes, causing interference with spermatogenesis. In addition, clotting of blood and formation of fibrin within clotting blood

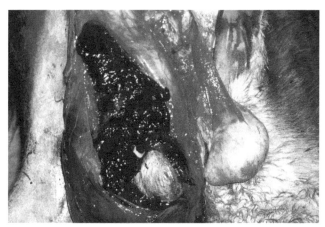

Figure 16-32 Massive bleeding, emanating from the testis through a rupture in the tunica albuginea, into the vaginal cavity, of a jack.

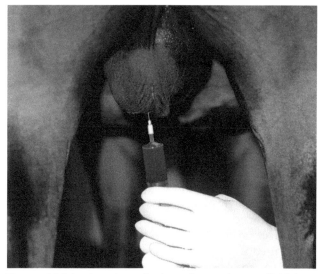

Figure 16-34 Aseptic aspiration of sanguineous fluid from the vaginal cavity of a stallion with hematocele.

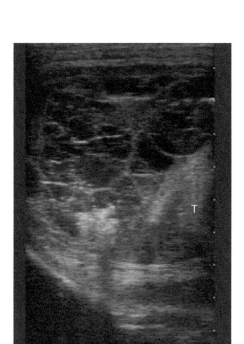

Figure 16-33 Transscrotal ultrasonographic image of a hematocele organizing into a clot adjacent to the testis *(T)* of a stallion.

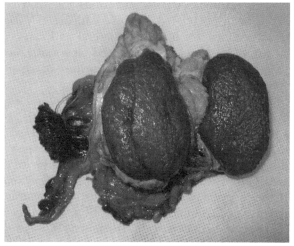

Figure 16-35 Chronic adhesions between common (parietal) and proper (visceral) tunics of the testis of a stallion that had suffered a scrotal injury and hematocele. The testicular tunics were thickened and completely adhered to each other and the epididymis. Semen quality was poor with many detached sperm heads.

may result in formation of thick adhesions between parietal and visceral tunics (Figure 16-35), preventing free movement of the testis within the tunics and leading to probable alteration in thermal regulation and constriction of epididymal tubules culminating in obstruction to sperm outflow. If the hematocele is relatively fresh and not too large, it may be advantageous to aseptically place a 16- to 18-gauge soft catheter into the vaginal space for aspiration of bloody fluid and for lavage of the vaginal cavity with sterile lactated Ringer's solution, in the hope of preventing adhesion formation. If the hematocele is large, the hemorrhage

should be evacuated surgically from the vaginal cavity, and the testis and epididymis should be carefully inspected to identify the source of hemorrhage. A tear in the tunica albuginea should be sutured, and copious lavage of the vaginal cavity should be performed with sterile lactated Ringer's solution until remaining blood clots and fibrin strands have been removed. Orchiectomy is indicated if the testis or epididymis is badly damaged. The effect of testicular trauma on formation of antisperm antibodies and secondary subfertility in stallions is not known. Removal of the affected testis may be indicated to minimize the likelihood of such a complication and to prevent depression of spermatogenesis of the contralateral testis from increased temperature caused by inflammation of the damaged testis.

VARICOCELE

A varicocele is a dilation and tortuosity of the veins of the pampiniform plexus and the cremasteric veins. Varicoceles in men and rams have been associated with testicular atrophy and decreased semen quality, possibly caused by interference with normal exchange of heat from the testicular artery to the pampiniform plexus. Varicoceles occur uncommonly in stallions, and their effect on fertility is not documented. More than 50% of men with varicoceles have normal semen quality, but varicocele in some men is associated with a low total sperm count. We have noted varicocele in some stallions with normal semen quality.

Most varicoceles are idiopathic, but a defect in the valves of the spermatic vein where it empties into the vena cava or renal vein or a deficiency of elastic and fibrous tissue in fascia that surrounds the spermatic vein has been postulated to cause varicocele. Varicoceles of stallions are usually unilateral and cause no pain when palpated. The affected spermatic cord appears enlarged and may have the texture of a bag of worms.

Definitive treatment of horses affected with varicocele is removal of the affected cord and testis, but treatment is unnecessary if semen quality is unaffected. Men who are infertile or subfertile because of a varicocele are commonly treated with ligation of the dilated vasculature or high ligation of the spermatic vein, but no good evidence shows that such treatment improves the likelihood of conception. A hydrocele has formed in a small percentage of men after ligation of the spermatic vein.

TESTICULAR NEOPLASIA

Testicular neoplasms of the horse are rarely reported, probably because most horses are castrated at an early age and perhaps because testes removed from apparently normal stallions are seldom examined closely for the presence of neoplasia. Only primary testicular neoplasms (i.e., those that originate within the testis) have been reported, and those can be divided into germinal and nongerminal types. Germinal neoplasms arise from the germ cells of the seminiferous epithelium and are the most common type of testicular neoplasm. Germinal testicular neoplasms reported to occur in the horse include the seminoma, teratoma, teratocarcinoma, and embryonal carcinoma. The seminoma is the most commonly reported testicular neoplasm of the horse. Nongerminal testicular neoplasms arise from testicular stromal cells and include the Leydig cell tumor and Sertoli cell tumor. Nongerminal testicular neoplasms of the horse are less commonly reported than are germinal testicular neoplasms.

Although cryptorchidism has been shown by epidemiologic studies to increase the incidence of some forms of primary testicular neoplasia in men and dogs, the influence of cryptorchidism on the development of testicular neoplasia of horses has not been established definitively. A large percentage of testicular teratomas seem to be found in abdominally retained testes, but failure of descent of a testis may more likely be a result of the teratoma, rather than a predisposing factor in the formation of a teratoma. Whether cryptorchidism influences the development of Sertoli cell or Leydig cell neoplasms in horses is difficult to discern from the small number of reports, but the few Leydig-cell neoplasms of horses that have been reported have been found predominantly in retained testes.

Diagnosis

When a horse with a suspected testicular neoplasm is examined, the contralateral testis should be used for comparison, keeping in mind that testicular neoplasia can occur bilaterally. The normal testis is smooth and compliant, whereas a neoplastic testis is often enlarged and has either a soft or hardened texture (sometimes with a firm, lumpy texture). Neoplastic lesions located deep within the parenchyma may not be palpable. The neoplastic testis is often heavier than its normal counterpart. A neoplastic testis is usually painless when compressed and commonly remains freely movable within the scrotum. Scrotal enlargement caused by neoplasia must be differentiated from other causes of scrotal enlargement, such as torsion of the spermatic cord, orchitis, epididymitis, hydrocele, hematocele, and inguinal herniation or rupture. Careful external palpation and ultrasonographic examination of the contents of the scrotum and palpation of the vaginal rings per rectum can be used to differentiate these conditions from testicular neoplasia. Painless, scrotal enlargement that develops insidiously in older (>10 years of age) stallions is more likely to be caused by testicular neoplasia than by inflammation or ischemia.

Ultrasonographic examination may be helpful in determining whether a testis is neoplastic. Normal testicular parenchyma is homogeneously echogenic, but a neoplastic testis usually contains areas of decreased echogenicity and the affected testes may contain single or multiple tumors (Figure 16-36). However, advanced seminomas may occupy so much of the testicular parenchyma (Figure 16-37) that insufficient tissue interface exists to clearly differentiate neoplastic from normal tissue with palpation or ultrasonographic examination (Brinsko, 1998). Testicular neoplasia can be confirmed with cytologic examination of a needle

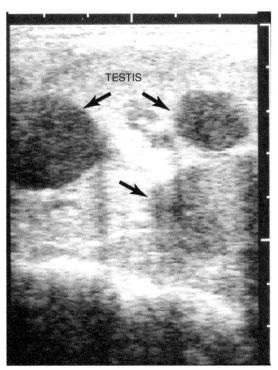

Figure 16-36 Transscrotal ultrasonographic image of a neoplastic stallion testis. Discrete hypoechoic areas *(arrows)* within the testicular parenchyma (testis) are typical of testicular tumors in the stallion.

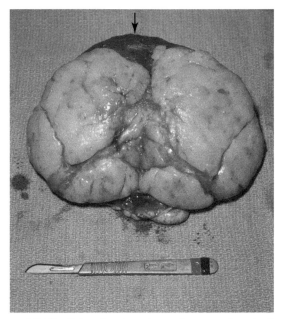

Figure 16-37 Extensive invasion of an equine testis by seminoma. The seminoma occupies most of the testis, leaving only a small area of normal parenchyma *(arrow)*. Differentiation of tumor and normal parenchyma via palpation or ultrasonographic examination may be difficult because of the lack of sufficient differential tissue interface.

aspirate or with histologic examination of a specimen obtained by punch or incision biopsy of the testis. Although testicular biopsy has been performed without noticeable side effects in normal stallions, the long-term effects of testicular biopsy have not been well studied. Biopsy of neoplastic testes of men has been associated with a high incidence of neoplastic invasion of extratesticular tissue. If testicular neoplasia is strongly suspected, the affected testis should be excised. Before a neoplastic testis is removed, the sublumbar lymph nodes should be examined via palpation per rectum for enlargement caused by metastatic spread of the tumor.

Surgical Removal

When a neoplastic testis is removed, the spermatic cord should be severed as proximally as possible. The spermatic cord should be examined grossly and histologically for evidence of metastasis. The scrotal incision should be sutured to reduce postoperative inflammation, which could interfere with thermal regulation of the remaining testis, but good hemostasis is necessary before the scrotal incision is sutured.

PENILE AND PREPUTIAL INJURIES

Penile and preputial injuries, such as lacerations and hematomas, are usually caused by kicks, especially to the erect penis; mounting of stationary objects; masturbation, particularly if a stiff brush has been placed to prevent masturbation; attempts to breed a mare across a fence; severe bending of the penile shaft caused by sudden movement of the mare during coitus; and improperly fitted or maintained stallion rings (Figures 16-38 and 16-39). Damage to the penile shaft, including the urethra, can be inflicted during castration performed by an inexperienced surgeon. Deep lacerations that extend into a corporeal body may result in impotence, and those that extend into the urethra may result severe necrosis of tissue from escape of urine.

Even superficial lacerations can result in severe penile damage if left untreated (Figure 16-40). An untreated laceration to the penile epithelium may result in cellulitis and preputial edema, which, in turn, lead to prolapse of the penis and internal preputial lamina from the preputial cavity. Prolapse of the penis and prepuce may lead to penile paralysis from damage to the penile nerves or to further damage to the exposed penile and preputial epithelium. Puncture or laceration of the glans penis may lead to severe hemorrhage during breeding when the corpus spongiosum becomes fully engorged (Figure 16-41).

Fresh lacerations to the penile and preputial epithelium should be sutured with soft absorbable or nonabsorbable suture material. An infected or heavily contaminated laceration should be left open to heal

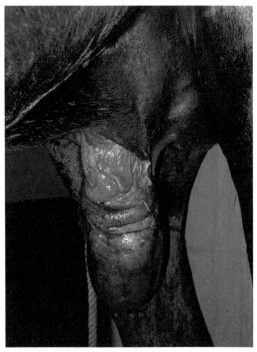

Figure 16-38 Laceration of the penis and prepuce of a stallion that was kicked while breeding.

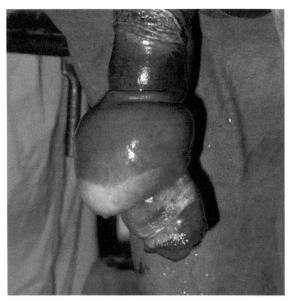

Figure 16-39 Prolapsed penis and prepuce of a stallion with an acute injury caused during breeding. The edema must be reduced to allow the penis to be returned to the preputial cavity.

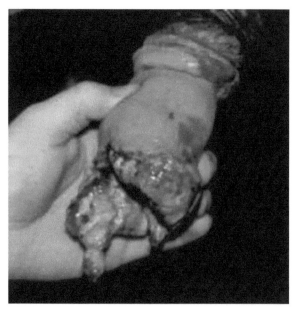

Figure 16-40 Chronic laceration from a kick to the penis resulting in extensive cellulitis and infection of the glans penis.

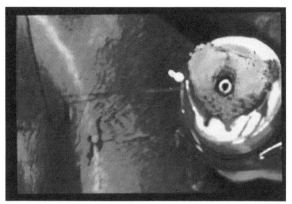

Figure 16-41 Perforation of the integument of the glans penis caused by a wire stallion brush (used to prevent masturbation) was postulated to cause a corpus spongiosal shunt that hemorrhaged when this stallion bred a standard artificial vagina. An open-ended, artificial vagina was used to permit visualization of the site of hemorrhage, which was evident as a spray of blood once the glans penis became engorged.

completely by second intention, or when it shows no signs of inflammation, it can be sutured. If the wound is left open, it should be dressed often with a nonirritating, antimicrobial ointment, preferably with a petrolatum base. If the laceration is accompanied by severe preputial edema, the penis and prepuce should be retained within the preputial cavity with use of a retainer bottle, nylon netting, or nylon hosiery suspended at the preputial orifice with a crupper and surcingle made of rubber tubing (Figures 16-42 and 16-43). The penis can be restrained within the preputial cavity for several days with sutures placed across the preputial orifice (Figure 16-44), but sutures can exacerbate the preputial trauma. If the penis cannot be retained in the preputial cavity, an enclosing abdominal support bandage (Figure 16-45) can be used in an attempt to decrease dependent edema sufficiently within a few days to allow the penis to return to the preputial cavity.

Penile hematomas that continue to expand should be explored to determine whether the origin of the hemorrhage is a rent in the tunica albuginea. Lacerations to the

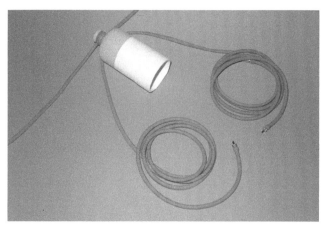

Figure 16-42 Device fabricated for retaining the penis within the preputial cavity of stallions with penile prolapse. (From Varner DD, Schumacher J, Blanchard TL, et al: *Diseases and management of breeding stallions,* St Louis, 1991, Mosby.)

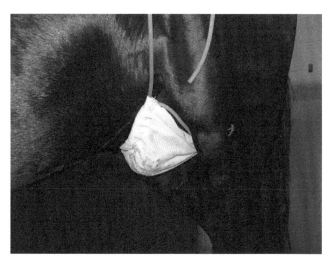

Figure 16-43 Nylon mesh, with attached tubing, fitted over the preputial orifice of a stallion to provide support of the penis of a stallion with paraphimosis. (From Brinsko SP, et al: How to treat paraphimosis. *Proc 53rd Ann Mtg Am Assoc Equine Pract* 580-582, 2007.)

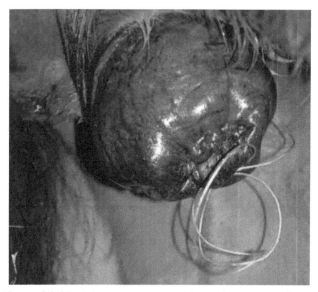

Figure 16-44 A temporary purse string suture can be placed in the prepuce, or preferably at the sheath orifice, to retain a prolapsed penis/prepuce. The suture should be tightened until a one-finger opening is left to prevent prolapse from recurring, yet to allow urine to be voided. The suture should be removed as soon as possible to prevent infection or scarring. (From Brinsko SP, et al: How to treat paraphimosis. *Proc 53rd Ann Mtg Am Assoc Equine Pract* 580-582, 2007.)

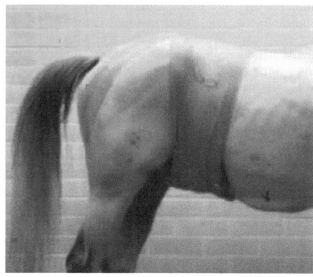

Figure 16-45 After the prolapsed penis and prepuce were cleansed and medicated with an emollient antimicrobial salve, the swollen penis and prepuce of this stallion still could not be returned to the sheath. The swollen penis and prepuce were placed in a support wrap to elevate the organ to reduce pendent edema and allow subsequent return to the preputial cavity after swelling subsided.

tunica albuginea should be sutured. Lacerations to the urethra should also be sutured, and if the laceration is transverse, the urethra should be stented with a large-bore catheter to prevent the formation of a stenosing cicatrix. A stallion whose prepuce or penis has been traumatized should be isolated from mares (to avoid erection) until the wound has healed.

PARAPHIMOSIS/PENILE PROLAPSE

Paraphimosis, or the inability of the horse to retract its penis into the preputial cavity, is usually caused by preputial edema (see Figure 16-39) that occurs from trauma, such as preputial laceration or preputial hematoma, or from preputial edema that accompanies systemic disease. It most commonly occurs in stallions as a result of breeding trauma, but geldings can also be affected. Penile prolapse occurs initially and then results in excessive edema and swelling of the penis and prepuce, thereby precluding the ability of the horse to fully retract the penis and prepuce and maintain them within the preputial cavity. Although trauma is usually the first suspected cause of the condition, other causes should also be considered, particularly when a traumatic incident is absent from the history. These include but are not limited to the use of phenothiazine tranquilizers; systemic diseases such as equine herpesvirus 1 infection, purpura hemorrhagica, and dourine; or severe debilitation. Priapism (discussed subsequently) and penile paralysis are commonly complicated by secondary paraphimosis.

Prolonged penile and preputial prolapse, regardless of the cause, impairs venous and lymphatic drainage of these tissues, leading to edema and excessive swelling. As the internal preputial lamina swells, the preputial ring can constrict, resulting in a further decrease in drainage (Figure 16-46). The penis distal to the ring becomes larger, heavier and more swollen, and a vicious cycle ensues. In longstanding cases, the pendulous weight of the prolapsed penis and prepuce can damage the internal pudendal nerves, resulting in permanent penile paralysis. Even in the short term, if not protected, the exposed epithelium of the penis and prepuce becomes excoriated, and areas can slough from pressure necrosis. Fibrosis can result, with loss of the normal telescoping action of the penis.

For initial examination, the penis and prepuce should be thoroughly cleansed and inspected to help determine the extent of injury. Ultrasonographic examination can be helpful in determining whether the swelling is solely a result of edema or whether other accumulations (e.g., seroma, hematoma, fibrin clot, or abscess) may be present that could impede the ability to reduce the penile/preputial prolapse (Figure 16-47). Drainage of large fluid accumulations or removal of

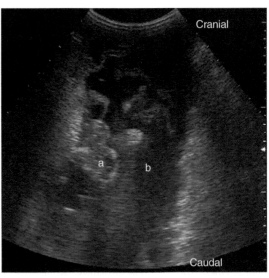

Figure 16-47 Ultrasonographic image of a hematoma in the prepuce of a stallion with paraphimosis shows blood clots *(a)* with free blood and serum *(b)*. (From Brinsko SP, et al: How to treat paraphimosis. *Proc 53rd Ann Mtg Am Assoc Equine Pract* 580-582, 2007.)

clots is often helpful in reducing otherwise refractory prolapses (Figures 16-48 and 16-49).

After the penis and prepuce are cleaned and inspected, reduction of penile and preputial swelling can often be readily accomplished with an elastic, compressive Esmarch bandage. The bandage is applied beginning at the glans penis and wrapped tightly toward the base of the penis (Figure 16-50). The bandage is left in place for 10 to 15 minutes, after which the penis is unwrapped and attempts at replacement in to the preputial cavity are made (Figure 16-51). Repeated application of the Esmarch bandage can be performed if necessary. Once the penis and prepuce can be replaced into the preputial cavity, a retention device or technique is usually successful in preventing reprolapse. If the

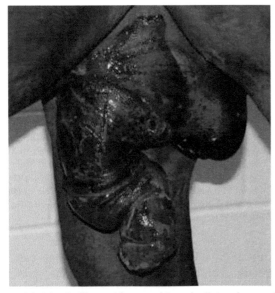

Figure 16-46 Stallion with paraphimosis. Extensive swelling of the penis and prepuce prevent retraction into the preputial cavity. (From Brinsko SP, et al: How to treat paraphimosis *Proc 53rd Ann Mtg Am Assoc Equine Pract* 580-582, 2007.)

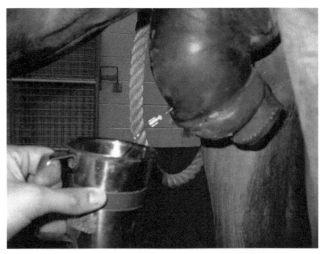

Figure 16-48 Drainage of fluid accumulation from the prepuce of a stallion with paraphimosis.

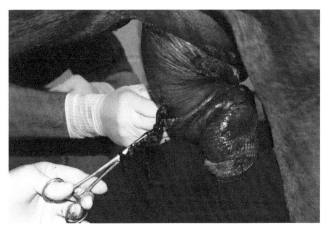

Figure 16-49 Removal of clotted blood from the prepuce of a stallion with paraphimosis.

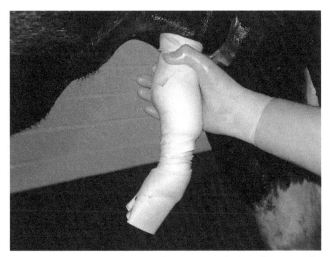

Figure 16-50 Application of an Esmarch bandage to the penis and prepuce of a horse with paraphimosis. The bandage is progressively wrapped from the tip toward the base of the penis to gradually force edematous fluid out of the tissues. The bandage is left in place for 10 to 15 minutes before removal. (From Brinsko SP, et al: How to treat paraphimosis. *Proc 53rd Ann Mtg Am Assoc Equine Pract* 580-582, 2007.)

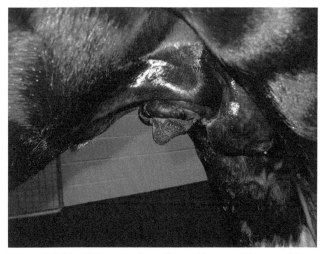

Figure 16-51 Edema and swelling of horse with paraphimosis has been reduced with application of Esmarch bandage and can now be withdrawn into the sheath. (From Brinsko SP, et al: How to treat paraphimosis. *Proc 53rd Ann Mtg Am Assoc Equine Pract* 580-582, 2007.)

penis and prepuce cannot be replaced into the preputial cavity, they should be held close to the ventral body wall with a support bandage to prevent further swelling, and daily attempts at application of a retention device are made until successful. Support devices such as a homemade surcingle or mesh sling (see Figures 16-42 and 16-43) can be used for this purpose. If penile prolapse cannot be corrected, the penis may have to be amputated (see section on penile amputation). Alternative support devices such as a mesh sling or narrow necked plastic bottle with elastic tubing can also be used. The bottom of the bottle is removed, and the edges are padded with several layers of tape. Two lengths of rubber tubing (approximately 5 feet in length) are tied around the neck of the bottle at their midpoints. The penis is then inserted into the bottle so that the

urethral orifice is aligned with the opening at the neck of the bottle. The penis and the overlying plastic bottle are then placed as far as possible within the preputial cavity. The bottle is held in place with the tubing running over the lumbar area and on either side of the scrotum up over the tail head. Voiding of urine occurs through the bottle. The bottle should be cleaned and replaced twice daily until the penis can be self retained in the retracted position.

Before the penis and prepuce are replaced into the preputial cavity or a sling is applied, the tissues should be well lubricated with an emollient, antimicrobial ointment. Products such as silver sulfadiazine cream or a compounded product consisting of dexamethasone (80 mg) and oxytetracycline (3.88 g) per pound of lanolin base are efficacious for this purpose. When these products are applied, it is also helpful to begin application distally and work proximally, massaging the dressings onto the penis and prepuce to further reduce edema and swelling. Adjunct therapies include use of nonsteroidal antiinflammatory drugs such as phenylbutazone or flunixin meglumine, daily exercise, and hydrotherapy (10 to 20 minutes once or twice daily. Systemic antimicrobials, although not always necessary, can be added to the treatment regimen at the discretion of the veterinarian; however, antimicrobials are indicated if surgical drainage was attempted. The duration of treatment varies but can often take a week to 10 days until the penis can be maintained in the preputial cavity without support; some cases may take several weeks.

If paraphimosis is caused by or has caused permanent penile paralysis, the stallion is unlikely to be able to achieve erection. If a stallion with penile paralysis can ejaculate into an artificial vagina, and if the stallion's breed registry permits artificial insemination, the stallion's breeding life can be extended with collection of semen for artificial insemination of mares. The stallion can be salvaged for uses other than breeding with amputation of its penis or with permanent retraction of the paralyzed penis into its prepuce after the horse is castrated. The penis can be permanently retracted into the preputial cavity with sutures placed through the annular ring (i.e., the reflection of the internal preputial lamina onto the free body of the penis) and anchored to tissue behind the scrotal area (i.e., the Bolz technique of phallopexy). The penis can also be retained within the preputial cavity with segmental posthectomy (i.e., reefing, Adam's procedure) of the entire internal lamina of the prepuce.

PHIMOSIS

Phimosis, or the inability to completely protrude the penis from the prepuce, occurs naturally in foals because the internal preputial lamina is fused to the free part of the penis for about the first month after birth. Excluding this normal physiologic condition, phimosis is usually the result of constriction of the external preputial orifice or the preputial ring caused by trauma or neoplasia (Figure 16-52). When the horse is unable to protrude its penis, it urinates within the preputial cavity, causing excoriation of the preputial epithelium, which leads to more inflammation and irritation, thereby compounding the problem (Figure 16-53).

A constricting external preputial orifice can be enlarged with removal of a triangular segment of external lamina, whose base is the preputial orifice. The cut edge of the external lamina is sutured to the cut edge of the internal preputial lamina. Removal of a similar triangle from the preputial fold can enlarge a constricting preputial ring, or the constricting preputial ring can be removed with segmental posthectomy after the preputial ring is incised to allow the penis and internal lamina to protrude. (See following section, "Neoplasia of the Penis and Prepuce," for a description of the reefing operation.)

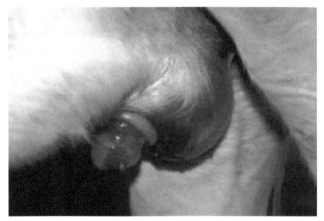

Figure 16-52 Phimosis in this stallion was caused by extensive melanomas arising from peripreputial tissues.

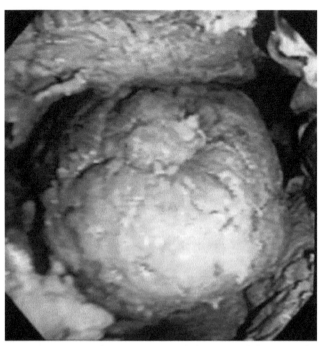

Figure 16-53 Endoscopic view of the preputial cavity of a stallion with phimosis. Urinary scalding contributes to the local infection and cellulitis when the horse cannot extend its penis to urinate.

NEOPLASIA OF THE PENIS AND PREPUCE

Any cutaneous neoplasm can affect the integument of the external genitalia, but the most common neoplasm of the penis and prepuce is squamous cell carcinoma. Lesions of squamous cell carcinoma are typically multiple and usually involve the glans penis or the internal lamina of the prepuce (Figure 16-54). Geldings develop squamous cell carcinoma of the penis and prepuce more often than do stallions, and horses with nonpigmented genitalia such as Appaloosas and American Paint Horses are more commonly affected than are horses with pigmented genitalia. The malignancy of squamous cell carcinomas of the penis, and prepuce of the horse is usually low, and lesions tend to remain localized; however, metastasis has been reported, so treatment should not be neglected.

Horses with small cancerous or precancerous lesions (i.e., 2- to 3-mm in diameter and superficial) can be treated with application of 5-fluorouracil cream to the lesions at 14-day intervals. Rubber examination gloves should be worn during application of this drug. The cream should not be applied more often because of its irritating capabilities. If the cream is effective, usually no more lesions are noted after two to three applications.

If larger, deeper lesions are present, a more aggressive treatment method (freezing, surgical excision) is necessary. Preputial and penile neoplasms that are superficial (do not invade deeper tissues) and less than 2 to 3 cm in diameter can be excised or destroyed with

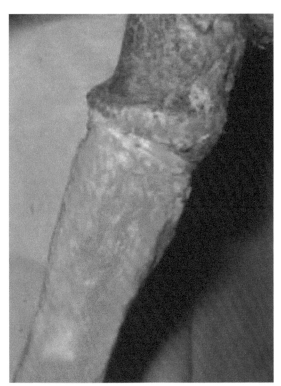

Figure 16-54 Multiple, pale, slightly raised lesions of squamous cell carcinoma on the penis and prepuce of a stallion.

cryotherapy. Cryotherapy can be performed with liquid nitrogen administered as a spray or through a cryoprobe or with carbon dioxide applied through a cryoprobe (Figure 16-55). Lesions should be frozen to a depth of 2 to 3 mm with two or three freeze-thaw cycles. A rapid freeze coupled with a slow thaw produces the most cellular damage. A thermocouple can be used to monitor the size and depth of the area affected by the cryogen. The penis and prepuce should be reexamined at 1- to 2-month intervals, and any recurring or new lesions should be frozen again (Figure 16-56). Horses with extensive lesions of the prepuce may need segmental posthectomy (i.e., reefing).

For reefing of the internal lamina of the prepuce (Figure 16-57), the horse is anesthetized, positioned in dorsal or lateral recumbency, and prepared for aseptic surgery. The penis is extended with traction, and the urethra is catheterized. If desired, a tourniquet can be placed proximal to the surgical site. Parallel, circumferential cutaneous incisions are made proximal and

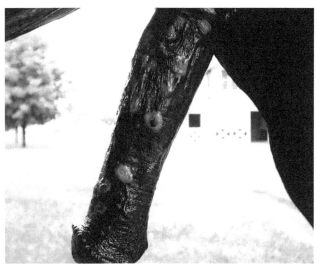

Figure 16-56 Healing lesions 2 weeks after use of cryoprobe to freeze diffuse, superficial lesions of squamous cell carcinoma on the penis of a breeding stallion. Within 2 months, only depigmented areas of skin remained visible.

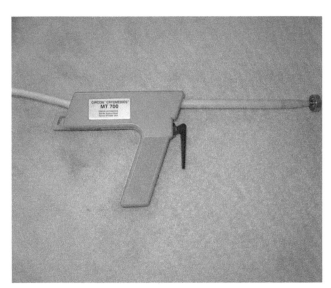

Figure 16-55 A 2-cm-diameter cryoprobe attachment for a CO_2 cryosurgery instrument that can be used to freeze superficial squamous cell carcinomas of the penis and prepuce. Tissue should be frozen and thawed two or three times to a depth of 2 to 3 mm.

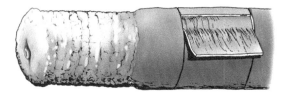

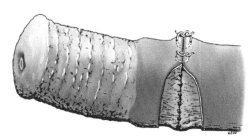

Figure 16-57 A reefing operation, or circumferential excision of a length of the prepuce, with subsequent closure of the preputial defect. (From Varner DD, Schumacher J, Blanchard TL, et al: *Diseases and management of breeding stallions,* St Louis, 1991, Mosby.)

distal to the preputial lesions, and these incisions are connected by a longitudinal incision. The diseased segment of prepuce between the circumferential incisions is excised from the penis with scissor dissection. Bleeding vessels are ligated with absorbable sutures, and loose fascia is apposed with interrupted, 2-0 absorbable sutures. Care must be taken to maintain the prepuce in proper alignment; placement of a suture in the fascia at four equidistant points around the circumference of the penis at each circumferential incision, before the segment of integument is excised, may aid in orientation. The integument is apposed with interrupted no. 0 or 2-0 absorbable or nonabsorbable sutures. The amount of prepuce that can be removed from a stallion without disruption of normal copulatory function is not known. To prevent disruption of sutures caused by penile erection, the stallion should be isolated from mares for at least 2 weeks; application of a stallion ring to the penis may be necessary to prevent erection. The horse should be exercised daily to reduce postsurgical edema. Nonabsorbable sutures should be removed at 10 to 12 days. Phallectomy (Figure 16-58) may be indicated if neoplasia has invaded the tunica albuginea, but phallectomy in stallions should be considered to be a salvage procedure. A stallion should be castrated at least 2 weeks before phallectomy and separated from other horses for 2 weeks after phallectomy to decrease the likelihood

of a sexually induced erection and disruption of sutures.

CUTANEOUS HABRONEMIASIS

Summer sores (i.e., cutaneous habronemiasis) are pruritic, pyogranulomatous lesions caused by aberrant cutaneous migration of the larvae of the equine stomach worm, *Habronema*. Summer sores can be found anywhere on the integument, and when the genitalia are involved, the urethral process and preputial ring are the most common sites of infestation (Figure 16-59). Summer sores appear in warm months when flies, which are the nematode's intermediate host, are prevalent. Summer sores of the genitalia may disappear with the advent of cold weather. Horses that are prone to protruding the penis are particularly vulnerable to cutaneous habronemiasis of the genitalia. Migration and encystment of *Habronema* larvae cause formation of exuberant granulation tissue that contains small, yellow, caseous granules. Skin surrounding the granulation tissue may be depigmented. Lesions of the preputial ring interfere with the normal telescoping action of the prepuce, and lesions of the urethral process may involve the corpus spongiosum penis, resulting in hematuria or hemospermia.

Summer sores may resemble lesions of pythiosis, carcinoma, the fibroblastic form of sarcoid, or exuberant granulation tissue caused by trauma. The presence of small granules in the lesion usually enables the condition to be differentiated from other diseases with similar appearance. With squeezing of the lesion, larvae can occasionally be extruded onto a slide and identified microscopically. Histologic characteristics of lesions are granulation tissue infiltrated with eosinophils, granules,

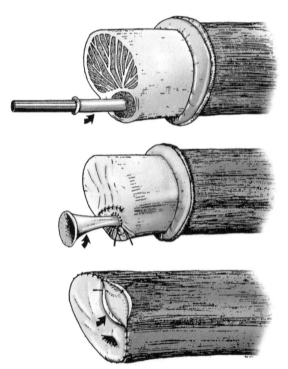

Figure 16-58 Amputation of the equine penis, with separate closure of the corpus cavernosum penis and the corpus spongiosum penis, followed by fixation of the flared urethral mucosa *(arrows)* to the skin of the penis. (From Varner DD, Schumacher J, Blanchard TL, et al: *Diseases and management of breeding stallions*, St Louis, 1991, Mosby.)

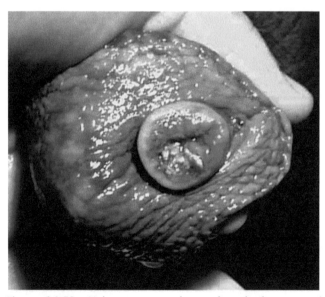

Figure 16-59 *Habronema* granuloma of urethral process of a stallion that resulted in profuse bleeding (hemospermia) when corpus spongiosum was fully engorged.

and larvae; affected horses often have a marked eosinophilia. Examination of multiple areas of tissue from biopsied lesions is advisable because combinations of habronemiasis and squamous cell carcinomas can occur when fly vectors have been feeding and depositing infective larvae on neoplastic lesions.

Administration of ivermectin (systemically) or an organophosphate (systemically or topically) has been effective in resolving lesions by eliminating the migrating larvae. Smaller urethral process granulomas (1- to 2-mm diameter) that tend to bleed, but are not large enough to justify amputation of the urethral process, can be injected with a mixture of long-acting corticosteroid (Depomedrol, Upjohn Co, Kalamazoo, MI) and liquid ivermectin (mixed in 1:1 ratio). In some cases, repeating the injection in 1 month is necessary. Systemic administration of a corticosteroid or diethylcarbamazine has also been reported to be successful in resolving lesions by eliminating the horse's response to the larvae.

Lesions of the internal lamina of the prepuce can be surgically excised. Small lesions can be removed with elliptical excision, but large or multiple lesions are often best removed with reefing. Lesions of the urethral process may necessitate amputation of the process (Figures 16-60 and 16-61). The urethral process can be amputated with the horse anesthetized or with the horse standing and sedated. A male urinary catheter is passed into the urethra, and if surgery is performed with the horse standing, the base of the urethral process is infiltrated with local anesthetic solution. The urethral process is circumferentially excised proximal to the lesion, and the epithelium

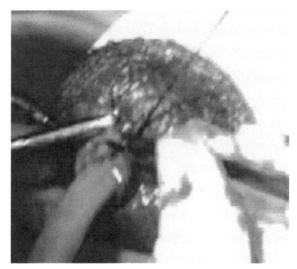

Figure 16-61 The urethral granuloma is excised, and the inner urethral mucosa is sutured to the outer integument of the urethral process with a simple interrupted pattern.

of the stump is sutured to the urethral mucosa, with 2-0 or 3-0 absorbable suture material in an interrupted pattern, to close the exposed corpus spongiosum penis. It is important to "roll" the skin inward (toward the urethral mucosa) when suturing; otherwise the mucosa will be everted and exposed to injury when the penis is fully erect after healing. Fibrous tissue at the suture site may also tear during subsequent breeding, contributing to further hemospermia.

PRIAPISM

Priapism, or persistent erection without sexual arousal, occurs when detumescence of the engorged corpus cavernosum penis (CCP) fails because of disturbances of arterial inflow or venous outflow (Figure 16-62). Priapism occurs uncommonly in horses but is economically devastating when a valuable breeding stallion is affected. Impotence is the usual outcome, and phallectomy may be necessary.

Priapism is categorized as low-flow when primary vascular or hematologic disease mechanically interferes with venous drainage or when the α-adrenergic impulses that bring about detumescence are blocked. It is categorized as high-flow when the venous outflow of the penis is overridden by an increase in arterial inflow to the cavernous tissue. High-flow priapism in men is nearly always a consequence of penile trauma that causes an arterial-cavernosal shunt. Men are much more commonly affected by low-flow priapism than by high-flow priapism, and the same appears to be true of horses.

Priapism in stallions is caused primarily by administration of a phenothiazine-derivative tranquilizer that blocks the sympathetic impulses that initiate detumescence. When detumescence fails, blood in the CCP stagnates, and partial pressure of CO_2 in the stagnant

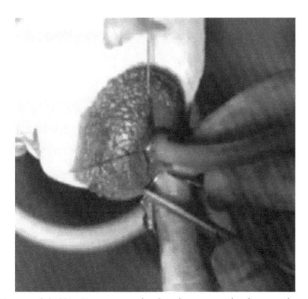

Figure 16-60 For removal of a large urethral granuloma caused by *Habronema* larvae unresponsive to medical therapy, the penis and prepuce are scrubbed with a disinfectant and dried. A sterile stallion catheter is passed into the urethra and held in place by retention needles passed through the urethral process proximal to the lesion.

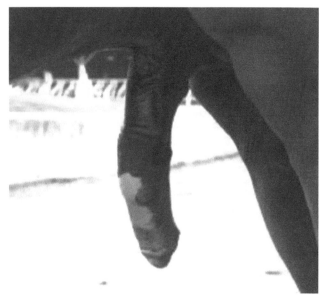

Figure 16-62 Persistent erection (priapism) in a stallion after administration of acepromazine.

blood rises, causing erythrocytes to sickle. The sickled erythrocytes obstruct venous outflow from the CCP, and the collecting veins eventually become irreversibly occluded. Arterial supply to the CCP is still patent in the early stages of priapism, but if priapism persists, it too becomes irreversibly occluded. Eventually, the trabeculae of the cavernosal tissue become fibrotic and lose their expansile capacity necessary for normal erection (Figure 16-63). In addition to damaging erectile

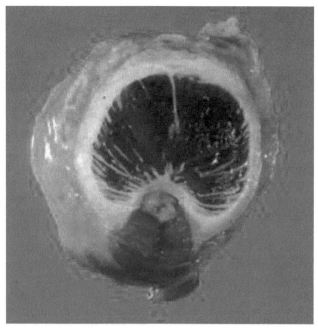

Figure 16-63 Cross section of an amputated penis from a stallion with chronic priapism unresponsive to treatment. Blood within the corpus cavernosum penis was clotted, and cavernosal trabeculae were thickened and fibrotic.

tissue, prolonged erection may also result in penile paralysis by damaging the pudendal nerves, perhaps by compressing the nerves against the ischium. The weight of the pendant penis may also damage the retractor penis muscles.

Horses with priapism have been treated empirically with administration of diuretic and corticosteroid drugs, general or regional anesthesia, penile and preputial massage, application of an emollient dressing, and slings. Although such treatments usually fail to resolve priapism, some, such as massage and application of an emollient dressing, are beneficial because they prevent damage to the integument of the exposed organ. Benztropine mesylate (Cogentin, Merck and Company Inc, West Point, Pa.), a cholinergic blocker administered systemically (8 mg via slow intravenous injection), and 1% phenylephrine HCl (GensiaSicor Pharmaceuticals Inc, Irvine, Calif.), a sympathomimetic drug injected aseptically directly into the CCP (2 to 10 mg), have been used successfully to bring about detumescence in horses affected with priapism. These drugs should not be given if the horse has ventricular tachycardia or high blood pressure, and the horse's heart rate should be monitored after administration.

When the horse does not respond to medical treatment, the CCP should be irrigated to evacuate sludged blood. Heparinized, physiologic saline solution (10 U heparin/mL physiologic saline solution) is injected through a 14- or 12-gauge needle inserted into the erect CCP proximal to the glans penis. Sludged blood and saline solution are evacuated 10 to 15 cm caudal to the scrotum through a small stab incision in the tunica albuginea of the CCP or through one or two 14- or 12-gauge needles inserted into the CCP. The CCP is irrigated until fresh hemorrhage appears in the efflux (Figure 16-64). If a stab incision is made in the tunica albuginea of the CCP, it should be sutured after irrigation. If arterial blood fails to appear after irrigation, the arteriolar supply to the CCP is probably permanently damaged, and impotence is likely. Failure of erection to subside after irrigation indicates that arteriolar inflow is patent and that venous outflow is still occluded. If erection recurs after irrigation of the CCP, the CCP can be anastomosed to the corpus spongiosum penis (CSP) to create a shunt for blood trapped within the CCP (Figure 16-65). This shunt is unlikely to interfere with subsequent erection and ejaculation.

HEMOSPERMIA

Hemospermia, a cause of infertility in stallions, has been attributed to bacterial and viral urethritis, improperly applied stallion rings, habronemiasis of the urethral process, and wounds to the glans penis. Hemospermia is also commonly caused by a pelvic urethral rent of unknown etiology. Regardless of the cause of hemospermia, the source of hemorrhage is probably the CSP.

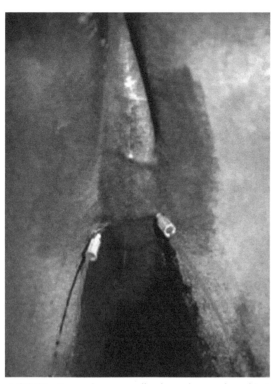

Figure 16-64 Large-bore needles have been placed into the corpus cavernosum penis (caudal to the scrotum; effluent sites) of a stallion with priapism for irrigation of the corpus cavernosal tissue with heparinized physiologic saline solution. Another large-bore needle (not shown) was placed distally (just proximal to the glans penis) into the corpus cavernosum penis for infusion of heparinized saline solution.

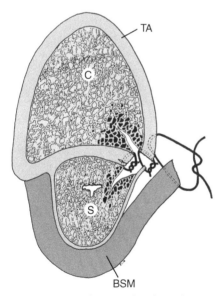

Figure 16-65 Creation of a vascular shunt between the corpus cavernosum penis (CCP) *(C)* and the corpus spongiousum penis (CSP) *(S)* as a surgical treatment for priapism in stallions. After incising of the CCP and CSP, the incised tunica albuginea *(ta)* of the CSP is sutured to the incised tunica albuginea overlying the lateral aspect of the CCP. The incised bulbospongiosus muscle *(bsm)* is then resutured to the tunica albuginea of the CCP. (From Varner DD, Schumacher J, Blanchard TL, et al: *Diseases and management of breeding stallions,* St Louis, 1991, Mosby.)

Hemorrhage occurs at the end of ejaculation, when contraction of the bulbospongiosus muscles causes pressure within the CSP to increase from 17 to 1000 mm Hg. Blood in the ejaculate, even in amounts than cannot be detected grossly, might contribute to infertility.

Hemospermia from a pelvic urethral rent may occur more commonly in frequently bred stallions. Affected stallions are sometimes slow to ejaculate, and ejaculation sometimes appears to cause pain. Hemospermia is usually diagnosed with gross examination of semen that has been collected with an artificial vagina. The site of hemorrhage can often be determined with examination of the urethra with a sterilized, flexible endoscope that is at least 100 cm long. Endoscopic examination of the urethra of such affected stallions reveals a longitudinal defect, 5 to 10 mm long, on the caudal surface of the urethra at the level of the ischial arch (Figure 16-66); no gross signs of inflammation surround the defect.

The fertility of stallions that have a slight amount of hemorrhage in the ejaculate can sometimes be preserved by adding an extender to the semen to dilute the concentration of red blood cells in the ejaculate. Horses infertile or subfertile because of hemospermia have been treated with sexual abstinence and with systemic administration of formalin, methenamine, or antimicrobial drugs. Enforcing sexual abstinence for a protracted time (e.g., many months) is often unsuccessful in resolving hemospermia. Horses with hemospermia seem to be most effectively treated with temporary urethrotomy performed at the level of the ischial arch (Figures 16-67 and 16-68). Urethrotomy is performed with the horse standing, with use of sedation and epidural anesthesia. For facilitation of identification of the urethra during dissection, a urethral catheter or small foal stomach tube is inserted into the urethra and advanced until it is

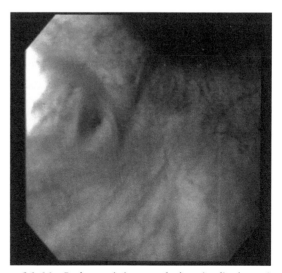

Figure 16-66 Endoscopic image of a longitudinal rent in the mucosa of the caudal aspect of the urethra at the level of the ischial arch of a stallion with hemospermia.

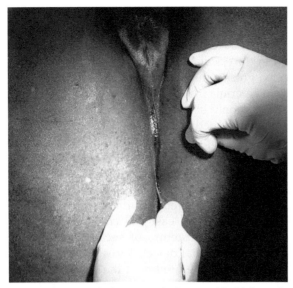

Figure 16-67 Surgical approach for a subischial urethrostomy. A longitudinal incision 8 to 10 cm long is centered on the perineal raphe at the level of the ischial arch.

proximal to the ischial arch. A longitudinal incision, 8 to 10 cm long, centered on the ischial arch, is made on the perineal raphe (Figure 16-67). The incision extends through skin, retractor penis and bulbospongiosus muscles, CSP, and urethral mucosa to expose the lumen of the urethra (Figure 16-68). Incising the urethral mucosa may be unnecessary for resolution of hemospermia. Opening the CSP without entering the urethra (spongiotomy) may reduce the risk of complications associated with urethrotomy, such as urethral fistula or stricture. The wound is allowed to heal by second intention. Daily installation of suppositories composed of an antimicrobial drug and a corticosteroid into the urethral

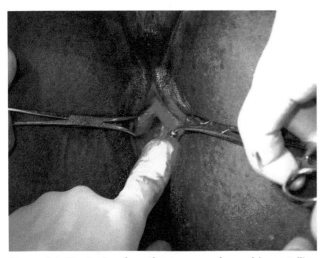

Figure 16-68 Perineal urethrotomy performed in a stallion for treatment for hemospermia resulting from a urethral tear. Caudal epidural anesthesia is used to provide analgesia. After the glans penis is scrubbed with disinfectant, a sterile urethral catheter is passed beyond the level ischium to aid in identification of the urethra during urethrotomy.

lumen has been advocated but is unnecessary. Stallions should receive sexual rest for at least 3 months after surgery. Horses may bleed at the urethrotomy for more than a week after surgery, especially at the end of urination when the bulbospongiosus muscles contract. The ischial wound generally heals within 3 to 4 weeks.

Incising the CSP at the level of the ischium may decrease cavernosal pressure at the end of urination, and this decreased pressure in the CSP may be responsible for the apparent success of temporary urethrotomy in eliminating hemospermia. When the bladder has emptied, the bulbospongiosus muscles contract to expel urine that remains in the urethra, and these contractions increase pressure within the CSP and may prevent healing of a urethral lesion that communicates with the CSP. The incision into the CSP converts this semiclosed, vascular space into an open space, and during urination, blood flow is diverted from the urethral lesion to the urethrotomy/spongiotomy, thus permitting the lesion to heal.

Because the urethral rents are typically located at the caudal surface of the urethra near the ischial arch and are accessible through ischial urethrotomy, primary closure of the defect may be indicated. Urethral endoscopy aids the surgeon in identifying the exact location of the defect. For confirmation of the location of the defect, a hypodermic needle can be inserted percutaneously into the lumen of the urethra at the level of the ischial arch during endoscopic examination. The urethral rent is sutured in an interrupted pattern with 3-0 absorbable suture. The perineal wound is left unsutured to heal by second intention.

HEMATURIA

A urethral defect of geldings, identical to the urethral defect at the ischial arch of stallions that causes hemospermia, also causes hematuria in geldings. Hematuria occurs typically at the end of urination when the intraluminal urethral pressure suddenly decreases while the pressure in the CSP remains high. Hemorrhage was once thought to be caused by a sudden increase in pressure in the CSP caused by contraction of the bulbospongiosus muscle at the end of urination, but the increase in pressure within the CSP associated with contraction of the bulbospongiosus muscle is slight. Occasionally, the affected horse shows sign of pain at the end of urination. Geldings with hematuria caused by a urethral rent are treated with temporary urethrotomy, the same treatment received by stallions with hemospermia caused by the identical urethral lesion. The ischial incision needs to penetrate only into the CSP to be effective. With incising of the CSP, vascular pressure at the end of urination is reduced, and with the reduction in pressure, blood no longer flows through the defect at the end of urination, allowing the defect to heal.

BIBLIOGRAPHY

Blanchard TL, Schumacher J, Edwards JF, et al: Priapism in a stallion with generalized malignant melanoma, *J Am Vet Med Assoc* 198:1043-1044, 1991.

Blanchard TL, Varner DD, Brinsko SP: Theirogenology question of the month: seminal and hormonal parameters in a stallion with hematocele, *J Am Vet Med Assoc* 209:2013-2014, 1996.

Brinsko SP: Neoplasia of the male reproductive tract. In Savage CJ, editor: Neoplasia, *Vet Clin North Am Equine Pract* 14(3):517-533, 1998.

Fortier AL, Mac Harg MA: Topical use of 5-fluorouracil for treatment of squamous cell carcinoma of the external genitalia of horses: 11 cases (1988-1992), *J Am Vet Med Assoc* 205:1183-1185, 1994.

McKinnon AO, Voss JL: Hemospermia and urospermia. In McKinnon AO, Voss JL, editors: *Equine reproduction*, Philadelphia, 1993, Lea & Febiger.

Schumacher J, Varner DD, Schmitz DG, et al: Urethral defects in geldings with hematuria and stallions with hemospermia, *Vet Surg* 24:250-254, 1995.

Varner DD, Schumacher J, Blanchard TL, et al: *Diseases and management of breeding stallions*, St Louis, 1991, Mosby, 140-340.

Walker DF, Vaughan JT: *Bovine and equine urogenital surgery*, Philadelphia, 1980, Lea & Febiger, 115-176.

Wilson DV, Nickels FA, Williams MA: Pharmacologic treatment of priapism in two horses, *J Am Vet Med Assoc* 199:1183-1184, 1991.

Embryo Transfer

17

CHAPTER

Aside from semen collection and artificial insemination, embryo transfer has become the most widely recognized assisted reproductive technique used in the horse. This brings to the equine practitioner an exceptional opportunity for practice expansion but also entails tremendous responsibility. What started about 25 years ago as a novel method of producing a foal from aged nonproductive broodmares has now expanded to become an elective procedure that is applicable to virtually all mares of reproductive age. This transition to a widely used elective procedure carries the responsibility commonly known as "above all else, do no harm" to the involved veterinarian.

Embryo transfer now lends itself to (1) obtaining foals from performance and show mares while they are competing; (2) multiple foals from the same mare in 1 year; (3) mares with nonreproductive health or musculoskeletal problems; and (4) mares with reproductive problems. In addition, through embryo transfer procedures, a mare that foals late in the year can be allowed early entry into the following breeding season without the loss of a foal. The use of embryo transfer has also enabled the development of more sophisticated advanced reproductive techniques such as intracytoplasmic sperm injection (ICSI) and nuclear transfer (cloning). Opportunities seem to be restricted only by our imagination.

Expectations for success have risen dramatically since the adoption of commercial embryo transfer. Results that were unimaginable just a few years ago are now achievable. For the sake of discussion, embryo recovery rates equal to or above the per-cycle pregnancy rate of a given stallion are expected. This translates to recovery of 100% of embryos in the uterus at the time of embryo retrieval. With regard to embryo-transfer success, the author (Hartman) contends that practitioners should set a goal of a 90% pregnancy rate at 12 days and 85% at 30 days after ovulation. One of the deceptive aspects of embryo transfer is that some degree of success may be achieved with relatively poor technique. The end result of this is an ever-present temptation to "cut corners" (i.e., to perform a uterine flush or embryo transfer in less-than-optimal conditions or using less-than-optimal supplies or media).

Conventional methods of embryo transfer have been described elsewhere by Colorado workers. This chapter discusses what has worked well in our practice and also some of the more controversial topics related to embryo transfer.

RECIPIENT MARE MANAGEMENT BEFORE TRANSFER

Management of a recipient herd is a daunting and labor-intensive task. This task begins in the fall of the previous year. During this period, it is important to acquire the total number of mares that are needed for the coming breeding season. New mares that may introduce contagious disease into the herd should not be added during the breeding season; the risk is too great among both the nonpregnant and pregnant mares. All individual mares should have a means of permanent identification to avoid any confusion regarding which mare is pregnant with which foal.

One of the most common complaints among mare owners concerns the quality of the recipient mares; therefore, selection of recipients that are reproductively sound is important, as is musculoskeletal soundness, dental health, vision, and behavior. The examination should include evaluation of udder health, because the ability to provide sufficient milk is a requisite for raising a healthy well-grown foal. All mares should pass a standard with regard to temperament and disposition. At the least, mares should be halter broke and gentle enough to catch in a small pen or stall. Fall and winter are also good times to manage vaccination, deworming, and Coggins tests, before mares are admitted into the recipient herd. Testing and vaccination for equine arteritis virus should be addressed where geographically indicated.

It is always a challenge to have sufficient mares with normal reproductive cyclicity in February (in the Northern Hemisphere) when the commercial breeding season begins. A good artificial lighting program is the most reliable method for ensuring early seasonal entry into reproductive cyclicity. For this protocol, mares are exposed to a total of 16 hours of light each 24-hour

period beginning in the middle of November (see Chapter 3). The challenge centers on a good method of artificial lighting that can be used with large numbers of mares. The most common system involves holding the mares in large pens during the artificial lighting period. This holding can be stressful to the mares because they may be crowded and unable to access feed or water and are often exposed to inclement weather during confinement. Some studies discount the effect of stress on mares (Baucus et al., 1990); however, such studies generally examine a single stress insult rather than assessing cumulative stressors over time. Considerable anecdotal evidence points to the detrimental effect high stress has on such factors as maintenance of a corpus luteum (CL) and the mare's ability to maintain early pregnancy.

With the onset of breeding season, the goals for management of open recipient mares are twofold. First, knowledge of the precise day that each mare ovulates is necessary. This is best established with transrectal palpation and ultrasound of the reproductive tract during behavioral estrus. Examination should be done daily as the mare approaches ovulation and, oftentimes, for at least 1 day after ovulation. For record-keeping purposes, the day of ovulation is always considered day 0. The next day after ovulation, the mare becomes "+1", the second day "+2", and so forth. The commonly accepted window of synchrony between donor and recipient mares is such that recipient mares that are +4 to +8 days after ovulation are considered to be eligible to receive embryos (McCue et al., 2001; Vanderwall, 2000). An alternative method of describing synchrony is in regard to the recipient's day of ovulation relative to that of the donor (Figure 17-1). The important concept here is that during this time the mare can respond to early signals involving maternal recognition of pregnancy and should also have adequate levels of circulating progesterone. Workers in the United Kingdom (Wilsher et al., 2005) successfully lengthened this window of synchrony, thereby enabling the use of recipients that were +9 to +10 days from ovulation. This was accomplished with the administration of meclofenamic acid (1 g per os, once daily) starting on day 9 after ovulation and continuing until day 7 after embryo transfer. With this protocol, the investigators were able to suppress the normal cyclical luteolytic response.

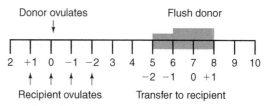

Figure 17-1 Schematic representation of synchrony between donors and recipients for successful embryo transfer.

If determination of the day of ovulation becomes the primary focus, then a difficult aspect of recipient mare management, which is endometritis, is easily overlooked. Therefore, a second, equally important goal of management of open recipient mares is to ensure that they are reproductively sound and ready to receive an embryo. Begin by considering only mares that are 3 to 12 years of age for admission into the recipient herd. This should eliminate most mares with substantial chronic endometritis that would interfere with the ability to maintain a pregnancy to term. Next, evaluate the anatomy of the perineum and vulva. Very thin mares often have poor perineal anatomy, which is improved when they gain weight. If indicated, a Caslick's operation should be performed. The importance of this cannot be overstated because bacterial contamination at the time of embryo transfer is a frequent cause of embryonic loss. It is apparent, then, that *transrectal* palpation and ultrasound examinations during estrus serve not only to establish the day of ovulation but also to evaluate the condition of the uterus. If indicated, uterine swabs should be procured for microbial culture. In our view, cultures should be taken only when the mare is in advanced estrus. The mare should have at least a 35-mm follicle that is beginning to mature, and the uterus should demonstrate substantial edema at the time of uterine culture. If these conditions are not met, false-negative culture results may be obtained. In addition, care should be taken not to contaminate the uterus during the process of obtaining the culture. Concurrently, control of delayed or inadequate uterine clearance is important. Florida workers recommend repeated oxytocin (20 IU given intravenously) injections to eliminate intrauterine fluid, but not more often than every 4 hours. These mares should be monitored for at least 1 day after ovulation to be certain no fluid is present in the uterus as they enter diestrus.

DONOR MARE MANAGEMENT BEFORE THE UTERINE FLUSH

Proper management of donor mares centers on the ultimate goal of recovering as clean an embryo as possible that is of a size that transfers well. With this in mind, practitioners should realize that contrary to conventional thought, donor mares with endometritis become pregnant on a regular basis and an embryo is commonly found in a very dirty flush. Regardless of the number of times the embryo is washed, getting these embryos to thrive after embryo transfer is difficult. Therefore, a prudent practice is to make sure the donor mare's uterus is free of microorganisms at the time of insemination. Once-daily transrectal palpation and ultrasound examinations allow the practioner to follow follicular development and ovulation and, just as important, to monitor the conditions of the uterus. The time and effort spent keeping the donor mare's uterus

clean are rewarded with increased rates of successful embryo transfer. Keep in mind that bacterial contamination of the donor's uterus can come from many sources. Among these are inadvertent contaminations during the breeding process, contaminated semen, and, increasingly commonplace, residual infection and endometritis from previous reproductive procedures.

Multiple embryo transfers on the same mare during a breeding season, oftentimes at different farms and by different veterinarians, are becoming more common. Colorado workers (Carnevale et al., 2005) analyzed the effects of repeated inseminations and embryo transfer attempts on uterine health and found an association with increased chronic inflammatory changes. These workers concluded that mares were susceptible to the additive effects of repeated uterine insults. In clinical practice, substantial evidence shows that repeated breeding and embryo transfer attempts yield an increased likelihood of acute bacterial endometritis, in addition to chronic inflammation. Therefore, proper donor mare management necessitates continued vigilance to guard against endometritis. Donor mares may need uterine cultures on a regular basis throughout the breeding season. However, the overuse of intrauterine antibiotic therapy should be discouraged because this may lead to overgrowth of yeasts or fungi. One of the most effective ways to keep a mare's uterus in a hygienic state is through effective uterine lavage along with ecbolics to aid in uterine clearance.

One factor that affects embryo transfer success is the size of the embryo at the time of transfer to the recipient mare. Large embryos present their own set of problems. For example, they are somewhat more fragile, and a transfer apparatus that can accommodate the larger embryos is sometimes difficult to find. On the other hand, if a donor mare's uterus is flushed too early, the embryo may still be in the oviduct and not available to traditional recovery attempts. In fact, it is not uncommon for a mare to end up pregnant after being flushed for embryo retrieval. Therefore, selecting the correct flush day is of paramount importance. The ideal embryo size is usually achieved by 7 days after ovulation, at which time its diameter is approximately 400 to 500 μm. However, the optimal approach is not so simple as to automatically flush all mare uteri at 7 days after ovulation. The timing of embryo entry into the uterus has been established to be somewhat variable (Battut et al., 2000), ranging between 144 hours (6 days) and 156 hours (6.5 days) after ovulation is first detected. Examination of the CL in the periovulatory period is important in that scheduling a 7-day flush date from a recent ovulation often results in a smaller-than-expected embryo. Several factors seem to influence this variability in embryo size: (1) the age of the donor mare; (2) the inherent fertility of the stallion; (3) the timing of breeding relative to the time of ovulation; and (4) variation in time between ovulation and fertilization. In our practice, most reproductively normal mares are flushed 7 days after ovulation is detected. A simple way to plan is to consider the day of the week when planning for the embryo flush attempt. For example, if Monday is the day ovulation is first detected (day 0), the mare's uterus is flushed on the following Monday for a 7-day flush. Among the exceptions to this are old mares (18 years or older), mares bred to subfertile stallions or older stallions, and mares bred with frozen semen, which are all flushed on day 8.

During the week between ovulation and the uterine flush, donor mares should be kept as stress-free as possible. Evidence shows that performance mares in training may have reduced embryo recovery rates (Mortenson et al., 2009). These reduced rates may result, in part, from the fact that some mares have a significant increase in body temperature during strenuous physical activity that can have an adverse affect on embryonic development or survival.

Older mares and mares that ovulate small follicles may benefit from progesterone supplementation during the first week after ovulation. The most practical way to do this is with administration of altrenogest (0.044 mg/kg orally, once daily) until the embryo recovery attempt is performed. Other candidates for progesterone supplementation are the mare that has multiple follicles with asynchronous ovulations (separated by 3 to 4 days) and the mare that does not develop a prominent CL after ovulation.

UTERINE FLUSH FOR EMBRYO RECOVERY

Methods used for embryo recovery have been described previously (McCue et al., 2001; Vanderwall, 2000). In general, recovery is accomplished with three to four transcervical uterine lavages, with the effluent fluid passed through a filter that captures the retrieved embryo.

A wide variety of embryo transfer supplies are readily available from commercial distributors for equine embryo-transfer procedures (Figure 17-2; Table 17-1). Product selection is largely based on personal choice. Most of these supplies have been sterilized with γ-irradiation before sale. After use, the decision of whether to reuse these supplies for subsequent embryo-transfer procedures is again up to the individual. Resterilization of supplies can be problematic. Only the most expensive catheters may be steam autoclaved. Gas sterilization presents a problem with regard to the amount of time after the sterilization that is safe before exposure of an embryo to sterilized supplies. Any disinfectants that are used in a washing program may also be potentially harmful to an embryo. For these reasons, all supplies in our practice are used only once for embryo transfer procedures and then reused thereafter for therapeutic uterine lavage.

The type of flush medium used is again a matter of personal preference. It may be ordered with or without

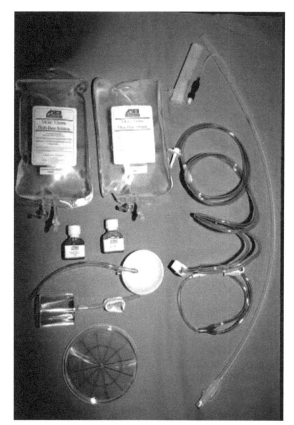

Figure 17-2 Equipment used for nonsurgical uterine flushing to retrieve embryos in the mare. *Clockwise from upper left:* Bags of commercially prepared flush media; syringe for inflating balloon of flushing catheter; flushing catheter and tubing with Y junction; search dish; two types of commercially available flush filters to catch embryo; commercially available neonatal calf serum to be added to flush media.

antibiotics. If antibiotics are desired, the most common media that are available contain kanamycin. Most flush media also contain ingredients that aid in preventing embryo adherence to the tubing and plastic ware. The time-tested ingredient for this purpose is bovine serum albumin (BSA). The primary drawback of BSA is its propensity to form bubbles or froth on the top of the recovered medium. If bubble formation is extensive, the search for embryos becomes more difficult. More recently, polyvinyl alcohol has been used to replace the BSA. With this alternative ingredient, bubble formation is minimized.

To begin, a Foley-type balloon-tipped catheter of sufficient length is needed to extend from the uterus externally to a Y junction that connects one end to the flush media and the other end to the filter (Figures 17-3 and 17-4). The flush procedure is performed as a transcervical uterine lavage. The exact methodology varies among individuals. However, several principles should be followed to ensure embryo recovery.

Immediately before the uterine flush, the donor mare should be examined with transrectal palpation and ultrasound. The ovaries should be examined for

TABLE 17-1

Sources for Embryo Transfer Equipment

Full Line of Embryo Transfer Products and Supplies

Agtech Inc, USA
8801 Anderson Avenue
Manhattan, KS 66503
Toll-Free: 800-367-4016
Direct: 785-776-3863
Fax: 785-776-4295
www.agtechinc.com

Bioniche Animal Health
1551 Jennings Mill Road,
Suite 3200A
Bogart, GA 30622
Toll-Free: 800-265-5464
Fax: 613-966-4177
www.bionicheanimalhealth.
com

**Exodus Breeders
Corporation**
5470 Mount Pisgah Road
York, PA 17406
Toll-Free: 877-396-3874
Fax: 717-252-4221
www.exodusbreeders.com

IMV USA
11725 95th Avenue North
Maple Grove, MN 55369
Toll-Free: 800-342-5468)
Fax: 763-488-1888
www.imv-technologies.com

Har-Vet
PO Box 39
Spring Valley, WI 54767
Toll-Free: 800-872-7741
Fax: 800-227-1324
www.har-vet.com

**Pets Professional Embryo
Transfer Supply Inc**
PO Box 188
Canton, TX 75103-0188
Phone: 903-567-4536
www.pets-inc.com

Partner Animal Health
3560 Pine Grove Avenue
#227
Port Huron, MI 48060

Veterinary Concepts
PO Box 39
Spring Valley, WI 54767

General Laboratory and Chemical Supplies

Fisher Scientific
711 Forbes Avenue
Pittsburgh, PA 15219
Toll-Free: 800-766-7000
www.fisherscientific.com

Sigma Chemical Co
PO Box 14508
St Louis, MO 63178-9916
Toll-Free: 800-325-3010
Fax: 800-325-5052
www.sigma-aldrich.com

VWR Scientific
PO Box 7900
San Francisco, CA 94120
Toll-Free: 800-932-5000
www.vwrsp.com

the presence of a CL. If more than one CL is present, the chance of finding multiple embryos is increased, regardless of the breeding information that may have been provided. In addition, the uterus should be examined for the presence of fluid. However, intrauterine fluid accumulation does not preclude the possibility of recovery of an embryo.

The disposition of the mare is evaluated at this time to determine the amount of sedation that will initially be used for the uterine flush procedure. Sedation of the mare is important because the uterus is distended with fluid, which often leads to discomfort. Oversedation of

the mare can be detrimental if the mare cannot stand evenly on both hind legs. The urinary bladder should be evaluated and emptied if it is full because a full bladder displaces the uterus to one side of the distended bladder. When this occurs, the uterine horn that is adjacent to the bladder does not fill or empty well because of interference from the lateral ligament of the full bladder, which is stretched and tight.

After this initial examination, the mare's tail should be wrapped and secured to one side. Thorough cleansing of the perineal area, vulva, and vestibule is essential to prevent contamination of the catheter as it is passed into the uterus, which could result in a failed embryo transfer attempt. Once the mare's hindquarters have been prepared, the flush generally requires 15 to 20 minutes to complete, depending on the number of flushes performed. Ideally, sedatives should not be administered until immediately before beginning the uterine flush because pneumorectum commonly occurs after sedation, making per rectum manipulation of the uterus difficult or impossible.

The flush medium may be prewarmed if so desired, but it is not mandatory. The author uses room-temperature (20°C to 25°C) media because embryos are quite tolerant of temperature changes that are not extreme. If the medium is prewarmed, care should be taken not to exceed body temperature (37°C). All tubing, the filter, and the catheter should be prefilled with medium before insertion of the catheter through the cervix to eliminate air from the system. The catheter should be placed through the cervix just to the level of the internal os where the balloon is inflated with either air or flush medium. The amount of inflation needed to ensure a proper seal against the internal cervical os varies with the mare. A mare whose cervix does not close well needs a larger balloon to prevent the catheter from slipping back through the cervix. Conversely, if the balloon is too large, the catheter cannot be moved around in the uterus easily. In most mares, 30 to 40 mL of inflation is adequate.

Once the catheter is in place, the fluid is allowed to flow by gravity into the uterus. From this point on, the practitioner's skill at palpation per rectum is critical. The entire uterus is palpated during the fluid instillation to ensure that both horns fill completely, which is easily accomplished in young, nonlactating mares but can be more difficult in older mares and all lactating mares. Regarding lactating mares, it becomes evident during the first flush that only the previously gravid uterine horn tends to fill. To prevent this, on successive flushes, this uterine horn is manually occluded at the bifurcation to force fluid into the other (previously nongravid) uterine horn until it fills. When both horns are palpably full, the inflow is stopped, and fluid recovery is accomplished by reversing the flow at the Y junction and directing the outflow through the filter. The amount of medium used for each mare is altered depending on individual mare's uterine characteristics. The uteri of young maiden mares may hold only 750 to 1000 mL, and older mares and lactating

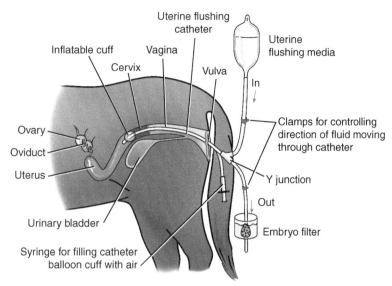

Figure 17-3 Illustration of catheter placement in uterus of a mare before flushing procedure. After insertion of the catheter through the cervix, the balloon is distended with air or fluid and the catheter pulled gently backward to seal the balloon at the internal cervical os.

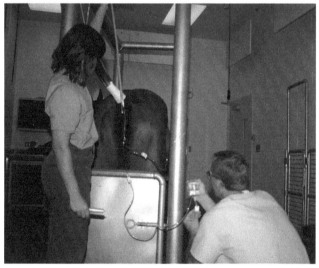

Figure 17-4 Nonsurgical uterine flushing procedure to recover embryos from a donor mare.

mares can easily hold 2 L or more. If the uterus cannot be filled with 2 L of medium, oxytocin (20 IU, intravenously) is administered to contract the uterus and thereby reduce its size. Once recovery of the fluid begins and the pressure on the cervix is reduced, the catheter is advanced into one of the uterine horns (alternate sides with successive flushes). Fluid is easily moved from the opposite horn into the horn with the catheter tip to empty the uterus completely. If the catheter is left at the internal os of the cervix, it is often not possible to empty the uterus completely. This entire process should be repeated for at least three complete flushes. Colorado workers (Hudson and McCue, 2004) described a fourth flush in which the medium was allowed to remain in the uterus for at least 3 minutes. Then, oxytocin was administered and the uterus was vigorously manipulated per rectum before recovery of the fluid. In that study, a significant number of embryos were recovered in the fourth (extra) flush attempt, when no embryo was recovered during the first series of three flushes. Failure to completely empty the uterus, especially on the last flush, can also predispose the donor mare to endometritis. Examination of the mare with transrectal ultrasonography may be helpful when finished to ensure that all fluid has been recovered.

Several different types of filters are available. Most require that the medium be transferred into a search dish for examination, necessitating rinsing of the filter into the search dish with flush medium. Our preference is to use a round dish with a grid on the bottom to aid the search process. Embryos that are 6 to 9 days of age sink to the bottom; therefore, the focus of the microscope should be on the bottom of the dish. This is most easily accomplished by initially focusing on the grid lines or on debris that has settled to the bottom. A small embryo can easily be missed by focusing at an incorrect depth. Often a significant amount of debris is found in the recovered flush fluid, especially with older and lactating mares. This finding is considered normal. However, if the recovered flush fluid is cloudy (not transparent), this generally indicates an active endometritis is present. An argument could be made that medium recovered from the first flush should always be cultured to give a starting point on therapy for the recipient mare, if needed.

Once the embryo has been identified, it should be evaluated for developmental stage (Figure 17-5; Table 17-2), graded for quality (Figure 17-6; Table 17-3), and transferred to a wash dish. Embryos may be handled with a 0.25- or 0.5-mL semen freezing straw (Figure 17-7). Several methods can be used to wash an embryo. Commercially available multiwell dishes provide the most practical approach. In 2007, Bielanski reviewed the most recent recommendations for washing

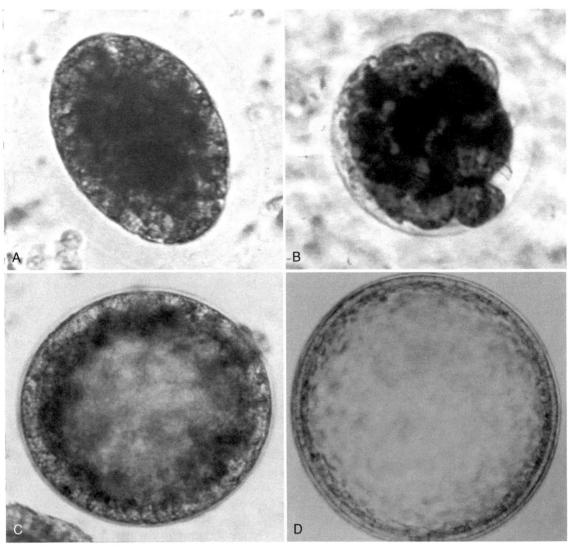

Figure 17-5   Developmental stages of the equine embryo. **A,** Unfertilized oocyte. **B,** Compacting morula. **C,** Early blastocyst. **D,** Expanded blastocyst (see Table 17-2 for typical sizes).

TABLE 17-2

Characteristics of Recoverable Embryos Based on Days after Ovulation

Day after Ovulation	Approximate Size (μm)	Approximate Size Range (μm)	Expected Stages
6	200	130-750	Morula to early blastocyst
7	400	135-1460	Morula to expanded blastocyst
8	1000	120-4000	Blastocyst to expanded blastocyst
9	2000	750-4500	Expanded blastocyst

Adapted from Vanderwall DK: Current equine embryo transfer techniques. In Ball BA, editor: *Recent advances in equine reproduction,* Ithaca, NY, 2000, International Veterinary Information Service, A0204-0400.

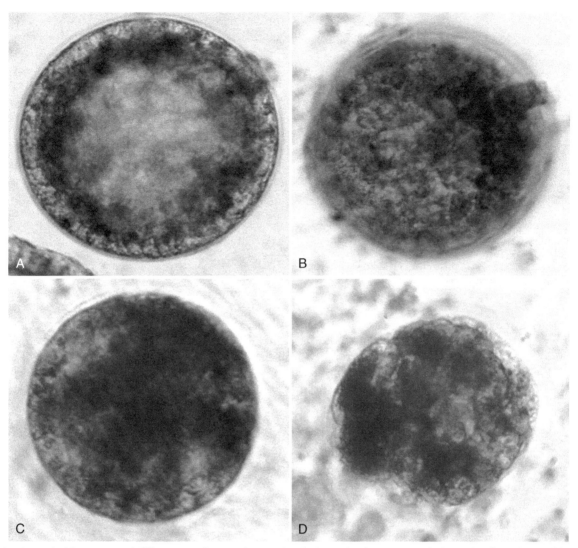

Figure 17-6 Early blastocysts of different-quality grades. **A,** Grade 1. **B,** Grade 2. **C,** Grade 3. **D,** Grade 4. (See Table 17-3 for typical descriptions.)

TABLE 17-3

Ordinal Scale for Grading and Description of Embryos

Grade	Category	Appearance	Characteristics
1	Excellent	Spherical	Uniform cell size, color, and texture
2	Good	Minor imperfections	Few extruded blastomeres; irregular shape; trophoblastic separation
3	Fair	Obvious problems	Extruded blastomeres; degenerate cells; collapsed blastocoele
4	Poor	Severe problems Oblong or irregular	Collapsed blastocoele; many extruded blastomeres; degenerate cells

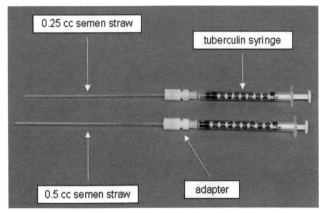

Figure 17-7 Embryo handling equipment consisting of tuberculin syringes with 0.25-mL or 0.5-mL semen freezing straws and adapter. (From Vanderwall DK: Current equine embryo transfer techniques. In Ball BA, editor: *Recent advances in equine reproduction*, Ithaca, NY, 2000, International Veterinary Information Service, A0204-0400.)

and disinfecting embryos. Simple transfers of the embryo from one well to another with clean medium, with a dilution factor of at least 1:100, is standard procedure. This should be repeated up to 10 times for optimal results. Most microorganisms are removed by this process, but some microorganisms may remain bound to the embryo.

After the washing procedure, embryos may be transferred immediately if the recipient mare is on site, or the embryos may be transported (same day or overnight) to an alternate location for transfer to a recipient mare. For transportation, embryos can be placed into one of several types of commercially available holding media. The customary method for embryo transport is to cool the embryos in the same systems that are used for cooled, transported semen. Colorado workers found no difference in pregnancy rates between good-quality embryos that were transferred fresh and those that were cooled and transported before surgical transfer. However, in our experience, about a 5% loss may be associated with transportation and cooling over a 4- to 8-hour period of time.

NONSURGICAL TRANSFER OF EMBRYOS

In the early years of equine embryo transfer, most embryos were transferred surgically through a standing flank laparotomy. In the last decade, results obtained with nonsurgical transfer have surpassed the success rates with the surgical method. The philosophical approach to nonsurgical transfer can be summarized as follows: use aseptic technique, with minimal insult to the cervix when depositing the embryo into the lumen of the uterus of a suitable recipient.

As stated previously, the accepted window of synchrony is to use recipient mares at +4 to +8 days from ovulation, with +5 and +6 days (i.e., in recipients that

have ovulated 1 to 2 days after the donor) generally providing the best results. Before transfer, the recipient mare should be examined via palpation and ultrasonography per rectum. The mare should have good uterine tone and a tightly closed cervix indicative of an acceptable circulating progesterone concentration. On ultrasound examination, a demonstrable CL and preferably some follicular development should be found. The echotexture of the uterus should be uniform with no edema or fluid. The disposition of the mare is evaluated to determine the level of sedation that is necessary before the embryo transfer is performed. Once again, sedation is delayed until immediately before the transfer to minimize air entry into the rectum. The mare's tail is wrapped and tied or held to the side. A through cleansing of the perineum, vulva, and vestibule is mandatory.

The exact apparatus used to transfer the embryo is not as important as the technique. A number of instruments are available, but the author prefers a stainless steel instrument (modified Cassou gun) (Figures 17-8 and 17-9) with a disposable, steel-tipped, side-delivery sheath (IMV, Maple Grove, Minn.). Two sizes are available: one accepts a 0.25-mL straw, and the other a 0.5-mL straw. The embryo should occupy no more than 60% to 70% of the internal diameter of the straw, and preferably less. A standard system of loading the straw is to place the embryo in the middle fluid bubble of a three-bubble system (Figure 17-10). The first bubble of fluid pulled into the straw is the last one out and is therefore the "push" bubble. This should be the largest of the three bubbles to help clear and carry the embryo away from the tip of the sheath. Jasko (2002) reported that embryos may remain stuck in the tip of a side-delivery sheath. For this reason, the tip should always be checked after the transfer and flushed under the dissection scope to observe if embryo retention has occurred. This problem can be minimized with use of a large "push" bubble in the straw and by ensuring that the tip of the sheath is free inside the lumen of the uterus (i.e., not pushed into the uterine wall to occlude the openings). If the embryo is too large for a 0.5-mL straw, a standard insemination pipette may be used, with the pipette loaded in the same manner as for the straw. Regardless of the system used, the transfer gun or pipette should be enclosed within a sterile plastic sleeve (see Figure 17-9) to protect the sterility of the transfer apparatus as it is passed through the vestibule and vagina.

Once the mare has been prepared and sedated, the embryo transfer gun or pipette is guided to the cervix. At this point, the external os may be encircled by the practitioner's thumb and fingers to provide stabilization. The gun is then advanced first through the plastic sleeve and then through the cervix. Once this is accomplished, the practitioner transfers the palpation arm to the rectum. The tip of the gun or pipette is then guided through the uterine body. When the tip is located in a

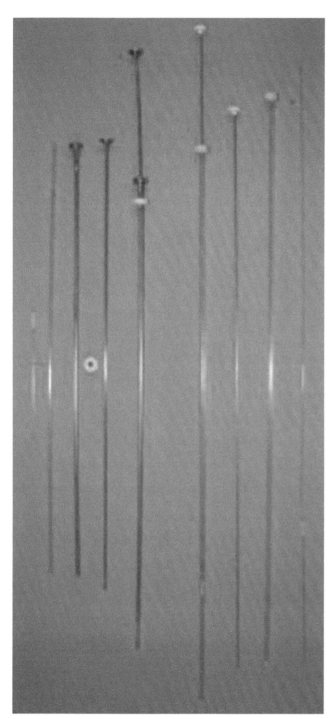

Figure 17-8 Two types of insemination guns used for nonsurgical transfer of embryos. *From top:* 0.5-mL straw, protective sheath, metal cannula, O-ring for holding the protective sheath on the metal cannula, metal plunger for pushing the fluid and embryo through the straw, and assembled unit: assembled disposable unit, inner metal plunger for pushing the fluid and embryo through the straw, outer plastic cannula, 0.25-mL straw *(bottom left)* and inner plastic guide *(bottom right)* to be placed behind the straw when it is loaded into the outer plastic cannula.

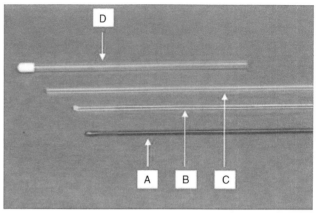

Figure 17-9 Nonsurgical embryo transfer equipment: *A*, stainless steel re-useable "insemination gun"; *B*, plastic disposable "insemination gun"; *C*, standard insemination pipette; and *D*, outer protective guard. (From Vanderwall DK: Current equine embryo transfers techniques. In Ball BA, editor: *Recent advances in equine reproduction,* Ithaca, NY, 2000, International Veterinary Information Service, A0204-0400.)

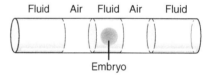

Figure 17-10 Drawing of embryo in a transfer straw positioned between air and fluid columns.

position that is free within the lumen at the base of the uterine horn (near the bifurcation), an assistant can slowly push the plunger of the apparatus and expel the embryo into the uterus. The embryo transfer gun or pipette is then withdrawn. This entire process should take only 1 to 2 minutes and should be as atraumatic as possible to the cervix and uterus. Any accidental passage of bacteria from the vagina to the uterus could result in endometritis. Recently, another method of nonsurgical transfer has been described (Wilsher and Allen, 2005). For the interested reader, this offers other perspectives.

MANAGEMENT OF THE RECIPIENT MARE AFTER TRANSFER

The optimal method of management for recipient mares after transfer is controversial. Fortunately, considerable research has been done in this area.

Originally, transcervical transfer of embryos was thought to be less successful because of release of prostaglandin-$F_2\alpha$ ($PGF_2\alpha$), which results in premature luteolysis. More recent studies (Handler, 2005; Handler et al., 2006) have examined the effect of cervical dilation on day 7 in recipient mares with a balloon catheter. This procedure resulted in the release of oxytocin but not

PGF$_2\alpha$. Oxytocin administered on day 7 after ovulation was also shown to not affect progesterone secretion, pregnancy rate, or embryonic growth. Further manipulation of the cervix itself was unlikely to contribute to varying success rates of transcervical transfer of embryos. The investigators concluded that other factors (i.e., window of synchrony, endometrial irritation, and bacterial contamination) were more likely to contribute to luteolysis.

The possibility of luteal compromise after transcervical transfer is also controversial. Stout et al. (2005) concluded that embryo transfer–induced luteolysis was not a significant cause of failed embryo transfer because luteal function did not differ between pregnant and nonpregnant mares until the onset of cyclical luteolysis. In contrast, Foss and Crane (2004), in a retrospective study involving a large number of mares, examined circulating progesterone levels at the time of transfer and then again 7 days later. Their data indicated that lower levels of circulating progesterone are likely, even in pregnant recipient mares, especially after the transfer of morula-stage embryos. Foss and Crane also found that the window of synchrony had no effect on progesterone levels. Most investigators agree that transcervical transfer of embryos carries with it the inherent risk of bacterial contamination with resultant endometritis. This endometritis may be the more common cause of luteolysis and lower progesterone levels. Although no controlled studies have been published documenting either the beneficial or adverse effects of exogenous progestins, supplementation of recipient mares with progestins is a common practice in many embryo-transfer programs.

Much remains to be learned about maternal recognition of pregnancy in the mare. A failure or delay in this important aspect of early pregnancy could account for some of the embryonic loss incurred after transfer. Possible therapeutic options in this area have yet to be discovered. However, this concept could support the use of supplemental progesterone at this time. Arruda and Fluery (2005) reported that the administration of human chorionic gonadotropin (hCG) (3000 IU, intramuscularly) on the day of transfer resulted in greater serum circulating progesterone concentrations and an increase in pregnancy rates when compared with other treatment and control groups. The hCG was thought to have a luteotrophic effect, promoting an increase in the number of large luteal cells and a resultant increase in progesterone secretion by the CL.

The following protocol is currently used by the author. At the time of transfer, routine medication includes flunixin meglumine (500 mg, intravenously), hCG (3000 IU, intramuscularly), and antibiotic therapy (sulfamethoxazole and trimethoprim, 24 mg/kg per os, twice daily). The antibiotic therapy is continued until the first pregnancy examination, which is usually 4 days later (i.e., 11 days after ovulation). At this time,

a decision is made regarding any continued therapy based on examination findings. A pregnant recipient mare should be monitored frequently. The mare is normally examined at 11, 13, 17, 23, and 29 days after ovulation, and more often if potential problems exist. With each examination, the uterus is evaluated for signs of endometritis (i.e., mild edema, small amounts of fluid, or thickening of the uterine wall). In addition, the CL function is also monitored for any signs suggestive of low circulating progesterone (e.g., decreasing uterine tone or softening of the cervix). If indicated at any time, alternative antibiotic therapy is initiated. Treatment options may also be based on the donor mare's uterine culture after transfer. Progesterone supplementation is initiated if any signs of low circulating progesterone concentration are detected. If any doubt exists, a serum progesterone sample is submitted for analysis. Pregnancies that would otherwise be lost can be rescued with supportive therapy. Our experience has been that most pregnancies that are maintained to 60 to 70 days are maintained to term. Usually, but not always, supplemental progesterone can be discontinued about this time. An important concept is to treat each pregnant recipient as an individual rather than with a herd-based mentality.

DONOR MARE MANAGEMENT AFTER THE FLUSH

The veterinarian may not always have control of the donor mare after her uterus is flushed for embryo recovery. However, several potential problems can arise, most of which can be avoided with proper precautions. The first problem, and potentially greatest liability, is for the donor mare to become pregnant. This pregnancy may go undiscovered and become a serious problem later, as in the case of a performance mare that is 10 months pregnant at the time of a competitive event. Most veterinarians are in the habit of administering PGF$_2\alpha$ immediately after the flush, but this may not always have the desired effect. The mare may have had a second delayed ovulation that resulted in an embryo still in the oviduct at the time of attempted embryo recovery. The second ovulation could also result in a CL that is refractory to the PGF$_2\alpha$ at the time of the uterine flush. The donor mare could also remain pregnant simply from an inadequate uterine flush technique (e.g., failure to completely fill the uterus with fluid during the uterine flush procedure). In recent years, some veterinarians have had a tendency to flush mares on day 8 or 9 so that the embryo may be visualized in the filter, enabling the flush to be stopped after just one flush rather than the three that are generally recommended. This practice can result in a twin embryo left in the uterus.

Another common mistake is to leave flush medium in the uterus at the end of the flush; this can predispose the mare to endometritis. In an ideal situation, the donor mare should be examined the day after her uterine flush to check for any signs of endometritis. Any mare with even a small amount of uterine fluid should be subjected to uterine lavage. The mare should then be examined again in a few days to determine that she is in estrus. A uterine culture should be performed at the appropriate time on all donor mares after the uterine flush.

In summary, embryo transfer can be a tremendously rewarding part of equine practice. If the veterinarian strives for excellence and is diligent in optimizing all aspects of the procedure, success will follow.

BIBLIOGRAPHY

Arruda RP, Fleury DC: Pregnancy rates and plasma progesterone concentrations in embryo recipient mares receiving hormone treatment, *Havemeyer Foundation Monograph Series* No. 14:95-96, 2005.

Battut I, Grandchamp des Raux A, Nicais JL, et al: When do equine embryos enter the uterine cavity?, *Havemeyer Foundation Monograph Series* No. 3:66-68, 2000.

Baucus KL, Ralston SL, Nockels CF, et al: Effects of transportation on early embryonic death in mares, *J Anim Sci* 68:345-351, 1990.

Bielanski A: Disinfection procedures for controlling microorganisms in the semen and embryos of humans and farm animals, *Theriogenology* 68:1-22, 2007.

Carnevale EM, Beisner AE, McCue PM, et al: Uterine changes associated with repeated inseminations and embryo collections in mares, *Proc 51st Ann Mtg Am Assoc Equine Pract* 51:202-203, 2005.

Foss R, Crane A: Serum progesterone changes in embryo transfer recipients, *Proc 50th Ann Mtg Am Assoc Equine Pract* 50:521-524, 2004.

Hudson JJ, McCue P: How to increase embryo recovery rates and transfer success, *Proc 50th Ann Mtg Am Assoc Equine Pract* 50: 406-408, 2004.

Handler J, Hoffmann D, Weber F, et al: Oxytocin does not contribute to the effects of cervical dilation on progesterone secretion and embryonic development in mares, *Theriogenology* 66:1397-1404, 2006.

Handler J: Cervical dilatation—a method for studying embryo-maternal interaction in mares, *Havemeyer Foundation Monograph Series* No. 16:5-7, 2005.

Jasko DJ: Comparison of pregnancy rates following nonsurgical transfer of day 8 equine embryos using various transfer devices, *Theriogenology* 58:713-715, 2002.

McCue PM, Squires EL, Bruemmer JE, et al: Equine embryo transfer: techniques, trends, and anecdotes, *Proc Ann Conf Theriogenol* 229-235, 2001.

Mortensen CJ, Choi YH, Hinrichs K, Ing N, Kraemer DC, Vogelsang SG, Vogelsang MM: Embryo recovery from exercised mares, *Anim Reprod Sci* 110:237-244, 2009.

Stout TA, Tremoleda JL, Knaap J, et al : Does compromised luteal function contribute to failure to establish pregnancy after nonsurgical embryo transfer, *Havemeyer Foundation Monograph Series* No. 14:8-9, 2005.

Vanderwall D: Current equine embryo transfer techniques. In Ball BA, editor: *Recent advances in equine reproduction 2000*, Ithaca, NY, 2000, International Veterinary Information Services, available at http://www.ivis.org/advances/Reproduction Ball/embryo transfer.

Wilsher S, Kölling M, Allen WR: The use of meclofenamic acid to extend donor-recipient asynchrony in equine embryo transfer, *Havemeyer Foundation Monograph Series* No. 18:56-57, 2005.

Wilsher S, Allen WR: A novel method for non-surgical embryo transfer in the mare, *Havemeyer Foundation Monograph Series* No. 14:110-111, 2005.

Evaluation of Breeding Records

18

CHAPTER

OBJECTIVES

While studying the information covered in this chapter, the reader should attempt to:
- Understand the costs associated with reduced fertility of stallions.
- Understand how to gather relevant information from breeding farm records.
- Understand how to evaluate data garnered from breeding farm records.
- Understand how to interpret the results of the breeding farm record evaluation.
- Understand how to use daily breeding records to aid with breeding management decisions for stallions.

STUDY QUESTIONS

1. Discuss economic losses associated with low pregnancy and foaling rates in equine breeding operations.
2. Define the term seasonal pregnancy rate, and explain its use and limitations for assessment of fertility.
3. Define the term cycles/pregnancy, and explain how it is used to assess fertility.
4. Explain the makeup of a stallion's book of mares, and discuss how it influences pregnancy rates.
5. Discuss factors that influence whether a mare becomes pregnant when bred to a given stallion.

ECONOMIC IMPACT OF LOWERED FERTILITY

A stallion that achieves suboptimal pregnancy rates greatly increases the cost of producing foals for mare owners and farm management. The increased costs associated with a stallion's lowered fertility arise from (1) increased mare expenses (e.g., extra covers, extra transport of mares to breeding sheds, extra veterinary examinations and treatments, and additional boarding fees for mares left at a breeding farm or facility over repeated estrous cycles); (2) wasted maintenance costs associated with support of mares that do not produce foals; (3) decreased income (e.g., from sale of penalized late-born foals that arise from mares not becoming pregnant early in the year, lost income from failure to produce a foal, and lost income from nonproductive stud fees); and (4) labor associated with rebreeding mares and potentially lost service opportunities for the stallion, which could have been breeding another mare. Thus, the economic impact associated with breeding of a stallion with lowered fertility can be substantial.

The following example is used to further illustrate the magnitude of losses that can occur with just a 20% difference in pregnancy rate (Table 18-1). If a stallion breeds a book of 100 mares (with an estimated 1.1 breedings per cycle; a conservative 10% double rate) and achieves a 60% pregnancy rate per cycle over a total of three estrous cycles, the stallion has a 93% seasonal pregnancy rate, necessitating a total of 172 covers. If 85% of the pregnancies (assuming a 15%

TABLE 18-1

Fertility Achieved per Cycle And per Season with Theoretical 40% and 60% Pregnancy Rates (PR) per Cycle

No. Mares Bred per Cycle × Theoretical PR/Cycle × Covers/Cycle = No. Mares Pregnant	**No. covers**
Lower Theoretical Fertility	
100 mares bred 1st cycle × 40% PR/cycle × 1.1 covers/cycle = 40 mares pregnant on 1st cycle	110 covers
60 mares bred 2nd cycle × 40% PR/cycle × 1.1 covers/cycle = 24 mares pregnant on 2nd cycle	66 covers
36 mares bred 3rd cycle × 40% PR/cycle × 1.1 covers/cycle = 14 mares pregnant on 3rd cycle	36 covers
Total mares pregnant after 3 cycles of breeding = 78	Total no. covers for season = 216 covers
No. foals produced = 78 − (78 × 15% loss rate) = 66	
No. barren mares = 34 mares	
Higher Theoretical Fertility	
100 mares bred 1st cycle × 60% PR/cycle × 1.1 covers/cycle = 60 mares pregnant on 1st cycle	110 covers
40 mares bred 2nd cycle × 60% PR/cycle × 1.1 covers/cycle = 24 mares pregnant on 2nd cycle	44 covers
16 mares bred 3rd cycle × 60% PR/cycle × 1.1 covers/cycle = 9 mares pregnant on 3rd cycle	18 covers
Total mares pregnant after 3 cycles of breeding = 93	Total no. covers for season = 156 covers
No. foals produced = 93 − (93 × 15% loss rate) = 79	
No. barren mares = 21	

Influence of two (40%, 60%) theoretical PRs/cycle on number of covers needed to complete three estrous cycles of breeding and seasonal pregnancy rate (SPR) for a stallion mated to 100 mares with natural cover.

Assuming 1.1 covers (i.e., 10% double rate) are needed per estrus and 85% of pregnancies result in production of viable foals (i.e., 15% pregnancy loss rate), the lower level of fertility would result in 44 extra covers (40 extra cycles) throughout the season yet produce 13 fewer foals (i.e., 13 more barren mares).

embryonic and fetal loss rate) result in live foals, 79 foals are produced. By contrast, if only a 40% pregnancy rate per cycle is achieved, the stallion has a 78% seasonal pregnancy rate, necessitating a total of 216 covers. If 85% of the pregnancies result in live foals, 66 foals are produced. The lower fertility culminates in an extra 44 covers (40 estrous cycles × 1.1 covers/cycle) that necessitate board and veterinary expense over the course of the breeding season yet produce 13 fewer foals and an additional 13 years of nonproductive maintenance expense (13 additional barren mares). If the boarding fee at the breeding farm is $26/day, the 40 extra estrous cycles of breeding (21 days/cycle) result in an extra cost of $21,840 over that for the higher level of fertility. If veterinary fees average $250 for examinations and treatments per cycle, the 40 extra estrous cycles of breeding result in increased veterinary fees of $10,000 over that for the higher level of fertility. If transport fees for the mare to the breeding shed are $150 per round trip, the cost of transport fees for 44 extra trips totals $6,600. The added cost of the lower fertility in this example totals $38,440, yet does not include lost income from 13 stud fees, the maintenance expenses for 13 additional barren mares for 1 year, or lost income from 13 foals that are not produced or labor costs associated with the farm where the stallion is, or even the lost opportunity in breeding another mare when the stallion is heavily booked and may need separation of services to breed three times or more per day. Although expenses, fees, and sales prices vary, this example serves to stress the importance of maximizing reproductive efficiency of the stallion.

SOME FACTORS THAT AFFECT STALLION FERTILITY

Achievement of suboptimal pregnancy rates remains a serious problem within the horse industry. The veterinarian must remain cognizant that many factors contribute to the overall fertility of a stallion, including: inherent fertility of the stallion, inherent fertility of the mares bred by the stallion, and quality of management (e.g., nutrition and body condition, teasing and breeding management, level of veterinary care). Each contributing factor is capable of severely constraining the percentage and number of offspring produced each year by a given stallion. It should therefore not be assumed that lowered pregnancy rates must result from a problem with stallion fertility unless record analyses and examination findings, along with a thorough evaluation of mating practices, support this conclusion. To this end, examination of fertility from stallions on the same breeding farm during the same time period is often useful.

Investigation of suboptimal fertility achieved by a stallion should be directed toward identification and correction of contributing factors. In some cases, treatment of a disease condition (e.g., infection, ejaculatory dysfunction; see Chapter 16) may improve the stallion's fertility. In other cases, no treatment is indicated for the stallion, yet the reduced reproductive quality of the mares in his book precludes significant improvement in fertility. More commonly, recommendations for alterations in breeding management practices can be identified that might improve the stallion's fertility. The search for causes of suboptimal fertility should begin with record analysis to fully characterize a stallion's breeding performance.

Breeding records should be the most detailed, objective historic information that the clinician can obtain. Breeding records exist in many forms that range from poorly organized handwritten papers to highly organized computerized spreadsheets listing numerous mathematic parameters. However, even computerized record-keeping programs usually remain inadequate for summarizing and measuring relevant fertility endpoints, and further collation and analysis are needed for accurate assessment of breeding performance. Figures 18-1 and 18-2 are examples of breeding records that are sometimes used for Thoroughbred stallions; they can easily be adapted for stallions used in artificial breeding programs. They consist of a chronologic breeding sheet (see Figure 18-1) for recording of pertinent information obtained from each mating and a graphic summary of mares mated in a given month (see Figure 18-2). The monthly breeding sheet is used to summarize various reproductive endpoints as pregnancy outcome from breeding becomes known.

The clinician should not hesitate to request breeding records from previous breeding seasons and the current breeding season to facilitate determination of whether the fertility of a stallion has changed. A stallion's fertility can change from year to year simply because of the reproductive quality of the mares in his

Stallion _____

Date	Mare name	Farm name	Status	Cycle	Cover	Mounts	Double	Dismount	Reinforce	TQ	Other	Outcome

Figure 18-1 A manual recording system to be filled out chronologically with pertinent data for a given stallion after each cover is completed. Information to be filled in with each cover includes the following: date of cover, mare identification, farm of origin for the mare, beginning status of the mare (foaling, maiden, barren, not bred, slipped), cycle of breeding (1st, 2nd, etc.), cover of the day for the stallion (1st, 2nd, etc.), number of mounts necessary to complete service, whether or not the cover is a double during the same cycle, quality of the dismount sample (may include a scoring system for motility and concentration), whether or not reinforcement breeding was used on that cover, whether or not the mare had to be tranquilized to facilitate a safe cover, other comments thought to useful (e.g., whether the mare was difficult to cover and why, whether the mare tolerated a twitch, whether inflammatory cells were noted in the dismount, etc.), and the outcome of the cover (pregnant or not pregnant).

Monthly Breeding Activity

Farm: X Farm
Stallion: Mr. R
Month and Year: April, 2006

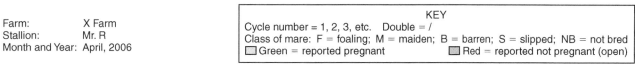

KEY
Cycle number = 1, 2, 3, etc.   Double = /
Class of mare: F = foaling; M = maiden; B = barren; S = slipped; NB = not bred
☐ Green = reported pregnant   ☐ Red = reported not pregnant (open)

Number of covers in 3 days preceding each given date

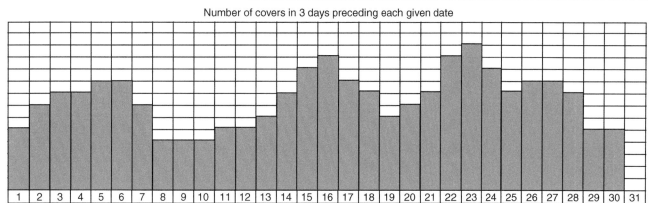

Covers on given dates

1	2	3	4	5	6	7	8	9	10	11	12	13	14	15	16	17	18	19	20	21	22	23	24	25	26	27	28	29	30	31
		F2										F2	B1					F3	F1	F1/										
F1		F2	NB1									F2	F1	F1		F1		F1	F1/	F1	M3		F1	F1/	B2			F1	F1	
F1	M2	M1	M1	M1			F1		F1	F1	F2	F1	M2	F1	F2	M1		M3	F1	M1	F2	F1/	F2	M1/	F1	S1		M1/	F2	
F1	F1	F1	F1	F1	F1	M2	F2	M2	F1	F1	F1	F1	F1	B1	F1	F2	M2	F1	F1	NB3	F1	F1	F2	F1	B3	F1		F1	M1	
1	2	3	4	5	6	7	8	9	10	11	12	13	14	15	16	17	18	19	20	21	22	23	24	25	26	27	28	29	30	31

Total covers: 76   Total cycles: 73   Number of doubles: 3
Overall pregnancy rate (PR)/cycle for month: 67%
1st cycle PR: 64%
PR/cycle by class of mare: foaling 38/52 = 73%; maiden 10/14 = 71%; barren 0/4 = 0%; slipped 0/1 = 0%; not bred 1/2 = 50%

PR/cycle when ≤ 3 covers in preceding 3 days: 0/0
PR/cycle when 4-6 covers in preceding 3 days: 15/22 = 68%
PR/cycle when 7-9 covers in preceding 3 days: 25/37 = 68%
PR/cycle when ≥ 10 covers in preceding 3 days: 8/13 = 62%

PR/cycle on 1st cover of day: 19/29 = 66%
PR/cycle on 2nd cover of day: 20/24 = 83%
PR/cycle on 3rd cover of day: 7/15 = 47%
PR/cycle on 4th cover of day: 3/5 = 60%
PR/cycle on 5th cover of day: 0/0

Figure 18-2 A summary record system for stallion matings that graphically presents pregnancy outcome. Matings are recorded in order of occurrence, by class of mare. When pregnancy outcome is known, matings that result in pregnancy are highlighted *green,* and matings that fail to result in pregnancy are highlighted *red.* The graph can be used to examine effects of mating frequency, beginning status of mares covered and their cycle of the year, and the cover of the day for the stallion (see lower blanks to be filled in with calculations). Evaluation of reproductive performance at regular intervals throughout the season not only provides confidence that a given stallion's fertility is good but also can alert the cognizant manager to potential problems that may require prompt intervention to restore reproductive performance to an acceptable level.

book (Table 18-2). A decrease in the quality of mares bred commonly follows a decline in the stallion's popularity. As the stallion's stud fee drops, the owner or manager must accept mares of lesser reproductive quality to fill the stallion's book (Table 18-3).

EVALUATION OF BREEDING FARM RECORDS

This exercise is intended to introduce the reader to the breeding records that may be available on breeding farms that have stallions standing at stud. Keep in mind that the stallion owner or the manager may not keep data regarding each mating, leaving a conclusion to be drawn about a stallion's "subfertile" condition solely from results of semen evaluation. Analysis of

the breeding records should be considered as much a part of the breeding soundness evaluation as other components of the examination.

Table 18-4 provides an example of a typical breeding record. Records may also be provided as day-to-day worksheets that have not been tabulated. The information that is commonly recorded is listed across the top of the table and includes the following:

- Mare: Identification of the mare.
- Begin status: The reproductive status of the mare before the current breeding season.
- Mares are classified as the following:
  - **Maiden:** Usually a young mare that has not been bred in previous years and thus has not produced a foal.

TABLE 18-2

Influence of Declining Quality in Mare Book on Fertility Achieved by a Thoroughbred Stallion in Two Consecutive Years

Year	Class of Mare	No. Bred	No. Pregnant	No. Cycles	PR/Cycle	PR/Season
1	Barren	6	6	9	67%	100%
	Foaling	49	42	59	71%	86%
	Maiden	4	4	5	80%	100%
	Not Bred	3	3	4	75%	100%
	Slipped	9	6	15	40%	67%
TOTAL		71	61	92	66%	86%
2	Barren	10	5	18	28%	50%
	Foaling	16	13	18	72%	81%
	Maiden	9	8	11	73%	89%
	Not Bred	3	2	3	67%	67%
	Slipped	2	2	3	67%	100%
TOTAL		40	30	53	57%	75%

Seasonal pregnancy rate (PR/season) declined from 86% to 75%, and overall pregnancy rate/cycle (PR/cycle) declined from 66% to 57%. The lower than expected seasonal pregnancy rate in the second year most likely resulted from two problems that are apparent from examining the records: (1) low fertility in the barren mare group in year 2, which comprised one fourth of his book (note that the PR/cycle was quite good in other classes of mares in year 2 and comparable in foaling and maiden mares, typically the most fertile classes of mares, in both years); and (2) insufficient opportunity to rebreed mares that did not become pregnant. In this regard, note that only 53 cycles were used to cover the total book of 40 mares in year 2. The PR/cycle among other (than barren) classes of mares in year 2 varied from 67% to 73%; thus, if more opportunities had existed for covering those mares not becoming pregnant in the first cycle in those groups, seasonal pregnancy rate might not have been so low.

TABLE 18-3

Fertility Results from a 22-year-old Thoroughbred Stallion with a Book of 27 Mares

Class of Mare	PR/Season	PR/Cycle
Barren	2/3 (67%)	2/7 (29%)
Foaling	19/22 (86%)	19/32 (59%)
Slipped	2/2 (100%)	2/4 (50%)
All Classes	23/27 (85%)	23/43 (53%)

The book of mares is small, which limits conclusions that can be made about the stallion's inherent fertility. Although the overall pregnancy rate (PR) per cycle was only 53%, his first cycle PR achieved in foaling mares was 73% (14/19). Of the rest of his book of mares, only one (slipped) mare became pregnant on the first cover. This finding suggests if the stallion had a larger book of mares, of which more were known to be fertile (e.g., foaling mares), he could achieve better overall PRs per cycle and per season.

- **Barren:** A mare that was bred the previous year but is not pregnant. Several reasons besides reproductive unsoundness exist for mares to be classified as barren. For example, late-foaling mares may have only had one chance to become pregnant before the end of the breeding season.
- **Slipped:** A mare in which pregnancy was diagnosed in the previous breeding season but that failed to carry the pregnancy to term because of embryonic loss or abortion.
- **In-foal:** A mare that became pregnant the previous breeding season and is assumed to still be pregnant or has recently delivered a term foal at the time she is booked to be bred to the stallion.
- **Not bred:** A mare that was not bred the previous year, which is the owner's choice sometimes when the mare foals late in the year. Skipping breeding that summer allows early rebreeding the next year with the hope of producing an early-born foal in the following year. Some managers include "not bred" and "slipped" mares in the barren category.
- Date foaled: The date the mare foaled.
- Dates bred: The dates on which the mare was bred.
- Days since: The difference between the date the report was printed and the last breeding date. For

TABLE 18-4

Mares Bred Summary

Mare	Begin Status	Date Foaled	Dates Bred	Days since Last Breeding	Status after Last Examination
Betty	Slipped		2/26/00	258	In-foal
Suzy	Maiden		2/29/00	255	In-foal
Kelly	In-foal	2/14/00	3/20/00	235	Barren
			2/24/00		
			2/22/00		
Konnie	In-foal	3/12/00	4/20/00	204	In-foal
			4/1/00		

those mares found to be in-foal, this number can be considered the current gestation length.

▪ Status after last examination: The current pregnancy status, either in-foal, barren, or slipped.

The following list includes endpoints that should be measured (also summarized in Table 18-5). Although this list is not complete, the endpoints listed should be considered first. Computerized programs sometimes measure certain endpoints differently, and in some cases incorrectly, so the practitioner should not assume that a farm summary sheet of these measures is accurate. Instead, perform the calculations yourself to ensure accuracy.

▪ Total number of mares bred: Count the number of mares in the "Mare" column.

▪ Total number of mares pregnant: Count the number of mares identified as in-foal in the "Status After Last Examination" column.

▪ Seasonal pregnancy rate: Divide the total number of mares bred by the total number of mares in foal and multiply this figure by 100 to provide the seasonal pregnancy rate as a percentage.

▪ Cycles per pregnancy: Count the number of cycles a mare was bred in the "Dates Bred" column. The dates bred number assumes that each mare was in

normal estrus and was bred at the appropriate time relative to ovulation. Some mares are **doubled,** which means that they are bred more than once during a given estrous cycle, usually because the mare did not ovulate as planned. In general, if two dates are within 1 week of each other, assume they are the same estrous cycle. Do not count doubles as separate estrous cycles (see subsequent discussion in this chapter).

▪ Number of mares that are classified as barren, in-foal, or maiden before the breeding season: Count the individual classifications in the "Begin Status" column. Mares in the slipped category are usually included in the barren mare group. If the number of slipped mares is high, a separate group identifying this number should be included. After the number of mares in each group is assessed, the percentage of each category in the stallion's book should be determined.

▪ Pregnancy status of mares in each classification: Assess the pregnancy status of mares in each classification and determine the percentage pregnant in each classification (Table 18-6). This assessment is important because a stallion may achieve acceptable pregnancy

TABLE 18-5

Summary of Reproductive Endpoints to be Assessed from Stallion Breeding Records

Mare Status	No. of Mares	% of Book	No. Pregnant	% Pregnant	Cycles per Pregnancy	Seasonal PR
Barren						
Maiden						
In-Foal						
TOTAL						

TABLE 18-6

Pregnancy Status for Stallion 4 (see Figure 18-6) Based on Mare Status (Barren, Foaling, Maiden, Not Bred, or Slipped)

Mare Type	No. of Mares	No. of Mares Pregnant	% Pregnant
No. barren total	24	16	67
No. foaling total	43	32	74
No. maiden total	14	8	57
TOTAL	81	56	69

rates in mares expected to have normal fertility (i.e., in-foal and maiden mares) but poor pregnancy rates in mares with breeding problems (i.e., barren mares). The overall pregnancy rate achieved by such a stallion could appear to be unacceptable, but it could be entirely the result of inclusion of a predominant percentage of mares with breeding problems.

INTERPRETATION

Total Number of Mares Bred

This value determines the total number of different mares in a stallion's book and is used in the denominator when the clinician determines a seasonal pregnancy rate. The clinician should recognize that the inherent fertility and management are not the same for all mares in the book. One goal of evaluation of a stallion's book is to describe these differences. Maiden and barren mares are generally bred earlier in the breeding season and therefore should have more opportunities (more estrous cycles) to become pregnant. Foaling mares, because they cannot be bred until after parturition, are generally bred later in the breeding season and therefore have fewer opportunities to become pregnant. If the total number of mares becomes too great for a given stallion, the overall seasonal pregnancy rate may decrease with a concomitant increase in cycles/pregnancy (because the stallion is being "overbred," meaning he is bred so often that insufficient numbers of sperm are being produced in ejaculates to result in good pregnancy rates). On some well-managed farms, as the number of mares in the book increases, so does a stallion's fertility. This paradoxical increase in fertility results from the stallion's popularity (usually associated with a higher stud fee), which results in the ability of the stallion owner or manager being able to pick and choose the highest-quality mares for breeding. A secondary reason for the increased fertility with increasing book size is that the overall value of (and investment in) the mare is generally higher, resulting in more intense management to prepare the mare for breeding. The combination of high reproductive quality and intense management of mares can dramatically improve the pregnancy rate achieved by a given stallion.

Total Number of Mares Pregnant

This parameter can be defined in different ways depending on (1) when pregnancy examinations occur; and (2) how data are entered for mares that become pregnant yet later have embryonic death or abortion. We recommend that, for initial evaluation, the clinician consider the mare pregnant regardless of whether she maintains the pregnancy. The number of mares losing pregnancies tends to be low; however, some rare stallions may contribute to production of abnormal embryos that culminate in embryonic loss. For identification of such a stallion, determination of the number (and percentage) of mares that lose their pregnancy after a positive pregnancy diagnosis is warranted.

The clinician should also be aware of an economic fact in the Thoroughbred industry: the stud fee (guaranteed live foal) is contractually transferable from the mare owner to the stallion owner when the foal stands and suckles after it is born. Therefore, a seasonal pregnancy rate based on pregnancy diagnosed with ultrasound 14 days after ovulation is virtually always greater than the actual foaling rate on which the economic status of the farm depends. The 14-day pregnancy rate and the foaling rate can differ by 10% to 20%. The payment of stud fees for some breeds may be contractually due before the breeding season. In the Thoroughbred industry, stallions at stud with no contractually guaranteed live foal usually achieve high pregnancy rates (per cycle and per season) because only highly fertile mares are booked to these stallions with high stud fees.

Seasonal Pregnancy Rate

This parameter is based on the number of mares in which pregnancy is diagnosed at a particular point in gestation divided by the total number of mares in a stallion's book. This endpoint is important economically, but it is not a sensitive indicator of a stallion's fertility because it does not reflect the total number of cycles that a mare is bred to achieve the pregnancy. A stallion can achieve a relatively low pregnancy rate per cycle but end the season with a seasonal pregnancy rate similar to that of a stallion with a relatively high pregnancy rate per cycle. The only difference is that the stallion with a relatively low pregnancy rate per cycle must breed the mares in his book more times during the season to reach the same seasonal pregnancy rate.

Several factors that can alter seasonal pregnancy rate include the following:

1. The point at which the seasonal pregnancy rate is determined (i.e., during the breeding season, shortly after the breeding season, or many months after the breeding season). When this value is calculated near the start of the next breeding season, it more closely approximates the foaling rate.

2. The number of estrous cycles that a mare was bred. The stallion manager or owner commonly adds mares on to a stallion's book as the end of the breeding season approaches. The addition of mares onto a stallion's book is often done when mares are switched from one stallion to another for a variety of reasons. These mares are included in the total number of mares that the stallion breeds but in reality are given fewer opportunities to become pregnant (usually only one cycle) than other mares in the stallion's book. If mares added onto a stallion's book near the end of the breeding season do not become pregnant, the seasonal pregnancy rate for that stallion is lowered but does not truly represent the actual rate for the stallion. Therefore, if a stallion is presented because of a low seasonal pregnancy rate, it is important to determine that all mares were bred during an adequate number of estrous cycles to have a reasonable chance of becoming pregnant (see subsequent discussion in this chapter).

3. Inclusion or exclusion of mares that have early embryonic death. The assumption can be made that most embryonic deaths result from mare and not stallion factors. If an accurate seasonal pregnancy rate figure is to be created to describe the stallion's inherent fertility, all diagnosed pregnancies (which indicate that the stallion was able to accomplish fertilization in those mares) should be included in calculation of the rate. However, keep in mind that counting an embryonic death as a pregnancy when figuring seasonal pregnancy rate is of no economic relevance (i.e., stud fees are not transferred). If embryonic deaths are included as pregnancies in calculation of seasonal pregnancy rate, an inflated economic value for the seasonal pregnancy rate is created.

Cycles/Pregnancy (Pregnancy Rate/Cycle)

This measure is a more sensitive indication of a stallion's fertility because it measures how efficient a stallion is in establishing pregnancies. For determination of this value, count the number of cycles a mare was bred in the "Dates Bred" column. The assumption is made that all entries into the "Dates Bred" column were for mares in normal estrus and that mares were being bred near to the time of ovulation.

This assumption is not always correct, especially for breeding via artificial insemination on some farms where mares are either not in estrus or not near ovulation. Whenever it is typical for a high number of breedings per estrous period to occur, pregnancy rates may not reflect truly the fertility of either the stallion or the mares. This situation is unlikely to occur when breeding occurs with natural service because the mare must actually stand for breeding by the stallion (the best indicator of estrus).

Some mares are doubled, which means that they are bred more than once during an estrous period. Double entries occur because the mare does not ovulate as predicted, so another breeding is provided to ensure that the mare is bred near to the time of ovulation. The incidence of doubles is a reflection of the overall managerial (broodmare manager and veterinarian) ability to detect and breed mares at the proper time to maximize pregnancy rates. On well-managed farms, the double rate may range from 0 to 10%. A double does not count as a cycle. If two breeding dates are within 7 days of each other, breeding during only one estrous cycle is included in the calculation of cycles/pregnancy. An example of a double is that for "Kelly," the third mare listed in Table 18-4. She was bred on February 22 and February 24. Both matings occurred during only one estrous period and thus count for breeding on only one cycle. In rare instances for mating with natural service, but more commonly for mating via artificial insemination, breeding more than twice (e.g., triples or quadruples) during one estrous period may occur. Again, multiple matings in one estrous period should only be counted as one estrous cycle of mating. The total number of cycles can be determined by counting all dates bred excluding multiple matings during single estrous periods (usually doubles). To calculate the cycles/pregnancy, divide the total number of mated cycles in all mares bred by the total number of mares becoming pregnant (not by the total number of mares in the book).

Cycles/Pregnancy (Pregnancy Rate/Cycle) for Cycles 1 through 6

This parameter evaluates the per cycle pregnancy rate of the first through sixth cycles that mares were bred. All mares in the book are bred on at least one estrous cycle; therefore, the number of mares in this category should equal the total number of mares in the stallion's book. Ideally, if all mares are of equal and high fertility, the pregnancy rate achieved in mares bred during the last estrous cycle should be the same as that in the first estrous cycle; these pregnancy rates would accurately reflect the stallion's fertility. However, because fertility of individual mares varies, actual pregnancy rates for each successive estrous cycle of breeding are seldom the same. Mares that are subfertile tend to take more estrous cycles to become detectably pregnant. Table 18-7 reveals that pregnancy rates achieved during the first three estrous cycles are similar (for the stallion used) but dramatically decrease for breedings on the fourth estrous cycle (i.e., only one of seven mares bred on the fourth estrous cycle became pregnant). This decline in pregnancy rate per cycle as mares in the stallion's book are bred over successive estrous cycles indicates that those mares are themselves subfertile.

Whether all mares that do not become pregnant after breeding on a particular estrous cycle get rebred on the following estrous cycle can also be determined from this type of table. In Table 18-7, 32 of 81 mares became pregnant on the first cycle; therefore, 49 should have returned for a second cycle breeding, yet only 44 were bred a second time. Thus, five mares were bred only one time; the mares were not given adequate opportunity to become pregnant.

Barren, Foaling, and Maiden Mares

Barren
This group contains nonpregnant mares coming into the breeding season of interest. Mares in this group usually have lower fertility than in the other groups. Several reasons why a mare might be barren are discussed in the following paragraphs.

Not Bred the Previous Season
This can occur because the owner simply decided not to breed the mare, or the mare may have foaled late in the previous season and did not have ample opportunity to become pregnant. Mares classified as barren for these reasons have normal fertility. Some managers and computer programs include these mares in a separate category from barren mares.

Subfertile
These mares have intrinsic fertility problems that contributed to failure to become pregnant during the previous breeding season and are commonly older than the rest of the mare population. In most cases, the subfertile mares account for most of the mares classified as barren.

Aborted
These mares have aborted since the previous breeding season. Some managers and computer programs use the term **"slipped"** instead of "aborted" and include these mares in a separate category from the barren mares. Once they recover, they tend to have fertility similar to the Not Bred group.

Foaling
These mares have produced a foal in the current breeding season and will be rebred during the same season. One should expect high fertility in this group of mares because they recently conceived and carried a foal to term. Reduced fertility may be seen in this group if a predominant proportion of the mares foaled late in the breeding season, thus having only one to two estrous cycles available for rebreeding. Fertility in this group may also be reduced if some event (injury/illness to the stallion) prematurely shortens the breeding season.

Maiden
Mares that have never been bred. Mares in this group are generally young; however, occasional maiden mares are older because their owner has elected not to breed them when young (usually because of a continuing performance career). Older maiden mares are generally less fertile than young maiden mares, which typically have high fertility rates. Mares that have been recently retired from strenuous performance careers may not have regular cycles when they first become available for mating (typically in February) and thus may need more breedings to become pregnant. However, because maiden mares are generally

TABLE 18-7

Pregnancy Rate for Stallion 4 (see Figure 18-6) Based on Cycle Number

Cycle No.	No. of Cycles	No. of Mares Pregnant	% Pregnant/Cycle
1st cycle	81	32	40
2nd cycle	44	15	34
3rd cycle	18	7	39
4th cycle	7	1	0
5th cycle	3	1	0
6th cycle	0	0	0
TOTAL	153	56	37

available for breeding early in the season, their chances of becoming pregnant are high.

Pregnancy Status for Each Mare Class

The pregnancy status can reveal important information about stallion fertility. As a general rule, breeding of maiden and foaling mares should result in the highest fertility achievable by a stallion and represents a stallion's intrinsic fertility. Breeding of barren mares may result in similar or lesser fertility. If a large proportion of the barren mares in a stallion's book are nonpregnant because of intrinsically lower individual mare fertility, measures of stallion fertility that reflect the entire mare group are lower than that achieved in the foaling and maiden mare groups. Conversely, mares may be barren because they were not bred the previous year, in which case their fertility may be similar to that of foaling and maiden mare groups, resulting in the stallion achieving high fertility measures for the entire mare book.

In some cases, foaling mares may represent the group of lowest fertility. This may be due to a large proportion of foaling mares delivering their foals late in the season, leaving an insufficient number of estrous cycles available in the remainder of the season to truly test their fertility (i.e., only one or perhaps two estrous cycles before the breeding season ended). In this case, neither the stallion nor the foaling mares are at fault.

Number of Covers or Breedings (Matings) in a Cycle

The number of matings in a cycle refers to the average number of natural covers or inseminations performed per estrus. This value is a reflection of management ability to time breeding near to ovulation. Excessive covers or inseminations per cycle can result in overuse of a stallion (i.e., semen is essentially being wasted). Intense mare management to minimize the number of covers or inseminations per cycle results in more ejaculates (semen) available to breed more mares.

MATHEMATICS OF HORSE BREEDING

Although many factors are involved in the breeding process, perhaps the most critical is the realization that mares need adequate exposure to the stallion for high fertility to be achieved (i.e., a 100% pregnancy rate per cycle is not achievable, so mares not becoming pregnant on the first service must be bred a sufficient number of times to afford a realistic opportunity to become pregnant during the season). To illustrate this principle, if a stallion achieves a 50% pregnancy rate per cycle, mares must on average be bred at least two estrous cycles to yield a 75% seasonal pregnancy rate, yet a 75%

seasonal pregnancy rate is considered to be low on well-managed breeding farms. Evaluation of breeding records reveals whether the low seasonal pregnancy rate is simply from insufficient exposure to the stallion or whether other factors explain the low seasonal pregnancy rate.

EVALUATION OF THE EFFECT OF BREEDING FREQUENCY ON FERTILITY

One factor that modulates fertility during the breeding season is how often stallions are used. For a farm that is using natural cover, the breeding frequency represents the number of times a stallion is bred in a given time period (i.e., the number of times bred in a day or week). On farms where artificial breeding is used, the breeding frequency represents the number of mares bred with an individual ejaculate. No stallion will have mares presented for breeding at even intervals throughout the breeding season. Therefore, pregnancy rates achieved by the stallion when used for different breeding frequencies can be used to evaluate whether overuse of the stallion has occurred (i.e., whether he has been bred too frequently for ejaculates to contain sufficient numbers of sperm to effect good fertility). Use of breeding frequencies to evaluate this phenomenon is presented in Figures 18-3 to 18-6; this method relies on the following parameters:

1. Number of mares bred in last week: This identifies the number of mares bred in the week before the day in question. This parameter is an evaluation of the long-term effect of frequent breedings, with the intent to determine whether there is a threshold breeding frequency above which fertility of the stallion declines. This phenomenon occurs in many stallions; if periods of too high breeding frequency are numerous during the season, reduced fertility becomes apparent.
2. Number of mares bred the previous day: This identifies the number of mares bred (with either natural or artificial breeding) on that day.
3. Pregnancy differential: For each date every mare is bred, a pregnancy score is given (+1 if pregnancy results, −1 if no pregnancy results, or a zero for all double dates except for the last one of the cycle). The scores are summed for the week previous to a particular date and graphically indicate the fertility of a stallion for the previous week.
4. Cumulative pregnancy value: This value represents the summed pregnancy scores (+1 or −1) for the entire breeding season leading up to the date of interest. The zero line represents a 50% pregnancy rate per cycle.

To illustrate the effects of breeding frequency, the reader is referred to Figure 18-3. The arrow (March 7) represents the date for recording the following breeding

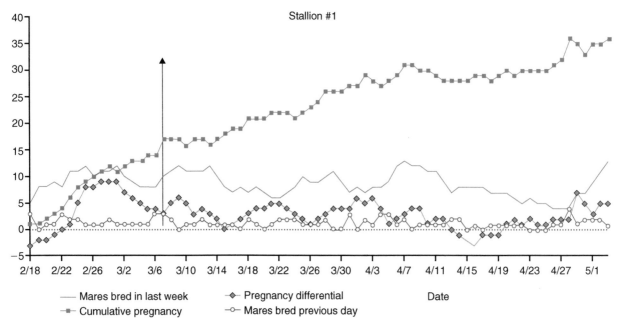

Figure 18-3   Stallion 1. This figure graphically represents an example of a highly fertile Thoroughbred stallion bred by natural cover. Note that the cumulative pregnancy value continues to climb regardless of preceding breeding frequencies. No indication shows that a threshold breeding frequency, above which fertility declines, has been reached. Although peaks and valleys are found in the pregnancy differential, they are probably related to nonstallion factors. This stallion is expected to achieve a 90% seasonal pregnancy rate, requiring less than an average of 1.5 estrous cycles per pregnancy, in a book of 100 mares bred with natural service.

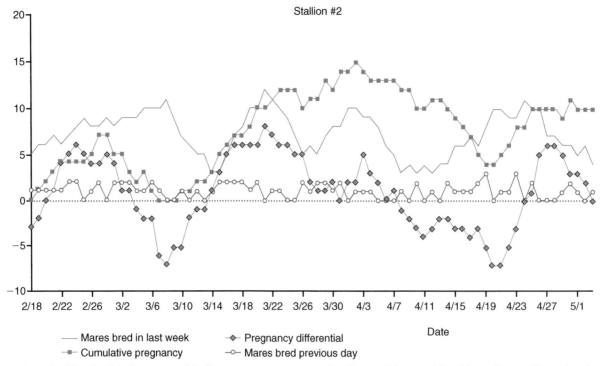

Figure 18-4   Stallion 2. This figure graphically represents an example of many Thoroughbred breeding stallions that breed a large book of mares. Note that a steep decline in pregnancy differential occurs from February 28 to March 8, which probably corresponds to the increase in breeding frequency during the previous week to 11 mares. Breeding frequency again rises to this level at times later in the season, but it is not maintained for as long a period as that from February 6 to March 8. Other declines in pregnancy differential and cumulative pregnancy value occur during the breeding season, but the declines are more gradual and are not associated with peaks in breeding frequency. This figure is representative of most breeding stallions that do reach threshold levels of breeding frequencies at times in the breeding season. Such stallions typically achieve an 80% to 90% seasonal pregnancy rate, necessitating 1.5 to 2.2 estrous cycles per pregnancy in a book of 80 to 90 mares if bred with natural service.

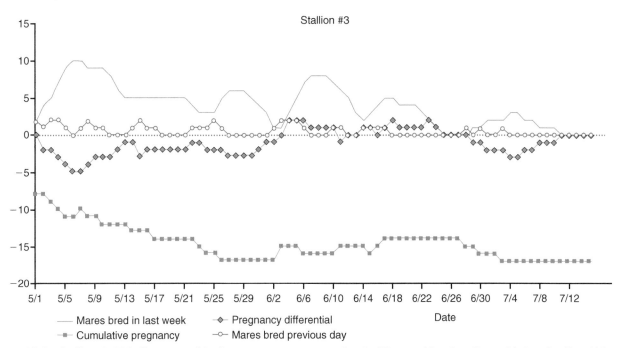

Figure 18-5 Stallion 3. This figure graphically represents an example of a Thoroughbred stallion with low fertility. Although breeding frequency remains low (zero to two mares per day), the pregnancy differential remains below the zero line (zero line: 50% pregnancy rate per cycle) and his cumulative pregnancy value is very low.

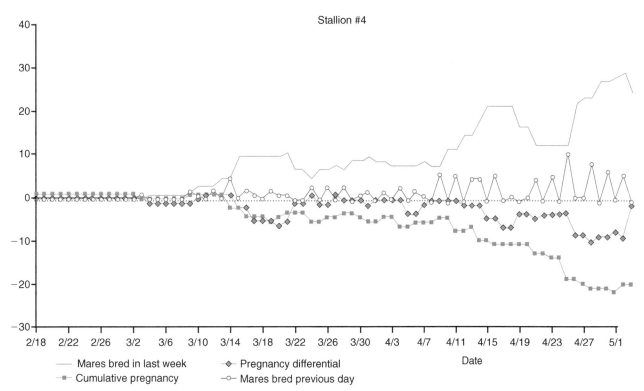

Figure 18-6 Stallion 4. This figure graphically represents an example of a Quarter Horse stallion with low fertility. The stallion was bred artificially to mares on the same farm, mares hauled to the farm (tailgate breeding), and mares at outside farms with transported, cooled semen (semen mailed overnight for breeding the next day or semen picked up at the farm for breeding the same day).

TABLE 18-8

Pregnancy Status of Mares Based on Location (On-Farm with Fresh Semen or Off-Farm with Shipped Semen) for Stallion 4 (see Figure 18-6)

Location of Mare	BARREN			FOALING			MAIDEN			Pregnant Overall	
	No. Pregnant	No. Bred	Percent Pregnant	No. Pregnant	No. Bred	Percent Pregnant	No. Pregnant	No. Bred	Percent Pregnant		
Mare and stallion on farm	3	11	27	14	21	67	7	10	70	24/42	(57%)
Overnight	2	2	100	4	6	67	0	1	0	6/9	(67%)
Pick-up	10	10	100	9	10	90	2	3	67	21/23	(91%)
Trailer-bred	1	4	25	5	6	83	1	3	33	7/13	(54%)
TOTAL	16	27	59	33	43	77	10	17	59	58/87	(67%)

frequency values: number of mares bred in last week, 10; number of mares bred previous day, 3; pregnancy differential, 3; and cumulative pregnancy value, 17. Interpretation of these data reveals that on March 7: 10 mares were bred in the previous week, 3 more mares became pregnant than were nonpregnant (pregnancy differential), and for the breeding season on this date, 17 more mares were pregnant than nonpregnant. With this approach, the reader should study Figures 18-3 to 18-6, while referring to the following interpretations.

For breeds that use artificial insemination, additional factors influence overall fertility. For example, mares may be inseminated with fresh semen immediately after collection, with stallions and mares being managed on the same farm. Assuming good management, this method of artificial breeding is expected to result in high fertility. Tailgate breeding may also occur, in which case the mare is moved to the farm by trailer, is inseminated in the trailer, and is immediately returned to the farm of origin. Because with tailgate breeding mares and stallions are under different management, pregnancy rates achieved in mares bred in this manner are sometimes lower than those achieved for mares managed at the farm where the stallion stands at stud. For mares bred with transported, cooled semen, each mare is again under different management from that for mares maintained on the farm where the stallion stands at stud. Additional factors that may adversely affect pregnancy rates when mares are bred with transported, cooled semen are that insemination timing in relation to ovulation can be more variable and that for some stallions the same level of fertility is not achieved with cooled semen as with fresh semen. Pregnancy rates achieved with frozen semen tend to be substantially lower for most stallions than those achieved with fresh or cooled semen. Therefore, in addition to those factors outlined for evaluation of the Thoroughbred breeding operation, additional parameters must be considered in evaluating the fertility achieved by a stallion used for artificial insemination. An example of one such evaluation is illustrated with Figure 18-6 and Tables 18-6 to 18-9.

Figure 18-6 shows several points regarding a stallion's lower-than-expected fertility when used in an artificial insemination breeding program. This stallion did not begin the breeding season until March 8, instead of February 15. The loss of almost a month of breeding season resulted in lost opportunities for barren and maiden mares to become pregnant. During March 10 through April 10, this stallion was bred

TABLE 18-9

Summary of Stallion 4 (see Figure 18-6) Fertility Parameters

Cycles/Pregnancy	Cycles/Mare	Covers/Cycle
2.73	1.89	1.79

infrequently, yet achieved only an approximate 50% pregnancy rate per cycle. When the number of inseminations per week exceeded 10 (March 11), the pregnancy rate declined. This graphic presentation is typical of the effect of overbreeding, in that pregnancy rates decline when the stallion is bred to too many mares; however, other factors contribute to the reduced fertility (see Tables 18-6 to 18-9).

Table 18-6 lists the fertility of differing mare groups bred to this stallion. The reader should note that the lower fertility in maiden than in barren mares is not typical. The overall seasonal pregnancy rate is low (69%). Evaluation of Table 18-8 reveals extreme variation in fertility achieved by different methods of breeding for this same stallion. Mares inseminated as soon as possible with semen that was picked up at the stud farm had a 91% pregnancy rate per season, whereas other methods of breeding resulted in pregnancy rates per season of only 54% to 67%. This finding suggests that, in the right conditions (i.e., intense mare management for prompt insemination at a time near to ovulation—the method used for breeding with transported, cooled semen), this stallion has the potential to be very fertile and raises the question of whether the low pregnancy rates were primarily due to inadequate breeding management.

Table 18-9 summarizes this stallion's fertility endpoints. The value for cycles per pregnancy was high, whereas that for cycles per mare was low, indicating that mares were not bred often enough when the pregnancy rate per cycle was so low. The number of covers per cycle was also quite high, which indicates that mares were often being bred too soon during the estrous period, long before ovulation occurred. Because the stallion's pregnancy rate declined dramatically when 10 or more mares were bred in the previous week, intensive mare management to constrain breeding to near the time of ovulation should increase pregnancy rates per cycle.

Assisted Reproductive Technology

19

CHAPTER

OBJECTIVES

While studying the information covered in this chapter, the reader should attempt to:

- Acquire a working understanding of assisted reproductive technologies, including oocyte transfer, intracytoplasmic sperm injection, gamete intrafallopian transfer, in vitro fertilization, and nuclear transfer.
- Acquire a working understanding of types of infertility in the mare that may benefit from assisted reproductive techniques.

STUDY QUESTIONS

1. Describe the principles used in performing the following techniques, and explain circumstances that may favor use of one technique over the other:
   a. Oocyte transfer
   b. Intracytoplasmic sperm injection
   c. Gamete intrafallopian transfer
   d. In vitro fertilization
   e. Nuclear transfer (cloning)

2. Describe procedures for harvesting ovaries from a mare after an untimely death and for transporting those ovaries to a laboratory for oocyte retrieval for assisted reproductive technology.

The term **assisted reproductive technology** (ART) covers a broad range of procedures but is most commonly used to refer to those procedures that use isolated oocytes to produce offspring. The ARTs most important in equine reproduction include oocyte transfer (OT), intracytoplasmic sperm injection (ICSI), gamete intrafallopian transfer (GIFT), in vitro fertilization (IVF), and nuclear transfer (NT; cloning).

With the exception of NT, these ARTs offer methods to obtain foals from mares that cannot provide embryos for transfer, or from reserves of stallion semen that are not adequate to achieve good pregnancy rates after standard intrauterine insemination. The main drawback to these techniques is that they require collection of oocytes from the valued donor mare, which is a semiinvasive procedure that requires specialized skill and equipment to perform. The technique of NT, or cloning, requires collection of only a skin biopsy sample from the donor animal and produces a foal with the same genetics as the donor. Major advances have been made in almost all fields of ART in horses over the last 10 years, making many of them commercially applicable.

The emphasis of this chapter is on the concepts behind these procedures and the potential for their application in equine practice.

OOCYTE RECOVERY

Recovery of Oocytes from the Dominant Preovulatory Follicle

In the live mare, oocytes may be efficiently recovered from the dominant preovulatory follicle after gonadotropin stimulation, via either transvaginal ultrasound–guided follicle aspiration (TVA), or puncture of the follicle via a needle placed through the flank. Aspiration of the stimulated preovulatory follicle provides a chance at only one or perhaps two oocytes per cycle but gives an oocyte with optimal developmental competence. Recovery rates from stimulated preovulatory follicles are high (70% to 80%) because the oocyte-cumulus complex has loosened from the wall of the follicle in preparation for ovulation (Carnevale and Ginther, 1995; Hinrichs et al., 1998).

The major drawbacks to aspiration of the stimulated dominant preovulatory follicle are the necessity for monitoring of follicular growth, and accurate timing of gonadotropin administration in the mare, and the fact that only one or sometimes two follicles are available for aspiration. Superovulation regimens appear to be only minimally useful to increase the number of preovulatory follicles available for aspiration, as the ovary becomes flaccid after the first follicle is aspirated, and aspiration of subsequent follicles may be difficult (Maclellan et al., 2002). Limited superstimulation (of one or two additional follicles) may be useful but also may be difficult to achieve. Oocyte recovery from the dominant follicle may be performed simply with use of a 13- to 15-gauge, 20-cm needle guided through a cannula placed through the flank (Hinrichs et al., 1998). The ovary is manipulated with one hand per rectum, while the other hand manipulates the needle to puncture the follicle. The contents of the follicle are aspirated using a 50-mL all-plastic syringe and extension tubing (Figures 19-1 and 19-2).

Because the follicle has received gonadotropin stimulation, the oocytes recovered from aspiration of the stimulated, dominant preovulatory follicle have already resumed nuclear maturation and thus need only to be supported in culture to the time of predicted ovulation to mature completely.

Recovery of Oocytes from Immature Follicles

Oocytes may be recovered from nonmature follicles present on the ovaries of live mares; because of their small size, ultrasound–guided aspiration (TVA) is necessary to visualize the follicles. Oocytes recovered from these follicles are immature and must be cultured in the presence of gonadotropins to induce maturation in vitro (Figure 19-3). When all follicles on the ovary are aspirated, some oocytes are recovered from juvenile follicles, some from growing follicles, and some from follicles undergoing atresia.

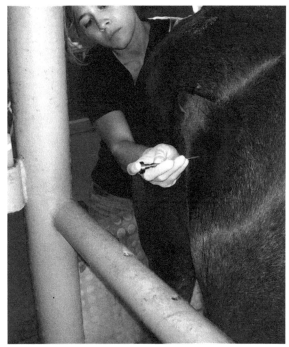

Figure 19-1 A large-bore (12-gauge) needle with a trocar has been inserted through the upper flank of a mare with a dominant preovulatory follicle. The mare was sedated with detomodine and burophanol and was administered a rectal tocolytic (Buscopan, Boehringer Ingelheim Pharmaceuticals, Ridgefield, Conn.). The hand in the rectum is used to position the surface of the ovary with the large preovulatory follicle next to the upper abdominal wall. The needle with trocar is advanced through the skin, muscular layers, and peritoneum until the trocar is felt per rectum. The trocar is pulled back, and the ovarian follicle is pushed over the advancing needle.

Thus, only 50% to 60% of recovered oocytes may be expected to mature on in vitro culture. Those that do mature in vitro have lower development rates after fertilization than those for oocytes obtained from stimulated preovulatory follicles. In addition, the recovery rate on aspiration of immature follicles has historically been low (typically 15% to 30%). For these reasons, most clinical ART programs have used aspiration of the stimulated preovulatory follicle to obtain oocytes for commercial oocyte transfer or ICSI (Hinrichs et al., 2000; Carnevale et al., 2005, 2007).

Recently, however, a good recovery rate (>50%) has been reported in a clinical program in which TVA of immature follicles was performed for oocyte collection. Oocytes were matured in vitro, fertilized with ICSI (see subsequent discussion), cultured to the blastocyst stage, and transferred to recipient mares. In this program, the increase in oocyte number per aspiration session overcame the effect of oocyte quality and resulted in a higher pregnancy rate per cycle (~48%) (Colleoni et al., 2007) than was reported with a program that used ICSI with oocytes recovered on aspiration of only the dominant follicle (approximately 20% per cycle) (Carnevale et al., 2007). After the report of

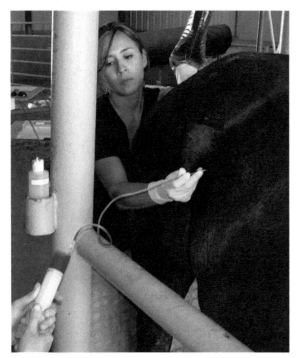

Figure 19-2 Aspiration begins, usually yielding serum-like clear fluid initially. As the follicle is evacuated, massage of the follicular walls per rectum is performed; the other hand manipulates the needle to effectively scrape the follicular wall free of cellular contents. The aspirated fluid becomes bloody at this point. Some practitioners infuse fluid into the follicular cavity after it is first drained to allow repeated flushing to occur, with the hope of increasing the chance of obtaining the oocyte.

Colleoni and coworkers, our laboratory at Texas A&M performed TVA of immature follicles on Quarter Horse–type research mares every 2 weeks throughout the breeding season of 2008, for an average of 9 follicles aspirated and 5 recovered oocytes per mare per session. In vitro blastocyst production after ICSI averaged 63% per aspiration session (Jacobson, et al., in press).

Transvaginal aspiration is performed with a transvaginal probe handle into which the ultrasound probe is mounted. The probe handle has within it a channel for the needle (see Figure 5-9). In the tranquilized mare, the probe is placed in the vagina, and the ovary is manipulated via palpation per rectum. A specialized needle, typically a 12- to 17-gauge double-lumen needle, is placed through the guide channel of the probe handle. The ovary is imaged through the vaginal wall (Figure 19-4) and manipulated by the hand per rectum so that the follicle is placed in the path of the needle as visualized on the ultrasound screen. The needle is then guided forward through the vaginal wall into the follicle (Figure 19-5), and the contents of the follicle are aspirated, typically with a vacuum pump (Figure 19-6). Obtaining a high recovery rate on aspiration of immature follicles necessitates manipulation of the follicle and needle during aspiration, to attempt to scrape the follicle walls, and repeated (up to 10 times) filling and emptying of the follicle with flush fluid. Recovery rates on aspiration of immature follicles with TVA appear to be technician-dependent; different laboratories consistently report very different recovery rates (from <15% to >50%) with this procedure.

Oocyte Recovery Post Mortem

If a mare dies or must be euthanized for medical reasons, then the ovaries may be removed and oocytes collected from them for ART. The ovaries are shipped to a laboratory equipped for oocyte collection and maturation. At the laboratory, the follicles are opened with a scalpel blade, and the interior tissue of the follicle (the granulosa cell layer) is scraped from the follicle wall with a bone curette. With use of a medium, the cells are washed into a Petri dish and the oocyte is located in the recovered cells. Oocyte recovery rates with this technique can be more than 80% with careful attention;

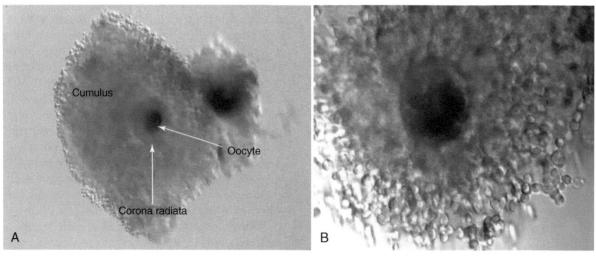

Figure 19-3 Equine oocytes. **A,** After recovery with follicular aspiration. **B,** After in vitro maturation (note that the corona radiata and cumulus are now expanded).

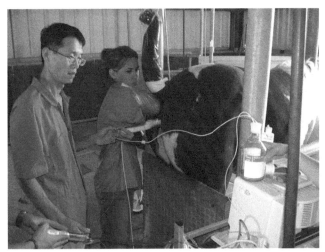

Figure 19-4 An ultrasound machine with a transvaginal curvilinear probe attached is used per vagina to visualize ovarian follicles for transvaginal aspiration. The ultrasound unit has a needle guide that prelineates the pathway the needle will follow when advanced past the end of the probe. The ovary is positioned with the hand in the rectum until the desired follicle underlies the needle pathway. The transvaginal needle, with an etched echogenic end, is advanced through the vaginal wall, fascia, and peritoneum and into the ovarian stroma. When the needle is located within the center of the follicle, aspiration in a closed system begins. Refilling and reaspiration is repeated up to seven times to increase the chance of obtaining an oocyte.

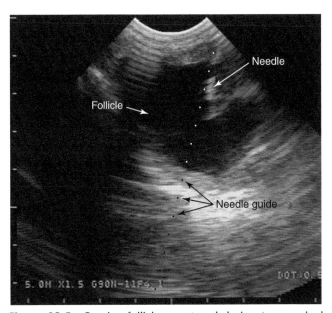

Figure 19-5 Ovarian follicle punctured during transvaginal aspiration procedure. The etched tip of the special needle is echogenic, allowing visual confirmation that the tip is within the follicle lumen.

typically, an average of 10 oocytes per mare are recovered from the ovaries of commercial mares processed post mortem. As for oocytes recovered from immature follicles ex vivo with TVA, these oocytes must be matured by culturing them in vitro in the presence of gonadotropins.

The factors that affect embryo development from oocytes recovered postmortem are still unclear; little information is available in this area. Factors that are likely to have an effect on the potential to produce a foal from these oocytes are the age of the mare, the length and severity of the illness, treatments administered, the method of euthanasia, the length of time the ovaries remain in the mare post mortem before removal, the temperature at which the ovaries are transported, and the length of time between death of the mare and processing of the ovaries. In our postmortem ICSI program, chronic illness of the donor mare and prolonged transport time (>12 hours) are associated with both lower blastocyst development in vitro (12% to 14% per oocyte subjected to ICSI versus 23% for mares not in these categories) and increased embryo loss rates of resulting pregnancies after embryo transfer. Carnevale et al. (2004), using oocyte transfer with oocytes recovered post mortem, reported a 36% embryo development rate if ovaries were processed within 1 hour of the mare's death and a 10% development rate if the ovaries were processed 8 to 26 hours after death. With use of slaughterhouse tissue, we found a higher in vitro blastocyst development after ICSI in oocytes from ovaries processed within 6 hours postmortem than in those from ovaries processed 7 or more hours post mortem (Ribeiro et al., 2008). Cooling of ovaries to refrigerator temperature lowered maturation rates of recovered oocytes (Love et al., 2003).

On the basis of data from both clinical and research programs, current recommendations are to remove the ovaries from the mare with anesthesia (e.g., ketamine and xylazine) if possible; if not, then removal of the ovaries as soon after death as possible is recommended. We suspect that use of KCl for euthanasia may lower development rates but do not have controlled data on this. Ovaries should be transported to the laboratory at room temperature, preferably in less than 6 hours.

Clients should be informed that the rate of viable pregnancy from oocytes collected from mares post mortem is low. In the oocyte transfer program at Colorado State University, with oocytes collected post mortem, foals or pregnancies ongoing more than 70 days were obtained for six of 25 mares (24%; Carnevale et al., 2004). In our postmortem ICSI program at Texas A&M, from 2006-2009 we have obtained a total of 21 blastocysts from 16 mares, of which 13 produced pregnancies after transcervical transfer and 10 (63% per mare) have produced foals or currently ongoing pregnancies.

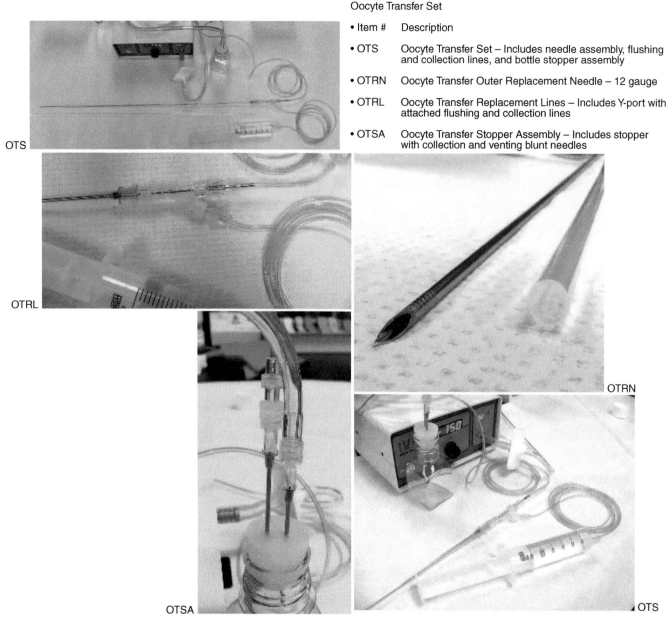

Oocyte Transfer Set

- Item #   Description

- OTS   Oocyte Transfer Set – Includes needle assembly, flushing and collection lines, and bottle stopper assembly

- OTRN   Oocyte Transfer Outer Replacement Needle – 12 gauge

- OTRL   Oocyte Transfer Replacement Lines – Includes Y-port with attached flushing and collection lines

- OTSA   Oocyte Transfer Stopper Assembly – Includes stopper with collection and venting blunt needles

Figure 19-6 Commercial oocyte aspiration sets for transvaginal follicle aspiration are available with needles, needle guides, tubing, stoppers, bottles, connecting tubes, and vacuum pumps.

OOCYTE TRANSFER

OT is currently the most effective method to obtain a foal from a mare's single isolated oocyte. It is conducted on a commercial basis in two centers (Colorado State University and Texas A&M University) and in a few clinical practices in the United States.

The basic techniques for OT start with synchronization of follicle growth in the donor and recipient mares so that each mare has a follicle that is receptive to gonadotropins (e.g., human chorionic gonadotropin [hCG] or deslorelin) on the same day. Gonadotropins are administered to both mares at approximately the same time. The follicles of both mares are aspirated 24 to 35 hours after gonadotropin administration. We aspirate the donor mare's follicle first to ascertain that an oocyte is available for transfer. If an oocyte is collected from the donor, we then aspirate the follicle of the recipient mare to remove her oocyte. The recipient mare is typically inseminated with semen from the desired stallion after follicle aspiration, when we know that the oocyte has been recovered from the mare and she is a good candidate as a recipient.

Alternatively, recipient mares may be nonovulatory mares (mares in anestrus, early transition, or early estrus [no follicle >25 mm]) treated with estrogen before the transfer and progesterone after the transfer. This eliminates both the requirement for synchronization of follicle growth between donor and recipient mares and the necessity of performing follicle aspiration on the recipient. Many different hormonal regimens have been effective for preparation of nonovulating mares as oocyte recipients (Hinrichs et al., 1999, 2000; Carnevale et al., 2001).

The donor mare's oocyte is transferred to the oviduct of the recipient mare at the time the donor mare would have been expected to ovulate (i.e., 36 to 40 hours after hCG or injectable deslorelin administration, or 40 to 44 hours after deslorelin implant administration). The transfer is done surgically through a standing flank laparotomy. After the incision is made through the abdominal musculature, the ovary is exteriorized; the infundibulum of the oviduct is attached to the ovary and so is available for cannulation (Figure 19-7). The oocyte is loaded into a pipette or tomcat catheter and is transferred to the ampulla of the oviduct. The ovary is then replaced into the abdomen, and the incision closed.

Reported success rates with clinical oocyte transfer are a 77% oocyte recovery rate from the donor mare's preovulatory follicle and a 38% initial pregnancy rate after transfer of a single oocyte, with an overall pregnancy rate at day 50 of 32% per transferred oocyte

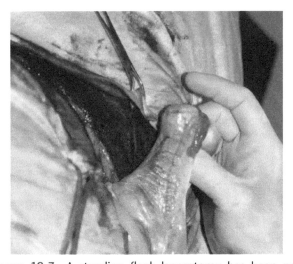

Figure 19-7 A standing flank laparotomy has been performed for oocyte transfer in this recipient mare. The surgeon brings the ovary to the incision site and exteriorizes the infundibulum. A second operator cannulates the infudibulum, passing the cannula 2 to 3 cm into the tubular oviduct. The oocyte is deposited, and the ovary is gently dropped back into the abdominal cavity. The recipient mare is then inseminated either before or after the transfer, with the goal of fertilization of the donor mare's oocyte occurring normally within the oviduct of the recipient mare.

(24% per follicle aspirated) (Carnevale et al., 2005). An average of 1.2 follicles were aspirated per mare per cycle due to growth of two dominant follicles. The pregnancy rate is lower in clinical cases than in research studies (in which it is typically ~75%) because of variable semen and oocyte quality in clinical cases. Oocytes from older mares (>20 years old) produce lower pregnancy rates after OT than those with oocytes from younger mares (Carnevale and Ginther, 1995).

Selection of Mares for Oocyte Transfer

Mares should be selected for OT only if standard embryo transfer is not an option because of problems with the cervix, uterus, or oviducts that preclude fertilization or cause embryonic loss before day 7, the time at which embryos would be recovered with standard uterine flushing technique. Common reasons to consider OT include chronic endometritis, pyometra, and uterine or cervical damage from dystocia. In addition, some mares appear to have idiopathic infertility (often attributed to failure of sperm or embryos to pass through the oviduct), and these mares may be able to produce foals via OT. OT is best used when only one or two oocytes are recovered from the donor mare, as would be obtained from aspiration of the dominant preovulatory follicle. Therefore, mares selected for OT should show normal follicle growth and ovulation.

OT may not be the technique of choice if multiple oocytes are harvested, such as after transvaginal aspiration of all follicles on the ovary or after recovery of oocytes from mares post mortem. These techniques result in recovery of a large number of oocytes of relatively low developmental competence. If used for OT, multiple oocytes necessitate either multiple surgeries (and recipient mares) to transfer single oocytes of unknown competence to individual recipient mares or alternatively, transfer of multiple oocytes to the oviducts of fewer mares, which may result in multiple conceptuses within one recipient mare and thus loss of potential foals. The number of recipient surgeries performed for OT is typically governed by the number the client wishes to pay for. Carnevale et al. (2004) reported transfer of up to 14 oocytes to the oviducts of single recipient mares and presence of up to 8 embryonic vesicles within the uteri of individual recipient mares after transfer (in this case, all conceptuses were subsequently lost). Therefore, if multiple oocytes are obtained from a mare, ICSI followed by individual transcervical transfer of resulting in vitro-cultured blastocysts may be preferable to transfer of multiple oocytes to one oviduct, to allow the maximum number of viable pregnancies possible.

When OT is performed, the recipient mare is bred by standard insemination, so this technique should be used only when the desired sire has sperm with normal fertility. If semen stores are low or sperm quality is poor, then ICSI should be considered.

INTRACYTOPLASMIC SPERM INJECTION

ICSI is a method to fertilize mature oocytes in vitro. With ICSI, one sperm is picked up with a micropipette under a micromanipulator microscope and is injected into the oocyte (Figure 19-8). This technique has been well developed in the horse because a method for standard IVF (incubating sperm and eggs together for fertilization) has not been repeatably successful (see subsequent section on IVF).

For performance of ICSI, sperm is prepared using a swim-up or density-gradient separation technique. This is done to ensure that the best-quality sperm is available for the procedure, rather than just any sperm picked from a semen sample. The mature oocyte is denuded of its cumulus and is placed in a droplet of medium under oil on a Petri dish lid. A second droplet on the lid holds medium for the sperm; this medium contains polyvinylpyrrolidone, which slows the sperm movement. An aliquot of the prepared sperm is added to the sperm medium droplet. Manipulation is performed on a microscope equipped with a micromanipulator with a Piezo drill. The Piezo apparatus provides minute vibrations to the injection pipette, allowing it to actually drill into the substrate rather than to be pushed into it, and its use appears to be associated with better embryo development after equine ICSI than when standard micromanipulation is used. When the Piezo drill is used, the accompanying pipette is cut straight, rather than pulled to a point as for standard micromanipulation. The oocyte is held in place with a holding pipette,

and one sperm from the sperm droplet is aspirated, tail first, into the injection pipette. The sperm is immobilized, and its membrane is disrupted by a few pulses with the Piezo drill. The sperm is then injected into the cytoplasm of the oocyte, again with use of the Piezo drill to ensure that the oocyte plasma membrane has been disrupted.

After the oocytes are fertilized, three options exist for transfer of resulting zygotes/embryos to recipient mares: (1) immediate surgical transfer to the oviduct of a recipient mare; (2) culture for 24 to 48 hours, with surgical transfer of cleaved embryos to the oviduct; or (3) culture for 7 to 8 days, with transcervical transfer of resulting blastocysts to the uteri of recipient mares, as for standard embryo transfer. If multiple oocytes have been obtained (as for aspiration of all follicles on the ovary with TVA, or collection of oocytes post mortem), the first two options again have the drawback of surgical transfers needed of multiple zygotes/embryos of unknown developmental competence. Culture to the blastocyst stage in vitro, followed by transcervical transfer, is the logical method of choice when multiple oocytes are obtained, because this allows individual transfer of each developed embryo to a separate recipient mare and maximizes the number of foals obtained from a given number of oocytes.

Complicating this choice, however, is the fact that it is not yet clear whether culture in vitro reduces the developmental capacity of the oocyte (whether a fertilized oocyte is more likely to develop to a successful pregnancy after transfer to the oviduct rather than after culture to blastocyst in vitro). Currently, ART methods preferred by different laboratories reflect their results on culture for blastocyst development. Blastocyst development rates in vitro range from less than 10% to 40%, depending on the source of the oocytes (in vitro

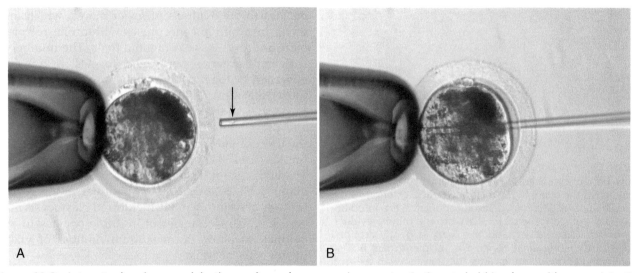

A   B

Figure 19-8 Intracytoplasmic sperm injection performed on an equine oocyte. **A,** Oocyte held in place, with sperm injection pipette *(arrow)* adjacent to the zona pellucida. **B,** The zona pellucida has been punctured by the pipette, and sperm is being deposited within the oocyte cytoplasm.

matured versus in vivo matured; normal fertile mares versus subfertile commercial [client] mares) and the culture system used. In our laboratory, in vitro blastocyst development rates after ICSI of in vitro matured oocytes from normal mares, recovered with TVA, are currently 33%, and pregnancy rate after transcervical transfer of these embryos is 80%.

Because the technique of ICSI has only recently been applied clinically, limited data are available on success rates in commercial practice. In one clinical program in which ICSI was used with oocytes recovered from the dominant preovulatory follicle, followed by surgical transfer of cleaved embryos to the oviduct, cleavage rates were 68% and pregnancy rates at 50 days were 31%, for an overall 21% pregnancy rate per oocyte subjected to ICSI; oocyte recovery rates per cycle were not given (Carnevale et al., 2007).

Results have also been presented from a clinical program in which oocytes were collected with TVA of all immature follicles on the ovary, followed by in vitro maturation, ICSI, in vitro culture to the blastocyst stage, and transcervical transfer (Colleoni et al., 2007). In this program, an average of 10 oocytes was recovered per mare (these were Warmblood mares with a high number [average of 17] of follicles present on the ovaries). After maturation culture, 66% of oocytes matured and were fertilized with ICSI. Thirteen percent of fertilized oocytes developed to the blastocyst stage in culture. Pregnancy rates 60 days after embryo transfer were 55%, resulting in an estimated 48% pregnancy rate per mare per aspiration session.

Selection of Mares and Stallions for Intracytoplasmic Sperm Injection

Intracytoplasmic sperm injection is applicable to mares from which multiple oocytes will be recovered, such as when all follicles are aspirated with TVA or when oocytes are recovered post mortem. ICSI and in vitro culture to the blastocyst stage may also be used when the dominant preovulatory follicle is aspirated to avoid the need for surgery as for OT; however, the chance of a resulting pregnancy is lower than with oocyte transfer (for normal mares, approximately a 40% chance of pregnancy after ICSI and transfer of the resulting blastocyst versus a 75% chance of pregnancy after OT).

A major reason for use of ICSI clinically is that only one viable sperm is needed to fertilize each oocyte. No difference is found in embryo development after ICSI with fresh or frozen-thawed sperm (Choi et al., 2002). Frozen sperm may be thawed, diluted 1:100, aliquoted, and refrozen, with no difference in blastocyst development when used for ICSI from that of the original frozen semen (Choi et al., 2006). Immotile sperm can be used for ICSI, but blastocyst develop-

ment is lower than that with motile sperm (Choi et al., 2006). Lazzari et al. (2002) reported that if motile sperm were selected for ICSI, no difference was found in embryo production among stallions with differing conception rates in the field. Thus, ICSI is especially useful with stallions for which low sperm numbers are available, such as when only a few frozen straws of semen are available from a stallion that has died or when sperm quality is inadequate for standard insemination.

GAMETE INTRAFALLOPIAN TRANSFER

GIFT is the technique of transferring both oocytes and sperm to the oviducts. This is performed with essentially the same procedures as for OT, through a standing flank laparotomy; however, the sperm are loaded into the pipette with the oocyte and instilled into the oviduct. The potential advantages of this procedure include use of lower-quality or lower numbers of sperm for OT and a decrease in the possibility of postbreeding endometritis in oocyte recipients. OT recipient mares inseminated with standard techniques appear to have a higher incidence of postbreeding endometritis than that in the typical embryo recipient mare, probably because the tranquilizers and smooth muscle relaxants used for oocyte aspiration interfere with uterine muscle contractility, thus suppressing clearance of semen and debris from the uterus.

GIFT has been shown in one research study to work well (pregnancy rate of 82%) with fresh, nonextended semen (Coutinho da Silva et al., 2004). The semen in that study was processed through a density gradient before insemination directly into the oviduct. However, pregnancy rates with either frozen semen or transported, cooled semen were low, which suggests that this technique may not be commercially feasible unless the desired stallion is available to produce fresh semen for the procedure.

IN VITRO FERTILIZATION

IVF (incubating oocytes with sperm for fertilization) is the standard method for fertilization of isolated oocytes in most species other than the horse. In the horse, success rates with IVF have been low because of an inability of the sperm to penetrate the zona pellucida in vitro. Thus, ICSI has been developed for fertilization of horse oocytes in vitro. Recent research indicates that problems with induction of sperm hyperactivated motility may underlie the failure of IVF in the horse. When hyperactivated motility was chemically induced in horse sperm, fertilization rates exceeding 50% were achieved on several occasions (McPartlin et al., 2009). This development opens the door for a less expensive and less labor-intensive alternative to ICSI for fertilization of horse oocytes in vitro. Much further research in this area is anticipated.

NUCLEAR TRANSFER (CLONING)

Production of foals via NT appears to be a repeatable procedure in the horse. The first cloned equids were reported in 2003; these were a mule that was produced from fetal cells (Woods et al., 2003) and a horse that was produced from adult somatic cells (Galli et al., 2003). Only the following three laboratories have reported the birth of cloned horse foals resulting from NT with adult somatic cells: (1) the laboratory of Dr. Cesare Galli, in Italy, reported the birth of three cloned foals, of which two survived, including one foal carried to term by the same mare that provided the cells for NT (Galli et al., 2003; Lagutina et al., 2005); (2) Texas A&M reported the birth of 14 cloned foals, of which 12 have survived; and (3) a commercial laboratory, ViaGen (Austin, Tex.), reported the birth of cloned foals in the popular press.

The efficiency of production of cloned horse foals in our laboratory at Texas A&M has been relatively high. As an overall average from the last three studies, the pregnancy rate after transfer of cloned embryos has been 66%, with 50% of the pregnancies resulting in birth of viable foals, for a 33% live foal rate per embryo transferred (Hinrichs et al., 2007; Choi et al., 2009; Johnson et al., in press). This rate is notably higher than the 5% to 10% rate of production of viable offspring per transferred embryo reported in other species (Wells, 2005).

Procedures for cloning begin with collection of a tissue sample from the donor animal. This sample is typically a small (0.5-cm^2) piece of subcutaneous connective tissue. The tissue is placed immediately into chilled culture medium and shipped to the laboratory for culture. Culture of the tissue over the next few weeks results in growth and proliferation of fibroblasts, which are then frozen for future use. When cloning is to be performed, mature oocytes are needed as host ooplasts for the donor cell nuclear material. These typically have been recovered from slaughterhouse tissue, but our laboratory has used oocytes recovered with TVA from immature follicles.

NT is performed with a micromanipulator microscope. The metaphase plate and polar body, containing the chromosomes of the mature oocyte, are removed, and a cell from the desired donor animal is either injected directly into the oocyte cytoplasm or placed into the perivitelline space and its membrane fused with that of the oocyte with electrical pulse. Once the donor cell and oocyte have fused, the oocyte is stimulated to start embryo development, typically by triggering calcium influx or inhibiting activity of specific cell-cycle proteins. The oocyte divides, forming an embryo in which the nuclei contain the chromosomes of the transferred donor cell. Thus, a foal is produced with the genetics of the donor animal.

After the NT procedure, the embryo is cultured in vitro to the blastocyst stage. In our laboratory, the blastocyst development rate for cloned embryos (~5% to 10%) is much lower than that for ICSI embryos (~25 to 35%). The pregnancy rate after transcervical transfer of NT-derived blastocysts to recipient mares is also somewhat lower than that for ICSI-derived blastocysts (66% versus 80%).

Pregnancy loss of cloned embryos produced in our laboratory is approximately 50%; these losses are distributed throughout gestation. At birth, cloned foals have an increased incidence of maladjustment, enlarged umbilical remnant, and contracted tendons and valgus deformity of the front legs. However, these conditions all appear to respond to treatment, and health of cloned foals, once they are beyond the first 2 weeks, appears to be normal. Three of 17 live-born cloned horse foals reported in the literature have died post partum (one of septicemia, one of pneumonia, and one after a hypotensive episode during induction of anesthesia for exploration for a possible ruptured bladder). (Johnson et al., in press)

Selection of Horses for Cloning

Cloning should be regarded as a method to preserve genetics for breeding, rather than as a method to produce individuals of a given genotype. As noted previously, at this time, cloned foals have a higher incidence of problems at birth that could affect their performance as adults. Although cloned foals have the same genetics as the donor horse, they may use these genes differently (have different epigenetic patterns) and thus may be phenotypically slightly different from the original animal. However, when cloned horses are used for breeding, their offspring should be completely normal.

The selection of a horse for cloning is largely a decision of the owner, similar to other breeding decisions. Cloning is an option when a horse of a valued bloodline cannot produce offspring or when an owner desires more offspring from this horse's genetics. A major application of cloning is to rescue the genetics of geldings that have proven themselves to be outstanding individuals; the resulting cloned colt, left entire, will sire foals that should be identical to the foals that the original gelding would have produced if he had been left a stallion.

Currently, major breed associations in the United States do not recognize foals produced with NT. However, the American Quarter Horse Association held its first open forum on the subject in the spring of 2009, so it is possible that recognition of foals produced with NT by this registry may follow at some point in the future. Cloned horses are allowed to compete in National Cutting Horse Association competitions in the United States, and other competition organizations that require only identification of competitors are likely to follow suit. Some sport horse registries in Europe will register cloned foals. The effect of registration status on the value of the cloned animal and its offspring must be weighed in the decision to perform cloning.

Clones have the chromosomal DNA of the donor horse. However, the cells of the clone do have the mitochondria and mitochondrial DNA of the oocyte used as a recipient for the NT. This has no effect on the offspring of a male clone because the mitochondria of the sperm are eliminated after fertilization. However, because the eggs of the female clone contain the same mitochondria that the clone's somatic cells do (i.e., the mitochondria originating from the recipient oocyte used for cloning), a female clone passes these mitochondria onto her offspring. Thus, the foals of a cloned mare are not 100% genetically identical to the foals of the original mare unless the oocytes used for cloning have been selected for mitochondrial identity. The impact of this mitochondrial heterogeneity on the performance or phenotype of the offspring is currently unknown in the horse; however, in cattle, no difference is found in growth rate or in milk composition or production between donor cattle and clones of those cattle produced with slaughterhouse-derived oocytes (Wells et al., 2004; Norman and Walsh, 2004; Watanabe et al., 2008). More information on mitochondrial identity among horse breeds and effects of mitochondrial DNA on horse phenotype should be available in the near future.

SUMMARY

Equine assisted reproduction techniques have moved from the research laboratory to the clinic in the last 10 years. Methods including OT and oocyte recovery, ICSI, and transfer of resulting embryos are now available to enable production of foals from mares that cannot carry their own foal to term or provide an embryo for transfer. These methods may also be used to produce foals from oocytes recovered from mares post mortem. ICSI allows production of foals from stallions with sperm reserves incompatible with pregnancy after standard insemination. NT presents an option for preservation of valuable genetics or rescue of genetics from an otherwise sterile animal, such as a gelding. These methods provide the veterinarian with additional options to offer clients faced with difficult reproductive problems in valuable animals.

BIBLIOGRAPHY

Carnevale EM, Coutinho da Silva MA, Preis KA, et al: Establishment of pregnancies from oocytes collected from the ovaries of euthanized mares, *Proc Am Assoc Equine Pract* 50:531-533, 2004.

Carnevale EM, Ginther OJ: Defective oocytes as a cause of subfertility in old mares, *Biol Reprod Mono* 1:209-214, 1995.

Carnevale EM, Maclellan LJ, Coutinho da Silva MA, et al: Equine sperm-oocyte interaction: results after intraoviductal and intrauterine inseminations of recipients for oocyte transfer, *Anim Reprod Sci* 68:305-314, 2001.

Carnevale EM, Stokes J, Squires EL, et al: Clinical use of intracytoplasmic sperm injection in horses, *Proc Am Assoc Equine Pract* 53:560, 2007.

Carnevale EM, Coutinho da Silva MA, Panzani D, et al: Factors affecting the success of oocyte transfer in a clinical program for subfertile mares, *Theriogenology* 64:519-527, 2005.

Choi YH, Hartman DL, Fissore RA, et al: Effect of sperm extract injection volume, injection of PLCæ cRNA, and tissue cell line on efficiency of equine nuclear transfer, *Cloning Stem Cells* 11:301-308, 2009. In press, 2009.

Choi YH, Love CC, Love LB, et al: Developmental competence in vivo and in vitro of in vitro-matured equine oocytes fertilized by intracytoplasmic sperm injection with fresh or frozen-thawed sperm, *Reproduction* 123:455-465, 2002.

Choi YH, Love CC, Varner DD, et al: Equine blastocyst development after intracytoplasmic injection of sperm subjected to two freeze-thaw cycles, *Theriogenology* 65:808-819, 2006.

Colleoni S, Barbacini S, Necci D, et al: Application of ovum pick-up, intracytoplasmic sperm injection and embryo culture in equine practice, *Proc Am Assoc Equine Pract* 53:554-559, 2007.

Coutinho da Silva MA, Carnevale EM, Maclellan LJ, et al: Oocyte transfer in mares with intrauterine or intraoviductal insemination using fresh, cooled, and frozen stallion semen, *Theriogenology* 61:705-713, 2004.

Galli C, Lagutina I, Crotti G, et al: A cloned horse born to its dam twin, *Nature* 424:635, 2003.

Hinrichs K, Choi YH, Varner DD, et al: Production of cloned horse foals using roscovitine-treated donor cells and activation with sperm extract and/or ionomycin, *Reproduction* 134:319-325, 2007.

Hinrichs K, Matthews GL, Freeman DA, et al: Oocyte transfer in mares, *J Am Vet Med Assoc* 212:982-986, 1998.

Hinrichs K, Provost PJ, Torello EM: Birth of a foal after oocyte transfer to a nonovulating, hormone-treated mare, *Theriogenology* 51:1251-1258, 1999.

Hinrichs K, Provost PJ, Torello EM: Treatments resulting in pregnancy in nonovulating, hormone-treated oocyte recipient mares, *Theriogenology* 54:1285-1293, 2000.

Jacobson CC, Choi YH, Hayden SS and Hinrichs K.: Recovery of mare oocytes on a fixed biweekly schedule, and resulting blastocyst formation after intracytoplasmic in sperm injection. *Theriogenology* (in press).

Johnson AK, Clark-Price SC, Choi YH, Hartman DL, and Hinrichs K: Physical and clinicopathologic findings in foals produced by somatic cell nuclear transfer—14 cases (2005-2008). *J Amer Vet Med Assoc* (in press).

Lagutina I, Lazzari G, Duchi R, Colleoni S, Ponderato N, Turini P, Crotti G and Galli C. Somatic cell nuclear transfer in horses: effect of oocyte morphology, embryo reconstruction method and donor cell type. *Reproduction* 130:559-567 (2005).

Lazzari G, Crotti G, Turini P, et al: Equine embryos at the compacted morula and blastocyst stage can be obtained by intracytoplasmic sperm injection (ICSI) of in vitro matured oocytes with frozen-thawed spermatozoa from semen of different fertilities, *Theriogenology* 58:709-712, 2002.

Love LB, Choi YH, Love CC, et al: Effect of ovary storage and oocyte transport method on maturation rate of horse oocytes, *Theriogenology* 59:765-774, 2003.

Maclellan LJ, Carnevale EM, Coutinho da Silva MA, et al: Pregnancies from vitrified equine oocytes collected from super-stimulated and non-stimulated mares, *Theriogenology* 58:911-919, 2002.

McPartlin LA, Suarez SS, Czaya CA, et al: Hyperactivation of stallion sperm is required for successful in vitro fertilization of equine oocytes, *Biol Reprod* 81:199-206, 2009.

Norman HD, Walsh MK: Performance of dairy cattle clones and evaluation of their milk composition, *Cloning Stem Cells* 6:157-164, 2004.

Ribeiro BI, Love LB, Choi YH, et al: Transport of equine ovaries for assisted reproduction, *Anim Reprod Sci* 108:171-179, 2008.

Watanabe S, Nagai T: Health status and productive performance of somatic cell cloned cattle and their offspring produced in Japan, *J Reprod Dev* 54:6-17, 2008.

Wells DN: Animal cloning: problems and prospects, *Revue Scientifique et Technique* 24:251-264, 2005.

Wells DN, Forsyth JT, McMillan V, et al: The health of somatic cell cloned cattle and their offspring, *Cloning Stem Cells* 6:101-110, 2004.

Woods GL, White KL, Vanderwall DK, et al: A mule cloned from fetal cells by nuclear transfer, *Science* 301:1063, 2003.

Index

Note: Page numbers followed by f indicate figures; t, tables; and b, boxes.

Colpotomy, 6
Combined uteroplacental thickness
    (CUPT), 120-121, 121f-122f
Complete abdominal cryptorchid, 250-251
Complete blood count (CBC), 146
Computerized motility analysis, 193, 193f
Conceptus, early equine, 86. *See also*
    Embryos.
Condoms, 164, 164f
Congenital cataracts, 150
Contagious equine metritis, 77, 186-187
Control panel, ultrasound scan system, 55,
    55f
Cooling semen, 214-215, 211f-214f.
    See also Semen, cooled.
Corpora lutea, supplementary, 86-89,
    88f-89f
Corpus hemorrhagicum, 13f
Corpus luteum (CL), 13, 13f
    in early pregnancy, 85
    primary, 86-88, 88f-89f
    transrectal ultrasonography of, 58-59,
        59f, 61
Cortex, ovarian, 3f, 4
Corticosteroids
    for cutaneous habronemiasis, 271
    for endometritis, 83-84
    for parturition induction, 129
    for shock, 140
Covers or breedings/cycle, 297, 301, 301t
Cream-gel extender, 169t, 208
Creatinine, neonatal serum, 146
Cryopreservation media, 217t-218t
    adding, 217-218
    for epididymal sperm, 225
Cryopreservation of semen, 208, 215-225
    adding medium for, 217-218, 217t-218t
    centrifugation for, 216-217, 217f
    cooling semen before, 223
    epididymal sperm in, 223-225, 224f-226f
    freezing process for, 219, 220f
    insemination in, 221-223
    packaging for, 217f, 218-219, 219f-220f
    processing form for, 222f
    storage after, 220-221, 221f
    thawing after, 221
Cryotherapy for penile neoplasia, 268-269,
    269f
Cryptorchidectomy, 253-255, 254f-255f
Cryptorchidism, 250-255
    castration for, 253-255, 254f-255f
    causes of, 251
    diagnosis of, 251-253, 252f-253f
    hormone levels in, 203
    testicular neoplasia and, 262
CSU model artificial vagina, 162-163,
    162f-163f
Culture
    oocyte, 303-305, 304f, 308-309
    for stallion genital infections, 187, 187f
    uterine, 46-47, 47f, 76-77, 278
Cumulative pregnancy value, 297-301,
    298f-299f
Curettage, uterine, 82
Cutaneous habronemiasis, 270-271,
    270f-271f
Cycles/mare, 301, 301t
Cycles/pregnancy. *See* Pregnancy rate/cycle.

Cyclooxygenase inhibitors, 137
Cystorelin. *See* Gonadotropin-releasing
    hormone (GnRH).
Cysts, parovarian, 42-43, 43f. *See also*
    Uterine cysts.
Cytogenetics, 201
Cytology, uterine, 47-51, 48f-51f, 76-77
Cytotec. *See* Misoprostol; Prostaglandin E₁.

D

Daily sperm output (DSO), 180-181, 192
Dam-foal interaction, 152, 153f
Deep-horn insemination, 174-175, 174f, 223
Delivery. *See* Parturition.
Densimeter, 167f, 192, 192f
Density-gradient centrifugation, 170-171,
    171f
Dental examination of pregnant mare, 118
Deslorelin, 21-27t
    for advancing ovulatory estrus, 30
    for oocyte transfer, 306-307
    for ovulation induction, 31-33, 33f,
        34t-35t
Detomidine hydrochloride, 109
Deworming of pregnant mare, 118, 119b
Dexamethasone, 83-84, 109, 129
Diarrhea, rotavirus, 117-118
Diestrous ovulation, 12
Diestrus, 10-11, 11f
    follicular size and, 14
    hormonal control of, 12f
    ovarian characteristics in, 59
    staging, 16t
    uterine characteristics in, 64-65, 64f-65f
Diethylcarbamazine, 271
Diff-Quick stain, 48, 48f-49f, 77
Digestible energy (DE) requirements for
    pregnant mare, 118-119
Dimethyl sulfoxide, 81-82t
Dinoprostin. *See* Prostaglandin E₂.
Dinoprost tromethamine, 21-27t, 36
Direct hernias, 255
Disinfectant
    intrauterine infusion of, 80-82
    for umbilical stump, 151
Display monitor, 55, 55f
Dominant preovulatory follicle, oocyte
    recovery from, 303, 303f-304f
Domperidone, 20-28, 113
Donor mare
    for embryo transfer
        management of, 278-279, 286-287
        recipient-donor synchrony and, 277,
            277f, 284
        uterine flush in, 279-284, 279f,
            281f-284f, 282t-283t
    for oocyte transfer, 306-308
Dopamine D2 antagonists, 20-28, 28f, 113
Doppler ultrasonography, color, 55-56, 65,
    66f
Doubled mares, 293t, 295
"Double emasculation," 247
Dr. Kenney Ready Mix Extender, 170t
DSO. *See* Daily sperm output (DSO).
Ductus deferens
    culturing secretions from, 187-188
    harvesting sperm from, 223-225,
        224f-226f

Dummy, breeding, 160-161, 166-167, 166f
Dummy foal, 110, 148, 148f
Dysmature fetuses, 102, 103f
Dysmaturity, 114-115
Dystocia, 131-135
    delivery via mutation and traction for,
        133
    examination for, 127, 132-133
    malposture correction for, 133-134, 134f
    obstetric equipment for, 132, 132f
    uterine torsion and, 134-135

E

Eastern equine encephalomyelitis, 117, 154
Eastern tent caterpillars, 96, 99, 101f
Ecbolics, uterine
    for endometritis, 75, 79-80, 79f
    postpartum use of, 37
eCG. *See* Equine chorionic gonadotropin
    (eCG).
Echogenic tissues, 55
Ectopic testis, 250-251
Edema
    scrotal, 188-189, 188f
    uterine, 98, 98f
EDTA-Tris, 81-82t
eFSH. *See* Equine follicle-stimulating
    hormone (eFSH).
EHV-1. *See* Equine herpesvirus 1 (EHV-1).
Electrolytes
    neonatal serum, 146
    in udder secretions, 124, 124f
Electron microscopy of sperm, 198,
    198f-199f
Emasculators, 243, 245-246, 243f, 246f. *See
    also* Castration.
Embryonic death. *See also* Pregnancy loss.
    counting as pregnancy, 294-295
    diagnosis of, 96-98, 96f-98f
    incidence and causes of, 95-96
    return to estrus after, 99-100
Embryonic period, 95
Embryonic vesicles
    anembryonic, 96, 96f, 99f
    examination of, 65-67, 66f-68f
    migration and fixation of, 86
    small-for-age, 96, 96f
Embryos
    abnormal location and orientation of,
        97, 97f
    characteristics of recoverable, 282t
    development of, 85-87, 282f
        abnormal, management of, 98, 99f
        retarded, 97, 97f, 112-113
    endometrial cysts adjacent to, 97-98,
        97f-98f
    examination of, 65-67, 66f-68f
    handling procedures for, 281-284, 284f
    quality grading of, 283f, 283t
    recovery of, 279-284, 279f, 281f-284f,
        282t-283t
    size of, 278-279
    in transfer straw, 285f
Embryo transfer (ET), 276-277
    donor mare management for, 278-279,
        286-287
    embryo recovery for, 279-284, 279f,
        281f-284f, 282t-283t

Rectovaginal or rectovestibular fistulas, 228-229, 229f, 237-239, 238f-239f
Rectovestibular lacerations, 228-229, 229f, 234-237, 236f-237f
Red bag delivery, 110f, 125
Red blood cell count, neonatal, 146
Reefing operation, 268-270, 269f
Registration of cloned foals, 310-311
Regu-Mate. *See* Altrenogest.
Relaxin, 89f
Reproductive anatomy and physiology. *See* Breeding soundness examination (BSE); Mares; Pregnancy; Stallions.
Reserpine, 113
Respiratory rate, neonatal, 145t, 148
Respiratory system of foal
   evaluation of, 144, 144f, 145t, 148-149, 149f
   resuscitation procedure for, 144-146, 145f
Restraint
   during breeding, 165-166, 166f
   for examination of mare, 7-8, 8f, 42, 42f, 56
   for examination of stallion, 182-185
Resuscitation, neonatal, 144-146, 145f
Retained placenta, 135-137, 135f-137f
Retractile testis, 250-251
Retrograde flush for harvesting epididymal sperm, 224-225, 225f-226f
Rhinomune, 116
Rhodococcus equi hyperimmune plasma, 158, 158f
Rib fractures, 147, 147f
Roanoke artificial vagina, 163
Rotavirus diarrhea, 117-118
Rupture
   abdominal wall, 112
   of chorioallantois and amnion, 125-127, 125f-126f
   inguinal, 255-257
   prepubic tendon, 112, 112f
   uterine, 138-139, 139f
   of uterine or iliac artery, 140

S

Saline solution for uterine lavage, 78-79
Salpingitis, 74
Scanning electron microscopy of sperm, 198, 198f
Scirrhous cord, 248
Scrotal edema, 188-189, 188f
Scrotal herniation. *See* Inguinal herniation.
Scrotal width, 180-181, 181f, 181t
Scrotum, 180-181, 181f-182f, 181t
Seasonal anestrus, 16-18, 59, 60f
Seasonal endometrial atrophy, 50f
Seasonality
   of gestation length, 115
   of mare reproductive performance, 16-18
Seasonal polyestrous animal, 10-11
Seasonal pregnancy rate, 288-289, 289t, 292t, 293-295
Secondary corpora lutea, 88-89
Secondary follicular waves, 12
Second-degree perineal laceration, 234-235
Sedation
   for castration, 243, 247
   for embryo transfer, 284
   for penile examination, 179
   for uterine flush, 279-280

Segmental posthectomy, 267-268
Semen. *See also* Sperm.
   cooled, 207-210, 226
      chilling for storage, 210-215, 211f-214f
      extenders for, 208-210, 210t
      fertility of, 301
      for transport before cryopreservation, 223
      transport form for, 208, 209f
   evaluation of, 190-191
      acrosome reaction in, 198-199, 198f-199f
      electron microscopy in, 198, 198f
      gross quality in, 190-191, 191f
      pH in, 192-193
      seminal plasma analysis in, 197
      sperm chromatin in, 201, 202f
      sperm compartments in, 199, 199f-200f
      sperm concentration in, 191-192, 191f-192f
      sperm morphology in, 195-197, 195f-197f
      sperm motility in, 193-195, 193f-195f
   frozen, 207-208, 226
      cryopreservation procedure for, 215-225, 217f, 217t, 218-219, 218t, 219f-220f
      fertility of, 301
      insemination with, 221-223
      processing form for, 222f
      storing, 220-221, 221f
      thawing, 221
   handling techniques for, 167-169, 167f-168f, 169t-170t
   for low-dose insemination, 169-171, 171f
   volume of gel-free, 190-192
Semen collection, 160-171
   artificial vaginas for, 161-163, 161f-163f
   for bacterial culture, 187-188, 188f
   condoms for, 164, 164f
   for evaluation, 190
   stallion mount for, 165-167, 165f-166f
Semen extenders, 160-161
   commercial, 170t
   common, 169t
   for cooled semen, 208-210, 210t, 223
   for cryopreservation, 217-218, 217f, 217t-218t, 225, 226f
   pre-breeding infusion of, 75
   preparation and use of, 167-169, 168f
   for sperm motility evaluation, 194-195, 195f
Semen preservation, 207-208, 226
   considerations for, 208
   cooling method of, 208-210, 209f, 210-215, 210t, 211f-214f
   cryopreservation method of, 215-225, 217f, 217t-218t, 219f-222f, 224f-226f
Seminal pH, 192-193
Seminal plasma
   chemical analysis of, 197
   removing excess, 194-195, 194f-195f, 209-210, 216-217, 217f
Seminal vesicles, 186f, 187-188, 188f
Seminal vesiculitis, 199-200, 191f, 200f-201f
Seminoma, 262-263, 263f
Semiquantitative immunoassays, 156-157
Sepsis score, 154

Septicemia
   metritis and, 74
   neonatal, 154
   retained placenta and, 136-137
Septic peritonitis, post-castration, 249
Serologic examination
   for abortion, 103
   for neonatal foal, 146-147
Sertoli cells, 201-203, 203f
Sertoli cell tumor, 262
Serum/milk progesterone assay, 89
Settle. *See Mycobacterium phlei* immunomodulator.
Sexual behavior in stallion, 185-186, 186f, 242-243, 250
Shock
   hemorrhagic, 139-140
   to sperm, 197, 207-208
Silent estrus, 35-36
Skim milk-based centrifugation medium, 218t
Skim milk extender, 169t, 208
Skim Milk Extender (Lane), 170t
Sleeping sickness, 117, 154
Slipped mares
   breeding records for, 292-293, 292t-293t
   fertility of, 40, 296
Slusher, Steven, 231, 231f
Smegma, 179-180, 180f
Sodium, in udder secretions, 124
Sodium bicarbonate, 146
Sound waves, high-frequency, 55
Specific gravity of colostrum, 155, 155f
Specimens for abortion diagnosis, 103
Speculum. *See* Vaginal speculum.
Sperm. *See also* Intracytoplasmic sperm injection (ICSI); Semen.
   acrosome reaction in, 198-199, 198f-199f
   antibodies against, 201, 258-259, 260-262
   cryopreserved, 216
   daily output of, 180-181, 192
   electron microscopy of, 198, 198f-199f
   environmental factors affecting, 175, 207-208
   freezing epididymal, 223-226, 224f-226f
   insemination number of, 172
   seminal plasma effects on, 197
   total number of, 192
SpermaCue, 192
Spermatic cords, 182
   hemorrhage from, 247-248
   infection of, 248
   torsion of, 182, 257-259, 258f-259f
Spermatogenesis, 201-204, 203f-205f, 251
Sperm chromatin structure assay (SCSA), 201, 202f
Sperm compartments, 199, 199f-200f
Sperm concentration
   increasing, 169-171, 171f, 194-195, 194f-195f, 210, 216-217, 217f
   measuring, 167-168, 167f-168f, 190-192, 191f-192f
Sperm morphology, 195-198, 195f-198f
Sperm motility, 167-168, 168f, 193-195, 193f-195f
   in cooled semen, 215
   postthaw, 220-221
Sperm pellet, 169-171, 171f, 194-195, 195f

Transrectal ultrasonography *(Continued)*
of mare *(Continued)*
procedural considerations for, 56-58,
56f-58f
for staging estrous cycle, 13-16, 59
for tubular tract evaluation, 64-65,
64f-65f
for twins, 108-109, 108f-109f
for uterine pathology diagnosis,
69-71, 70f-80f
of stallion
in breeding soundness examination,
185, 185f-186f
for cryptorchidism, 252, 252f
Transscrotal ultrasonography
in breeding soundness examination,
180-182, 182f-184f
for hematocele, 260, 261f
for hydrocele, 259, 260f
for inguinal hernia, 256, 256f
for spermatic cord torsion, 258, 258f-259f
for testicular neoplasia, 262-263, 263f
Transvaginal ultrasonography, 55, 58
equipment for, 58f, 306f
for oocyte recovery, 58f, 303-304,
303f-305f
for twin reduction, 109, 109f
Transverse fold, 2f, 6
Transverse presentation, 134
Trophoblast, 87
Trophoblastic microvilli, 87
Truss for inguinal hernia, 256-257,
256f-257f
Trypanosoma equiperdum, 190
Tubular tract of mare, evaluation of, 64-65,
64f-65f
Tumors
granulosa cell, 42-43, 42f, 63-64, 63f
Leydig and Sertoli cell, 262
ovarian, 42-43, 42f, 63-64, 63f-64f
uterine, 43, 44f, 53f
Turner's syndrome, 62-63
Twinning, 106-109, 108f
abortion and, 100, 103-107, 106f-107f
diagnosis and reduction of, 67, 108-109,
108f-109f
fetal viability monitoring for, 122, 123f
Two-bladed speculum, 45, 46f, 239-240,
240f

U

Udder
examination of, 151
precocious development of, 121-122
prefoaling secretions from, 123-124
Ultrasonography. *See also* Transcutaneous
ultrasonography; Transrectal ultrasonography; Transscrotal ultrasonography; Transvaginal ultrasonography.
for cryptorchidism, 252, 252f-253f
for paraphimosis, 266, 266f
real-time, 55-56, 55f
Umbilical cord
care of, 125-127, 151-152, 151f, 152f
delivery of, 125-127, 127f
evaluation of, 67, 68f
Unilateral (unicornual) twins, 107-108

Unopette system, 191-192
Urachus, patent, 151, 151f-152f
Urethral culture, 187, 187f
Urethral endoscopy, 199-200,
200f-201f
Urethral extension technique, 233-234,
233f-234f
Urethral granuloma, 270-271, 270f-271f
Urethral laceration, 200f
Urethral process of penis, 179-180, 180f
Urethral rents, 272-274, 273f-274f
Urethrotomy, 273-274, 274f
Urinary bladder, uterus vs., 71, 71f, 91
Urination, stimulation of, 179
Urine, estrogen detection in, 92-93
Urine scalding, 233, 233f
Urovagina
examination for, 47f, 229
in pregnancy, 120
surgery for, 233-234, 233f-234f
Uterine artery, 2f, 5, 140
Uterine body pregnancy, 97, 104-106t,
109-110
Uterine culture, 46-47, 47f
for embryo transfer, 278
for endometritis, 76-77
Uterine curettage, 82
Uterine cysts, 43, 44f
diagnosis of, 69-71, 70f
embryo adjacent to, 97-98, 97f-98f
endoscopic view of, 52f
removal of, 240-241, 241f
Uterine cytology, 47-51, 48f-51f, 76-77
Uterine edema, 98, 98f
Uterine fluid
for abortion diagnosis, 103
intraluminal, 76
diagnosis of, 71, 71f-72f
management of, 74-75, 79-80, 79f
Uterine flush
for culture, 47
for cytology, 48
donor mare management for, 278-279,
286-287
for embryo recovery, 279-284, 279f,
281f-284f, 282t-283t
Uterine hematoma, 140-141, 141f
Uterine horns, 2f, 3f, 5
in early pregnancy, 86f
endometrial folds in, 4f
endoscopic views of, 51-52, 51f
insemination at, 174-175, 174f, 223
invaginated, 138, 138f
palpation of, 9f
rupture in, 139
transrectal ultrasonography of, 56, 57f,
64, 64f-65f
Uterine involution, 37, 129
Uterine lavage, 77-79, 78f
postbreeding, 75
for retained placenta, 136, 137f
Uterine lumen
endoscopic views of, 52f-53f
fluid in, 71, 71f-72f, 74-75,
79-80, 79f
Uterine prolapse, 137-138,
137f-138f
Uterine rupture, 138-139, 139f

Uterine torsion, 110-111, 111f, 134-135
Uterine tubes. *See* Oviducts.
Uterine tumors, 43, 44f, 53f
Uterotubal junction (UTJ), 4-5
Uterus, 1-2, 2f, 4f, 5
air in, 50f, 71, 72f, 75-76
in early pregnancy, 86-87, 86f
examination of
for breeding soundness, 42-43, 44f,
51-52, 51f-53f
palpation per rectum for, 8-9, 9f
for pathologic conditions, 69-71,
70f-72f
for pregnancy diagnosis, 86f, 90-91,
90f-92f
for staging estrous cycle, 13-14, 16t,
64-65, 64f-65f
transrectal ultrasonography for, 56-58,
56f-57f, 64-65, 64f-65f
postparturient hemorrhage in, 140-141,
141f

V

Vaccination
for equine viral arteritis, 190
against gonadotropin-releasing and
luteinizing hormones, 250
neonatal, 154
of pregnant mare, 115-116, 115b, 119b,
154
preoperative tetanus, 229, 243
Vagina. *See also* Artificial vagina (AV);
Pneumovagina; Urovagina.
anatomy of, 2-3, 2f, 6, 6f
postparturient hemorrhage in, 141,
141f
Vaginal artery, 5
Vaginal fornix, 5-6
Vaginal hemorrhoids, 120, 120f
Vaginal process, everting inverted, 253-254,
254f
Vaginal rings, 185, 185f
Vaginal speculum
for artificial insemination, 173, 174f
Caslick's, 45, 46f
for cervical laceration repair, 239-240,
240f
two-bladed, 45, 46f, 239-240, 240f
Vaginal speculum examination
for breeding soundness, 45-46,
45f-46f
for endometritis, 76
of genital discharge, 120
for pregnancy diagnosis, 89-90
Vaginal varicosities, 46f
Vaginitis, 74
Vaginocele. *See* Hydrocele.
Varicocele, 262
Vascular shunt for priapism,
272, 273f
Venereal disease, 186-190, 187f-189f
Venezuelan equine encephalomyelitis,
117
Ventilation, assisted, 145-146, 145f
Ventipulmin Syrup. *See* Clenbuterol.
Vesicovaginal reflux, 233. *See also*
Urovagina.
Vestibule, 2-3, 2f, 6

Vestibuloplasty
    for perineal lacerations, 235
    for pneumovagina, 231-232, 231f-232f
Vestibulovaginal ring, 2-3, 6, 42
Viability assessment
    fetal, 55-58, 57f-58f, 120-122, 120f-123f
    neonatal, 144-146, 145t
Videoendoscope, 174, 174f
Vinegar, 81-82t
Viral arteritis, equine. *See* Equine viral
    arteritis (EVA).
Viral genital infections, 189-190, 189f
Vulva, 2-3, 2f, 6-7, 7f
    examination of, 42
    postparturient hemorrhage of, 141,
      142f
    sunken, 7f

Vulvar lips, 6-7, 7f, 42, 68
Vulvoplasty, Caslick's
    for perineal lacerations, 235-237, 237f
    for pneumovagina, 229-231, 230f-231f

W

Waxing, of teat ends, 123, 123f
Western equine encephalomyelitis, 117, 154
West Nile virus, 117
Window of synchrony for embryo transfer,
    277, 277f, 284
"Wind sucking." *See* Pneumovagina.
Winter anestrus, 16-18, 59, 60f

X

Xylazine, 132

Y

YAG-laser surgery, 240-241, 241f
Yeast infection, 48-49, 49f, 77
Yolk sac, 66-67, 67f-68f
Y-sutures of lens, 150

Z

Zinc sulfate turbidity test, 156, 157